KIELHOFNER'S
RESEARCH *in* OCCUPATIONAL THERAPY

Methods of Inquiry for Enhancing Practice

SECOND EDITION

Renée R. Taylor, PhD
Professor, Department of Occupational Therapy
University of Illinois at Chicago

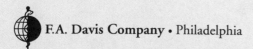 F.A. Davis Company • Philadelphia

F. A. Davis Company
1915 Arch Street
Philadelphia, PA 19103
www.fadavis.com

Printed in the United States of America

Last digit indicates print number: 10   9   8   7   6   5   4   3   2   1

Senior Acquisitions Editor: Christa Fratantoro
Director of Content Development: George W. Lang
Developmental Editor: Nancy J. Peterson, Laura S. Horowitz
Art and Design Manager: Carolyn O'Brien

Library of Congress Cataloging-in-Publication Data

Names: Kielhofner, Gary, 1949– author. | Taylor, Renee R., 1970– author.
Title: Research in occupational therapy : methods of inquiry for enhancing practice / Renee R. Taylor, Gary Kielhofner.
Description: Second edition. | Philadelphia : F.A. Davis Company, [2017] | Gary Kielhofner's name appears first in the
  previous edition. | Includes bibliographical references and index.
Identifiers: LCCN 2016053438 | ISBN 9780803640375 (alk. paper)
Subjects: | MESH: Occupational Therapy | Research Design
Classification: LCC RM735 | NLM WB 555 | DDC 615.8/515–dc23 LC record available at https://lccn.loc.gov/2016053438

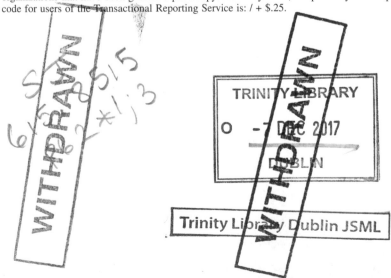

Dedication

This book is dedicated to the memory of Dr. Gary Kielhofner (b. 2/15/1949, d. 9/2/2010). By nature a humanitarian, by identity a pacifist, and by profession an occupational therapy practitioner, researcher, and scholar, Professor Kielhofner stood as the foremost theorist in his day, and arguably to this day, in the field of occupational therapy. As exemplified by his Model of Human Occupation (MOHO) (Kielhofner, 2008), Professor Kielhofner's work epitomized evidence-based practice. This is supported by a developing body of research that points to MOHO as being the most evidence-based, client-centered, and occupation-focused conceptual practice model in the world (Haglund, Ekbladh, Thorell, & Hallberg, 2000; Law & McColl, 1989; Lee, 2010; National Board for Certification in Occupational Therapy, 2004). Most importantly, Professor Kielhofner put the priorities of occupational therapy clients, students, and practitioners before all other professional priorities, as was evident across all of his scholarly works. It is hoped that these priorities have shined through within this second edition of his work, written in his honor.

Author Note

Deciding to assume editorship of the second edition of Gary Kielhofner's original text, *Research in Occupational Therapy,* was as difficult as it was daunting. The first edition of this text was highly informative, at the cutting edge of science, easy to read, and occupational therapy (OT) relevant, and it contained continuous examples derived from OT practice. Dr. Kielhofner selected contributing authors who stood at the top of their respective fields within occupational therapy, and their expertise in the various approaches to OT research was well portrayed. From my perspective, the first edition did not need much in the way of improvement.

At the same time, I recall a conversation that I had with Dr. Kielhofner early in 2010, before either of us knew he would leave the profession, and indeed this world, far too early. At that time, we decided that if a second edition were to be requested, we would work on it together. Thus, in this second edition, I retained as much of the original content and as many of the original contributors to the first edition as possible. At the same time, this edition reflects a combination of ideas for improvement the second time around. With all of this said, I truly hope that you will find that this edition lives up to its expectations and to its title, *Kielhofner's Research in Occupational Therapy.*

References

Haglund, L., Ekbladh, E., Thorell, L. H., & Hallberg, I. R. (2000). Practice models in Swedish psychiatric occupational therapy. *Scandinavian Journal of Occupational Therapy, 7,* 107–113.

Kielhofner, G. (2008). *Model of Human Occupation: Theory and application* (4th ed.). Philadelphia, PA: Lippincott, Williams and Wilkins.

Law, M., & McColl, M. A. (1989). Knowledge and use of theory among occupational therapists: A Canadian survey. *Canadian Journal of Occupational Therapy, 56,* 198–204.

Lee, J. (2010). Achieving best practice: A review of evidence linked to occupation-focused practice models. *Occupational Therapy in Health Care, 24,* 206–222.

National Board for Certification in Occupational Therapy. (2004, Spring). A practice analysis study of entry-level occupational therapist registered and certified occupational therapy assistant practice. *OTJR: Occupation, Participation, and Health, 24* (Suppl. 1), S1–S31.

Contributors

Beatriz C. Abreu, PhD, OTR, FAOTA
Clinical Professor
Department of Occupational Therapy
School of Allied Health Sciences
University of Texas Medical Branch
Director of Occupational Therapy
Transitional Learning Center at Galveston
Galveston, TX

Marian Arbesman, PhD, OTR/L
President, ArbesIdeas, Inc.
Consultant, AOTA Evidence-Based Literature
    Review Project
Clinical Assistant Professor, Department of
    Rehabilitation Science
University at Buffalo
Buffalo, NY

Nancy A. Baker, ScD, OTR/L
Assistant Professor
School of Health and Rehabilitation Sciences
University of Pittsburgh
Pittsburgh, PA

Brent Braveman, PhD, OTR/L, FAOTA
Director
Department of Rehabilitation Services
University of Texas
M.D. Anderson Cancer Center
Houston, TX

Mary A. Corcoran, PhD, OTR, FAOTA
Research Professor
The George Washington University
Department of Health Care Sciences
School of Medicine and Health Sciences
Washington, DC
Professor
Department of Occupational Therapy
Shenandoah University
Winchester, VA

Wendy J. Coster, PhD, OTR/L, FAOTA
Professor and Chair
Department of Occupational Therapy and
    Rehabilitation Counseling
Sargent College of Health & Rehabilitation
    Sciences
Boston University
Boston, MA

Anne Cusick, BAppSc(OT), Grad Cert Bus
    Admin, Grad Dip Beh Sc, MA(Psych),
    MA(Interdisc Stud), PhD
College of Science and Health
University of Western Sydney
Richmond NSW, Australia

Anne E. Dickerson, PhD, OTR/L, FAOTA
Professor and Chair
Department of Occupational Therapy
East Carolina University
Greenville, NC
Co-Director of Research for Older Adult Driver
    Initiative (ROADI)
Editor of *Occupational Therapy in Health Care*

Jean Crosetto Deitz, PhD, OTR/L, FAOTA
Professor and Graduate Program Coordinator
Department of Rehabilitation Medicine
University of Washington
Seattle, WA

M. G. Dieter, MLIS, MBA, PhD
Program Director, Health Informatics
Clinical Assistant Professor, Biomedical and Health
    Information Sciences
Department of Biomedical and Health Information
    Sciences
University of Illinois at Chicago
Chicago, IL

Heather Dillaway, PhD
Professor, Sociology
Wayne State University
Detroit, MI

Marcia Finlayson, PhD, OT(C), OTR/L
Associate Professor
Department of Occupational Therapy
College of Applied Health Sciences
University of Illinois at Chicago
Chicago, IL

Kirsty Forsyth, PhD, OTR
Professor
Occupational Therapy Department
Queen Margaret University College
Edinburgh, Scotland

Ellie Fossey, DipCOT (UK), MSC (Health
    Psychol), PhD
Professor and Head
Occupational Therapy Department
Monash University
Adjunct Professor
La Trobe University
Melbourne, Australia

Patricia C. Heyn, PhD
Associate Professor
Physical Medicine and Rehabilitation Department/
    School of Medicine
University of Colorado Health Sciences Center
Denver, CO

Gary Kielhofner (Deceased)
Professor and Wade-Meyer Chair
Department of Occupational Therapy
College of Applied Health Sciences
University of Illinois at Chicago
Chicago, IL

Frederick J. Kviz, PhD
Professor
Community Health Sciences
School of Public Health
University of Illinois at Chicago
Chicago, IL

Mark R. Luborsky, PhD
Professor of Anthropology and Gerontology
Director of Aging and Health Disparities Research
Institute of Gerontology
Wayne State University
Detroit, MI

Cathy Lysack, PhD, OT(C)
Associate Professor, Occupational Therapy and
    Gerontology
Wayne State University
Detroit, MI

Annie McCluskey, PhD, MA, DipCOT
Lecturer in Occupational Therapy
School of Exercise & Health Sciences
University of Western Sydney
Richmond NSW, Australia

David L. Nelson, PhD, OTR, FAOTA
Professor Emeritus
Occupational Therapy Program
Department of Rehabilitation Sciences
College of Health Sciences
Medical University of Ohio at Toledo
Toledo, OH

Kenneth J. Ottenbacher, PhD, OTR/L
Professor and Director
Division of Rehabilitation Sciences
University of Texas Medical Branch
Galveston, TX

Amy R. Paul-Ward, PhD, MSOT
Assistant Professor
Department of Occupational Therapy
Florida International University
Miami, FL

Nadine Peacock, PhD
Associate Professor
Community Health Sciences
School of Public Health
Adjunct Associate Professor
Department of Anthropology
University of Illinois at Chicago
Chicago, IL

Geneviève Pépin, PhD, OTR
Senior Lecturer
Deakin University
School of Health & Social Development
Victoria, Australia

Yolanda Suarez-Balcazar, PhD
Professor
Department of Occupational Therapy
Associate Director, Center for Capacity Building for
    Minorities With Disabilities Research
University of Illinois at Chicago
Chicago, IL

Pimjai Sudsawad, ScD, OTR
Knowledge Translation Program Coordinator
National Institute on Disability, Independent
    Living, and Rehabilitation Research (NIDILRR)
Administration for Community Living
U.S. Department of Health and Human Services
Washington, DC

Renée R. Taylor, PhD
Associate Professor
Department of Occupational Therapy
University of Illinois at Chicago
Chicago, IL

Hector W. H. Tsang, PhD, OTR
Associate Professor
Department of Rehabilitation Sciences
The Hong Kong Polytechnic University
Hong Kong

Toni Van Denend, MS, OTR/L
Staff Therapist
RehabWorks
Aurora, IL

Elizabeth White, PhD, DipCOT
Head of Research and Development
College of Occupational Therapists
London, England

Don E. Workman, PhD
Clinical Psychology Subject Matter Expert
Triple-I
Deployment Health Clinical Center
Silver Spring, MD

Reviewers

Jane Davis, MSC, OT Reg. (Ont.), OTR
Lecturer and Curriculum Coordinator
Department of Occupational Science and
    Occupational Therapy
University of Toronto
Ontario, Canada

Lorna Hayward, EdD, MPH, PT
Associate Professor
Physical Therapy
Northeastern University
Boston, MA

Lynne Jaffe, ScD, OTR/L
Professor Emeritus
Department of Occupational Therapy
Augusta University
Augusta, GA

Margaret Wittman, EdD, OT/L, FAOTA
Professor
Occupational Therapy
Eastern Kentucky University
Richmond, KY

Andrea Gossett Zakrajsek, OTD, MS, OTRL
Associate Professor
Occupational Therapy Program
Eastern Michigan University
Ypsilanti, MI

Preface

Choosing to become an occupational therapist involves a commitment from each and every one of us to ensure that the profession's practice and scholarship stand at the cutting edge of rehabilitation science and innovation. This responsibility carries with it an effortful and disciplined practice of applying the theoretical underpinnings, infrastructural requirements, scientific methods, and practical means of disseminating research findings. Contributions represented within this second edition represent a collective effort on the part of many occupational therapy educators to make the process of learning and utilizing research in occupational therapy one that is relevant to practice, unintimidating, and, most importantly, motivating.

By definition, research represents a disciplined and systematic approach to the development, identification, and verification of new knowledge. It is governed by ethics and rules of conduct and is structured and rational in nature. In the field of occupational therapy, research involves testing theories and theoretical concepts as they are reflected in practice frameworks and in conceptual practice models. Moreover, research involves using assessments and other approaches to data collection to generate knowledge and to test innovative devices, technologies, and approaches to practice.

The focus of this book is the concepts, methods, and common practices that comprise the act of conducting research in the field of occupational therapy. Content in this text is balanced to ensure equal coverage from both quantitative and qualitative perspectives. The two original themes binding the first edition were retained in this volume. First, the chapters illustrate how research is fueled by creativity, represented in the ongoing development and discovery of new knowledge. The development of this knowledge and any associated skills or technologies contributes to the field's mandate to approach practice using the most humane, inclusive, contemporary, rigorous, and engaging methods possible. Second, specific efforts were made to demonstrate how research is both essential to and can support and improve occupational therapy practice. To this end, all of the examples and cases contained in this book emanate directly from the field of occupational therapy. Additionally,

the chapters emphasize the usefulness of research in terms of building practitioners' knowledge base and credibility within and outside of our field.

Organization and Scope

This book offers a comprehensive guide to conducting applied research in the field of occupational therapy from quantitative, qualitative, and mixed perspectives. It is organized in terms of six sections. Given the breadth of material covered, the content is targeted toward a student–practitioner audience, and most topics are covered at a foundational level. Each of the six sections and chapters within each section may be read in isolation. However, readers will gain the most by reading the sections and chapters in the order in which they are presented.

The first section, *Research in Occupational Therapy: Basic Elements for Enhancing Practice,* emphasizes every therapist's professional responsibility to conduct practice that is informed by research and stresses the importance of evidence-based practice to advancing the field of occupational therapy. Basic content on what to look for when reading a published research study, including how to critically appraise research, is included. This section provides an overview of the aims and classifications of research and a discussion of the philosophical foundations of research. The importance of theory in the development of research and testing of concepts, assessments, and interventions is also emphasized.

The second section, *Laying the Groundwork for Evidence-Based Practice: The Steps of the Research Process,* covers six broad components of the research process: conducting a literature review, generating research questions and defining specific aims and hypotheses, selecting the research method, writing the research proposal, ensuring ethical review, and securing samples and performance sites.

The third section, *Qualitative Approaches: First Steps in Communicating With Language,* describes design considerations, approaches to the collection of qualitative data, contemporary methods for analyzing qualitative data, and approaches to interpreting and reporting qualitative data.

The fourth section, *Quantitative Approaches: First Steps in Communicating With Statistics and Measures,* focuses on the same topics, but from a quantitative perspective. Chapters emphasize selection of the appropriate research design; measurement approaches; data collection; techniques for entering, storing, and managing data; statistical analysis; and meta-analytic studies.

The fifth section, *Descriptive, Exploratory, and Pilot-Study Research,* covers single-subject, and survey research.

The sixth section, *Additional Topics for the Developing Investigator,* covers needs assessment research, program evaluation research, participatory research approaches, the process for writing a literature review and writing up one's research findings, approaches to obtaining grant funding for research, mixed-methods designs, and outcomes research for evidence-based practice.

Conclusion

Each contribution to this book not only represents a level of expertise within the relevant topic area, but more importantly envelops the passion and dedication required for the conduct of science within the field of occupational therapy. The book was designed to offer a clear and comprehensive approach to conducting occupational therapy research at any level that is directed at improving our practice. After having read this edition, it is my sincere hope, and that of all of the contributors, that its contents will inspire a similar sense of passion, commitment, and dedication to the continual improvement of our field through the rigors involved in the application of science and discovery.

Renée R. Taylor

Acknowledgments

I wish to thank Christa Fratantoro, Senior Acquisitions Editor at F. A. Davis, who believed in my work enough to support my assuming the sole editorship of the second edition of this text. Additionally, I wish to thank Roxanne Klaas, for her excellence and good sense in copy editing. I wish to thank all of the contributors to this second edition. Without their experience and excellence, this book would not have been possible. I also wish to thank three former University of Illinois at Chicago (UIC) occupational therapy students—Baily Zubel, Mary Pearson, and Phoebe Kinzie-Larson—for their editorial contributions, including some of the photography and figures. Finally, I wish to thank Nancy Peterson, Dana Bataglia, and Laura Horowitz for assisting with the editorial production of this text.

Contents

CHAPTER 1

Occupational Therapy as an Evidence-Based Practice Profession

Renée R. Taylor • Gary Kielhofner • Nancy A. Baker

Learning Outcomes

- State why research is an obligation of the profession.
- Define the role of evidence-based practice in occupational therapy.
- Explain why evidence-based practice is necessary to the profession.
- Explain the importance of clinical expertise in evidence-based practice.
- Identify major ways in which research supports occupational therapy practice.
- Describe the major types of research that provide evidence about the nature and outcomes of occupational therapy.

Introduction

Why and to what extent is research important to a practice-based profession such as occupational therapy? If you are like many of us, this is a question that you have asked yourself at some time during the course of your development as a student or occupational therapist.

The Case Example in this chapter provides just one illustration of why research is important to the occupational therapy field overall. Research provides insight into:

- The resolution of practice dilemmas
- The means to test innovations that improve people's well-being and functioning in a wide range of contexts
- Knowledge and guidelines that direct therapists in their everyday work

- A means of growth through developing new approaches to understanding and treating people with impairments
- Evidence that assures others (e.g., family members, employers, insurance companies, and other public institutions) about the impact of occupational therapy services, thus increasing public credibility

For greatest relevance to practice and to the profession, research should be conducted according to a theoretical framework. Figure 1.1 summarizes the dynamic relationships among theory, research, and practice. Each of these key elements of the profession influences the other elements. Theory and research evidence guide practice. Practice raises problems and questions to be addressed in theory and research. Research tests theory and practice, providing information about their validity and utility, respectively.

This chapter explores the role of research in supporting the theories that form the basis of the occupational therapy profession. You will learn the importance of research to clinical reasoning and other types of decision-making in practice. This involves defining evidence-based practice, explaining why it is necessary to the profession, describing the predominant ways in which research supports the profession, and emphasizing the importance of student and clinician involvement in and support of research-related activities.

A Profession's Research Obligation

Every health profession asks its clients and the public to have a level of confidence in the worth of its services. To justify that confidence, the

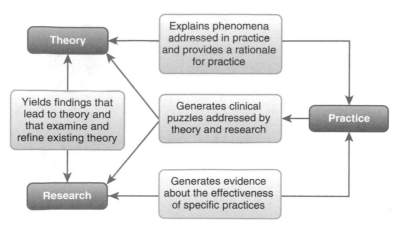

Figure 1.1   The dynamic relationship among theory, research, and practice.

profession must enable its members to offer high-quality services that will benefit clients. Thus, when health-care professionals provide services to clients, the knowledge and skills they use should be "justified in terms of a systematic and shared body of professional knowledge" (Polgar & Thomas, 2000, p. 3). This knowledge includes the underlying theory that informs practice and the tools and procedures that are used in practice.

Research is the means by which the profession generates evidence to test and validate its theories and to examine and demonstrate the utility of its practice tools and procedures. Therefore, our profession has an ongoing obligation to support occupational therapy professionals who choose to undertake systematic and sustained research.

Research for Professional Recognition and Support

The occupational therapy profession depends on societal support. This support ranges from subsidizing educational programs that prepare occupational therapists to reimbursing occupational therapists for their services. Societal support for the health-care professions cannot be assumed; the individuals who make public policy and decide what health-care services are needed increasingly rely on scientific evidence to determine where limited public and private resources should be directed. As a result, research is increasingly necessary to ensure that resources will be available to support the profession. Christiansen (1983) notes, "It seems clear that as administrators and policy-makers render decisions about how health care

providers are used and reimbursed, those disciplines with objective evidence of their effectiveness and efficiency will have a competitive advantage" (p. 197). He concludes that research is an economic imperative for the profession.

Without the development of a research base to refine and provide evidence about the value of its practice, occupational therapy simply will not survive, much less thrive, as a health profession (Christiansen, 1983; Christiansen & Lou, 2001; Cusick, 2001).

Evidence-Based Practice

The obligation of the profession to conduct research that refines and validates its knowledge base is paralleled by an obligation of individual therapists to engage in **evidence-based practice (EBP)** (Taylor, 2000). Evidence-based practice is an approach to practice that assumes the active application of current, methodologically sound research to inform practice decisions and treatment options in light of a client's preferences, expectations, and values (Sackett, 2002).

The process of evidence-based practice begins with a clinical situation that poses a unique question or challenge for the practitioner (Sackett, 2002). Using evidence-based practice, the practitioner engages in a highly deliberate, publicly transparent, and well-reasoned use of clinical research findings to inform decision-making about an individual client in an actual practice situation (Sackett, 2002). Those who approach clinical decision-making from an evidence-based perspective consider what clients value, prefer, and expect

CASE EXAMPLE

Dr. Kerstin Tham is an occupational therapist who specializes in the neurorehabilitation of individuals who have had a cerebrovascular accident (CVA), or stroke (Fig. 1.2). After working with a number of clients with many different kinds of impairments resulting from their CVAs, Kerstin observed that unilateral neglect was one of the most difficult and frustrating impairments to treat in occupational therapy.

Unilateral neglect is an impairment in which people no longer recognize half of their own bodies or perceive half of the world around them. As a consequence, people neglect these regions of the self and the world, for example, washing only one side of the body, eating only the food on one-half of a plate, and bumping into objects that they do not perceive to be present.

For answers, Dr. Tham turned to the existing evidence base, which consisted of a number of published journal articles citing research findings about various training approaches to treat people with unilateral neglect. The common finding, however, was that these approaches had *not* been shown to be very successful in improving the overall functioning of people with this problem.

Dr. Tham became convinced that the research describing unilateral neglect had one major flaw: It always examined how neglect appeared from the outside, that is, how it appeared to clinicians and researchers. The researchers never asked the individuals with CVA what it was like to experience the impairment. So, she decided to undertake research that would describe neglect **phenomenologically,** or from the point of view of the person who had it. Her goal was to provide insights into how to improve service provision to individuals with the impairment.

In a qualitative study in which she observed and interviewed four women over an extended period of time, Dr. Tham and her colleagues came to provide some startling insights into the nature of unilateral neglect (Tham, Borell, & Gustavsson, 2000). For example, they found that people with neglect felt that the neglected body parts were not their own or were not attached to their bodies. Their research described a natural course of discovery in which individuals with neglect came to understand that they had the impairment and were able to make sense of the strange and chaotic experiences of their bodies and the world.

In a subsequent investigation, Dr. Tham and a colleague went on to examine how the behavior of other people influenced the experiences and behaviors of a person with neglect (Tham & Kielhofner, 2003). She is continuing this line of research, which is providing a new approach to understanding and providing services to persons with unilateral neglect. Moreover, she and her doctoral students have expanded these ideas and are now examining the experience of persons with other types of perceptual and cognitive impairments following acquired brain injuries (Erikson, Karlsson, Söderström, & Tham, 2004; Lampinen & Tham, 2003).

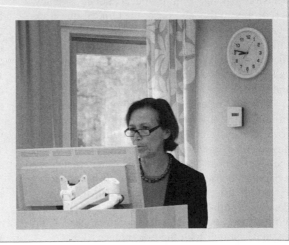

Figure 1.2 Kerstin Tham, OT, PhD, is an occupational therapist and researcher.

from the health-care encounter, alongside their own ever-growing clinical experience, practical skill sets, and educational backgrounds (Sackett, 2002). Evidence may be used to shed light on:

- The anticipated course and outcome of a particular impairment, symptom, or diagnosis
- The relevance and accuracy of a selected assessment tool
- The nature, conduct, and expected outcome of a chosen intervention

Accordingly, whenever possible, practitioners should select intervention strategies and tools that have been empirically demonstrated to be effective (Eakin, 1997). This process requires practitioners to remain up to date with new developments in their practice areas. It also requires practitioners to develop the ability to conduct thoughtful and efficient literature reviews and possess knowledge about how to evaluate published research in terms of its quality and level of methodological rigor (Sackett, 2002).

The Canadian Association of Occupational Therapists' position statement on evidence-based occupational therapy is available online (Canadian Association of Occupational Therapists, Association of Canadian Occupational Therapy University Programs, Association of Canadian Occupational Therapy Regulatory Organizations, & the Presidents' Advisory Committee, 2009). It defines evidence-based occupational therapy as the client-centered enablement of occupation, based on client information and a critical review of relevant research, expert consensus, and experience.

Bennett and Bennett (2000) describe the process of how evidence-based practice informs clinical decision-making within occupational therapy. According to this approach, the clinical questions being considered must address the nature of specific clients and client groups, as well as their treatment contexts. This definition stresses that the relationship between clinician and patient is centrally important in clinical decision-making.

After a clinical question is defined, the next step in the process involves conducting a literature review. During this review, practitioners must be cognizant of the quality and standards by which the research has been conducted. Then, match the evidence to each feature of the client's context, including the client as an individual, the client's desired occupation, and the client's environment. Within this process, the client acts as an active and engaged partner with the practitioner.

In 2002, Dysart and Tomlin surveyed 209 practicing occupational therapists to determine the extent to which they access, use, and apply clinically relevant research findings in practice (Dysart & Tomlin, 2002). Findings revealed that occupational therapy practitioners were using evidence in practice to a modest degree; more than one-half (57 percent) relied on one to five evidence-based treatment plans per year.

In sum, evidence-based practice requires an ongoing commitment from researchers to investigate problems and answer questions that emerge out of practice. Equally, it requires an enduring commitment from practitioners to access, evaluate, and use this research to inform their decision-making in everyday practice. It also requires the client's perspective and involvement (Bennett & Bennett, 2000). Evidence-based practitioners integrate their own expertise with the best available research evidence. The next section briefly examines some of the ways in which research provides evidence for practice.

Clinical Expertise and Evidence-Based Practice: A Collaborative Approach

Evidence-based practice integrates individual *clinical expertise* with the *best available external clinical evidence* from systematic research (Sackett, Rosenberg, Grey, Haynes, & Richardson, 1996). **Clinical expertise** refers to the proficiency and judgment that individual practitioners acquire through experience. Best available **external clinical evidence** refers to findings from highest available quality, clinically applied, research studies within the field's scientific literature.

It is clear from this definition that evidence-based practice relies on practitioners' clinical expertise when applying research evidence to practice. Sackett et al. (1996) state that neither clinical expertise nor the best available external evidence alone are enough for evidence-based practice; external clinical evidence can inform but can never replace individual clinical expertise. Clinical expertise is what determines whether the external evidence applies to the individual patient (i.e., whether and how it matches the client's clinical state, predicaments, and preferences).

Sackett, Straus, Richardson, Rosenberg, and Haynes (2000) later described evidence-based practice as the integration of *best research evidence* with *clinical expertise and patient values*. With this updated definition, the patient's values are acknowledged as an equally important and necessary ingredient in the practice of EBP as research evidence and clinical expertise (Fig. 1.3).

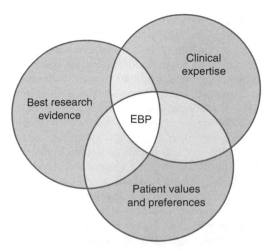

Figure 1.3 Evidence-based practice is the integration of best research practice, clinical expertise, and patient values and preferences.

The Role of Evidence-Based Practice in Occupational Therapy

Evidence-based practice evolved from the principles of evidence-based medicine (EBM), a concept that originated in the 1980s at McMaster University in Canada (Taylor, 1997). EBP emerged within health care and health education in the 1990s. It is now widely known that research evidence must be used as a primary foundation for informing occupational therapy practice (Stronge & Cahill, 2012).

Since the introduction of EBP in occupational therapy, there continues to be discussion about its implementation. There is an increasing recognition that the implementation of evidence-based practice is a complex process that may need to be adapted to ensure its applicability to occupational therapy. To implement EBP in occupational therapy, the synthesis of the available evidence with clinical expertise and judgment, as well as knowledge of the values and preferences of the clients, is critical (Graham, Robertson, & Anderson, 2013; Pighills, Plummer, Harvey, & Pain, 2013; Stronge & Cahill, 2012). Authors have also argued that the direct adoption of EBM and its established prescriptive guidelines may not adequately reflect the philosophical beliefs and the highly contextualized and dynamic nature of occupational therapy (Graham et al., 2013; Pighills et al., 2013; Stronge & Cahill, 2012).

Evidence-based occupational therapy is an offshoot of evidence-based practice that recognizes the range of sources and scope of evidence available to occupational therapists (Zimolag, French, & Paterson, 2002), including:

- Research evidence
- Information provided by the client for determining occupational priorities and capacities
- The knowledge that occupational therapists have gained from past experience

Based on those definitions, the essence of EBP may be summarized as follows:

- Evidence-based practice involves more than just the use of research evidence.
- Clinical expertise is as important to evidence-based practice as research evidence.
- Client input is vital to the decision-making process in evidence-based practice.
- Health-care decisions are also influenced by available resources.

For example, a client has had several acute episodes of low back pain that he states have led to decreased participation in work, play, and home activities. After assessment, it is clear that the client has low flexibility and endurance, and he reports high levels of pain. He has had several courses of physical therapy but continues to have problems. The client states that he would like to miss less work, improve his ability to play with his children, and improve his overall fitness level. The practitioner working with the client believes that a course of intensive work-related occupational therapy will benefit the client and provides him with the following information to help him make his decision: "Mr. Koifier, you have had chronic low back pain for 1 year now. Your physical therapy has helped some, but you continue to have trouble with home activities, and you feel that your overall fitness level is low. I would like to suggest a course of therapy in which you attend daily therapy lasting 4 hours a day. The therapy is designed to improve your flexibility, endurance, strength, and work ability. A recent study reported that this type of therapy was superior to a three-times-a-week physical therapy program in decreasing sick days, improving flexibility and endurance, and assisting people to getting back to leisure and sports activities. For example, there was a 17 percent greater decrease in sick days for people who received this type of therapy, a 29 percent increase in endurance, and a 17 percent decrease in pain. In addition, one in five clients in this type of intervention report the improved ability to participate in sports and leisure activities."

This type of evidence-based statement provides the client with information that will help him to make a more informed decision as to whether the additional time and effort required to attend the more intensive program will be worth it.

How Research Supports Practice

Research supports practice in many different ways, including:

- Generating foundational knowledge used by therapists
- Proving the need for occupational therapy services
- Developing and testing the theories that underlie practice
- Generating findings about the process and outcomes of therapy

The following section examines each of these ways in which research supports and advances practice.

Generating Foundational Knowledge

Much of the background information that occupational therapists use on a daily basis stems from research. Often, a long history of investigation is behind what has become common knowledge. Knowledge of musculoskeletal anatomy, neuronal transmission, the milestones of child development, the nature of personality, and the etiology and prognoses of diseases has resulted from thousands of studies.

Over decades, investigators examined these phenomena, providing analyses that were subsequently verified or corrected by others. In time, this knowledge was accumulated and refined until it became part of the repository of knowledge that informs occupational therapy practice. This knowledge is ordinarily generated by individuals who are not occupational therapists; however, their research is important to occupational therapy practice.

Proving the Need for Occupational Therapy Services

Without clear identification of need, one can neither decide what services to provide nor accurately evaluate the value of any service. **Needs assessment research** determines what clients require to achieve some basic standard of health or to improve their situation (Witkin & Altschuld, 1995). It focuses on identifying gaps between clients' desires and their situations (Altschuld & Witkin, 2000).

Needs assessment is particularly important in identifying the nature and consequences of new types of disabilities and new circumstances that affect persons with disabilities, and in identifying problems not previously recognized or understood. For example, studies have indicated that HIV/ AIDS increasingly affects individuals from underserved minority populations and individuals with histories of mental illness, substance abuse, poverty, limited education, and limited work experience (Centers for Disease Control and Prevention [CDC], 2001; Karon, Fleming, Steketee, & De Cock, 2001; Kates, Sorian, Crowley, & Summers, 2002). Research has also shown that although newer drug therapies have lowered AIDS mortality, the chronic and disabling aspects of the disease and its numerous associated conditions continue to pose challenges for those affected (CDC, 2001). Many people with HIV/AIDS struggle to overcome personal, financial, and social challenges that affect their desire to live independently and return to the workforce (McReynolds & Garske, 2001). In addition to these general characteristics of the AIDS population, a needs assessment study demonstrated that individuals' perceptions of needs differed by race, ethnicity, and gender (Sankar & Luborsky, 2003).

Together, these studies indicated that individuals with HIV/AIDS would potentially benefit from an individualized intervention designed to help them achieve independent living and employment as they envisioned it. These studies provided a foundation on which to propose a study of that type of occupational therapy intervention (Paul-Ward, Braveman, Kielhofner, & Levin, 2005).

Developing and Testing Occupational Therapy Theory

Every profession makes use of theories that underlie and explain its practice. By definition, the explanations offered by a theory are always tentative. By testing these explanations, research allows theory to be corrected and refined so that it provides increasingly useful explanations for practice. Ideas about how research refines and tests theory have evolved over the centuries, but research remains the primary tool by which a theory can be improved.

Practice theory research explains problems that therapists address and justifies approaches to solving them that are used in therapy. Consequently, the testing and refinement of such theories through research contributes to advancing practice. Therapists should always judge and place their confidence in the explanations provided by any theory in relation to the extent to which that theory has been tested and developed by research.

The motor control model provides one example of how research tests theory with implications for practice. Occupational therapy practice for individuals with central nervous system damage has been guided by the motor control model, which is a theory of how people control movement. Toward the end of the 20th century, this model, which previously saw the control of movement as being directed exclusively by the brain, began to change. A new conceptualization (Mathiowetz & Bass-Haugen, 1994, 2002) argued that movement is a result of the interaction of the human nervous system, the musculoskeletal system, and the environment. This theory emphasized the importance of the task being performed and the environment (e.g., the objects used) in influencing how a person moves. The implication of this theory was that the tasks chosen and the objects used in therapy would have an impact on recovery of coordinated movement.

Occupational therapists conducted research that illustrated clearly that the nature of the task being done and the environment do affect the quality of movement (Lin, Wu, & Trombly, 1998; Mathiowetz & Bass-Haugen, 1994; Wu, Trombly, & Lin, 1994). These and other studies (Ma & Trombly, 2002; Trombly & Ma, 2002) now provide evidence that tasks involving meaningful objects and goal-oriented activities positively influence performance and motor learning.

A wide range of research can be used to test and develop theory. In fact, no single study can ever test all aspects of a theory. The types of studies that are typically used to examine and develop theory include:

- Studies that aim to verify the accuracy of the concepts by asking whether there is evidence to support the way a concept describes and/or explains certain phenomena
- Studies that ask whether there are relationships between phenomena as specified by the theory
- Studies that compare different groups of participants on concepts that the theory offers to explain the differences between those groups
- Studies that examine the potential of the theory to predict what will happen

Over time, as the evidence accumulates from such studies, informed judgments can be made about the accuracy and completeness of a theory. Findings from such research typically lead to alterations in the theory that allow it to offer more accurate explanations. Because the theories used in occupa-tional therapy typically seek to explain problems that therapists encounter in practice and how therapists attempt to solve those problems, these types of studies directly inform practice.

Providing Evidence About the Nature and Outcomes of Therapy

Many types of studies examine the various aspects of occupational therapy practice and its outcomes. These are typically studies that:

- Are undertaken to develop and test assessments used in practice
- Examine the clinical reasoning of therapists when they are making decisions about therapy
- Determine the outcomes that result from therapy
- Examine the process of therapy (i.e., asking what goes on in therapy)
- Use participatory methods to investigate and improve services in a specific context

Studies That Test Assessments Used in Therapy

A number of interrelated forms of inquiry are used to develop and test assessments used in the field; the aim of **assessment research,** sometimes referred to as **psychometric research,** is to ensure the dependability of those methods (Benson & Schell, 1997). Dependable assessments are reli-able; that is, they yield consistent information in different circumstances, at different times, with different clients, and when different therapists administer them. A dependable information–gathering method must also be valid, providing the information it is intended to provide. Studies that examine whether an assessment is valid are typi-cally those that:

- Ask experts whether the content of an assess-ment is coherent and representative of what is intended to be gathered
- Analyze the items that make up an assessment to determine whether they coalesce to capture the trait they aim to measure
- Ask whether the assessment correlates with mea-sures of concepts that are expected to concur and whether it diverges from those with which no relationship is expected
- Determine whether they can differentiate be-tween different groups of people

In addition to studies that examine the reliabil-ity and validity of assessments, there are studies that examine their clinical utility. Such studies may ask therapists and/or clients whether they find the assessments informative and useful for identifying problems and making decisions about theory. The development of any assessment ordinarily involves a series of studies that contribute to the ongoing improvement of the assessment over time.

Studies of Clinical Reasoning

Occupational therapists work with clients to identify their problems and choose a course of action so clients may manage their problems and improve their functioning through engaging in occupations. Research that examines how occupational therapists identify problems and make treatment decisions is referred to as **clinical reasoning research** (Christiansen & Lou, 2001; Rogers, 1983; Schon, 1983). Investigations that examine clinical reasoning constitute an important area of research in occupational therapy.

One of the most influential studies of clinical reasoning, by Mattingly and Flemming (1994), identified different types of reasoning that characterized occupational therapy practice. Their research has served as a framework for understanding how occupational therapists make sense of and take action with reference to their clients' problems and challenges in therapy.

Outcomes Research

Outcomes research is concerned with the results of occupational therapy. Investigations that examine the outcomes of occupational therapy services include:

- Investigations of specific intervention strategies or techniques
- Studies of comprehensive occupational therapy programs
- Inquiries that examine the occupational therapy contribution to an interdisciplinary program of services (Kielhofner, Hammel, Helfrich, Finlayson, & Taylor, 2004)

The study of occupational therapy techniques and approaches helps refine the understanding of these discrete elements of practice. This type of research examines outcomes specific to an intended intervention. Such studies may also seek to determine the relative impact of different techniques or approaches, such as comparisons between individual versus group interventions.

Studies of comprehensive occupational therapy programs ask whether an entire package of services produces a desired outcome. Such studies typically examine the impact of services on such outcomes as independent living, employment, and

enhanced school performance. A well-known example of this type of research is a study by Clark and colleagues (1997), which documented the positive outcomes of an occupational therapy program for well elderly individuals. Finally, studies that examine the effect of interdisciplinary services can also document the impact of the occupational therapy component of such services.

Inquiry Into the Processes of Therapy: Mechanisms of Change

It is important not only to understand whether interventions work but also *why* they work or do not work. This approach is often referred to as **process research** or **formative research.** This approach involves understanding the **mechanisms of change,** that is, the processes by which an intervention creates change in a client. Studies that examine the effect of interventions are increasingly focusing on identifying the underlying mechanisms of change (Gitlin et al., 2000). Often, an important prelude to designing intervention outcome studies is to examine what goes into therapy in order to improve upon services before they are more formally tested.

An example is a study by Helfrich and Kielhofner (1994) that examined how clients' occupational narratives influenced the meaning they assigned to occupational therapy. This study showed how the meanings of therapy intended by therapists were often not received by or in concert with clients' meanings. The study findings underscored the importance of therapists having knowledge of their clients' narratives and organizing therapy as a series of events that enter into those narratives. Such studies of the process of therapy provide important information about how therapy can be improved to better meet clients' needs.

Participatory Research

A new and rapidly growing approach to investigation is **participatory research.** This approach involves researchers, therapists, and clients doing research together to develop and test occupational therapy services. Participatory research reverses the traditional role in which the occupational therapist decides on what research questions to answer and what procedures to use. Instead, it relies on the client to drive, or heavily influence, these decisions. Participatory research embraces the idea of partnership in which all the constituents work together and share power and responsibility to investigate, improve, and determine the outcomes of service. It also involves innovation in which new services are created to respond to problems that are mutually identified by researchers, therapists, and clients.

This type of research is especially useful for contributing knowledge that practitioners can readily use and that consumers will find relevant to their needs. An example of this kind of study involved developing and evaluating a consumer-driven self-management program for individuals with fatigue and other impairments associated with chronic fatigue syndrome. This program provided clients an opportunity to learn self-advocacy skills, energy conservation, and other ways to improve their quality of life, functional capacity, coping skills, and resource acquisition (Taylor, 2004).

Summary

This chapter introduces the necessity of research for the occupational therapy profession and emphasizes that research gives clients and the public reason to have confidence in occupational therapy services and outcomes. Research also provides the rationale for administrators and policymakers to support occupational therapy services.

The chapter also examines the evolution of evidence-based practice and its applications in occupational therapy. Additionally, this chapter covers the types of research most often conducted by occupational therapists, ranging from needs assessment to theory development, to psychometric research, to clinical outcomes studies and participatory research. Each of the key elements of the profession (research, theory, and practice) influences the others. Theory and research evidence guide practice. Practice raises problems and questions to be addressed in theory and research. Research tests theory and practice, providing information about their validity and utility, respectively.

Other chapters in this text explain the nature, scope, design, methods, and processes of research and illustrate the wide range of tools that researchers use for their inquiries. Throughout the text, as you encounter multiple discussions of how research is performed, it is important not to lose sight of *why* it is done. Remember Yerxa's (1987) observation that "Research is essential to achieving our aspirations for our patients and our hopes and dreams for our profession" (p. 415).

Review Questions

1. Describe three approaches to occupational therapy practice that have been informed by research. Provide specific examples.

2. What are some likely consequences if research is not conducted or used to enhance occupational therapy practice?
3. How did evidence-based practice originnate? What is the difference between evidence-based medicine and evidence-based practice in occupational therapy?
4. Compare and contrast participatory research and outcomes research in occupational therapy, describing the utility of each in context.
5. How does needs assessment research differ from practice theory research? Describe two different practice situations in which each of these approches would be appropriate, and explain why they would be appropriate.

REFERENCES

Altschuld, J. W., & Witkin, B. R. (2000). *From needs assessment to action: Transforming needs into solution strategies.* Thousands Oak, CA: Sage Publications.

Bennett, S., & Bennett, J. W. (2000). The process of evidence-based practice in occupational therapy: Informing clinical decisions. *Australian Occupational Therapy Journal, 47,* 171–180.

Benson J., & Schell, B. A. (1997). Measurement theory: Application to occupational and physical therapy. In J. Van Deusen & D. Brunt (Eds.), *Assessment in occupational therapy and physical therapy* (pp. 3–24). Philadelphia, PA: W.B. Saunders.

Canadian Association of Occupational Therapists, Association of Canadian Occupational Therapy University Programs, Association of Canadian Occupational Therapy Regulatory Organizations, & the Presidents' Advisory Committee. (2009). Joint position statement on evidence-based occupational therapy. *Canadian Journal of Occupational Therapy, 66,* 267–269.

Centers for Disease Control and Prevention (CDC). (2001). *HIV/AIDS surveillance supplemental report* (Vol. 7, No. 1). Atlanta, GA : Author.

Christiansen, C. (1983). An economic imperative. *Occupational Therapy Journal of Research, 3*(1), 195–198.

Christiansen, C., & Lou, J. (2001). Evidence-based practice forum. Ethical considerations related to evidence-based practice. *American Journal of Occupational Therapy, 55*(3), 345–349.

Clark, F., Azen, S. P., Zemke, R., Jackson, J., Carlson, M., Mandel, D., … Lipson, L. (1997). Occupational therapy for independent-living older adults: A randomized controlled trial. *Journal of the American Medical Association, 278*(16), 1321–1326.

Cusick, A. (2001). The experience of clinician-researchers in occupational therapy. *American Journal of Occupational Therapy, 55*(1), 9–18.

Dysart, A. M., & Tomlin, G. S. (2002). Factors related to evidence-based practice among U.S. practitioners. *American Journal of Occupational Therapy, 56,* 275–284.

Eakin, P. (1997). The Casson Memorial Lecture 1997: Shifting the balance—evidence based practice. *British Journal of Occupational Therapy, 60*(7), 290–294.

Erikson, A., Karlsson, G., Söderström, M., & Tham, K. (2004). A training apartment with electronic aids to daily living: Lived experiences of persons with brain damage. *American Journal of Occupational Therapy, 58*(3), 261–271.

Gitlin, L. N., Corcoran, M., Martindale-Adams, J., Malone, M. A., Stevens, A., & Winter, L. (2000). Identifying mechanisms of action: Why and how does intervention work? In R. Schulz (Ed.), *Handbook of dementia care giving: Evidence-based interventions for family caregivers* (pp. 225–248). New York, NY: Springer.

Graham, F., Robertson, L., & Anderson, J. (2013). New Zealand occupational therapists' views on evidence-based practice: A replicated survey of attitudes, confidence, and behaviors. *Australian Occupational Therapy Journal, 60*, 120–128.

Helfrich, C., & Kielhofner, G. (1994). Volitional narratives and the meaning of therapy. *American Journal of Occupational Therapy, 48*(4), 319–326.

Karon, J. M., Fleming, P. L., Steketee, R. W., & De Cock, K. M. (2001). HIV in the United States at the turn of the century: An epidemic in transition. *American Journal of Public Health, 91*(7), 1060–1068.

Kates, J. R., Sorian, J. S., Crowley, T. A., & Summers, T. A. (2002). Critical policy challenges in the third decade of the HIV/AIDS epidemic. *American Journal of Public Health, 92*(7), 1060–1063.

Kielhofner, G., Hammel, J., Helfrich, C., Finlayson, M., & Taylor, R. R. (2004). Documenting outcomes of occupational therapy: the center for outcomes research and education. *American Journal of Occupational Therapy, 58*, 15–23.

Lampinen, J., & Tham, K. (2003). Interaction with the physical environment in everyday occupation after stroke: A phenomenological study of visuospatial agnosia. *Scandinavian Journal of Occupational Therapy, 10*(4), 147–156.

Lin, K. C., Wu, C. Y., & Trombly, C. A. (1998). Effects of task goal on movement kinematics and line bisection performance in adults without disabilities. *American Journal of Occupational Therapy, 52*(3), 179–187.

Ma, H., & Trombly, C. A. (2002). A synthesis of the effects of occupational therapy for persons with stroke, part II: Remediation of impairments. *American Journal of Occupational Therapy, 56*(3), 260–274.

Mathiowetz, V., & Bass-Haugen, J. (1994). Motor behavior research: Implications for therapeutic approaches to central nervous system dysfunction. *American Journal of Occupational Therapy, 48*(8), 733–745.

Mathiowetz, V., & Bass-Haugen, J. (2002). Assessing abilities and capacities: Motor behavior. In C. A. Trombly & M. V. Radomski (Eds.), *Occupational therapy for physical dysfunction* (5th ed., pp. 137–158). Baltimore, MD: Lippincott Williams & Wilkins.

Mattingly, C., & Flemming, M. (1994). *Clinical reasoning: Forms of inquiry in a therapeutic practice*. Philadelphia, PA: F.A. Davis.

McReynolds C. J., & Garske, G. G. (2001). Current issues in HIV disease and AIDS: Implications for health and rehabilitation professionals. *Work: A Journal of Prevention, Assessment, and Rehabilitation, 17*, 117–124.

Paul-Ward, A., Braveman, B., Kielhofner, G., & Levin, M. (2005). Developing employment services for individuals with HIV/AIDS: Participatory action strategies at work. *Journal of Vocational Rehabilitation, 22*(2), 85–93.

Pighills, A. C., Plummer, D., Harvey, D., & Pain, T. (2013). Positioning occupational therapy as a discipline on the research continuum: Results of a cross-sectional survey of reseach experience. *Australian Occupational Therapy Journal, 60,* 241–251.

Polgar, S., & Thomas, S. A. (2000). *Introduction to research in the health sciences*. Edinburgh, UK: Churchill Livingstone.

Rogers, J. C. (1983). Eleanor Clarke Slagle Lectureship—1983; Clinical reasoning: The ethics, science, and art. *American Journal of Occupational Therapy, 37*(9), 601–616.

Sackett, D. L. (2002). *Evidence-based medicine: How to practice and teach EBM* (2nd ed.). Edinburgh, UK: Churchill Livingstone.

Sackett, D. L., Rosenberg, W. M., Grey, J. A., Haynes, R. B., & Richardson, W. S. (1996). Evidence-based medicine: What it is and what it isn't. *British Medical Journal, 312*(7023), 71–72.

Sackett, D.L., Straus, S.E., Richardson, W.S., Rosenberg, W., & Haynes, R.B. (2000). *Evidence-based Medicine: How to Practice and Teach EBM*, Second Edition. London: Churchill Livingstone.

Sankar, A., & Luborsky, M. (2003). Developing a community-based definition of needs for persons living with chronic HIV. *Human Organization, 62*(2), 153–165.

Schon, D. (1983). *The reflective practitioner: How professionals think in action*. New York, NY: Basic Books.

Stronge, M., & Cahill, M. (2012). Self-reported knowledge, attitudes, and behaviour towards evidence-based practice of occupational therapy students in Ireland. *Occupational Therapy International, 19*, 7–16.

Taylor, M. C. (1997). What is evidence-based practice? *British Journal of Occupational Therapy, 60*, 470–474.

Taylor, M. C. (2000). *Evidence-based practice for occupational therapists*. Oxford, UK: Blackwell Science Ltd.

Taylor, R. (2004). Quality of life and symptom severity in individuals with chronic fatigue syndrome: Findings form a randomized clinical trial. *American Journal of Occupational Therapy, 58*(1), 35–43.

Tham, K., Borell, L., & Gustavsson, A. (2000). The discovery of disability: A phenomenological study of unilateral neglect. *American Journal of Occupational Therapy, 54*(4), 398–406.

Tham, K., & Kielhofner, G. (2003). Impact of the social environment on occupational experience and performance among persons with unilateral neglect. *American Journal of Occupational Therapy, 57*(4), 403–412.

Trombly, C. A., & Ma, H. (2002). A synthesis of the effects of occupational therapy for persons with stroke, part I: Restoration of roles, tasks, and activities. *American Journal of Occupational Therapy, 56*(3), 250–259.

Witkin, B. R., & Altschuld, J. W. (1995). *Planning and conducting needs assessments: A practical guide*. Thousand Oaks, CA: Sage Publications.

Wu, C. Y., Trombly, C. A., & Lin, K. C. (1994). The relationship between occupational form and occupational performance: A kinematic perspective. *American Journal of Occupational Therapy, 48*(8), 679–687.

Yerxa, E. J. (1987). Research: The key to the development of occupational therapy as an academic discipline. *American Journal of Occupational Therapy, 41*(7), 415–419.

Zimolag, U., French, N., & Paterson, M. (2002). Striving for professional excellence: the role of evidence-based practice and professional artistry. *OTNow, 4*, 8–10.

CHAPTER 2

Classifications and Aims of Research

Renée R. Taylor • Gary Kielhofner • Ellie Fossey

Learning Outcomes

- Compare and contrast the three ways of classifying research: major methodological approach, research design, and research purposes.
- Describe the basic characteristics of quantitative research and the relevance of this approach to occupational therapy research and practice.
- Delineate the key aspects of qualitative research and explain their role in occupational therapy and practice.
- Explicate the utility and benefits of the following research designs, including their limitations: quasi-experimental studies, single-subject studies, field studies and naturalistic observation, survey studies, and psychometric studies.
- Differentiate among basic research, applied research, and transformative research.

Introduction

Research studies are almost as varied as they are numerous. Even within a specific field such as occupational therapy, there is considerable diversity in terms of the different topics and approaches to investigation. For example, studies may differ along such dimensions as:

- The sample size, or number of study participants (from one to hundreds or thousands)
- What participants are asked to do (being observed versus undergoing complex interventions)
- How information is gathered (following participants in their ordinary activities and context versus taking measurements in a laboratory setting)
- How the data are analyzed (identifying underlying narrative themes versus computing statistical analyses)

One way to appreciate the diversity of research is to examine the different ways it is classified and to understand the aims of the different approaches. Research may be classified in terms of major methodological approach, design, and the underlying purpose for the research.

Another important aspect of the diversity of research is the value system and worldview that underlies the selection of a particular approach. This underlying value system drives decisions about whether an approach to a particular research question is useful and valid. For example, is a study more valid if the researcher is blinded to the experiences of the subjects? Or is it more valid if the researcher personally identifies with the subjects' experiences? Depending on whom you ask, the answers to these questions are bound to be vastly different. These differences are deeply rooted in the underlying beliefs and traditions of knowledge discovery to which each researcher adheres. The belief system that underlies a researcher's data collection approach, measurement instruments, and orientation to analysis is often referred to as the philosophical foundation of research.

This chapter examines the three different ways to define and classify research: (1) by major methodological approach, (2) by design, and (3) by aim, or purpose, of the research.

Defining and Classifying Research

The three major ways in which to define and classify research are (Table 2.1):

- Major methodological approach
- Research design
- Research purposes

Major Methodological Approach

One of the broadest ways to classify research is to examine it in terms of the two major methodological approaches: qualitative and quantitative

CASE EXAMPLE

Kate is an entry-level student enrolled in a research methods course at a large, research-intensive university. She is working on an assignment in which she must explain the major types of research in occupational therapy and their aims. Then, she will choose one approach to research and explain the philosophical foundation that underlies that particular approach.

Kate visits the university library and retrieves various journal articles containing studies with vastly different experimental designs and approaches to data collection. In some studies, the researchers have made every effort to restrict the amount of information that both they and subjects have about the research process, so that there is no chance that the effects of any treatment that is given are influenced by advanced knowledge or expectations about the outcome.

In other studies that Kate encounters, researchers and subjects not only know the type of treatment that the subjects are receiving, but they are collaborators in producing the treatment. One example is a chronic illness self-management program in which participants helped develop a treatment protocol in order to manage their own chronic illnesses and symptoms. Still another study reveals how a researcher with a particular disability joins a focus group that includes other individuals with the same disability to detail and plan a persuasive way to document their experiences with environmental barriers within their communities.

After reading through the different studies and their approaches, Kate realized that some researchers designed their studies in such a way that subjectivity and personal bias were minimized by strict standardization procedures and careful distancing of themselves from the subjects. By contrast, others immersed themselves in the lives of those they studied and detailed how their personal histories and subjective experiences shaped and informed their investigations. Still other investigators invited study participants to be equal partners in the research enterprise. Previously Kate had stereotyped research as a dry and rather boring topic of study, but she immediately became enthused to learn more about the various ways to approach science within the field of occupational therapy. Her plan was to learn about the different classifications and purposes of research and then to examine her own thoughts and feelings about how these underlying worldviews and belief systems might correspond philosophically with the various approaches.

Table 2.1 Ways to Define and Classify Research

Classifications	Examples
Major methodological approach	Qualitative methods
	Quantitative methods
Research design	Experimental and quasi-experimental studies
	Single-subject designs
	Field studies and naturalistic observation
	Survey studies
	Psychometric studies
Research purposes	Basic research
	Applied research
	Transformative research

research methods. The terminology suggests these methods differ by the presence or absence of quantification. However, it is important to note that these two broad categories of research are also distinguished by important philosophical differences (Crotty, 1998). The following discussion describes the origins of these research methods and their differing assumptions, approaches to rigor, and research foci, as well as examines how researchers using these approaches gather, analyze, and interpret data.

Quantitative Research

Quantitative research is an approach to research that is characterized by objectivity. Researchers create and test theories using standardized and predetermined designs, measures, sampling approaches, and procedures. Quantitative approaches test one **hypothesis** (a structured statement of anticipated results of the study) or more and translate reports and observations into numerical data that are analyzed using statistical approaches. The aim of quantitative methods is to discover the rules or laws underlying the objective world as a basis for scientific prediction and control (Guba & Lincoln, 1994). Quantitative researchers make every effort to enforce rigor by limiting the influence of subjective bias and other actions and events that interfere with an accurate interpretation of the data. It is helpful to consider historical and contemporary examples of quantitative research in occupational therapy.

Historical Examples. Research in the occupational therapy field began to develop in earnest in the mid-20th century. At that time, occupational therapy practice was dominated by an approach that emulated medicine's emphasis on scientific methods developed in the physical and life sciences, such as chemistry and biology (Kielhofner, 2009). Not surprisingly, the research that began to appear around this time was quantitative in nature. The following two examples of research, reported in the *American Journal of Occupational Therapy,* are characteristic of the period:

- Drussell (1959) reported a descriptive study to investigate whether the industrial work performance of adults with cerebral palsy was related to their manual dexterity, as measured by the Minnesota Rate of Manipulation Test (MRM). The MRM is a standardized measure of manual dexterity originally used for testing workers' ability to perform semiskilled factory operations. Work performance was measured with a widely used industrial measure, the Service Descriptive Rating Scale. In this study, both tests were administered to 32 adults with cerebral palsy who were enrolled in an adult vocational training program. The results of the study indicated that the two measures were positively correlated. This finding was interpreted as indicating that the MRM could be a valuable tool in assessing vocational potential for this population.
- Cooke (1958) reported results of an experimental study that investigated whether adding a weight to the dominant upper extremity of patients with multiple sclerosis would improve their coordination. The rationale was that the addition of weight would mitigate patients' intention tremors and thus increase coordination. In this study of 39 patients in a physical rehabilitation program, the subjects were tested with and without a weighted cuff using the MRM (used in this study as the measure of coordination). The results of the study failed to support the hypothesis that the addition of a weight would improve coordination. In fact, the opposite was observed; subjects scored significantly lower when wearing the weighted cuffs. This author concluded that the addition of the cuff slowed the speed of movement, negatively affecting coordination.

The characteristics of these two studies—quantification of the variables under study through use of standardized measures, use of experimental conditions in the second study, and statistical analyses (descriptive in the first study; inferential in the second study)—are hallmarks of quantitative research. Since these studies were conducted, the use of more complex experimental designs, including pre- and postintervention testing, randomization of study participants, and test development, has developed in occupational therapy. Nevertheless, the underlying logic of the research designs used in these two historical studies is similar to that of contemporary quantitative research in occupational therapy.

Contemporary Example. Let's examine a contemporary example of a quantitative research study. The study is a randomized clinical trial involving clients with trigger finger, a painful condition affecting the flexor tendon of a digit in which the digit locks or catches, as if a finger were wrapped around the trigger of a gun. A particular splinting approach is being tested on an experimental group, and a placebo splint is given to a control group. This is considered a randomized clinical trial because subjects are assigned to either the experimental or control group without knowing the condition to which they are assigned. When a researcher is not allowed to know which kind of splint has been given to a particular subject, it is often referred to as **blinding.** When subjects are not allowed to know the kind of treatment they are receiving, it is also called blinding. When both researchers and subjects are not permitted to know which treatment a particular subject is receiving, it is referred to as a **double-blind study.** The hypothesis of this study is that subjects receiving the experimental splint will demonstrate a decreased frequency of trigger finger compared with controls within a 1-year period.

Qualitative Research

Qualitative research is an approach that aims to describe and explain individuals' subjective experiences, actions, interactions, and social contexts through various approaches involving interviewing, note-taking of events and actions, examining written and visual documents, and making audio and video recordings. Qualitative research is an umbrella term for a range of methodologies originating from the fields of anthropology, sociology, philosophy, and psychology. Today, these methods are widely used in the health sciences. Many researchers in occupational therapy have embraced these methodologies to study occupation and practice issues, viewing them as congruent with the profession's philosophical orientation (Hammell, 2002).

Qualitative research is generally divided into ethnographic, phenomenological, and narrative inquiry approaches, each of which represents a somewhat different standpoint. **Ethnography** emphasizes the societal and cultural context that shapes meaning and behavior. **Phenomenology** focuses on how people experience and make sense of their immediate worlds, using the people themselves as co-researchers, and **narrative inquiry** seeks to understand how people construct storied accounts of their and others' lives and of shared events (Rice & Ezzy, 1999). The following section provides historical and contemporary examples of these kinds of approaches to qualitative research.

Historical Examples. Qualitative research began to appear in occupational therapy literature during the 1980s. At that time, there was a resurgence of interest in ideas about occupation, its meanings and significance for health upon which occupational therapy practice was founded (Kielhofner, Braveman, et al., 2004). This led occupational therapists to seek relevant research designs for exploring the meanings and contexts of people's everyday lives, occupations, and experiences of illness, disability, and therapy, and to argue for the use of qualitative designs in occupational therapy (Kielhofner, 1982a; 1982b; Krefting, 1989; Yerxa, 1991). Early examples of qualitative research published in occupational therapy most commonly used ethnographic designs, originating in anthropological fieldwork methods, of which the following is an example.

This study examined the daily life experiences of 69 adults with developmental delay who were discharged from state hospitals to residential facilities as part of the deinstitutionalization movement. In this study, the project team (anthropologists, sociologists, and clinicians) followed the study participants over a 3-year period, participating with them in their daily life events in the five residential facilities where they lived. Researchers recorded observational data in field notes, conducted ongoing open-ended interviews with the residents, and videotaped them.

Analysis of the data from this field study resulted in several publications (Bercovici, 1983; Goode, 1983; Kielhofner, 1979, 1981). Kielhofner

(1979) reported how the participants experienced and organized their behavior in time. He described how the participants did not progress through the usual life events that tend to demark maturation (e.g., graduating high school, marriage, and parenthood). Rather, their lives were largely unchanged over time, with the result that the participants tended not to be future oriented; they did not expect things to change, nor did they make plans for achieving change in their lives. Hence, he argued, among other points, the participants ". . . have ceased to become in the sense of the dominant culture, and from their own point of view, they are off the career time track. They are, in a sense, 'frozen in time.' " (Kielhofner, 1979, p. 163).

Another feature of how these study participants experienced their lives uniquely was that, unlike many other members of American culture, they had a surplus of time and a deficiency of things to do to fill up their time. As a result, they did not experience long periods of waiting for events to occur with the impatience or frustration that characterized the investigators' reactions. Rather, waiting was something that helped to fill time. These and other findings pointed out that these adults approached the organization of their daily activities and their lives in a radically different way from mainstream American culture (Kielhofner, 1981).

This study highlights the emphasis of ethnographic research on illuminating the social and cultural context of human action and its meaning. It also illustrates the use of this type of research in examining how changes in health policy and services can impact people. Since this study was conducted, qualitative research in occupational therapy has diversified, using phenomenological, narrative, and, more recently, participatory approaches. It has also expanded in focus to explore occupational therapists' clinical reasoning and practice issues in many settings, as well as the everyday lives and occupations of clients of occupational therapy services.

Contemporary Examples. One contemporary example of an ethnographic study involves perceptions of safety among 54 underserved children attending third grade at a public school within an impoverished neighborhood. In this study, the children are provided with cameras and asked to take photos of anything that makes them feel unsafe. Once the photos are printed, the children are asked to write captions under each photo describing the unsafe scene or object. The photographic data gathered in this study are then organized by themes representing the societal and cultural contexts that shape the children's perception of safety within their immediate neighborhoods.

An example of a phenomenological study involves a study of 14 parents of young children with past-year juvenile criminal records. In this study, a researcher seeks to understand the personal experiences and perceptions of the parents from their points of view. The central research question is: "Describe your experience as a parent of a child who has had a conviction within this past year." Subsequent interview questions include: "How has the conviction affected your relationship with your child? How has the conviction affected relationships within your immediate family? Within your extended family? Has the conviction affected you socially? In your community? Has it affected you at work? Has it affected you financially? What other effects have your child's conviction had on your life?"

In this study, data are analyzed from the perspective of Kornfeld (1988). The first phase is **epoche,** in which the researchers write down all of their personal assumptions, biases, and stereotypes of how the parent co-investigators might answer these questions and then throw them away. This symbolic process reminds the researcher to ignore preconceived notions and focus on striving to understand the participants' experiences. In the second phase, the questions are administered to the parents in a seamless interview fashion, recorded, and transcribed verbatim. Each interview is listened to in full and analyzed in depth, with the ultimate goal of clustering and synthesizing categories to discover themes for each participant and for all the participants together.

Ciuffetelli-Parker (2013) conducted a narrative inquiry of poverty in a primary school community in Canada. Conceptualizations of poverty were analyzed by gathering brief stories, referred to as small narrative discourses, about the experience of living in poverty from shared dialogues between teachers and community members. As anticipated, the stories reflected that many participants held what were referred to as deficit conceptualizations of the children served by the school district. In order to overcome this biased and unhelpful way of viewing the children, participants learned to challenge and cross-examine the meanings behind their own stories in order to create new awareness and new understandings of poverty and education (Ciuffetelli-Parker, 2013).

Comparing Quantitative and Qualitative Research

Although they share the similar objectives of developing and evaluating new knowledge about one or more phenomena, quantitative and qualitative research differ in some fundamental ways. Table 2.2 summarizes these differences, which are also depicted in Figure 2.1.

Research Design

Research can also differ by its basic design. **Research design** refers to the fundamental strategy or plan of how the research will be structured. Research designs each have their own inherent logic. Although an exhaustive list of all research designs would not be practical, this discussion addresses the most common designs

Table 2.2 Key Differences Between Quantitative and Qualitative Research Methods

Characteristic	Quantitative Research	Qualitative Research
Origin	Physical and life sciences	Study of people different from the investigator (e.g., anthropology, philosophy, sociology)
Assumptions	Objective reality contains stable, preexisting patterns or order that can be discovered	Social reality is dynamic, contextual, and governed by local meanings
Aims	To discover natural laws that enable prediction or control of events	To understand social life and describe how people construct social meaning
Approach to Rigor	Maintain objectivity	Authentically represent the viewpoints of the individuals studied
Data Presentation	Numbers (statistics)	Textual, "thick" descriptions in language of participants
Data Analysis	Describes variables and their relationships and tests hypotheses in order to test theory	Identifies meaning, patterns, and connections among data; describes experience/social scene; produces theory "grounded" in the data

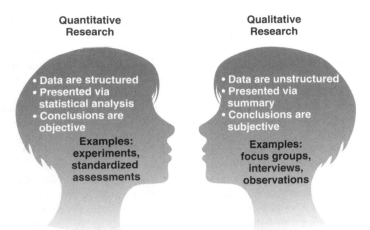

Quantitative Research
- Data are structured
- Presented via statistical analysis
- Conclusions are objective

Examples: experiments, standardized assessments

Qualitative Research
- Data are unstructured
- Presented via summary
- Conclusions are subjective

Examples: focus groups, interviews, observations

Figure 2.1   The fundamental differences between quantitative and qualitative research.

found in occupational therapy investigations. They include:

- Experimental and quasi-experimental studies
- Single-subject studies
- Field studies and naturalistic observation
- Survey studies
- Psychometric studies

Experimental and Quasi-Experimental Studies

Experimental and quasi-experimental studies fit within the quantitative research tradition. Studies using these designs seek to examine the effects of an experimental manipulation (e.g., an occupational therapy treatment approach) of some characteristic or set of characteristics of the research subject. The basic characteristic of all experimental research is that the investigator manipulates an **independent variable** (the antecedent variable that is expected to produce an effect) in order to affect a **dependent variable** (the variable in which a specific outcome or effect is observed, or not observed). Experimental and quasi-experimental designs aim to provide evidence that the independent variable is the cause of changes or differences in the dependent variable.

Experimental and quasi-experimental designs are specific blueprints for how to conduct an experiment (Campbell & Stanley, 1963). The fundamental aim of experimentation is to control, as much as possible, for extraneous influences (**confounding variables**) that could lead to an incorrect conclusion about the influence of the independent variable on the dependent variable. For example, in the study described earlier that compared the

effects of an experimental splint with a control-condition splint on the past-year frequency of trigger finger in a sample of hand therapy clients, the amount of fine motor activity performed when wearing and not wearing the splint is one confounding variable that could affect the findings. It is possible that individuals performing excessive activity would experience more symptoms, irrespective of treatment condition. Similarly, it is possible that individuals performing significantly less activity with the affected hand would show different effects from the splint than those performing an average amount of activity.

In a true **experimental design,** two or more groups of participants are randomly assigned to different levels (or experimental conditions) of one or more independent variables. A **level of an independent variable** is an experimental condition that reflects the degree to which the variable is introduced to the subject.

Let's consider a study of the effects of one independent variable on one dependent variable. In this scenario, we will examine the effects of three different doses of a particular medication on spasticity. The independent variable would be represented as the medication, and the three levels (or conditions) of that variable would be represented as "high dose," "low dose," or "no dose." Accordingly, subjects would be divided into three respective groups, with the first group receiving a high dosage of the medication, the second receiving a low dosage, and the third group (control group) receiving no medication. Each condition represents a level, or dose, of the medication variable.

An important characteristic of all experimental studies and many quasi-experimental studies is the inclusion of a **control group.** A control group is an experimental condition to which a group of subjects is assigned as a basis for comparison with the **experimental group** (or groups). Subjects in the experimental groups receive the condition of primary interest (in this example, medication). Subjects in the control group do not receive the condition of primary interest. Sometimes subjects in the control group receive a **placebo** (a substitute for the condition or treatment that is intended to have an effect, but in reality has no effect). Groups of subjects receiving a placebo condition are referred to as **placebo control groups.** When used in an appropriate context, placebo controls offer a more rigorous test of an independent variable because they rule out **expectancy effects,** or the possible psychological effects of knowing one is receiving a treatment, on actual treatment outcomes.

A simple example of an experimental study in occupational therapy is a study in which one group of clients on an inpatient neurorehabilitation unit is randomly assigned to receive therapy focusing on self-care training using serial repetition and rehearsal of the tasks. A second group does not receive any hygiene training. In this study, the dependent variable would be represented as the level of independent self-care performance. The independent variable would be the presence or absence of the self-care training (two levels). The aim of the experiment would be to attribute any differences in self-care independence (dependent variable) between the two groups to the independent variable (receipt of training).

In this example, it is important to consider a potential confounding variable: The dependent variable may have been influenced by the initial level of functioning of participants. If one group was generally better functioning than the other group at the beginning of the experiment, the difference in functioning could account for differences in self-care independence, raising questions about whether the training had any effect. We might find this difference between the two groups whether or not they received occupational therapy services.

Thus, the primary difference between an experimental study and a quasi-experimental study is that in an experimental study, subjects are randomly assigned to the different conditions to achieve equivalent groups. **Random assignment** to groups means that neither the subjects nor the researchers are allowed to choose the group to which subjects are assigned. Instead, a specific statistical or mathematical method is used to assign subjects to groups. Depending on the number of groups and on other issues involving demand for

rigor, random assignment to groups may be completed using a number of different strategies, ranging from tossing a coin to sophisticated computer-generated techniques.

Quasi-experimental designs follow the same logic as experimental designs but lack the degree of rigor found in true experimental designs (Shadish, Cook, & Campbell, 2002). Both designs typically involve the experimental manipulation of an independent variable of interest in order to measure the effects on a dependent variable. In terms of rigor, however, the primary difference between experimental and quasi-experimental designs is that of randomization. In a quasi-experimental study, subjects are not randomly assigned to a condition. Instead, subjects either remain in a single group and are studied at various time points before and after the experimental manipulation (**time-series designs**) or they end up in different groups as a matter of convenience (i.e., **pretest–posttest nonequivalent group designs**) or for other practical purposes, such as the need to test two groups known to differ on the characteristic of interest even before the study begins.

Following is an example of the pretest–posttest nonequivalent group design: A researcher compares two groups of subjects to test the effects of a year-long self-management program for individuals with chronic pain combined with a new medication versus the effects of the self-management program alone. A pain self-rating scale is administered prior to and after the intervention. The researcher chooses not to blind subjects to the condition but instead provides full disclosure to subjects and allows them to select in which condition they would like to participate. As a result, subjects with higher levels of pain more often choose the self-management program with the new medication. Thus, the researcher begins the study with two groups that are not equivalent in terms of the outcome to be measured, which is pain severity.

Occupational therapy researchers sometimes undertake less rigorous quasi-experimental research because true experimental research can be difficult to undertake in real-life contexts. This is often the case in community-based research, such as the study undertaken by Professor Gary Kielhofner and his colleagues (Kielhofner, Braveman, et al., 2004) that compared the effects of a work rehabilitation program based on the Model of Human Occupation (Kielhofner, 2008) with a less intensive standard educational intervention; the researchers investigated the effects of the two programs on independent living and employment (dependent variables).

In this study, services were delivered to residents in the facilities where they lived. Random assignment was not feasible because delivering different types of services to people living in the same house was likely to create other situations that would bias the results. For example, if a person in one group shared information and resources he received from services with a roommate who was not receiving those services, it would lead to **contamination effects** (an unanticipated confound in which subjects in an experimental condition share aspects of a treatment with subjects in a control condition, influencing outcomes for subjects in the control condition). Similarly, a human subjects review board might determine that it would be unethical to administer services that are expected to be superior to one group of individuals but not to another group, particularly when both groups are living in the same household, making the potential injustice of the situation apparent to everyone involved.

Consequently, for this study, a quasi-experimental design was chosen. All residents in one setting received the same services (the work rehabilitation program based on the Model of Human Occupation) and were compared with residents of another setting who received usual services (a standardized educational intervention). This type of design opens the experiment to alternative explanations for any differences in independence or employment found other than the services received, such as group personality, types of people in each house, and house staff. However, it was the most rigorous design practicable in this context. Thus, despite their limitations, quasi-experimental designs are valuable when demands and constraints within the health-care system prevent the use of random assignment.

Single-Subject Studies

Experimental and quasi-experimental designs rely on comparisons of averages in groups. Individual variation in response to an intervention is not a focus of such studies. For that reason, practitioners sometimes find large-group experiments to have limited relevance to decision-making about what services or strategies would be best for an individual client. **Single-subject designs** follow the logic of experimentation but examine the impact of interventions on single subjects who serve as their own controls. Single-subject designs allow a researcher to measure changes in single subjects as they undergo varying treatment conditions within an actual practice setting.

Single-subject designs generally involve two major strategies that allow the subject to represent both a control and an experimental condition(s):

- Gathering baseline data over time during which the experimental condition is absent and then gathering data over time during which the experimental condition is present
- Gathering data during alternating periods in which the experimental condition is present or withdrawn

Quantitative data are gathered on the dependent variable during the different experimental and control phases, and the data are analyzed both visually and using statistics designed for single-subject experimentation.

For example, consider a researcher who wants to study the dosing effects of an antiviral medication commonly used to treat HIV/AIDS on the signs, symptoms, and viral load associated with a much less common and relatively new virus. Because of the low incidence of the novel virus, the researcher only has access to small groups and must study one subject at a time. The researcher might choose to employ a single-subject design that begins with an observational baseline period of no medication, followed by a period of high-dose medication, then by a period of low dosage, and finally by a follow-up period of no medication. This design would offer the researcher the opportunity to measure viral load, signs, and symptoms in the presence and absence of the medication at four different time points: time 1 (observational baseline), time 2 (high dosage), time 3 (low dosage), and time 4 (observational follow-up).

Because single-subject designs follow an experimental logic, they should not be confused with qualitative studies that may involve a single participant. Both types of studies are characterized by a sample of one, but their underlying logic is different. Qualitative research that includes only one study participant follows the logic of qualitative methodology. In this instance, the judgment is made that one participant is of sufficient interest or adequately characterizes the phenomena under question. Thus, additional participants are not necessary to inform the qualitative goals for the study.

Field Studies and Naturalistic Observation

Field studies and naturalistic observation are forms of research that take place in actual settings. Investigators study events as they happen and individuals in their natural context. Both qualitative and quantitative research methods make use of this type of design.

In qualitative **field studies,** investigators seek to gain an insider's view of the phenomena under study through intensive and extended immersion. Field study is a broad term referring to data collection outside of the laboratory and in a naturalistic setting. Investigators typically collect data in multiple ways (e.g., gathering documents and artifacts; informal interviewing and observation) over an extended period of time. Researchers also use their growing appreciation of the phenomena under study to continuously evolve the types of data collected, the methods for acquiring data, and who is sought out as a source of data.

Naturalistic observation refers to quantitative research that takes place in natural settings. Such research aims to study the phenomena "undisturbed" by laboratory conditions or experimental procedures. For example, naturalistic observation can be used to study specific behaviors as they occur in classrooms, hospitals, or nursing homes. In naturalistic observation studies, the observer seeks to make "unbiased" observations of how events or behaviors actually take place. The investigator does not participate in the events under study but rather seeks to be as unobtrusive as possible. Data are typically collected using a coding procedure determined prior to beginning the research, which enables the behavioral observations to be recorded in a manner that can be enumerated. Naturalistic observations generally seek to determine the kinds of behaviors that occur, their frequency, the conditions under which they occur, and so forth. Investigators may use a time-sampling approach in which observations are recorded at specific time intervals that are chosen randomly or according to some logical schema. For example, in a naturalistic observation of aggressive behavior among adolescents living in a group home to treat conduct disorder, a researcher might choose to record observations of aggression during times when the aides have reported that the aggressive behavior is most likely to occur: during group sports games, during mealtimes, and before bedtime.

Survey Studies

Survey studies investigate unknown characteristics in a defined population according to a nonexperimental design. They are often conducted with large samples (i.e., hundreds or thousands of subjects). Survey studies are used to investigate such things as conditions or needs within a defined community or the extent of disease or disability in a population. Generally, survey research aims to randomly select the sample so the findings can be generalized to the population from which the sample was chosen.

Survey research is implemented either through the use of mailed questionnaires or electronic technologies such as the Internet. For example, surveys can be conducted through web-based survey sites to which selected subjects are directed using an e-mail or other type of invitation to participate. Questionnaires are usually designed to gather quantitative data, although open-ended questions may be asked to elicit qualitative responses that are used to supplement quantitative findings.

Other survey research methods include telephone and face-to-face interviews. When surveys follow the logic of quantitative research, the investigator uses a structured interview protocol so that all the participants respond to the same standardized questions. In qualitative surveys, the investigator is more likely to use an interview guide that allows participants to influence the direction of the interview but also emphasizes strategies for probing in order to elicit the respondents' perspectives.

Psychometric Studies

Psychometric studies are specifically designed to investigate the properties of clinical assessment tools or data collection instruments that are intended for use in research. Psychometric research is largely quantitative, although qualitative methods are sometimes used to determine the type of content that should go into an assessment before it is developed as well as to examine its clinical utility. Strictly speaking, this type of research is aimed at determining the validity and reliability of these instruments. Following quantitative logic, instruments with known validity and reliability provide objective measurement of the variables under study.

Validity refers to whether an instrument measures what it is intended to measure. Because instruments are designed to operationalize an underlying concept or construct, this aspect is often referred to as **construct validity.** For example, construct validity would define the likelihood that an assessment that was intended to measure empathy in parents of children with disabilities accurately estimated all of the parental values, communications, and behaviors associated with empathy. There are many methods of determining validity, including concurrent validity and predictive validity.

Concurrent validity follows the logic that an instrument designed to capture a variable should show an association with another variable that is theoretically expected to be related to it. Returning to the example of the assessment of empathy in parents of children with disabilities, concurrent validity would be estimated if the researcher elected to compare the strength of the relationship between scores on this measure with scores on another general measure of empathy among adults within the general population.

Predictive validity asks whether a measure of some characteristic (e.g., ability to perform activities of daily living) is able to predict some future outcome, such as whether a person is able to perform those activities with or without assistance. Thus, studies designed to test expected associations, or predictions, provide evidence on behalf of the validity of an assessment tool or data collection instrument.

Reliability refers to whether a given instrument provides stable information across different circumstances. Thus, studies designed to test reliability might examine whether a given instrument is reliable, for instance, when multiple raters use the instrument to gather data and when data are gathered on more than one occasion (referred to as **interrater reliability** and **test–retest reliability,** respectively).

There are a number of examples of psychometric research in occupational therapy. Some of these include but are not limited to the development of observation-based performance measures such as the Assessment of Motor and Process Skills (Assessment of Motor and Process Skills, 2012; Fisher, 1997) and interview-based tools such as the Canadian Occupational Performance Measure (COPM; Carswell et al., 2004) and the Occupational Performance History Interview II (Kielhofner, Mallinson, et al., 2004).

Research Purposes

Research can be differentiated according to its underlying purpose. There are three underlying purposes of research: (1) basic, (2) applied, and (3) transformative. Within the field of occupational therapy, each purpose reflects a different viewpoint regarding how information generated from research informs practice and advances the science of our field.

Basic Research

Basic research, sometimes referred to as basic science, includes investigations that are under-

taken, primarily in a laboratory or other controlled setting, for the purposes of understanding some phenomena or testing a model or theory that explains some phenomena. For example, a basic research study may aim to test a hypothesis about a specific genetic polymorphism associated with a neurological disease. Alternatively, a basic research study may aim to test the mechanism of action that allows a medication commonly used for depression to also be helpful in alleviating chronic pain. Basic research is undertaken for the sake of generating new knowledge without direct concern for its applicability or practical significance. The full range of research methods and designs previously described may be used in basic research. However, basic research traditionally emphasized the importance of value-free science that was disinterested in questions of application in order to avoid undue bias. It was thought that basic science would inform practice by identifying the underlying laws that governed phenomena thus providing the logic for professions that applied that knowledge (Schon, 1983). This approach has been criticized by some scholars who argue that basic science knowledge does not translate readily into practice (Peloquin, 2002).

Occupational Science. Prior to the late 1980s, occupational therapy relied on basic research conducted by other disciplines to inform much of its practice. For instance, research studies that identified the anatomy of the musculoskeletal system and the physiology of nerve conduction are two examples of information generated from basic research in the fields of anatomy and physiology that form part of the foundation of occupational therapy knowledge.

Many occupational therapists now support the development of the field's own basic science that is concerned with the study of occupation, referred to as **occupational science.** Its proposed purpose is to generate explanations of humans in everyday life circumstances behaving within occupational contexts (Yerxa et al., 1989). Like other basic research, the role of occupational science is envisioned as describing, explaining, and predicting events as part of the search for knowledge and truth (Primeau, Clark, & Pierce, 1989).

Today, occupational science has grown into an academic discipline in itself, with a growing number of master's and doctoral degree programs around the world that reflect this unique perspective. Additionally, an academic journal, the *Journal of Occupational Science,* has been developed to publish research that focuses on the form, function, performance, and meaning of human occupations, or everyday activities in which people engage. The overarching goal of occupational science is to explicate the complexity of everyday occupations (Clark et al., 1991; Wilcock, 1991). Additionally, occupational science emphasizes the understanding of people as occupational beings who have the capability and need to participate in activities that shape their humanity (Yerxa et al., 1989). Moreover, the linkage of occupation and health serves as a central emphasis in occupational science because occupational scientists believe that occupations serve to enable or disable health and health serves to enable or disable people's participation in occupation (Wilcock, 1993; Yerxa, 1998). Another foundational concept behind occupational science is the understanding that occupations occur within cultural, spiritual, social, environmental (physical and natural), and economic contexts (Yerxa et al., 1989).

Hocking and Wright-St. Clair (2011) conceptualize occupational science in terms of its two major components: occupation and science. According to the occupational science perspective (Hocking & Wright-St. Clair, 2011) occupations are defined as the everyday activities in which people engage. Numerous scholars have reflected on how these occupations are enacted. From this perspective, occupation may be compartmentalized in terms of patterns, routines, and roles (Christiansen, 1991; Yerxa, 1998) and as having personal significance or symbolism (McGlaughlin Grey, 1997). Additionally, occupation has been viewed as promoting development and self-efficacy (Yerxa et al., 1989; Yerxa, 1998). Occupational scientists refer to science as the intention to develop new knowledge through quantitative and qualitative studies demonstrating adequate methodological rigor (Hocking & Wright-St. Clair, 2011).

Mosey (1992b, 1993) questioned the legitimacy of basic science in occupational therapy on the grounds that the allocation of human and other resources to basic inquiry would detract from badly needed applied inquiry. Its proponents, nevertheless, argue that occupational science will likely influence how occupational therapists perceive and approach their work (Zemke & Clark, 1996).

Basic research may vary in how closely it relates to practical problems and practice issues on which applied research focuses. Hocking and Wright-St. Clair (2011) summarized the relevance of occupational science to occupational therapy with a cluster of studies, including an international study of the meaning of preparing food for a special holiday among older women. The researchers asked fundamental questions about the occupations in which the women engaged in order to prepare the holiday meal. For example, the researchers asked the women when they began to prepare the meal, how they organized meal preparation, who else was involved, what each person did, how everyone knew what to do, and where the preparation took place. Hocking and Wright-St. Clair found that the older women drew upon local traditions, historical knowledge, and values passed down from honored people to inform their meal preparation, while at the same time accommodating the preferences of those being served.

The linkage to occupational therapy practice was made by Thibeault (2002), who then used the concept to unite and organize women ravaged by war and internal conflict in Sierra Leone to restore civility, trust, and organization within their community. The activity of meal preparation, with all of its associated traditions and personal, historical meanings, served as a cornerstone for future projects aimed to bring perpetrators and victims within the same community or families together, to rebuild their sense of community.

Applied Research

Investigations that seek to solve a practical problem or generate information specifically to inform practice are referred to as **applied research.** Many important research problems or questions generated in the health and human service environments are applied in nature. Applied research generally seeks to investigate the merits of practice strategies, such as assessments and interventions. In occupational therapy, applied research addresses issues such as:

- Whether an assessment used in practice provides dependable and useful information to guide practice
- How therapists reason in the context of practice
- What outcomes are achieved by providing particular services as part of therapy

Applied research is often viewed as particularly important for achieving external credibility (i.e., influencing the individuals who make policy and economic decisions that affect the delivery of occupational therapy services). Indeed, Mosey (1992a) argued that this type of research is critical to occupational therapy because it provides information about the value of what the profession does. However, practitioners have critiqued applied research for testing practice strategies under ideal conditions that cannot be reproduced in practice (Dubouloz, Egan, Vallerand, & Von Zweck, 1999;

Dysart & Tomlin, 2002). Applied research in occupational therapy ranges from psychometric studies to qualitative investigations of the therapy process to controlled experiments that compare different therapeutic approaches.

Transformative Research

Transformative research is a broad classification for inquiry that is designed to bring about change in a practical situation or a specific context. Its emphasis is on transforming social realities so that people's lives are improved. Transformative research aims to foster self-reflection, mutual learning, participation, and empowerment (Letts, 2003; Reason, 1994; Wadsworth & Epstein, 1998). Hence, this type of research has been used to enable groups of people who are in some way marginalized, deprived, or oppressed to bring about change in their lives and communities (Rice & Ezzy, 1999).

Examples of transformative research are growing in occupational therapy (Hocking & Wright-St. Clair, 2011). The efforts initiated by Thibeault (2002) to use a group meal preparation to initiate a series of projects that would eventually transform mistrust and animosity between perpetrators and victims of violence in Sierra Leone serves as one example. The most common form of research with a transformative purpose in health care and in occupational therapy is participatory research. Participatory research is an approach that involves the participants as co-creators and co-investigators who shape the research questions, methods, and outcomes while at the same time transforming themselves and others within their immediate contexts in significant and enduring ways. Some common features of participatory types of research are that it:

• Is always grounded in a practical context
• Involves people not simply as data sources but as partners in the research process
• Emphasizes power sharing between the researchers and local stakeholders (e.g., therapists and clients)
• Is action-oriented, focusing on making changes in the practice setting and on examining the impact of that change from the perspectives of those who are most influenced by it

Participatory approaches and other forms of transformative research are newer than either basic or applied research. Transformative research calls for embedding the research process in the practice setting and giving stakeholders a voice in shaping the research process. It aims to alter and

empirically examine services while empowering the stakeholders and embedding change processes within the context to which they are relevant. In this way, it attempts to combine research, education, and action; in other words, it links theory (knowing) with practice (doing) (Rice & Ezzy, 1999).

On the face of it, transformative research has special relevance to practitioners and clients in fields such as occupational therapy because it is much more directly driven by their agendas and is aimed at having a positive impact on their circumstances (Crist & Kielhofner, 2005). Proponents argue that research grounded in and directly helping to evaluate practice in natural contexts should be given high priority in the field.

Summary

Research is a complex and multifaceted endeavor. Because there are so many approaches, it would be unrealistic to easily or quickly develop expertise across all areas. However, knowing the basic classifications and purposes of research offers a good beginning. This chapter provides an overview of how research is defined and classified. It delineates the major differences between quantitative and qualitative traditions and describes some of the most commonly used research designs in occupational therapy that lie within these traditions. These include experimental and quasi-experimental studies, single-subject studies, field studies and naturalistic observation, survey studies, and psychometric studies. The chapter also summarizes the purposes and relevance of basic, applied, and transformative research to occupational therapy. This includes coverage of the historical and contemporary foundations of occupational science as the field's most celebrated approach to basic science. Future chapters will provide greater detail on the various quantitative and qualitative approaches to research discussed in this chapter.

Review Questions

1. Define the three central purposes of research in occupational therapy according to research classifications.
2. Provide an example of a study that uses an experimental design, and justify why the study would be realistic/feasible to conduct.
3. Describe a circumstance under which using a single-subject design would be appropriate to answer an occupational therapy research question.
4. Provide an example of a naturalistic study and describe one benefit of the approach.

5. What is a central characteristic of transformative research? How is transformation achieved?
6. Explain the unique contributions of occupational science to the broader field of occupational therapy.

REFERENCES

Assessment of Motor and Process Skills. (2012). *What is the AMPS?* Retrieved from http://www.ampsintl.com/AMPS/index.php

Bercovici, S. (1983). *Barriers to normalization.* Baltimore: University Park Press.

Campbell, D., & Stanley, J. (1963). *Experimental and quasi-experimental designs for research.* Chicago, IL: Rand-McNally.

Carswell, A., McColl, A., Baptiste, S., Law, M., Polatajko, H., & Pollock, N. (2004). The Canadian Occupational Performance Measure: A research and clinical literature review. *Canadian Journal of Occupational Therapy, 71*(4), 210–222.

Christiansen, C. (1991). Occupational therapy: Intervention for life performance. In C. Christiansen & C. Baum (Eds.), *Occupational therapy: Overcoming human performance deficits* (pp. 3–43). Thorofare, NJ: Slack.

Ciuffetelli-Parker, D. (2013). Narrative understandings of poverty and schooling: Reveal, revelation, reformation of mindsets. *International Journal for Cross-Disciplinary Subjects in Education, 4*(1), 1117–1123.

Clark, F. A., Parham, D., Carlson, M. E., Frank, G., Jackson, J., Pierce, D., ... Zemke, R. (1991). Occupational science: Academic innovation in the service of occupational therapy's future. *American Journal of Occupational Therapy, 45,* 300–310.

Cooke, D. M. C. (1958). The effect of resistance on multiple sclerosis patients with intention tremor. *American Journal of Occupational Therapy, 12*(2), 89–92.

Crist, P., & Kielhofner, G. (2005). Editors' overview. *Occupational Therapy in Health Care, 19*(1/2), 1–5.

Crotty, M. (1998). *The foundations of social research: Meaning and perspective in the research process.* Thousand Oaks, CA: Sage Publications.

Drussell, R. D. (1959). Relationship of Minnesota rate of manipulation test with the industrial work performance of the adult cerebral palsied. *American Journal of Occupational Therapy, 13,* 93–105.

Dubouloz, C. J., Egan, M., Vallerand, J., & Von Zweck, C. (1999). Occupational therapists' perceptions of evidence-based practice. *American Journal of Occupational Therapy, 53*(5), 445–453.

Dysart, A. M., & Tomlin, G. S. (2002). Factors related to evidence-based practice among U.S. occupational therapy clinicians. *American Journal of Occupational Therapy, 56*(3), 275–284.

Fisher, A. G. (1997). Multifaceted measurements of daily life task performance: Conceptualizing a test of instrumental ADL and validating the addition of personal ADL tasks ... first International Outcome Measurement Conference, co-sponsored by Rehabilitation Foundation, Inc., and the MESA Psychometric Laboratory at the University of Chicago. *Physical Medicine & Rehabilitation, 11*(2), 289–303.

Goode, D. (1983). Who is Bobby? Ideology and method in the discovery of a Down's syndrome person's competence. In G. Kielhofner (Ed.), *Health through occupation: Theory & practice in occupational therapy* (pp. 237–255). Philadelphia: F.A. Davis.

Guba, E. G., & Lincoln, Y. S. (1994). Competing paradigms in qualitative research. In N. K. Denzin & Y. S. Lincoln (Eds.), *Handbook of qualitative research* (pp. 105–117). Thousand Oaks, CA: Sage Publications.

Hammell, K. W. (2002). Informing client-centred practice through qualitative inquiry: Evaluating the quality of qualitative research. *British Journal of Occupational Therapy, 65*(4), 175–184.

Hocking, C., & Wright-St. Clair, V. (2011). Occupational science: Adding value to occupational therapy. *New Zealand Journal of Occupational Therapy, 58*(1), 29–35.

Kielhofner, G. (1979). The temporal dimension in the lives of retarded adults: A problem of interaction and intervention. *American Journal of Occupational Therapy, 33,* 161–168.

Kielhofner, G. (1981). An ethnographic study of deinstitutionalized adults: Their community settings and daily life experiences. *Occupational Therapy Journal of Research, 1,* 125–142.

Kielhofner, G. (1982a). Qualitative research: Part One— Paradigmatic grounds and issues of reliability and validity. *Occupational Therapy Journal of Research, 2*(2), 67–79.

Kielhofner, G. (1982b). Qualitative research: Part Two— Methodological approaches and relevance to occupational therapy. *Occupational Therapy Journal of Research, 2*(2), 67–79.

Kielhofner, G. (2008). *Model of human occupation: Theory and application* (4th ed.). Baltimore, MD: Lippincott Williams & Wilkins.

Kielhofner, G. (2009). *Conceptual foundations of occupational therapy practice* (4th ed.). Philadelphia: F.A. Davis.

Kielhofner, G., Braveman, B., Finlayson, M., Paul-Ward, A., Goldbaum, L., & Goldstein, K. (2004). Outcomes of a vocational program for persons with AIDS. *American Journal of Occupational Therapy, 58*(1), 64–72.

Kielhofner, G., Mallinson, T., Crawford, C., Nowak, M., Rigby, M., Henry, A., & Walens, D. (2004). *Occupational Performance History Interview II (OPHI-II) version 2.1.* Chicago, IL: MOHO Clearinghouse.

Kornfeld, A. S. (1988). *Sixth grade girl's experience of stress: A phenomenological study.* Unpublished doctoral dissertation, Union Experimenting Colleges and Universities, Cincinnati. OH.

Krefting, L. (1989). Disability ethnography: A methodological approach for occupational therapy research. *Canadian Journal of Occupational Therapy, 56,* 61–66.

Letts, L. (2003). Occupational therapy and participatory research: A partnership worth pursuing. *American Journal of Occupational Therapy, 57*(1), 77–87.

McGlaughlin Gray, J. (1997). Application of the phenomenological method to the concept of occupation. *Journal of Occupational Science: Australia, 4*(1), 5–17.

Mosey, A. C. (1992a). *Applied scientific inquiry in the health professions: An epistemological orientation.* Rockville, MD: AOTA Press.

Mosey, A. C. (1992b). Partition of occupational science and occupational therapy. *American Journal of Occupational Therapy, 46*(9), 851–853.

Mosey, A. C. (1993). Partition of occupational science and occupational therapy: Sorting out some issues. *American Journal of Occupational Therapy, 47*(8), 751–754.

Peloquin, S. M. (2002). Confluence: Moving forward with affective strength. *American Journal of Occupational Therapy, 56*(1), 69–77.

Primeau, L., Clark, F. A., & Pierce, D. (1989). Occupational therapy alone has looked upon occupation: Future applications of occupational science to the health care needs of parents and children. *Occupational Therapy in Health Care, 6*(4), 19–32.

Reason, P. (1994). Three approaches to participative inquiry. In N. Denzin & Y. Lincoln (Eds.), *Handbook of qualitative research* (pp. 324–339). Thousand Oaks, CA: Sage Publications.

Rice, P. L., & Ezzy, D. (1999). *Qualitative research methods: A health focus.* Oxford, UK: Oxford University Press.

Schon, D. A. (1983). *The reflective practitioner: How professionals think in action.* New York, NY: Basic Books.

Shadish, W. R., Cook, T. D., & Campbell, D. T. (2002). *Experimental and quasi-experimental designs for generalized causal inference.* Stamford, CT: Wadsworth Publishing.

Thibeault, R. (2002, September). *Occupation at the edge: Fostering healing and resilience in war and trauma victims.* Paper presented at the New Zealand Association of Occupational Therapists Conference, Auckland, New Zealand.

Wadsworth, Y., & Epstein, M. (1998). Building in dialogue between consumers and staff in acute mental health services. *Systemic Practice and Action Research, 11*(4), 353–379.

Wilcock, A. (1991). Occupational science. *British Journal of Occupational Therapy, 54,* 297–300.

Wilcock, A. (1993). A theory of the human need for occupation. *Journal of Occupational Science, Australia, 1*(1), 17–24.

Yerxa, E. J. (1991). National speaking: Seeking a relevant, ethical, and realistic way of knowledge for occupational therapy. *American Journal of Occupational Therapy, 45,* 199–204.

Yerxa, E. J. (1998). Health and the human spirit for occupation. *American Journal of Occupational Therapy, 52,* 412–418.

Yerxa, E. J., Clark, F., Frank, G., Jackson, J., Parham, D., Pierce, D., … Zemke, R. (1989). An introduction to occupational science. A foundation for occupational therapy in the 21st century. *Occupational Therapy in Health Care, 6*(4), 1–17.

Zemke, R., & Clark, B. (1996). *Occupational science: An evolving discipline.* Philadelphia, PA: F.A. Davis.

CHAPTER 3

Philosophical Foundations of Research

Renée R. Taylor • Gary Kielhofner

Learning Outcomes

- Identify the four time periods that formed the philosophical foundations for the understanding of science, including the unique contributions of each.
- Describe linkages between contemporary research traditions and their philosophical foundations.
- Analyze one's own preferences toward knowledge generation and how they influence the choice of a research approach.

Introduction

Although the philosophical foundations of studies are rarely described in research publications, they inevitably have had an influence on their design and execution. Such differences in the conduct of research are not simply incidental to the methods used; they reflect fundamentally different ideological stances on reality, objectivity, and human knowing. Individuals who participate in research and/or consume research should appreciate the philosophic underpinnings that shape the fundamental attitudes and beliefs of the researchers. In the end, these may be as important and consequential as the researchers' adherence to accepted methods and protocols (Kaplan, 1964). This chapter introduces the major historical traditions of thought that form the philosophical foundations of research, describes how these philosophical approaches link to contemporary research traditions, and helps guide individuals to identify their own preferences toward knowledge generation and the impact of those preferences on a research approach.

Philosophical Foundations for Understanding Science

An examination of the philosophical foundations of research begins by examining four periods marking the philosophy of science:

- Classicism
- Modernism
- Critical modernism
- Postmodernism

Each of these periods offers a different understanding of the aims and consequences of conducting inquiry. Note that this is not a comprehensive discussion of the philosophy of science. Rather, the following sections describe key concepts and highlight the different perspectives for understanding knowledge and the process of knowing that are likely to be implied in the range of research found in occupational therapy. Table 3.1 outlines these

CASE EXAMPLE

As a postdoctoral fellow working for a well-known occupational therapy researcher, Radhika is fortunate to receive a scholarship to study abroad. The first part of the scholarship involves interning for a 1-month period with each of the research faculty at the host university. During her internship, Radhika has the opportunity to study with researchers who are conducting inquiry according to a wide range of approaches. Each of these approaches reflects a distinct philosophical orientation toward the application of science. For her final assignment, Radhika is required to link each researcher's study designs and methods to an underlying philosophical orientation. Then, she is required to disclose her own preference toward a philosophical orientation and corresponding research tradition and to state the strengths and limitations of her choice.

Table 3.1 A Continuum of Ideas in the Philosophy of Science

	Classicism	Modernism	Critical Modernism	Postmodernism
The Nature of Theory	Theory is built on first principles that are self-evident (i.e., revealed by the world).	Theory is a logical system that explains and can predict events in the world.	Theory is a product of creative imagination that enables scientists to appreciate the world in a particular way.	Theory is a meta-narrative that falsely claims privileged status over other possible narratives.
The Role of Empiricism	Theory can be proved by deducing empirically demonstrable statements.	Theory can be disproved through empirical tests of logically derived hypotheses.	Theory can only be improved by empirical testing.	Empirical testing proves nothing; it only reinforces claims to power/ legitimacy.
View of Scientific Knowledge	Scientific knowledge represents truth.	Scientific knowledge is tentative but can be made increasingly true over time.	Scientific knowledge is one possible version of the world, which must be critically judged for its consequences.	All knowledge, including scientific knowledge, is socially constructed and relative.

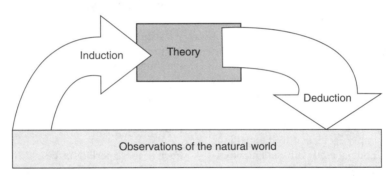

Figure 3.1   Aristotle's inductive–deductive method. *(From* Research in Occupational Therapy: Methods of Inquiry for Enhancing Practice, *by Gary Kielhofner, 2006, Philadelphia, PA: F.A. Davis Company, p. 11.)*

four periods in the philosophy of science and their major arguments concerning theory, empiricism, and scientific knowledge. It represents not only the evolution of ideas about research, but also a continuum of perspectives—some of which are embraced, either implicitly or explicitly, by researchers today.

Classicism: The Origins of the Scientific Method

Aristotle and other early philosophers of science were fundamentally concerned with separating scientific knowing from the fallibility of ordinary knowing. The truthfulness of any knowledge, they believed, depended on logic. The supporters of **classicism** reasoned that if pure logic was used to

connect the natural world to scientific knowledge, the latter could be demonstrated to be true. Thus, they critically examined how logic was used in both the **inductive** (i.e., generating explanations and theory from specific observations of the natural world) and **deductive** (i.e., deriving predictions from existing theory to see if those predictions hold in the natural world) phases of research (Fig. 3.1).

For Aristotle and many philosophers who followed, the deductive stage readily conformed to rigorous logic; that is, the specific statements that were tested through research could be deduced from the larger theory following strict logical principles. However, the inductive phase was problematic because it involved an intuitive leap. In arriving at explanations, a scholar had to invent "first principles," which were the foundation of the explanation that any theory provided. These first principles could only be assumed to be true because they couldn't be proved. Aristotle argued that they were self-evident.

In the late 15th and early 16th centuries, Galileo criticized Aristotle's self-evident first principles as being too metaphysical and therefore unscientific. Galileo sought, instead, to ground scientific explanations in the "obvious truth" of mathematical descriptions that perfectly fit the natural world (Klee, 1997; Losee, 2001). Nonetheless, like Aristotle, Galileo was ultimately confronted with the fact that the process of induction involved intuition. He made extensive use of imagining phenomena that he could not observe (e.g., free fall in a vacuum) to arrive at explanations. In the end, this imaginative process also required him to use certain unavoidable nonmathematical assumptions to construct his explanations. Thus, a complete logical connection between the natural world and theory was still not achieved for the inductive process.

Descartes, a contemporary of Galileo, was not convinced that mathematical correspondence was sufficient to constitute the truth of theoretical first principles. He sought to resolve the problem by doubting all potential first principles in search of those that were beyond doubt (Watson, 2002). His search for principles beyond all doubt resulted in the famous dictum "*Cogito, ergo sum*" ("I think, therefore I am"). Like Aristotle and Galileo, Descartes also was unable to avoid the fact that he made intuitive leaps in his inductive reasoning. He referred to these intuitive leaps as using analogies (e.g., inferring that planetary movement had to be circular based on observations of other naturally occurring phenomena such as whirlpools). Although he sought to defend the logic of analogical thinking, like those before him, Descartes was unable to reduce induction to pure logic. It remained a creative act that went beyond logical thought.

In the end, philosophers of science were unable to avoid the conclusion that induction involved more than pure logic. Even today it is understood that induction is an intuitive and creative process. Moreover, they were also unable to resolve the problem that the first principles that were generated through induction could not be proven. Early philosophers attempted to justify the first principles that resulted from induction on the grounds of self-evidence, mathematical correspondence, and truth beyond doubt. No matter how well argued these justifications, the bottom line was that they each demanded some type of belief that went beyond logic. The fact that intuition and faith remained unavoidable parts of induction eventually led philosophers to search for truth in the deductive phase.

Modernism: From Absolute Truth to Positivistic Science

A critical turning point in the philosophy of science was ushered in by Newton and his contemporaries in the 17th century (Cohen, 1978; Klee, 1997; Losee, 2001). The early researchers who supported the ideas of **modernism** replaced the concern for absolute truth with concern for how to correct errors in knowledge. They envisioned science as a process of testing and verification of the theory created through inductive reasoning. Newton accepted the idea of intuition and creativity in generating theory as a necessary process because he made extensive use of such thinking in his own theorizing. Thus, to establish confidence in his theories, Newton focused on the deductive phase.

To specify how error could be identified in theory through testing, he outlined an axiomatic method (Cohen & Smith, 2002) involving three steps:

1. Identifying within the theory those first principles that could not be deduced from any others that were, therefore, ultimately not provable. These first principles were labeled *axioms,* and the other theoretical principles that could be deduced from the first principles were labeled *theorems.*
2. Specifying how the theorems were correlated with the empirical world so that they could be systematically tested.
3. Testing the theorems through observation of the natural world.

Although this approach admitted that the first principles could not be proved, the principles had to yield theorems that did not contradict the natural world. Hence, first principles that yielded incorrect theorems would ultimately be understood to be false and therefore could be eliminated (Cohen, 1978).

Logical Positivism

This approach to research meant that theories had to be contingent and subject to revision because the evidence generated in research required it. Thus, the approach of Newton and his contemporaries did not seek to claim that their theories were true. Rather, they asserted that any theory was a possible, but not necessarily infallible, explanation. A theory's plausibility depended on whether statements that could be logically deduced from it held up in the natural world. If observations of the natural world did not bear out what was logically deduced from a theory (i.e., were disproved), then the theory would ultimately be rejected. Within this framework, although truth was not immediately at hand, scientists could make progress toward it. Research could systematically identify what was false through empirical testing. What survived the test of time and evidence would be increasingly closer to the truth.

This view that research allowed theory to progress toward truth came to be known as **logical positivism.** Subsequent philosophers of science in the logical positivist tradition focused on improving the logical rigor of methods through which researchers induced theory from observation and then went about testing the fit of theoretical explanations with the empirical world.

Logical positivism contained an important idea of progress that is also a cornerstone of modernism. Born out of 18th-century Enlightenment, modernism included not only faith in science as a method, but also a belief that true human progress would result from science. That is, science was expected to continually improve the human condition as knowledge accumulated and was used for the betterment of society and its institutions. Thus, modernism optimistically sought "universal human emancipation through mobilization of the powers of technology, science, and reason" (Harvey, 1990, p. 41).

The Critique of Positivism

Logical positivism underscored the importance of deriving hypotheses logically from theory so that they could be tested by research and, when incorrect, shown to be false. However, a major problem with this approach was whether a hypothesis, much less a theory, could actually be demonstrated to be false. The whole foundation of logical positivism was based on the falsifiability of hypotheses, which allowed research to correct theories.

The popular notion was that a crucial experiment could be designed for each hypothesis that would, once and for all, determine whether it was false. However, the idea of the crucial experiment came to be strongly criticized. For instance, Grunbaum (1971) argued that no hypothesis derived from a theory could be sufficiently isolated from the theory so as to provide an absolute test of the theory. This was, in part, because the meaning of any hypothesis was not contained solely in the statement of that hypothesis but also in the entire matrix of concepts from which the hypothesis was

deduced. This means that the understanding of the hypothesis, including what evidence could constitute its falsity, also depends on the theory from which it is derived.

Therefore, evidence that contradicts a particular hypothesis can easily be explained away. A convenient shift in the sense of the hypothesis will suffice to protect the theory from which the hypothesis was derived. Grunbaum's argument led to the conclusion that there could be no logic of proof or disproof external to any theory. Rather, any proposed test of a theory depends on the theory for its sensibility. For instance, Hesse (1970) pointed out that all observational terms contained in hypotheses are theory-dependent. That is, their meaning cannot stand apart from the theory. Therefore, any attempt to capture the empirical world in the language of a hypothesis irrevocably commits the researcher to the theory that makes sense of the hypothesis in the first place.

These were not small problems for logical positivism. If the very observational terms necessary to generate evidence about a theory are themselves reliant on the theory for their meaning, then:

- A theory can never truly be shown to be false.
- Evidence cannot be used to show that one theory is better than another (Hesse, 1970; Scriven, 1970).

These two conclusions basically undermine the whole idea of a progressive, self-correcting science that incrementally eliminates error and thereby moves toward truth. Instead, these arguments point out that a theory, at best, represents one possible explanation of the events it addresses (Hesse, 1970; Scriven, 1970).

Critical Modernism: Rethinking the Role of Empiricism

Criticisms of logical positivism ushered in an important new direction in the understanding of science. This perspective has been labeled **critical modernism** (Midgley, 2003). As noted, an earlier shift had redirected the ideal of science as achieving necessary truth toward a conception of science as progressing toward truth through self-correcting empiricism. Despite their differences, both of these views ultimately sought to identify logical principles and procedures that would emancipate science from the fallibility of ordinary human thinking and knowing.

However, the more philosophers attempted to isolate the logic of science from other psychological processes (e.g., intuition and creativity), the more apparent it became that this was not possible.

The logical principles that were once considered to specify the very nature of science came to be understood as only one property of science. Although logic is necessary, it is not sufficient for doing research. Within this new framework, the role of intuition in induction, the nonprobability of first principles, and the embeddedness of observations within their theoretical contexts were considered anew.

Philosophers of science came to see the incorrigibility of the first principles upon which all theories must be based not as a fundamental problem, but as an important clue about the nature of science. That is, if the most abstract components of a theory cannot be shown to be grounded in the empirical world, it is because theory imparts meaning to, rather than extracts meaning from, the natural world. Theory is a creation of the human mind that makes sense of the world. The creative process by which researchers originate ideas to make sense of their observations of the natural world is as much a part of the research process as the logic by which researchers link the theoretical with the observed (Bronowski, 1978).

These critics of logical positivism identified flaws in its assertion that research would advance theory toward truth. Moreover, they were able to give creative and meaning-making processes a place in the research process. Along with other critics of positivism, Kuhn (1977) argued that when investigators collect data, they do not directly test their theories. Kuhn argued that this was the case because "the scientist must premise current theory as the rules of his game" (p. 270). He further noted that all theories "can be modified by a variety of ad hoc adjustments without ceasing to be, in their main lines, the same theories" (Kuhn, 1977, p. 281). So, instead of testing theory, evidence generated in research allows the theory to be adjusted to better fit whatever phenomena it is designed to explain.

Kuhn's insights point out that research does not prove or disprove the theory. However, it does improve the theory. Research serves as the basis for generating theories and, thereafter, can be used to enhance the fit of that theory to the natural world. As noted earlier, theory serves as a way to impart meaning to observations made in research. Once in place, theory becomes a schema for guiding the systematic observation of the world. Finally, because theory explains the world in a particular way, it leads to investigations that refine that explanation. All of these processes result in the accumulation of knowledge. Studies thus add to the stockpile of information related to any theoretical system.

Over time, the knowledge accumulated through research does appear somewhat like the progression of knowledge envisioned by the logical positivists—with one important difference. Instead of progressing toward truth, critical modernism argues that theories progress by becoming better at the particular way they make sense of the world.

Postmodernism

Postmodernism represents the most recent set of ideas in the philosophy of science. It is not a coherent single argument, but rather a set of loosely related themes. Postmodernists are particularly critical of the logical positivist perspective in more extreme ways than the critical modernists (Harvey, 1990). The critique of modernism discussed earlier pointed out that it is impossible to disentangle the language of a hypothesis from the theoretical system in which it is embedded. The philosopher Wittgenstein (1953) went even further, asserting that language constructs reality. His argument leads to the conclusion that because language determines what humans perceive, science cannot escape its own linguistic blinders. In other words, the very language of science determines what the scientist can come to know.

Wittgenstein is generally attributed with beginning what has come to be known as **social constructivism,** a viewpoint that pervades postmodern thought. It asserts, in essence, that all knowledge, including scientific knowledge, is socially constructed and, therefore, relative. According to postmodernism, scientific knowledge is no more privileged than any other source of knowledge. It is the particular perspective of a particular group of people who have a particular purpose in mind.

Lyotard's (1979) critique of the state of scientific knowledge directly assaults the positivist approach of modernism. He argues that science is a form of meta-narrative. According to Lyotard, the scientific meta-narrative claims that science is a project of human enlightenment based on logic and empiricism, which promises to create a unified understanding of the word, work for the good of all, and improve the human condition. Lyotard and other postmodernists point out the many failures of science in this regard (e.g., contributions of science to the atrocities of modern warfare and ecological problems; the failure of modern science to address the needs of oppressed groups, women, ethnic minorities, and members of third-world countries).

Lyotard further argues that scientific disciplines are like games, with their own rules, boundaries, and permissible moves. Importantly, what is permissible in the game is determined by the power structure of any particular branch of science. Foucault (1970), in particular, emphasizes this relation between power and knowledge, arguing that the production of knowledge is closely tied to social control and domination. His work provides a basis for many postmodern critiques of how science serves to perpetuate oppression.

As a result of Lyotard's and Foucault's work, postmodernists are particularly critical of any broad theories, which they see as forms of meta-narrative. They argue that these meta-narratives privilege certain groups and certain perspectives, while they have no more validity than any other "story" that might be narrated. Postmodernists emphasize the right of groups to have their own voice and speak for their own reality (Harvey, 1990). For this reason, postmodern thinking has been used by scholars whose work has championed disenfranchised groups (e.g., women's studies and disability studies).

In the end, most postmodernists paint a negative view of science. They not only discount the methodological claims made by the logical positivists, but also call into question the value of much of the information science has created. The ultimate conclusion of postmodernism is that "there can be no universals, that absolute truth is an illusion" (Midgley, 2003, p. 48). Moreover, postmodernists have critiqued science as being ideologically biased, tied to power structures, and ultimately contributing to oppression by replacing local knowledge with falsely claimed universal knowledge. Consequently, postmodernists seek to "promote variety, undermine certainty, and promote local, critical thought" (Midgley, 2003, p. 55).

As with all of the philosophical foundations covered in this chapter, a number of severe critiques of postmodernism exist (Harvey, 1990; Midgley, 2003). Some of these are directed at apparent self-contradictory arguments within postmodernism. For example, the most frequently cited contradiction within postmodernism is that, while it disparages grand theories (meta-narratives), it proposes a grand theory that is supposed to supersede all previous theories. Or conversely, if one accepts the proposition that no universal claims about knowledge are true, then one has to reject the postmodernist claim that all knowledge is socially constructed. Postmodernists typically admit that there are ironic and self-contradictory elements of the postmodern argument, but they dismiss criticisms of this aspect of postmodernism as a misplaced concern for logic and coherence.

The most salient criticism of postmodernism, however, is that although it has successfully pointed out some of the limitations and failures of modernism, it has not offered any alternative (Midgley, 2003). In fact, extreme postmodernists argue that any attempt at creating universal knowledge is essentially pointless.

Application of Philosophical Foundations to Contemporary Research

This section reviews the major historical traditions of thought that comprise the philosophical foundations of contemporary science today. When applying the philosophical foundations of science to the practical situation of occupational therapy research, it is important to approach these foundational ideas with a sense of perspective. Few individuals today would embrace the classic idea that science produces truth. However, with the exception of extreme postmodernists, most would agree that science produces potentially useful knowledge.

Contemporary science has evolved in such a way that the research conducted by most scientists derives from one of the three later traditions of logical positivism, critical modernism, or postmodernism. Or, in the case of mixed-methods approaches, research is derived from a blend of these traditions. For example, most quantitative research employs logical methods developed in the logical positivist tradition. Many qualitative researchers embrace ideas represented in critical modernism and postmodernism. In some way, every study draws upon the kinds of ideas that originated in the philosophical foundations of science.

What lessons can researchers and practitioners who use research take from the continuum of philosophical perspectives described in this chapter? First, it is important to recognize that one's preferences in adhering to one research approach over another automatically reflect a particular **philosophical orientation,** or inclination toward approaching knowledge and knowledge development. Knowing one's philosophical orientation is important in terms of shaping one's path of study and eventual independence as a researcher. The following section describes the three most relevant orientations (logical positivism, critical modernism, and postmodernism) as they apply to selecting and applying various research approaches in everyday practice.

Logical Positivism and Quantitative Research

Quantitative approaches are consistent with the tradition of logical positivism. In practical terms, logical positivism supports a process of scientific inquiry that involves testing hypotheses that are rooted in theory. This process is undertaken by following a logical and rigorous methodology. There is an objective reality (represented by a study outcome) that can be replicated using a specific methodological approach. Thus, if one researcher adheres closely enough to the methodology outlined by a second researcher, she or he should be able to replicate the original findings—assuming the second researcher follows the same procedures as the original researcher and uses the same assessments and data collection approaches to collect data from a sample with similar characteristics from the same overall population of clients. Experimental and quasi-experimental approaches fall into this general category, as do other quantitative approaches discussed in this text.

Critical Modernism and Qualitative Research

Representing the view of critical modernists, Kuhn (1977) ultimately concluded that scientific efforts should be judged on their utility—that is, "the concrete technical results of [what is] achievable by those who practice within each theory" (p. 339). Kuhn's comments suggest that scientific efforts in occupational therapy should be judged on their ability to help therapists effectively solve the kinds of problems their clients face. Within the general domain of critical modernism, it is understood that theories can be created and developed as much as they can be confirmed.

This perspective is endorsed by qualitative research. Theories evolve by providing increasingly accurate estimates of the subjective world, and these perspectives are based upon observations of people interacting in natural contexts, as well as the perceptions and experiences of those who participate and live in the world (i.e., clients). In this way, critical modernism supports the most commonly utilized approaches to qualitative research and naturalistic inquiry in occupational therapy today.

For example, ideas from critical modernism are consistent with phenomenology, which emphasizes how people experience and make sense of their immediate worlds. These ideas are also consistent with ethnography, which emphasizes the societal and cultural context that shapes meaning and behavior. Moreover, there is consistency with narrative inquiry, which seeks to understand how people construct storied accounts of their and others' lives and of shared events (Rice & Ezzy, 1999).

Postmodernism and Research Perspectives

Postmodernism is generally not useful as a philosophical premise for doing research, although it can be useful as a critical stance from which to judge scientific efforts. In particular, it is useful in calling attention to how science can be shaped by ideology, power, and interest.

One of the most relevant examples for occupational therapy is disabilities studies, which use the postmodern social constructivist argument as a basis for critiquing much existing research on disability. As Rioux (1997) points out, the various research efforts to classify, count, and study relationships among variables associated with disability appear to be objective and scientific. However, this science is informed by an ideology about the nature of disability that focuses on disability as an individual deviation from norms. Importantly, the understanding of disability that has resulted from this approach is at variance with how people with disabilities experience their situation. Thus, the dominant modern understanding of disability is a social construction, not a fact. Scholars in disability studies have called for the voices of disabled persons to be added to the scientific discourse about disability in order to correct this prevailing misunderstanding of disability (Scotch, 2001).

A second important point to be taken from postmodernism is the need to contextualize knowledge in the circumstances of its production—that is, to place any claims to knowledge in the context within which the knowledge was generated. A number of investigators, especially those involved in qualitative research, carefully document their research efforts in the context of their personal and other relevant histories, because most qualitative research approaches rely upon the investigator's interpretation as a major analytic tool. By doing so, the investigator gives the reader an additional perspective from which to understand and judge the research findings.

Basic Foundations for Moving Forward

Although the ideas about the nature of research in the philosophy of science have changed dramatically over the centuries, each era has offered certain principles, ideas, and understandings that are useful to keep in mind regarding research. Irrespective of one's preferred approach to research, the following general insights and guidelines can aid researchers and consumers of research in understanding the foundations upon which contemporary science is built.

Insights Regarding Theory

Contemporary approaches to science understand theory in terms of shared knowledge rather than fact. Correspondingly, the following points apply:

- Theories are human creations that seek to impart meaning to the world.
- First principles, or underlying assumptions, are unavoidable and untestable parts of any theory.
- Theories always represent one way of explaining or making sense of things.
- Although theories cannot be disproved, their ability to explain the natural world can be improved through research.
- The ultimate worth of any theory is its ability to generate solutions to practical problems.
- It is not possible to undertake research, no matter how open-ended and free of presuppositions, without some underlying theory and first principles, even if they are not made explicit. Thus, whether a researcher is using only a handful of loosely connected assumptions and concepts or a complex theory, some conceptual context is necessary to any research.

Insights Regarding the Research Process

Irrespective of the tradition of inquiry, modern research requires clear articulation of the role of theory in the scientific approach and specification of the methods by which one plans to conduct inquiry. In turn, one should attend to the following points:

- Research is part of an inductive–deductive process in which theory is derived from and tied back to the world through empiricism.
- Logic is necessary to connect the concepts and propositions that make up a theory with each other and to connect them with the things in the world to which they refer.
- All research is embedded in theory (whether or not it is made explicit). The theory is what makes sense of the phenomena examined, the scientific problems addressed, and the way those problems are solved.

- Research does not advance theory toward truth; instead, it improves the way that any theory makes sense of the world.

Insights Regarding Researchers

Researchers must know their own philosophical orientations and biases in order to conduct sound research. This is recognized by the following observations:

- Researchers always impart meaning to what they have observed by creating theories.
- Investigators bring to bear all their characteristics (including personal history, training, theoretical understandings, and assumptions) on the research process.
- Researchers are part of a social community that shares a perspective that makes sense of what is studied as well as related norms and rules that set out what should be studied and how.

Insights Regarding the Impact of Research

It is important to accurately represent the meaning, impact, and limits of research findings, as outlined by the following:

- Research is not inherently value-free or benign.
- Research can be tied to particular ideologies and used to reinforce power structures and to disenfranchise or oppress groups.
- Research can be used for positive ends. By advancing understanding or a prediction of certain phenomena, it can inform practical action.

Summary

This chapter provides an introduction to the major historical traditions of thought that form the philosophical foundations of research: classicism, modernism, critical modernism, and postmodernism. Most scientific approaches in occupational therapy derive from the historical periods of modernism, critical modernism, and postmodernism. During these periods, the ideas behind logical positivism and the criticisms of such ideas through the traditions of critical modernism and postmodernism contributed to the perspectives and methods used in quantitative and qualitative research.

Logical positivism is associated with major quantitative traditions, such as quasi-experimental and experimental research, whereas critical modernism and conservative interpretations of postmodernist thought are associated with many qualitative and naturalistic approaches to inquiry, including, but not limited to, ethnography, phenomenology, and narrative inquiry. Conservative interpretations of postmodernist thought can be observed through the perspectives of disability studies and other relativistic approaches to knowledge generation.

Following an explanation of how these approaches articulate with the philosophical foundations, the chapter concludes with insights for researchers and consumers of research in applying the chapter content to understand more broadly the role of theory in research, the necessity of clarity in the research process, the inherent biases in the approach of any researcher, and the responsibility of all researchers to qualify and accurately represent the impact of findings.

Review Questions

1. Describe the early contributions of classism and why they were rejected in favor of modernism.
2. List two or more approaches to research that are consistent with the ideas of critical modernism. Draw specific linkages between these approaches and the ideas of critical modernism.
3. Explain the utility of postmodernist ideas to scientific inquiry today, delineating the potential contributions, as well as limitations, to a postmodernist orientation toward science.
4. Based on the various philosophical orientations toward science, describe your own preferences toward knowledge generation. How might those preferences influence your choice of a research approach?

REFERENCES

Bronowski, J. (1978). *The origins of knowledge and imagination.* New Haven, CT: Yale University Press.

Cohen, I. B. (Ed.). (1978). *Isaac Newton's papers & letters on natural philosophy and related documents.* Cambridge, MA: Harvard University Press.

Cohen, I. B., & Smith, G. (Eds.). (2002). *The Cambridge companion to Newton.* Cambridge, UK: Cambridge University Press.

Foucault, M. (1970). *The order of things: An archeology of the human sciences.* New York, NY: Pantheon Books.

Grunbaum, A. (1971). Can we ascertain the falsity of a scientific hypothesis? In E. Nagel, S. Bromberger, & A. Grunbaum (Eds.), *Observation and theory in science* (pp. 69–129). Baltimore, MD: John Hopkins Press.

Harvey, D. (1990). *The condition of postmodernity: An enquiry into the origins of cultural change.* Oxford, UK: Blackwell Publishers.

Hesse, M. (1970). Is there an independent observation language? In R. G. Colodny (Ed.), *The nature and function of scientific theories; Essays in contemporary science and philosophy* (pp. 35–77). Pittsburgh, PA: University of Pittsburgh Press.

Kaplan, A. (1964). *The conduct of inquiry: Methodology for behavioral science.* San Francisco, CA: Chandler.

Kielhofner, G. (2006). *Research in Occupational Therapy: Methods of Inquiry for Enhancing Practice* (p. 11). Philadelphia, PA: F.A. Davis.

Klee, R. (1997). *Introduction to the philosophy of science: Cutting nature at its seams.* New York, NY: Oxford University Press.

Kuhn, T. (1977). *The essential tension.* Chicago, IL: University of Chicago Press.

Losee, J. (2001). *A historical introduction to the philosophy of science* (4th ed.). New York, NY: Oxford University Press.

Lyotard, J. (1979). *The postmodern condition: A report on knowledge.* Minneapolis, MN: University of Minnesota Press.

Midgley, G. (2003). Five sketches of postmodernism: Implications for systems thinking and operational research. *International Journal of Organizational Transformation and Social Change, 1*(1), 47–62.

Rice, P. L., & Ezzy, D. (1999). *Qualitative research methods: A health focus.* Oxford, UK: Oxford University Press.

Rioux, M. H. (1997). Disability: The place of judgment in a world of fact. *Journal of Intellectual Disability Research, 41,* 102–111.

Scotch, R. K. (2001). *From goodwill to civil rights: Transforming federal disability policy* (2nd ed.). Philadelphia, PA: Temple University Press.

Scriven, M. (1970). Explanations, predictions and laws. In H. Feigl & G. Maxwell (Eds.), *Minnesota studies in the philosophy of science* (pp. 51–74). Minneapolis, MN: University of Minnesota Press.

Watson, R. (2002). *Cogito, ergo sum: The life of René Descartes.* Boston, MA: Godine Press.

Wittgenstein, L. (1953). *Philosophical investigations.* Oxford, UK: Basil Blackwell.

CHAPTER 4

Reading and Understanding Published and Presented Research

Renée R. Taylor • Nancy A. Baker • Pimjai Sudsawad

Learning Outcomes

■ Identify the major types of research articles.
■ Describe the contents of the major sections of a peer-reviewed research article.
■ Differentiate the major types of presented research.
■ Compare and contrast the objectives and contents of presented and published research.

Introduction

Researchers are not the only professionals who need to develop expertise in reading and understanding published and presented research. Occupational therapy (OT) practitioners, OT managers, insurance agents, granting agency officials, policymakers, legislators, advocates, and clients should also possess these skills (to varying degrees). Assurances related to client safety, quality and efficiency of care, and evidence-based practice continually influence ongoing changes in the health-care system. A fundamental skill for all occupational therapists is the ability to understand and critically appraise the field's evidence. Whether you are a manager who needs to update a treatment approach within a practice setting or a practitioner attending a conference or paging through a professional journal to remain up to date on therapeutic approaches, knowing how to read, interpret, and evaluate published and presented research is a crucial part of evidence-based practice.

Evidence-based practice (covered in Chapter 1) involves using existing published or presented research to inform decision-making, rather than conducting it anew. In occupational therapy, evidence from research can be used in a wide range of ways (Tickle-Degnen & Bedell, 2003). Uses include, but are not limited to:

• Development or revision of practice guidelines

• Development of economic analyses of different treatment approaches
• Evaluation of local clinical performance against published outcomes
• Dissemination of information to clients and other consumers about the effectiveness of a given intervention
• Shaping of clinicians' choices regarding the most appropriate intervention

Evidence-based practice (EBP) is defined as the reciprocal use of research evidence and clinical expertise in informing decision-making about the care of individual clients (Sackett, Straus, Richardson, Rosenberg, & Haynes, 2000). Honing your research-related reading skills will allow you to apply an EBP perspective and decide which approaches and technologies are most likely to be helpful to you and your clients in therapy and beyond.

For individuals who are engaged in advanced graduate work, reading and understanding research will assist you in writing a final project, thesis, literature review, and/or dissertation, including the ability to recognize the strengths and limitations of your own work. This chapter guides you through the process of reading and understanding published and presented research and serves as an enduring reference for the process of reading and writing research papers. Moreover, this chapter covers the different components of research articles. You will understand why each component of a research article is important to the overall findings and recommendations from the study. Additionally, you will learn how to read and listen for results when presented at conferences or in journals by understanding basic approaches to interpreting research findings.

Applying the Evidence

Evidence-based practice is not a unilaterally formulaic guide to intervention (Sackett, Rosenberg,

CASE EXAMPLE

Kim is an occupational therapist and research coordinator with the Spinal Cord Injury Program at an urban medical center. Because new technologies and other innovations in the field of spinal-cord-injury research evolve at such a rapid pace, Kim must ensure that she, her fieldwork students, and the other therapists on her unit are always up to date on the results of published research in this area. Justin, an advanced fieldwork student on her unit, was assigned to work with a 23-year-old woman with a spinal cord injury resulting from traumatic abuse. The client was badly beaten by her partner and thrown down a flight of stairs. In addition to her spinal cord injury, the client was also diagnosed with reactive major depression and posttraumatic stress disorder.

Kim decided that one of the best ways of mentoring this student was to show her a basic application of evidence-based practice as a means of preparing for her consultation in advance. Fortunately, Kim works for a medical center that is affiliated with a medical school. The school has a medical library that is accessible online. Kim and Justin sat down together at the computer with a plan to visit the online library (Fig. 4.1). Among numerous articles, Justin located two recently published articles that were of particular relevance to his assigned client. The first was a descriptive study of women with violently acquired spinal cord injury (Forchheimer & Mcade, 2011). The second was an article that discussed psychological contributions to functional independence in spinal cord injury and included recommendations for rehabilitation professionals (Kennedy, Lude, Elfstrom, & Smithson, 2011).

After a brief assessment of levels of evidence, Kim and Justin agreed that the articles were not intended or designed to offer exceptionally high levels of rigor and evidence. One was a descriptive study of data extracted from an existing database (i.e., Forchheimer & Meade, 2011), and the other was a longitudinal cohort study examining questionnaire data (i.e., Kennedy et al., 2011). However, the research practitioners agreed that both studies provided useful information, responsibly cited limitations, and presented data that would contribute to their preliminary therapeutic reasoning about this client. The two articles served as a starting point for an in-depth discussion between supervisor and student about the upcoming client on the student's caseload.

Additionally, Justin later discussed some findings from the articles during a conversation with the client. During one session following a visit from her abusive boyfriend, the client looked particularly demoralized and distracted. Justin asked whether she had been having any distressing thoughts about her relationship with her boyfriend. This occurred after several sessions had passed and the two had established a trusting relationship. The client began to discuss the nightmares she was having, and this led to an important discussion about the psychosocial aspects of the client's care and rehabilitation process, which later resulted in a referral for additional support and services.

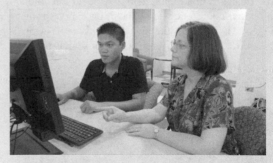

Figure 4.1 Advanced fieldwork student working with his research coordinator.

Gray, Haynes, & Richardson, 1996). The currently available best evidence must be used judiciously by skilled practitioners in combination with their knowledge of treatment principles and overall therapeutic skills. As covered in Chapter 1, part

of this skill is matching potential evidence-based interventions with the needs and values of clients (Sackett et al., 2000). In addition, practitioners should remember that there are "consumers" other than clients who are interested in the evidence for an intervention. For example, insurance companies, hospital administrators, policymakers, granting agencies, and OT managers are concerned about intervention options and choices. Practitioners can use evidence to justify their choices to clients, family members, policymakers, insurance companies, and other groups as necessary. Clinicians should be able to present the results to all of these groups, using different language and focus for each. Tickle-Degnen and Bedell (2003) suggest that when communicating the results of evidence, practitioners should:

- Use simple, concrete, nontechnical, culturally neutral language
- Keep the information brief
- Check frequently for confusion or lack of comprehension
- Suggest concrete actions related to the information (p. 229)

Research Articles and Conference Presentations

Many local, national, and international OT organizations publish magazines and/or professional journals that contain a range of articles relevant to our field. For example, within the United States, the American Occupational Therapy Association publishes a trade magazine, *Occupational Therapy Practice,* and a professional journal, *American Journal of Occupational Therapy* (Fig. 4.2).

Additionally, many organizations hold annual or periodic conferences where research is disseminated and discussed verbally. For example, the American Occupational Therapy Association holds an annual conference and exposition every spring (Fig. 4.3). Because the focus of this text is on research, this section emphasizes research-based

conferences and journals (as opposed to general articles about a topic or clinical continuing education presentations, for example).

When you open a professional journal, you will typically find two major types of research articles: **literature reviews** (i.e., articles that provide a summary of the scientific literature about a topic) and **experimental reports** (i.e., articles that provide a structured report of findings from a research investigation). Other types of research articles published in professional journals include, but are not limited to, **case reports** (i.e., articles that provide a structured description of a novel approach to assessment and/or intervention with a single client or a small number of clients) and **opinion papers** (i.e., articles that discuss novel or controversial information about a topic of broad impact within a profession).

Similarly, professional conferences offer five general formats for the verbal and visual dissemination of research. These include, but are not limited to:

- Individual paper presentations
- Symposia
- Workshops
- Poster presentations
- Roundtable discussions

The following sections describe and define the major types of research articles and presentations that are most commonly used by OT researchers and practitioners.

Peer-Reviewed Journal Articles

A **peer-reviewed journal article** is a research article that has undergone intensive review by at

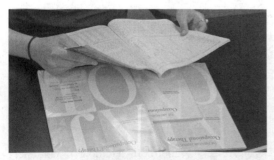

Figure 4.2 Cover of the *American Journal of Occupational Therapy.*

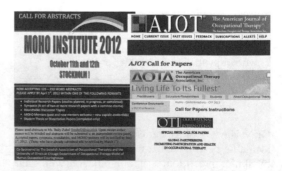

Figure 4.3 Call for papers for occupational therapy organizations from around the world.

least two other professionals who are considered peers of the authors in a given field of study. With some exceptions, there is a general format to a published, peer-reviewed research article, which makes reading and interpreting findings easier. This format, which is specified in publication manuals distributed by organizations such as the American Psychological Association (2010) and the American Medical Association (Iverson et al., 2009), is used by a wide range of research professionals who publish their findings in journals, including occupational therapists. Because many journals in which occupational therapists publish require papers to conform to the format specified by the *Publication Manual of the American Psychological Association* (American Psychological Association [APA], 2010), we will use these publication guidelines (**APA format**) to guide our discussion.

APA format is often discussed with respect to the specific order and format in which references are reported at the end of a research article. However, APA format refers to a very specific order in which an entire research article is presented, as well as how the contents of a study are reported and described. The order for literature reviews and experimental reports, which are the most common types of journal articles, is shown in Figure 4.4.

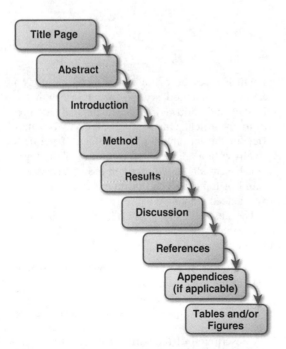

Figure 4.4   The sequence of sections in a peer-reviewed journal article.

The following section describes what goes into each of these parts in detail to guide you in your reading (and eventually in your writing) of a research article.

Title Page

At minimum, the **title page** typically contains the article title, running head, authors' names, and institutions with which the authors are affiliated. An example of a title page is provided in Figure 4.5.

When scanning through numerous articles during an online search for information, titles can be very informative at the preliminary stages. The title of a study should contain several key words that succinctly convey the topic, approach, and findings of the study. In the previous Case Example, the titles of the articles that Justin selected were very informative. For example, the first article was titled "Women With Violently Acquired Spinal Cord Injury: Characteristics of a Vulnerable Population." From this title, we understand that the topic is women who sustained spinal cord injuries as victims of violence. Moreover, we can hypothesize that it is a descriptive study because the title refers to the characteristics of these women. Finally, reference to the fact that these women are considered a vulnerable population suggests that the results, or findings from the data analysis, highlight the nature of vulnerabilities within this population of women.

The **running head** is an abbreviated title that appears on each page to remind readers of the title as they page through the particular study, which is one among many within a printed journal volume. (The running head becomes less significant with electronic dissemination because computer programs often do the job of only presenting a single article of interest at a time on the computer screen.)

Most title pages of journal articles also include the author names and **institutional affiliations.** An institutional affiliation gives the reader a general idea about the location and nature of the institution or institutions in which the research was developed, supported, and/or executed. Moreover, it allows readers to locate and contact authors if they have additional questions about the study or for other reasons, such as inviting them to serve as a collaborator on a grant or asking them how to obtain an assessment used in the study, for example.

Some title pages also include information such as word counts, acknowledgments, and contact information for the author who has agreed to receive and respond to any correspondence regarding the article (**corresponding author**). This

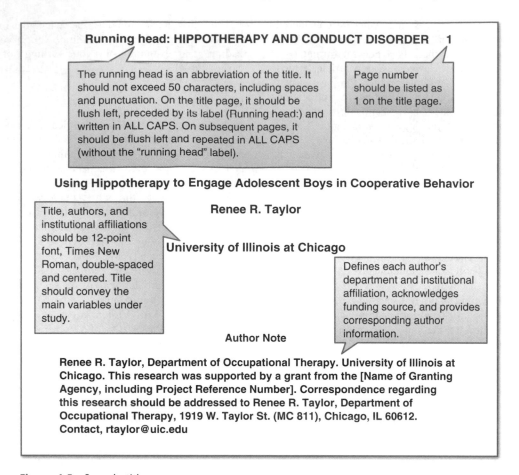

Figure 4.5   Sample title page.

individual may or may not be the first author of the article.

Abstract

An **abstract** is a concise summary (typically between 150 and 250 words) of key aspects of the study. This is an important component of the study because it is the first thing (and sometimes the only thing) that a busy practitioner may have time to read when determining whether to retrieve and read the entire article for more detailed information. A good abstract is clear, providing just enough information for a reader to navigate through the actual article. This is important to the experienced reader, who typically has been intellectually immersed in a topic area for a number of years and may only wish to read a certain part of the study. For example, a reader might be interested in a given article specifically because of a unique methodological approach that was used, in which case she or he would focus mainly on reading the method section, beginning with the abstract and followed by the main body of text within the article. Other readers may only be interested in the introduction, particularly if it offers a well-written and detailed overview of the topic area. Essentially, a well-written abstract serves as a kind of topical legend or reference point for an experienced reader.

The abstract is typically presented as a single paragraph. Most abstracts contain the following elements:

- A sentence or two of background information about the topic of the study
- The objectives of the study
- The research questions or hypotheses to be examined
- A description of the participants and the methodological approach (including data analysis)
- A description of the results and conclusions

HIPPOTHERAPY AND CONDUCT DISORDER   2

Abstract

Hippotherapy as an intervention for adolescent males with conduct disorder is an important but under-studied topic in occupational therapy. In this study, a quasi-experimental pretest-posttest design was used to test whether 50 1-hour group hippotherapy sessions focusing on cooperative behavior and delivered weekly over a 1-year period increased cooperative behavior among adolescent boys with conduct disorder. A sample of 28 boys with conduct disorder living in Group Home A, who received the intervention, was compared with a sample of 32 boys with conduct disorder living in Group Home B, who did not receive the intervention. A validated measure of cooperation was administered to both groups before and after the intervention. Results from an independent sample t-test (t [4] $= -5.51$, $p < .005$) revealed a significant effect of hippotherapy. The boys receiving hippotherapy ($M = .667$, $SD = 1.15$) scored higher on the measure of cooperation than the boys in the control group ($M = 8.99$, $SD = 2.00$). These findings provide preliminary evidence that a hippotherapy intervention focused on cooperative behavior improves cooperative behavior in adolescent males with conduct disorder.

KEY WORDS: hippotherapy, conduct disorder, cooperative behavior

The abstract summarizes the main objectives, methods, and findings of the study in 150–250 words. Findings from quantitative studies should be presented in statistical form, where possible. The first line of the abstract is not indented, but subsequent paragraphs in the paper are indented. The word *Abstract* should be centered at the top of the page. Key words may be listed at the end of the paragraph.

Figure 4.6 Sample abstract page.

Some journals request that abstracts include distinct headers for each section (e.g., objectives, methods, results, conclusions) followed by brief phrases describing each section, rather than full sentences. Many journals require a listing of three to five **key words** from the article that capture the main topics covered by the article but are distinct from the words used in the title. These are usually listed immediately after the abstract. An example of an abstract is presented in Figure 4.6.

Introduction

The **introduction** is an often underestimated, yet important aspect of a research article. It provides background evidence justifying the relevance and need for a given study. Many introductions are three to five pages in length. However, they may be as brief as one-half to two pages in some

medical journals or brief reports. A well-written introduction often begins with a strong **statement of impact.** A statement of impact references data that point to the importance of the topic under study. For example, consider a study with the objective of testing the outcomes of a work-rehabilitation program for women with HIV/AIDS. A statement of impact for this study would include a reference to a study about the high prevalence of HIV/AIDS among women, followed by a reference to additional studies citing the severity of symptoms, occupational consequences, and high rates of unemployment within this population.

The statement of impact would then be followed by a comprehensive and integrative review of current (i.e., from the past 5 to 10 years) literature specific to the topic under study. The most cohesive reviews include literature that relates as closely as possible to the central objectives of the topic under study. Thus, the study of women with HIV/AIDS would need to include a description of other studies that explain the barriers to and facilitators of employment for women with HIV/AIDS. The literature review would also include a description of any prior attempts at work rehabilitation with this population. Because the literature on this topic is relatively scant, one would want to include any relevant articles within and outside of the field of occupational therapy.

Additionally, strong introductions include an overview of the theory base upon which the research and methodological approach are rooted (Kielhofner, 2009). Returning to the example of a study on work rehabilitation for women with HIV/AIDS, the authors wish to ensure that their intervention is client centered and occupation focused and that it has been found to be successful with other populations. Moreover, they want to select outcome measures that reflect their theoretical orientation. After reviewing their options, they select the Model of Human Occupation (MOHO; Kielhofner, 2008). They select MOHO because it contains a range of work-rehabilitation assessments and evidence that prior work-rehabilitation programs based on this model were markedly successful with other populations.

Well-written introductions typically point out controversies or unanswered questions within the literature. Then they explain how the current study aims to respond to or provide new insight into those controversies or questions. For example, the study of women with HIV/AIDS might highlight the fact that prior intervention studies relying on biomechanical and cognitive disabilities approaches to rehabilitation have only shown modest outcomes because they were not tailored to the unique needs and capacities of the clients.

Finally, a strong introduction should end with a well-argued rationale for pursuing the particular question or hypothesis under study within that broader topic area. For example, the rationale might be that it is worth testing the outcomes of a client-centered, occupation-focused work-rehabilitation program because it is novel (i.e., has never been done before) and because its flexibility will better accommodate the unique and variable needs of the specific population. The rationale is often followed by a statement of the objectives, questions, and/or study hypothesis. This typically marks the end of the introduction, and it sets the stage for understanding the methods and results sections. More information about how to determine study objectives and write research questions and hypotheses is provided in later chapters of this text.

Method

The **method** section is often a good place to critically evaluate the level of evidence that a particular study contributes to knowledge about a given topic area. This section is where the approach that the researchers used to answer a particular practice question or solve a practice problem is described in detail. The method section is typically divided into a number of subsections that describe the ethical approvals, design, participants, procedures, measures, and data analysis approach. These headings are very helpful to readers who wish to learn more about a specific aspect of a study, such as the type of instrument used to measure a client's movement or the approach that an interviewer used when determining a client's treatment goals.

The **ethical approvals** section typically identifies the professional bodies that approved conduct of the research and describes how participants provided consent for the study. The **design** section describes the type of study that was developed and the way in which a research question or problem was examined. For example, if in the study of women with HIV/AIDS the researchers first conducted a work evaluation pretest and then compared outcomes from one group of women receiving the current standard of care for work rehabilitation with those from another group of women receiving an intervention based on the MOHO (Kielhofner, 2008), the study design would be described as a quasi-experimental pretest–posttest design; the study compared two groups of women (one receiving MOHO and one receiving standard care) and only measured work performance before and after intervention. The **participants** section describes the social and demographic characteristics of the sample, as well as the criteria by which the individuals in the study were selected for participation. It also describes the criteria by which certain individuals were excluded from participating in the study. For example, a researcher might choose to study occupational adaptation in a group of adolescent girls aged 13 to 18 with brachial plexus injury and those without such injury. The researcher would thereby exclude adolescents younger and older than this age range and would exclude males. Additionally, the participants section typically includes a description of the **recruitment and retention methods,** or means by which the authors were able to locate, access, enroll, and retain their sample over time and through the course of the study. Later chapters emphasize how important it is to develop a realistic and reliable recruitment strategy. If participants in the study were divided into subgroups and/or assigned to different conditions or treatments so that they could be compared with one another, the group assignment approach would also be described in the participants section of the article, as well as the means by which the groups were characterized.

The **procedures** section describes the sequence of actions taken to conduct the study, from beginning to end. Procedures include such actions as obtaining human subjects approval, obtaining consent from the subjects for study enrollment, and administering assessments.

The procedures section describes other approaches to collecting data, such as physical approaches to assessment (e.g., drawing blood, estimating grip strength, or obtaining a brain scan). Depending on the study, the description of the approach to data collection may be quite detailed. For example, a study that employs functional magnetic resonance imaging (FMRI) to look for changes in neuronal activity in the brain based on movement of the right upper extremity following a cerebrovascular accident may include the brand and model of the machine that was used to take the fMRI.

In a qualitative study, the procedures section may describe how field notes were recorded from observations and interactions with subjects. For example, a researcher interested in learning more about how small farming families living in remote rural areas create their own assistive devices and adaptations to accommodate a farming family member with a disability would describe exactly how, where, and for what duration the observations of this particular phenomenon took place.

When a study involves administering a treatment or other intervention to subjects or testing any other kind of experimental manipulation, the procedures section describes the treatment protocol or sequence of steps taken to carry out the intervention in detail. The procedures section is often a good place to include a sufficiently detailed description of the intervention so that it can be easily replicated by another research team. Often, **standardized interventions** (i.e., interventions that follow a structured format and do not deviate from implementation guidelines) are available in a manual that was created by a researcher or research team. That manual may be referenced in this section or appended to the paper, along with a description of how fidelity (faithfulness) to the procedures described in the standardized intervention was maintained by the person administering the intervention. The measurement of fidelity is often referred to as a **fidelity measure,** and it is similarly referenced or included in an article appendix.

The procedures section is also a good place to describe any **follow-up procedures,** or assessments undertaken after subjects have completed the intervention to follow their reaction to the intervention over time.

The **measures** section (sometimes referred to as the instruments section) is also included within the method section of the paper. This section describes the assessments and other data collection devices used to collect data. Descriptions of measures used should include any statistical or other evidence of the **dependability** of the measure, which often includes numeric data indicating the degree to which the measure was estimated as being reliable and valid. The **analytical approach** (or statistical analysis) section describes how the information or data collected in the study were coded, scored, summarized, analyzed, and interpreted. For quantitative data, this section often describes the sequence of statistical tests conducted to analyze the findings, including any details about particular variations of those tests that were used to best fit the data provided. For qualitative data, this section describes how data were coded, summarized, and interpreted in a way that tells a cohesive story about the findings to the reader.

Results

The **results** section of an article contains the statistical findings or qualitative summarization resulting from the data analyses that were conducted. The results section may be organized such that findings reflecting the sociodemographic characteristics of the sample or study groups are described, followed by the main findings from the study. Findings are typically presented in the order in which the study hypotheses, questions, or objectives were outlined in the introduction. The presentation of findings is typically limited to the direct results of the analyses undertaken and does not include an interpretation of or reflection on any of those findings.

Discussion

The **discussion** section provides an overview of study aims and findings. It typically begins with a summary of the central aim of the study and a general conclusive sentence about the corresponding central finding. An interpretation and reflective discussion about this central finding and a discussion of the other, related findings introduced in the results section typically follows. Often, the discussion of results includes a reflection on questions, controversies, and/or issues raised within the literature review, which is presented in the paper's introduction. The researchers may compare and contrast findings from the present study with findings from previous work that their team and other research groups studying the topic have completed. In the discussion section, the researchers may also reflect on how findings from this study can contribute to practice and how they can form a foundation for yet-to-be answered questions and future research.

Importantly, any discussion section should also include a **limitations section.** In this section, researchers acknowledge any flaws in study design, procedures, measures, and/or analyses, as well as any variables that were not examined but could have limited the interpretation and generalizability of the findings. If this section is well written, it is where one can find an abbreviated, critical appraisal of the study's methodological approach. If a study is not of the highest methodological rigor (the criteria for which are covered in Chapter 5), then the researchers must characterize the findings as preliminary and the conclusions as tentative and limited in scope.

References, Appendices, Tables, and Figures

Published articles always include a list of references that correspond to the literature cited within the paper. These references must be formatted in the style consistent with the requirements of the particular journal in which a study is being published. Typically, these styles include either APA style (the style recommended by the American Psychological Association) or AMA style (the style recommended by the American Medical Association). An example of an in-text citation and corresponding reference entry in APA style is presented in Figure 4.7.

Additionally, many studies include findings or other important data in tables, and concepts are often presented as diagrams, photographs, or other images in figures.

Reading the Various Sections: What to Look For

After one has read a number of peer-reviewed journal articles, one soon finds that they follow a specific format and pattern in terms of presenting the information to the reader. It is important to note that not all journals use the same headings as those presented here. Additionally, some are more inclusive and detailed in terms of subheadings. The following sections include the headings most often used and offer suggestions in terms of what to look for when reading each component of a peer-reviewed journal article.

The Abstract

In addition to the title, the abstract offers the most concise means of obtaining an overview of the approach and findings of a given research study. There may be circumstances in which reading only the abstract suffices in terms of serving a specific need, such as the need to be particularly time efficient while scrolling through numerous articles during an initial literature search. For example, when searching online databases to gather a specific subset of articles on a given topic, the reader does not typically search for and read each article one at a time. Instead, one enters the appropriate search criteria and then finds that the search screen is populated by numerous titles of articles. Once all of the articles appear (typically in a long list), reading the titles of all the articles serves as a good beginning in terms of weeding out irrelevant titles. However, this process, alone, does not typically provide enough information about the type or content of each article and its relevance to a reader's needs. In most, if not all, cases, one must also read the abstract of the article to understand the methodological approach and the results, which contribute to knowing whether the article is worth culling for further reading and analysis. A well-written abstract provides just enough information for this type of first-level screening and culling process to occur.

The Introduction

Sequentially, the next section of the paper is the introduction. In reading the introduction, the first part typically begins with a history and background of the scientific questions and findings in the area. It is important that the reader looks to the history and background to understand previous research questions and findings that provide a foundation for the questions to be answered in the current study. Also within the introduction, the reader will want to locate the rationale for the current study that outlines the unanswered questions in the scientific community that the current study addresses. Finally, toward the end of the introduction, the reader should find a statement of the study questions, objectives, and/or hypotheses. These anchor the reader when it comes time to read the study

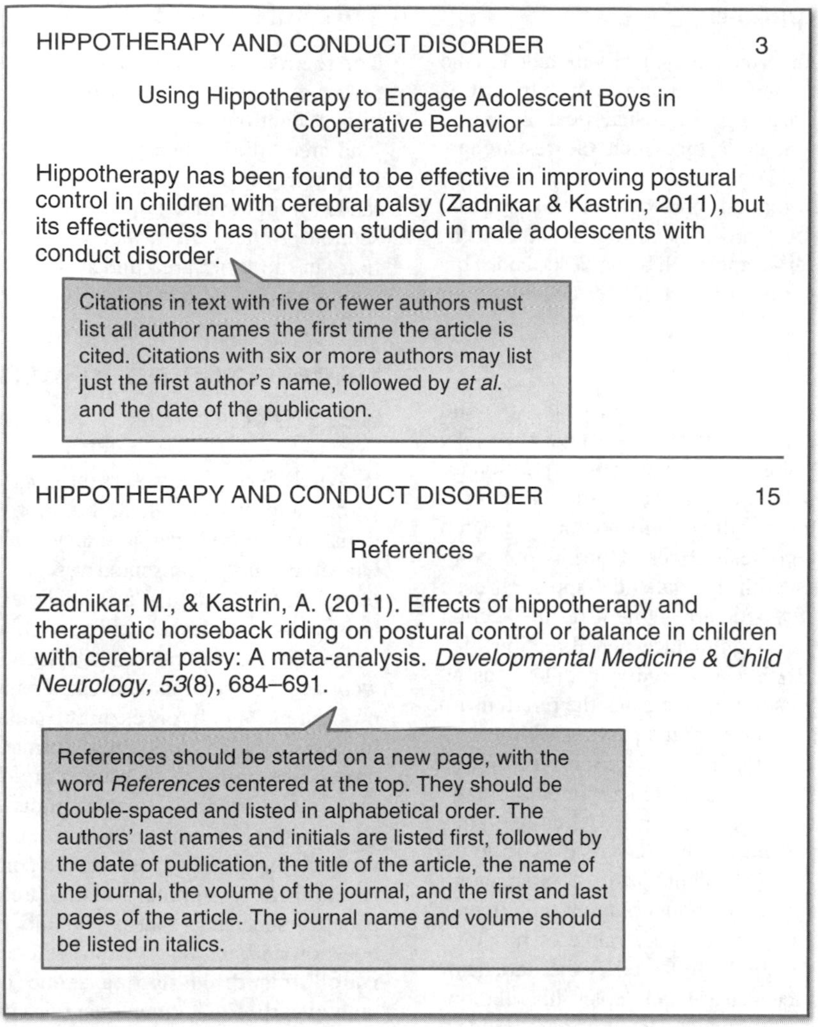

HIPPOTHERAPY AND CONDUCT DISORDER   3

Using Hippotherapy to Engage Adolescent Boys in
Cooperative Behavior

Hippotherapy has been found to be effective in improving postural
control in children with cerebral palsy (Zadnikar & Kastrin, 2011), but
its effectiveness has not been studied in male adolescents with
conduct disorder.

> Citations in text with five or fewer authors must
> list all author names the first time the article is
> cited. Citations with six or more authors may list
> just the first author's name, followed by *et al.*
> and the date of the publication.

HIPPOTHERAPY AND CONDUCT DISORDER   15

References

Zadnikar, M., & Kastrin, A. (2011). Effects of hippotherapy and
therapeutic horseback riding on postural control or balance in children
with cerebral palsy: A meta-analysis. *Developmental Medicine & Child
Neurology, 53*(8), 684–691.

> References should be started on a new page, with the
> word *References* centered at the top. They should be
> double-spaced and listed in alphabetical order. The
> authors' last names and initials are listed first, followed by
> the date of publication, the title of the article, the name of
> the journal, the volume of the journal, and the first and last
> pages of the article. The journal name and volume should
> be listed in italics.

Figure 4.7   An in-text citation and its corresponding reference presented in APA style.

results within the results section and their interpretation within the discussion section.

The Methods

Following the introduction is the method section. The method section should be written in a deliberately detailed way so that another research team will be able to replicate the study, if desired. If replication is not the reader's intention, it is important to know which aspects of this section to read and which to skim over. The general aspects of the method section to attend to include noting the study design, the number and nature of the participants, the types and quality of measures used to assess the study questions, the approach to data collection, and the interventions administered

and being tested (if any). The study design lends insight into the overall methodological rigor, or quality, of the study. The discussion of the nature and number of participants allows the reader to understand the general characteristics of the sample under study so that she or he may compare her or his own caseload (or sought sampling population) to the characteristics of the people under study. Larger sample sizes allow researchers to answer more complex questions with a greater degree of certainty. Knowing the types and quality of the measures used allows the reader to compare measurement outcomes across studies using the same measures. If different measures are used, the reader will know that findings may not be comparable across studies because of such differences.

Analytical Approach

The analytical approach is typically included in the method section, but some journals may treat it as a standalone heading. The analytical approach describes the methods by which the researchers examined the data collected in the study. To understand the information provided in this section, readers must be familiar with the statistics technique or qualitative approach being described. This information will be covered in later chapters.

The Results

When reading the results section, readers should pay closest attention to two key elements. The first is a reiteration of the research question or hypothesis. Each result in a study should be organized under a specific, corresponding research question or hypothesis. Even if one is not completely familiar with the statistical approach used in a given study, a clearly written results section should make the significance and direction of a finding clear. Let's use a study of athletes as an example. If this study investigates the relationship between the number of hours playing table tennis and the degree of upper extremity range of motion and the hypothesis is that a higher number of hours is associated with greater upper extremity range of motion, then the results may read as follows: "There was a significant positive association between the number of hours playing table tennis and degree of upper extremity range of motion." This would typically be followed by the statistic or statistics used to measure and depict this relationship and by the significance level of this finding.

The Discussion

The discussion summarizes the study objectives, approach, and findings and considers these findings in light of the existing literature. The discussion also includes a summary of the methodological limitations within the study. The limitations section is important to read because it qualifies the extent to which the findings are directly translatable into practice, or generalizable beyond the confines of the setting and circumstances during which the study took place. If a certain finding was expected and did not occur, the limitations section also explains possible methodological reasons as to why the result was not found. Toward the end of the discussion section, the reader will find recommendations for future research and, if it is an applied study, recommendations for prevention or practice.

The References

The references section follows the discussion and serves the reader in two primary ways. First, individual citations listed in the references section lend credibility to and provide source information regarding any informational claims or statements made throughout the paper. Second, the references section provides the reader with a list of publications in the topic area under study that she or he may wish to read and use in future research.

Understanding Presented Research

Research is typically presented in two formats, verbal and visual. Most, but not all, presentations contain both verbal and visual components. One may access presented research in a variety of contexts, including informal venues, such as brown-bag lunches and in-service presentations, grand rounds, conferences or teleconferences, and webinars. As summarized earlier in this chapter, professional conferences may include any combination of the following formats: individual **paper presentation** (a brief individual summary highlighting findings from an individual research study), **symposium** (a collection of individual research papers tied together by a common theme), **colloquium** (a summary of research papers by a panel of specialists that is typically followed by a question-and-answer session with the audience), **roundtable discussion** (a group of individuals with expertise in a given area raise and respond to questions that are focused on a specific topic; each expert in the group is typically seated at a different table with a different group of participants), **panel discussion** (a small group of people with special expertise are seated together at the front or in the center of the presentation room; interactive discussion among panel members and between panel members and audience members typically takes place, and audience members may pose questions to the panelists; the discussion is typically led by a facilitator, who poses thoughtful or provocative questions to the panel members), and/or **poster presentation** (experimental report or case study that is presented on a single poster with at least one author standing alongside to engage in discussion with the viewers).

Examples of conferences within the field of occupational therapy include the annual meeting of the American Occupational Therapy Association, the World Federation of Occupational Therapy conference, the annual conference of the British Association of Occupational Therapists and the College of Occupational Therapists, and the Annual Meeting of the European Network of Occupational Therapists. Every conference or presentation venue will have its own structure in terms of the types of verbal and visual presentations featured. Typically, a verbal presentation will be accompanied by some kind of visual aid, such as a digitally presented slide show using a popular software package such as PowerPoint or Prezzi. Alternative aids include paper handouts, videos, and photocopies of certain aspects that the presenters wish to highlight, such as a sample of an assessment used in the study or a picture of a device used for an intervention. A poster presentation relies on images, such as data visualization or photos of significant findings, and brief written phrases to present the same components of a research study discussed in the preceding section in a highly abbreviated and visually dramatic way. One or two presenters stand alongside the poster to invite viewers, provide a summary of the study, and respond to questions.

When attending any type of presentation, one should watch and listen for the presenter to structure the verbal presentation in the same way as a peer-reviewed journal article. The presentation should include all of the general sections of a written article but without as much detail as one would typically read in a full-length journal article. The presentation should begin with an introduction that includes a history and background on the topic and ends with a statement of the study questions, objectives, and/or hypothesis. A brief statement about the methodological approach and key features, including the sample size and characteristics, approach to data collection and assessment, and study design, should be included. This should be followed by an explanation of the findings and the conclusions drawn.

Summary

Evidence-based practice is an approach that requires the integration of several factors in decision-making, including knowledge gained through reading or hearing the research evidence, the practitioner's own clinical expertise, the client's values and preferences, and the available resources to incorporate all of these aspects into the treatment process. Evidence-based practice has become a norm and a standard for OT education throughout the developed world. Recent definitions of evidence-based practice emphasize the mutual,

bidirectional discourse between clients, practitioners, and researchers. This discourse is intended to contribute to the research questions that are raised and evaluated within this perspective.

This chapter covers the role of evidence-based practice in occupational therapy and the types of outputs that are considered as evidence in our field. Namely, it reviews the major types of research articles and conference presentations conducted by OT researchers, and it describes in detail the process of reading the major sections that comprise a typical peer-reviewed research article. Additionally, the chapter covers the basic aspects of attending professional conferences and understanding the ways in which research is typically presented in verbal and visual formats. Subsequent chapters in this section discuss how to evaluate the level of scientific rigor that characterizes a given research study and suggest resources for students and practitioners who must incorporate evidence into their work.

Review Questions

1. What is evidence-based practice, and what is its role in occupational therapy?
2. Why is clinical expertise important to evidence-based practice in occupational therapy?
3. What are the major types of presentations and research articles that allow for the dissemination (distribution) of evidence-based practice?
4. What are the major sections of a peer-reviewed research article?
5. What is one practical method of disseminating evidence to others in a given practice community?

REFERENCES

American Psychological Association. (2010). *Publication manual of the American Psychological Association* (6th ed.). Washington, DC: Author.

Forchheimer, M., & Meade, M. A. (2011). Women with violently acquired spinal cord injury: Characteristics of a vulnerable population. *Topics in Spinal Cord Injury Rehabilitation, 17,* 10–16.

Iverson, C., Christiansen, S., Flanagin, A., Fontanarosa, P.B., Glass, R.M., Gregoline, B., ... Young, R.K. (2009). *American Medical Association manual of style: A guide for authors and editors* (10th ed.). New York, NY: Oxford University Press.

Kennedy, P., Lude, P., Elfstrom, M. L., & Smithson, E. F. (2011). Psychological contributions to functional independence: A longitudinal investigation of spinal cord injury rehabilitation. *Archives of Physical Medicine and Rehabilitation, 92,* 597–602.

Kielhofner, G. (2008). *A Model of Human Occupation: Theory and application* (4th ed.). Philadelphia, PA: Lippincott Williams, & Wilkins.

Kielhofner, G. (2009). *Conceptual foundations of occupational therapy* (4th ed.). Philadelphia, PA: F.A. Davis.

Sackett, D. L., Rosenberg, W. M. C., Gray, J. A. M., Haynes, R., & Richardson, W. S. (1996). Evidence based medicine: What it is and what it isn't. B*ritish Medical Journal, 312,* 71–72.

Sackett, D. L., Straus, S. E., Richardson, W. S., Rosenberg, W. M. C., & Haynes, R. (2000). *Evidence-based medicine: How to practice and teach EBM* (2nd ed.). New York, NY: Churchill Livingstone.

Tickle-Degnen, L., & Bedell, G. (2003). Heterarchy and hierarchy: A critical appraisal of the "levels of evidence" as a tool for clinical decision-making. *American Journal of Occupational Therapy, 57,* 234–237.

CHAPTER 5

Critically Appraising and Classifying Published and Presented Research

Renée R. Taylor

Learning Outcomes

■ Articulate Cochrane's three criteria for evaluating the quality of a research study.
■ Differentiate among the levels of evidence as outlined by the Oxford Center for Evidence-Based Medicine.
■ Identify the major criteria used to evaluate published and presented research from the quantitative methodological perspective.
■ Differentiate the five dimensions of evidence used to evaluate qualitative research.
■ Describe how one would evaluate the quality of a mixed-methods study.

Introduction

When reading or listening to a presentation of research findings, it is important to evaluate the quality and relevance of those findings for your particular situation or need. If you are a student, you might consult a journal article as a basis for a paper you are assigned to write on a treatment topic (e.g., use of robotics in stroke rehabilitation). If you are an educator, you might update the readings you assign students, as well as your presentation slides, with current findings related to your lecture topic (e.g., latest developments in energy-conservation strategies for fatigue following cancer treatment). If you are a practitioner treating a child with hemiparesis of the right upper extremity, you might look to a systematic review article comparing constraint-induced approaches with bilateral-integration approaches to inform your practice. And if you are a researcher preparing a grant proposal involving posttraumatic stress disorder among combat veterans, you might search for articles that describe the prevalence and course of this disorder among different groups of veterans.

Whatever your role, as you are reading research or hearing a presentation, it is important to form your own judgments about the extent to which

the research findings can be considered applicable to a particular client, caseload, or setting. It is also important to evaluate the level of care and precision that the researchers took to ensure that the methods they used to evaluate the research question or problem were of the highest rigor possible. **Levels-of-evidence models** are heuristics (i.e., shortcuts or rules of thumb), such as rating systems and other frameworks, that allow consumers of research (i.e., students, educators, practitioners, and researchers) to determine the extent to which a particular study is methodologically rigorous and relevant to a particular client and/or practice setting. This chapter describes different approaches to evaluating quantitative and qualitative evidence and outlines the major criteria by which you may evaluate the level of rigor and quality of research.

This chapter's Case Example illustrates how to make a brief preliminary evaluation of the level of evidence from a quantitative perspective. However, this chapter also presents examples of levels-of-evidence models from the qualitative research tradition. In occupational therapy, no single model is held as the gold standard for determining whether a particular research study is valid and relevant to a specific client or practice setting.

Evaluating levels of evidence can be confusing if one does not consider the purpose and context of the research question. For example, a randomized trial would not answer the question of prognosis, or what would happen to a client if an impairment was left untreated. One research group studied the effect of applying different levels-of-evidence criteria to evaluate interventions for low back pain (Ferreira, Ferreira, Maher, Refshauge, & Latimer, 2002). As predicted, a comparison of four sets of levels-of-evidence criteria, in the absence of understanding the level of rigor required for the particular research question at hand, produced four different conclusions as to the efficacy of an ergonomically based "back school" intervention. For this reason, this chapter presents a balanced and practical perspective regarding the different standards by which evidence in our field may be judged.

It is important to recognize that there are numerous perspectives, critiques, explanations, and examples of models and approaches to appraising research in both the quantitative and qualitative literature. In this chapter, two of these perspectives are presented, an approach to appraising quantitative research and one for appraising qualitative research. These approaches are introduced at a foundational level and represent general overviews. More detail may be found in the sources cited within this chapter.

Additionally, it should be noted that **mixed-methodological studies**, which incorporate both quantitative and qualitative methodological approaches, may also offer the potential to produce a high level of evidence from both perspectives, depending on how the study is designed and executed. To date, there is no widely used levels-of-evidence model that rates mixed-methodological designs according to an established system. For mixed-methodological studies, it is recommended that rating systems from both perspectives be considered.

Levels of Evidence in Quantitative Research

In occupational therapy, a widely used levels-of-evidence model for evaluating the quality of treatment outcomes research is the **Cochrane levels-of-evidence model** (Cochrane Consumer Network, 2010). Similar to most models, the Cochrane model considers three major criteria to determine the credibility of findings from a treatment or intervention: strength of the evidence, size of the effect, and relevance of the evidence (Fig. 5.1). In considering the strength of the evidence of any research study, one must also assess the level of evidence offered by the research design. In this chapter, a basic outline of criteria put forth by a working group for the Oxford Center

for Evidence-Based Medicine (OCEBM) is used to define these levels (OCEBM Workgroup, 2011).

The Cochrane levels-of-evidence model and the OCEBM criteria offer just two examples of ways to assess levels of evidence in quantitative research. There are numerous levels-of-evidence models that one can reference when evaluating the quality of a research study. These include, but are not limited to, those offered by the field of evidence-based medicine and nursing (Carlson, Kruse, & Rouse, 1999; Cooke, 1996; Haughey, 1994; Le May, Mulhall, & Alexander,1998; Mitchell, 1999; Simpson & Knox, 1999). All of these models share an assumption that the highest level of evidence is represented quantitatively. However, much of what occupational therapists do and what they investigate requires a qualitative approach. It is possible to appraise evidence from research by taking both quantitative and qualitative approaches. This discussion begins with the Cochrane criteria concerning quantitative evidence, followed by a different perspective on levels of evidence offered by qualitative research.

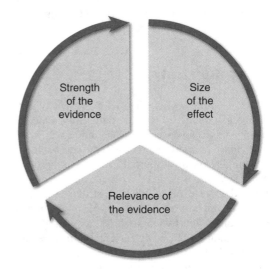

Figure 5.1 The Cochrane criteria for quality of evidence. (*From Cochrane Consumer Network, 2010.*)

CASE EXAMPLE

Lindsay is a practicing occupational therapist within a public school system. Recently, a popular approach to behavioral management has been introduced and promoted within her district, and all therapists in the district are required to attend a workshop on this topic and undertake specialized training. Lindsay completes the workshop and training and begins to use the approach with some of the children on her caseload. Soon, she realizes that it does not always work with highly introverted children who have features of autism. Moreover, she wonders if the new approach may be associated with the deterioration in behavior that she has recently noticed in some of the children with these kinds of problems. This causes Lindsay concern because there is an expectation for cohesion within the school, such that all therapists follow this approach at all times. She wants to say something about it during an upcoming staff meeting, but she does not want to appear uninformed or biased. She wonders whether she is not using the technique properly or is applying it to children for whom it was not originally intended, and she also wonders whether she is the only therapist who has found that it can occasionally produce negative effects.

Lindsay decides to turn to the research literature on this approach to answer these kinds of questions. Because this approach emanated from the field of behavioral medicine, she accesses her local university library on her tablet computer and selects three resources that are known to contain higher-quality, peer-reviewed, abstracted journal articles from this field: PsycINFO, CINAHL, and MEDLINE. When she searches each of these resources, she types in the search terms, which include the name of this particular behavioral management approach and the term "classroom."

Her search reveals one article that tested this approach and argued for its effectiveness within a highly specialized classroom setting for children with severe behavioral disorders. The research question associated with this study is stated as: "Is this approach to behavior modification effective in modifying misconduct within the classroom?" After Lindsay clicks the link to retrieve the article online, she scans the abstract to view the findings, which contend that the approach is effective. Next, she flips directly to the method section to get a preliminary evaluation of its **level of evidence**, or the extent of methodological rigor applied before asserting the conclusion that the intervention was effective.

First, Lindsay looks at the **study design,** which describes the method or experimental strategy with which the research question was approached. In this case, the design describes a within-groups study in which a behavioral assessment was conducted before the behavioral intervention was administered and immediately after it was terminated. When Lindsay looks at the **measurement approach** (i.e., the means by which the data were collected), she finds that the students' behavior was observed by an independent rater before and after the behavioral intervention, and these measures were corroborated with teacher self-reports on the classroom behavior of each child. Journal articles cited within the method section reveal that reliable and valid measures were used to make the self-report ratings. There was no evidence in the article that the observational rating scale used in the study had been subject to psychometric evaluation. However, the results indicate that the two measures produced similar results, so Lindsay is not very concerned about the fact that one of the two measures was not validated beforehand.

Next, Lindsay looks to the participants section to gather information on the characteristics of the population from which the sample of children was drawn and the number of children included in the sample. She learns that all 23 children in the sample met diagnostic criteria for externalizing types of behavioral disorders, such as conduct disorder or attention deficit-hyperactivity disorder, combined type.

In making this preliminary evaluation of the level of evidence of this study, Lindsay concludes that the strength and relevance of the evidence are low. The pretest–posttest design tells us that the study lacks a control group, so we do not know whether the effects of the intervention in improving the students' behavior were truly a result of the intervention itself or a result of some other unique feature of the study or setting. For example, the students and their parents might have known that the study was taking place and changed their behavior as a result of this knowledge. Moreover, in Lindsay's own school district, the sample on which the study was conducted was similar to the types of children for whom Lindsay found the intervention to be successful, but it differed significantly from the introverted children with features of autism for whom Lindsay found the intervention to be unsuccessful. Therefore, the relevance of the evidence for introverted children with features of autism was low. Because there was no other evidence in the literature concluding that the approach is effective for children with autism, Lindsay now had a basis for presenting her concerns about uniformly applying this approach to her colleagues from the school district.

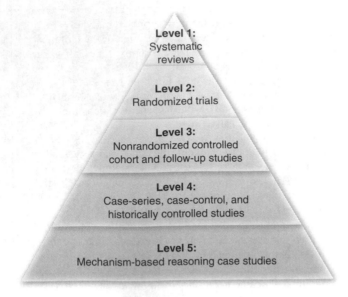

Figure 5.2   Levels of evidence from the quantitative perspective. *(Adapted from OCEBM, 2011.)*

Strength of the Evidence

The first of the Cochrane (Cochrane Consumer Network, 2010) criteria involves assessing the **strength of the evidence**. This is a broad term that is further determined by three criteria: the level of evidence of the study design, the quality of the evidence, and statistical precision.

Level of Evidence of the Study Design

The level of evidence of the study design provides an estimate of certainty that the identified evidence is a true measure of the benefits of an intervention. More information about study designs most often used in quantitative research is presented in Chapter 20.

Before embarking on this review, it is important to note that this chapter draws upon the OCEBM criteria (OCEBM Workgroup, 2011) to further explicate the levels of evidence for quantitative study designs. It should be noted that the hierarchical way in which the OCEBM levels are presented in this chapter is a simplification of the actual OCEBM approach to evaluating evidence, which considers the reason behind the evaluation of evidence in recommending an optimal study design (OCEBM Workgroup, 2011). For example, if one needed to evaluate the level of evidence pointing to the prevalence and incidence of HIV/AIDS, one would not look to local and current random-sample surveys and to systematic reviews of surveys that allow matching to local circumstances (OCEBM Workgroup, 2011). In this chapter, the OCEBM levels are described in the order that is typically applied to answer the question of whether an intervention or treatment is beneficial (Fig. 5.2).

Level 1: Systematic Reviews. In answering the question as to whether a given intervention is helpful, the systematic review provides an overview of all randomized controlled trials relevant to a given disorder and treatment topic. Systematic reviews are considered to represent the highest, or first, level of evidence. A **systematic review** is a literature review containing a synopsis of peer-reviewed publications focusing on a specific health problem or question. A single peer-reviewed journal article that summarizes and evaluates the statistical outcomes of 57 articles, some that point to evidence for the effectiveness of graded exercise in treating chronic fatigue syndrome, and some that do not find evidence in support of graded exercise, is one example of a systematic review. A systematic review applies rigorous, standardized methods that limit bias in the way the reviewed studies are selected, assembled, critically appraised, and synthesized. For a systematic review to be classified at the highest level of evidence, only studies that are true randomized controlled trials can be included. A **meta-analysis** is a subcategory of a systematic review, with one added feature: a meta-analysis presents a quantitative (i.e., statistical) summary of findings from all of the assembled studies on a given topic. More information about meta-analyses is provided in Chapter 25.

Level 2: Randomized Trials. The second level of evidence is a single randomized trial (also referred to as a *randomized controlled trial* or a *randomized* *clinical trial*). A **randomized trial** is a study in which participants from a given population are randomly assigned to groups (usually referred to as treatment or control groups) before a treatment (or other intervention, maneuver, or procedure) is applied. In a randomized trial, participants do not know the condition to which they are being assigned. For example, they do not know if they will be receiving a treatment versus a placebo control. Outcomes of the treatment are studied once the treatment has ended. Subjects do not have a choice as to which condition they are assigned, so individuals entering a study with an expectation of receiving a treatment must understand that they may or may not receive that treatment.

An example of a randomized trial is a study of the effects of a new acoustic training program as a means of assisting people who are blind and visually impaired in navigating while walking. The study hypothesis is that subjects who are blind and are provided with a specially engineered walking stick and corresponding acoustic training will walk with more speed and navigate with more accuracy while walking than those who are simply provided a typical walking stick. In this study, subjects who are blind are assigned to one of two conditions, a treatment group in which they receive the specially engineered walking stick plus the acoustic training or a placebo control group in which they receive a typical walking stick. Participants are measured on the speed at which they are able to walk and their accuracy while navigating before and after the treatment period.

Level 3: Nonrandomized Controlled Cohort and Follow-Up Studies. The third level of evidence includes **nonrandomized controlled cohort** and **follow-up studies**. Many of these studies utilize between-subjects designs and are also known as *pseudo-randomized trials* or *quasi-experimental studies*. **Between-subjects designs** compare two groups of subjects who are expected to change in different ways and at different rates, or they compare one group that is expected to change with another that is not. The common feature of these study designs that distinguishes them from randomized trials is that participants are not randomly assigned to a treatment or control group. Instead, they are assigned to groups based on convenience or some other criteria (such as geographical location, another demographic characteristic, or the time at which they enter the study and are available to participate).

A **nonrandomized controlled cohort study** is a study of subsamples from a given population who differ in terms of the extent to which they have been, are being, or will be exposed to something hypothesized to influence the outcome of a given impairment. The central feature of a well-designed cohort study is that it typically involves large numbers of subjects who are studied over a long period of time, with a comparison of rates or degrees of impairment outcomes based on original group membership and degree of exposure to the influential agent. For example, a controlled cohort study might involve a comparison of two group homes for adolescent teen mothers with a history of substance abuse problems. One home is open to placing an occupational therapy student with expertise in cognitive-behavioral therapy in the home to work with each of the teens as part of an assignment. The other home is not open to placing a study and is hence not able to offer an intervention consisting of cognitive-behavioral therapy.

Let's imagine that a professor of occupational therapy wishes to compare the teen mothers in terms of their scores on a well-validated measure of emotional distress. Knowing that she will be placing her student, a cognitive-behavioral therapy expert, in one home but not the other, she hypothesizes that the teens in the home that are exposed to the cognitive-behavioral therapy intervention will have higher scores on the measure compared with the teens in the home who are not exposed to this intervention. The professor cannot randomly assign the teens to a cognitive-behavioral therapy condition because they either live in the home that has the student expert on staff or they do not. Thus, she designs a study in which the measure of emotional distress will be administered to the teens in both of the homes 6 months before the student expert is placed in one of the homes, on the first day that the student expert is placed in one of the homes, and immediately after the student expert completes her placement in that home. Then, the professor analyzes whether placement of the student expert in the home had the anticipated effect of improving scores on the measure of emotional distress among teens in that home compared with teens in the home without the student expert.

A **follow-up study** is a controlled cohort study with a longitudinal element such that the outcomes of an intervention (or other experimental manipulation or exposure condition) are measured not only immediately upon completion of the intervention, but also at designated time points that occur after the intervention. Using our example, if the same professor wishes to study whether emotional distress scores continue to improve after the student expert has left the setting, she might administer the measure of emotional distress 6 months after the student's departure. This added time point

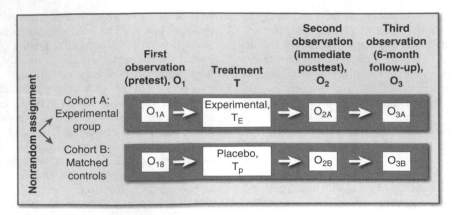

Figure 5.3   Diagram of a nonrandomized controlled cohort design with follow-up.

occurring after the immediate measurement of outcomes qualifies the study as a follow-up. A diagram of a nonrandomized controlled cohort design with follow-up is presented in Figure 5.3.

Level 4: Case-Series, Case-Control, and Historically Controlled Studies.
The fourth level of evidence includes case-series, case-control, and historically controlled studies. A **case-series study** is a longitudinal study of case-report information from a single group of subjects who were given a similar intervention. These reports typically contain detailed information about each of the subjects in the study, including demographic data (e.g., age, gender, race, and ethnicity) and information regarding the diagnosis, intervention, response to intervention, and follow-up after intervention. In this case, subjects act as their own controls and are measured before the intervention, immediately after the intervention, and at one or more follow-up time points. For example, let's examine a researcher who wants to measure the effects of graded exercise on autonomic symptoms in women with postural orthostatic tachycardia syndrome. Before comparing the effects of the graded exercise on the autonomic symptoms in a group of women without this diagnosis, the researcher feels that it is important to first understand whether exercise has an effect on the autonomic symptoms in this group.

A **case-control study** is an observational epidemiologic comparison of one group of subjects with a common diagnosis or problem (cases) with another group of subjects without this diagnosis or problem (controls). Cases and controls are compared in terms of the relationship of disease status and the presence, absence, or frequency/degree of that attribute to the disease. For example, if

a researcher wishes to examine the relationship between Epstein–Barr virus infection (the most common cause of mononucleosis) and the occurrence of chronic fatigue syndrome in adolescents, she might compare rates of Epstein–Barr virus infection in adolescents with and without chronic fatigue syndrome. This would allow her to determine the degree to which the attribute of having had an infection with Epstein–Barr virus is associated with the diagnosis of chronic fatigue syndrome.

A **historically controlled study** compares a group that received an intervention (treatment group) with a group that did not receive the intervention (control group). However, data collected on the group that did not receive the intervention are retrieved retroactively from records because they were collected before the data from the treatment group were collected. For example, a local hospital wants to reduce no-show rates and increase client attendance at appointments for occupational therapy (OT) services. In an effort to support this agenda, an OT researcher develops a smartphone-based educational program to remind clients about their appointment times, assist them in accessing transportation, and educate them about the services and supports offered through the OT service. She wants to test the effects of this program on attendance rates in the hospital. Knowing that money is being lost every time a client does not show for an appointment, she does not want to deprive any of the clients from receiving the program. Moreover, it is a small hospital, and she needs as many clients as possible to participate in the program (i.e., treatment group).

She considers accessing clients from another hospital in town, but there are a number of unique features about that hospital and the way in which OT services are delivered in that hospital that might

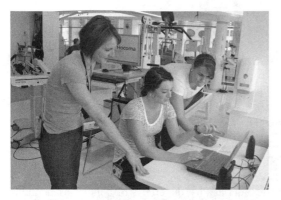

Figure 5.4 Occupational therapists conducting a review of medical records.

confound the comparison. For example, that particular hospital staffs twice as many occupational therapists, making appointment time slots easier to access, and its location is much closer to public transportation. Thus, attendance rates for OT services might be higher for these simple reasons. To avoid the potentially confounding effects of these extraneous variables, the researcher decides to utilize attendance records from the past 12 months for clients referred to OT services within her own hospital (Fig. 5.4). After ensuring that all of these clients were discharged and are no longer receiving services, these clients would serve as her historical control group.

Level 5: Mechanism-Based Reasoning and Case Studies. The fifth level of evidence involves **mechanism-based reasoning**. This includes studies that involve an inference from findings related to individual mechanisms to claim that an intervention leads to a particular outcome. A mechanism is a variable that drives the change process. For example, immobilization of the wrist may be a mechanism for healing and long-term functionality immediately following surgery. A case study examining the optimal length of immobilization in terms of healing and long-term functionality would involve mechanism-based reasoning.

These kinds of studies and reports may include, but are not limited to, expert opinion without explicit critical appraisal or mechanistic explanations that are based in physiological or bench research.

Additionally, **case-study research**, in which a researcher studies the effects of an intervention on a single individual over time with no control, is not considered to be randomized and also represents a lower level of evidence according to the Cochrane criteria. One example of case-study research involves measuring whether having an emotional support dog present during a painful shoulder manipulation leads to decreased pain ratings in an anxious client. A researcher might measure the client's pain and anxiety levels before, during, and after shoulder manipulation without the dog, then with the dog, and then without the dog again to determine whether the presence of the dog has only immediate effects versus long-term effects for that particular client.

Quality of Evidence

The second criterion by which strength of evidence is determined in the Cochrane model involves the **quality of the evidence** of an intervention study (Cochrane Consumer Network, 2010). This involves the extent to which the researchers minimize bias in the study design by controlling for variables that could bias the results or the interpretation of results. For example, one means of decreasing the effects of prejudice about whether a certain treatment will be effective or not is by not informing anyone of the condition to which subjects are assigned. This process of not informing participants of the condition to which they are assigned is referred to as **blinding**, and it is done to eliminate biases introduced by knowing one is receiving a treatment, such as the **placebo effect** (i.e., when a subject believes that a treatment is working and experiences positive effects that may be psychologically attributed to the belief in the treatment, rather than to an actual treatment). When researchers choose for not only subjects to be blinded but for the researchers not to know what condition a subject is in until the study is over, it is known as a **double-blinded** study. Double blinding can reduce other biases, such as **experimenter bias**, in which the researcher is testing a treatment that he or she believes will be effective. It may also reduce **observer bias**, which occurs when the researcher is looking for a physical cue or behavior to occur during an observation that follows a particular intervention or treatment.

Statistical Precision

Statistical precision is the third element that determines the strength of the evidence for a particular treatment or intervention. **Statistical precision** refers to the accuracy with which the outcome or effect of the intervention was measured and estimated using appropriate statistical analyses. More information about the accuracy of measurement and statistical analyses is given in Chapter 22, Chapter 23, and Chapter 24.

Size of the Effect

The size of the effect refers to the degree to which a positive (or negative) effect of an intervention exceeds the usual outcomes that would happen in the absence of the intervention. For a client of occupational therapy, it is important that the intervention demonstrates an apparent value that is above and beyond the current standard of care (**usual care**). The size of the effect of an intervention is typically measured statistically (i.e., a d-statistic, an r-statistic, or a binomial effect size display). It is important to note that effect size is different from statistical significance, which is typically determined by a statistic known as the *p*-**value**. **Significance testing** involves testing the **null hypothesis**, that is, that an intervention (or other experimental manipulation) has had no effect. Significance testing tells us whether the effect of an intervention is greater than 0.

Knowing that an intervention has had an effect beyond 0 is important, but it is often not enough because the size of the sample plays a role in this approach to estimating significance. There are cases in which an intervention may have been effective, but it was not demonstrated statistically because there were not enough people in the study to allow for the statistical analysis to have enough power to demonstrate this effect. The concepts of significance testing and p-values, along with their strengths and limitations, are described in more detail in Chapter 24.

Many researchers contend that the effect of an intervention is more accurately tested with a calculation know as effect size. **Effect size** determines that the effect of an intervention was greater than 0, and it provides a numerical estimate of how large the effect was. Additionally, effect size does not depend on sample size to the same extent. Thus, if an OT researcher wants to know the extent to which a bilateral movement intervention is more effective in engaging upper extremity movement than a usual care approach for young children with hemiplegia, effect size would establish whether the bilateral movement intervention increased movement of the affected arm 20%, 30%, or 40% beyond the usual care intervention.

Effect size is represented as a d-statistic, as an r-statistic, or as Rosenthal's **binomial effect size display** (BESD). The d-**statistic** is most commonly cited in published research, and it describes the effectiveness of an intervention as a range between 0 (negligible effect) and ≥ 1.00 (very large effect). The r-**statistic** is also referred to as Pearson's r or as a correlation coefficient. The r-statistic is a direct measure of effect size used when paired quantitative data are available. For example, if a researcher wanted to measure the relationship between body mass index and longevity, the researcher might expect a negative linear relationship indicating that as the body mass index decreases, longevity increases. By contrast, the BESD is often easier to understand because it converts the r-statistic into a percentage comparison of improvement between groups. For example, in considering a study comparing the effects of a yoga-based movement intervention for children with developmental discoordination disorder against the effects of a motor skills training intervention that involves working with one body segment at a time, one might find that 58.6% of the children improved on a global movement outcome measure in the yoga condition, whereas only 43.8% improved in the skills-training group.

Effect size is usually accompanied by a **confidence interval**, which is a statistical range that describes the lower and upper limits of the true effect size in the population. The confidence interval acknowledges that even under optimal conditions (i.e., when a study follows a random assignment of subjects to conditions and attempts to control for biases through blinding and other methods), the statistical findings of a study remain vulnerable to the circumstances of chance. The confidence interval defines the estimated range within which an intervention had a true effect. In many cases, studies utilize 95% as the estimated confidence interval. This means that the researchers are 95% certain that the effect size reported is a valid estimate. For example, if a study finds that 40% of participants benefitted from an intervention involving stretchable therapy bands, a 95% confidence interval would estimate the true effect of the bands as helping between 30% and 50% of the people.

Relevance of the Evidence

Relevance of the evidence refers to the degree to which the assessment used to measure the effectiveness (or harmfulness) of an intervention is appropriate and useful for the people and problem under study. For example, a study of the effects of a walking intervention for persons with unexplained chronic muscular pain might use a pain rating scale and dolorimeter (a probe that measures pain perception based on the extent to which pressure may be exerted with the probe before a subject reports pain). The degree to which these are appropriate and useful measures for persons with unexplained chronic pain would need to be evaluated to determine whether they would be relevant enough outcome measures to assess the effectiveness of the walking intervention.

Quality of Evidence in Qualitative Research: Five Dimensions

There are a number of well-cited, established methodological approaches to qualitative research that, if followed, produce studies that are considered to offer a high level of evidence within the qualitative perspective.

Qualitative researchers and occupational therapists share an important commonality: Similar to nurses, they both work from a worldview that is holistic and integrative (Cesario, Morin, & Santa-Donato, 2002). Within the field of nursing, Cesario and colleagues developed a levels-of-evidence model for qualitative research based on a detailed literature review of the qualitative studies within the obstetrics literature. According to this model (Cesario et al., 2002), quality of evidence is evaluated according to five dimensions:

I. Descriptive vividness
II. Methodologic congruence
III. Analytical preciseness
IV. Theoretical connectedness
V. Heuristic relevance

Unlike levels of evidence in quantitative research, qualitative research approaches the appraisal of quality from a nonhierarchical perspective. In this section, we apply Cesario et al.'s (2002) dimensions to the field of occupational therapy. Figure 5.5 offers a visual depiction of the criteria developed by Cesario et al. (2002).

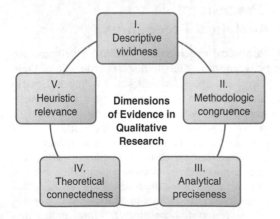

Figure 5.5 Dimensions of evidence in qualitative research. *(Adapted from Cesario et al., 2002.)*

Dimension I: Descriptive Vividness

Descriptive vividness refers to the degree to which the study methods and findings are clear, credible, complete, and valid (Cesario et al., 2002). To adequately respond to the requirements of this dimension, a study must include essential descriptive information about the study background, purpose, and research questions. This descriptive narrative must be written clearly. Details must be given about the characteristics of the participants, the observational setting, the methods for data collection, and the questions and approaches to assessment. These details and the vividness with which they are described are not possible unless adequate time is spent at the observational setting to gain familiarity with the participants. Additionally, this description must be credible and not so perfect so as to mask natural obstacles and missteps that occurred during the course of data collection. Part of this credibility involves what are sometimes referred to as **member checks**, in which the researcher approaches study participants to describe, cross-check, and thereby validate findings and interpretations. More information about data collection approaches in qualitative research are given in Chapter 17.

Dimension II: Methodologic Congruence

According to Cesario and colleagues (2002), **methodologic congruence** refers to the extent of rigor in documentation, procedures, and ethics. It also includes evidence of confirmability, such that another researcher would be able to replicate study methods and findings based upon the record-keeping, the description of the data collection process, and the decision rules and reasoning that went into decision-making and interpretation of the findings (Cesario et al., 2002). This requires a rigorous approach to documenting the essential elements of the study, including the consent procedures, the background literature review and introduction, a description of the research design, the approach to data collection, the approach to data analysis, and the findings and conclusions. Evidence of this level of procedural rigor may be detected in the type and quality of the questions asked to elicit participants' perspectives and experiences. Moreover, researchers should include a full description of the steps taken to ensure that participants represent themselves and their experiences accurately. In so doing, researchers should demonstrate an attempt to eliminate bias by placing equal weight on **high-status informant data** and **low-status informant data**. High-status informants are articulate, reflective, and observant. They have been in the culture long enough to provide an accurate report. They may have leadership positions in the community or hold similar positions of power. Their views may or may not represent those of the majority. Lower-status informants may not possess these qualities, and may even hold a minority viewpoint, but their perspectives and experiences must be considered against those of the higher-status informants for accuracy and representation of the experiences and perspectives of the community as a whole.

Researchers must also explain the steps that were taken to avoid the distortion of events resulting from the researcher's physical presence and/or equipment. In so doing, the researcher must be ethical and transparent with participants. Participants must willingly consent to participate in the study, and they must be informed of their rights of refusal and of the mechanisms that the researcher has put in place to protect participants' rights.

For example, if a researcher chooses to study the social behaviors of recovering alcoholics by attending a series of open support groups and getting invited to sober parties, whether the researcher is also a recovering alcoholic and a regular member of the support group would be an important variable to consider. For ethical reasons, it is important that participants know the researcher's status as a recovering alcoholic or as a person who does not struggle with alcohol addiction. It would not be ethical for the researcher to lie about her or his status as an alcoholic just to access the participants and gain entry into the group meetings and social events.

If a researcher is a regular member of an existing group and the researcher, acting as a **participant-observer**, discloses that she or he is a recovering alcoholic, the fact that she or he is conducting research may influence the disclosures and behaviors of the group members to a certain extent. Group participants may be a little more guarded, or they may seek reassurance about their confidentiality or have questions for the researcher about her or his loyalty as a group member. However, if the researcher is not a recovering alcoholic and not a regular member of the group, the likelihood that group members will self-disclose and interact naturally is even more questionable. In this case, the researcher would need to make extra efforts to integrate him- or herself into the group so that members would feel a mutual sense of trust, acceptance, comfort, and respect.

Another aspect of methodologic congruence (Cesario et al., 2002) is the requirement that participants are selected appropriately. Researchers are discouraged from selecting individuals out of convenience who do not fully meet the eligibility criteria intended for the study. For example, in a study of older women with severe fibromyalgia, it would not be appropriate for a researcher to recruit her mother simply because her mother has a few tender points and was told by her doctor that she would develop fibromyalgia if she did not continue exercising.

It is also important in qualitative research that sufficient amounts of data are collected from participants so that researchers are not lacking in information and left to guess at the missing information or fill it in on their own. Not only is this unethical (referred to as **data fabrication**, where one makes up one's own data), but it is also inaccurate. For data to be comprehensive enough to respond to detailed research questions, the researcher must invest a tremendous amount of time in pursuing data collection (Cesario et al., 2002).

A final aspect of methodologic congruence involves the requirement of confirmability and auditability of the data collection process (Cesario et al., 2002). This review must ensure that a sufficient amount of raw data was recorded and that the decision rules made to arrive at the ratings, judgments, and interpretations were described in sufficient detail. This process should ensure that another researcher would be able to arrive at the same ratings by following the same decision rules (Cesario et al., 2002). Additionally, it would be important to verify that the nature of the decisions, the data on which they were based, and the reasoning by which the decisions were made were all adequate.

Dimension III: Analytical Preciseness

Analytical preciseness is defined by congruence between study data, findings, interpretations, theoretical linkages, and conclusions drawn (Cesario et al., 2002). To meet requirements for this dimension, it is important that the study hypotheses or propositions are verifiable by the study data and presented as such in the research report. Moreover, any interpretive theoretical statements about the data must correspond closely with the findings. The set of themes, categories, or theoretical statements emerging from the analysis must form a cohesive narrative or picture. More information about analytical approaches in qualitative studies is given in Chapter 18.

Dimension IV:
Theoretical Connectedness

Theoretical connectedness defines the extent to which the theoretical constructs and their relationships with one another were validated by the data, clearly defined, comprehensive, and sufficient in contributing to the formation of a new theory or in confirming or linking to concepts within an existing theory (Cesario et al., 2002). This requires that theoretical concepts are adequately defined and/or validated by the data, that the relationships among the concepts are clearly described, and that these relationships are also validated by the data. For this to occur, theory developed from the data must yield an integrated story of the phenomenon under study. Unless new theory is being developed (or existing theory is being revised or expanded), a connection must be made between the data and an existing OT theory. More information about approaches to interpreting and integrating the findings from qualitative studies is given in Chapter 19.

Dimension V:
Heuristic Relevance

Heuristic relevance refers to applicability of the findings to practice, intuitive recognition of the described phenomena that is consistent with the field's knowledge base, and the necessity of these new findings and knowledge in relation to the existing knowledge base (Cesario et al., 2002). For this to occur, there must be evidence that the phenomenon under study would be recognized on an intuitive level by a practitioner. In turn, researchers must also be able to recognize the phenomenon easily, and the description of the phenomenon must be consistent with common meanings and experiences relevant to the field.

In addition to these requirements, heuristic relevance requires innovation and practicality. It is important that the researcher follows within a tradition of existing scholarship such that the new phenomenon or discovery acknowledges the existing evidence that came before it. At the same time, it is important to demonstrate that the new discovery is needed and relevant to OT practice because it fills a gap or sheds a new light on the understanding of a topic. A finding or study may not simply be a discovery for the sake of discovery itself, or a finding that replicates a past finding and does not acknowledge having done so. Finally, the findings must not only fill a gap, but they must be relevant to practice, important to the discipline of occupational therapy, and capable of pushing the science forward to a new level.

In summary, appraising qualitative research is a multidimensional effort that requires attention to description, methodology, analysis, theory, and relevance. It is important to understand that no single study will meet all of the requirements described in each of the five dimensions. Rather, a careful consideration of which aspects of which dimensions were fulfilled is what is required for such an appraisal.

Evaluating the Evidence: Issues to Consider

Standards of quality for evidence-based practice and the means for evaluating levels of evidence vary depending upon one's research approach and field of study. In this chapter, the standards set forth by the Cochrane Consumer Network (2010) and by the OCEBM Workgroup (2011) were selected as central reference points for quantitative research, and those described by Cesario and colleagues (2002) were utilized for qualitative research. With respect to evaluating quantitative studies, in particular, hierarchical levels-of-evidence models have come under significant criticism (Cook, Guyatt, Lupacis, & Sacket, 1992; Sacket, 1989). For example, some have argued that observational studies, case-series studies, and sometimes anecdotal studies may provide better evidence than other designs (Aronson & Hauben, 2006; Glasziou, Chalmers, Rawlins, & McCulloch 2007; Horwick, 2011). For this reason, it is important to consider the range of research questions in light of selecting an optimal way of evaluating the evidence. Table 5.1 presents examples of resources for evaluating evidence from both quantitative and qualitative perspectives. The evidence-based resources listed in Table 5.1 may be found online. Some are freely accessible, whereas others must be accessed through a university online library, hospital online library, or other online library with subscription services.

Summary

Whether one utilizes a quantitative, qualitative, or mixed-methodological perspective, conducting evidence-based practice involves knowing how to critically appraise the literature before applying it in a clinical practice situation. Reading and evaluating peer-reviewed journal articles and research presentations according to a levels-of-evidence

Table 5.1 Resources for Evaluating Evidence

Resource	Website
American Occupational Therapy Association: Evidence-Based Practice & Research	http://www.aota.org/Practice/Researchers.aspx
Agency for Healthcare Research and Quality: National Guideline Clearinghouse	http://www.guideline.gov/
Cochrane Consumer Network	http://consumers.cochrane.org/levels-evidence
Cochrane Reviewers' Handbook Version 3.0.2	http://handbook.cochrane.org
OTseeker	http://www.otseeker.com

perspective is a fundamental skill for all OT students and professionals. In this chapter, we explicate quantitative and qualitative rating systems commonly used to evaluate the level of rigor according to which research studies are conducted: the Cochrane levels-of-evidence model (Cochrane Consumer Network, 2010), the OCEBM levels of evidence for research designs (OCEBM Workgroup, 2011), and an adaptation of Cesario and colleagues' (2002) model applied within an OT context.

These systems are offered as examples of specific approaches to classifying a research study. Because numerous critiques, explanations, and examples of other models of levels of evidence exist in the literature, it is important to recognize that the examples provided in this chapter emanate from a larger body of work in this area. Furthermore, it is important to note that the overview of these approaches provided in this chapter is general and geared toward a foundational level of comprehension. The original cited sources from which these systems were summarized provide more detailed and nuanced descriptions.

Review Questions

1. What is an example of a quantitative research study design, and what criteria would you use for evaluating the study according to a levels-of-evidence model?
2. What is an example of a qualitative research study, and how would you evaluate the quality of the evidence from a multidimensional perspective?
3. What is a rationale for critically appraising a journal article according to a levels-of-evidence approach, and why would this be helpful to an OT practitioner?
4. How would you evaluate the quality of a mixed-methods study?
5. What are the limitations of evaluating quantitative designs according to a hierarchical levels-of-evidence model?

REFERENCES

Aronson, J. K., & Hauben, M. (2006). Anecdotes that provide definitive evidence. *British Medical Journal, 16*(333), 1267–1269.

Carlson, D. S., Kruse, L. K., & Rouse, C. L. (1999). Critiquing nursing research: A user-friendly guide for the staff nurse. *Journal of Emergency Nursing, 25*(4), 330–332.

Cesario, S., Morin, K., & Santa-Donato, A. (2002). Evaluating the level of evidence of qualitative research. *JOGNN: Principles and Practice, 31,* 708–714.

Cochrane Consumer Network. (2010). *Levels of evidence.* Retrieved from http://consumers.cochrane.org/levels-evidence

Cook, D. J., Guyatt, G. H., Lupacis, A., & Sacket, D.L. (1992). Rules of evidence and clinical recommendations on the use of antithrombotic agents. *Chest, 102,* 305S–311S.

Cooke, J. (1996). Cambodia–daring traditional birth attendants to change tradition. *Midwives, 109*(1299), 96–98.

Ferreira, P. H., Ferreira, M. L., Maher, C. G., Refshauge, R. F., & Latimer, H. J. (2002). Effect of applying different "levels of evidence" criteria on conclusions of Cochrane reviews of interventions for low back pain. *Journal of Clinical Epidemiology, 55,* 1126–1129.

Glasziou, P., Chalmers, I., Rawlins, M., & McCulloch, P. (2007). When are randomized trials unnecessary? Picking signal from noise. *British Medical Journal, 334,* 349–351.

Haughey, B. (1994). Evaluating research. *Clinical Nursing Specialization, 8*(4), 195–207.

Horwick, J. (2011). *The philosophy of evidence-based medicine.* Oxford, England: Wiley-Blackwell.

Le May, A., Mulhall, A., & Alexander, C. (1998). Bridging the research-practice gap: Exploring the research cultures of practitioners and managers. *Journal of Advanced Nursing, 28*(2), 428–437.

Mitchell, G. J. (1999). Evidence-based practice: Critique and alternative view. *Nursing Science Quarterly, 12*(1), 30–35.

Oxford Center for Evidence-Based Medicine Workgroup. (2011). The Oxford 2011 levels of evidence. Retrieved from http://www.cebm.net/index.aspx?o=5653

Sacket, D. L. (1989). Rules of evidence and clinical recommendations on the use of antithrombotic agents. *Chest, 95*(Suppl. 2), 2S–4S.

Simpson, K. R., & Knox, G. E. (1999). Strategies for developing an evidence-based approach to perinatal care. *MCN American Journal of Maternal and Child Nursing, 24*(3), 122–131.

CHAPTER 6

Managing Barriers to Evidence-Based Practice: An International Imperative

Annie McCluskey • Renée R. Taylor

Learning Outcomes

- Explain current research findings on barriers to evidence-based practice involving students and new graduates.
- Describe the international diversity in attitudes and approaches to evidence-based practice within the field of occupational therapy.
- Identify the major barriers to evidence-based practice for experienced occupational therapy practitioners.
- Describe strategies for managing barriers to evidence-based practice.

Introduction

The profession of occupational therapy (OT) produces important research that is relevant to what we do in practice every day. It is critical that we find ways to incorporate our findings into practice to improve client outcomes. We need to be able to discriminate between rigorous research and research that is of lower methodological quality. It is important that we utilize research critically so that we do not buy in to popular trends within our field that have not been adequately evaluated. Research is also meant to guide those of us who educate or wish to educate future practitioners. Although the process of change can be slow, individuals and organizations need to overcome the gap between research and practice and to understand the many benefits of evidence-based practice.

Previous chapters in this section have described the need for evidence-based practice and the process of classifying, reading, understanding, and appraising published and presented research that supports our practice. OT professionals are expected to appraise and classify studies according to methodological quality (Sackett, Straus, Richardson, Rosenberg, & Haynes, 2000; Taylor,

2000). Research evidence is not intended to be used in isolation. Rather, it should be combined with clinical experience, clinical reasoning, knowledge from formal education, and information about client needs and values (Pollock & Rochon, 2002).

This chapter reviews the history of the movement from experience-based to evidence-based practice. Additionally, a summary of the current international literature regarding common barriers to using research in practice is presented. The chapter concludes with a review of the research concerning how occupational therapists manage these barriers effectively to allow them to incorporate relevant research findings into their practice over time.

Moving From "Experience-Based" to "Evidence-Based" Practice

Until the mid-1990s, it was reasonable for practice to be based primarily on experience, hence the term **experience-based practice** (Redmond, 1997). When guidelines for clinical reasoning and standards for the education of practitioners were developed, research was not typically the primary source of information. Instead, guidelines were developed based on **expert opinion** (i.e., a person or convened group of people having specialized knowledge about a topic based on education, experience, or certain achievements that are not possessed by the average person) and **anecdotal evidence** (i.e., stories based on nonspecific observations, personal interviews, or other public statements). Research references were an optional "extra" in such standards and guidelines.

Today, evidence-based practice in occupational therapy has become a worldwide priority (Garner, Meremikwu, Volmink, Xu, & Smith, 2004; Hocking & Ness, 2002; Ilott, Taylor, & Bolanos, 2006). In 2004, the World Federation

CASE EXAMPLE

Veronica is a new graduate from a highly accredited professional doctorate (OTD) program in occupational therapy. Recently, she has been promoted to the position of manager of the rehabilitation unit at a large urban medical center. One of the primary expectations of her role is to encourage therapists on her unit to incorporate more evidence from the field of rehabilitation into their practice.

Many of the therapists on Veronica's unit are highly experienced, with 10 to 30 years of practice following OT school. During her initial orientation to the unit, Veronica notices that many are practicing using outdated techniques, with the explanation that they had learned these approaches from their much revered mentors in school. Another issue that Veronica quickly identifies is that much of the rehabilitation equipment on the unit is outdated and only utilized by a small portion of the staff.

Veronica knows that it would be fruitless to abruptly insist or try to convince the therapists on her unit to change their current practices, learn to utilize new equipment, and take an entirely new approach to incorporating research into practice. She decides to take a positive approach by initiating a series of mandatory lunch meetings on the unit. She reasons that these will be well attended not only because they are mandatory, but because they would be a welcome change for therapists who typically eat lunch at their desks because of heavy caseloads and a lack of time. For each lunch, one therapist would be asked to print out the abstracts from five research articles, published within the previous 5 years, and pertinent to an issue of interest within his or her area of practice. The group would then discuss the research over lunch.

Veronica recognizes that this activity is a modest starting point in terms of introducing evidence-based practice to the rehabilitation unit. However, she plans to increase the level of involvement and sophistication of lunchtime assignments over the course of the year once she knows that all of the therapists have gained competence in the basic skills of locating and retrieving peer-reviewed journal articles.

Moreover, Veronica plans to provide workday incentives for therapists who involve themselves in suggesting topics for research for OT students and faculty in the OT school affiliated with the hospital. Her hope is that the commitment to evidence-based practice among therapists on her unit will grow endogenously and become an embedded and self-perpetuating approach to practice among all therapists on staff.

of Occupational Therapists assembled an advisory group of OT scholars from a wide range of nations to inform the field's incorporation of this imperative. Different professional and regulatory groups from the United States (e.g., Coster, 2005; Coster, Gillette, Law, Lieberman, & Scheer, 2004), Canada (e.g., von Zweck, 1999), the United Kingdom (e.g., College of Occupational Therapists, 2003, 2005; Health Professions Council, 2003), Scandinavia (e.g., Van Bruggen, Renton, Ferreira, le Granse, & Morel, 2000), and Australia (e.g., McKenna et al., 2004) have created formal structures, resources, and guidelines to facilitate the incorporation of evidence-based practice into occupational therapy. Ilott and colleagues (2006) proposed a 10-year strategy for implementing evidence-based practice into the global practice of occupational therapy worldwide.

This strategy involves an effort on the part of all OT professionals to create more evidence through research. There is also an imperative to share research findings and knowledge in an equitable way using free-access, Internet-based avenues (Ilott et al., 2006). Moreover, professional and statutory organizations throughout the world need to continue to prioritize evidence-based practice in their standards for education and practice (Ilott et al., 2006).

This change from experience-based practice to evidence-based practice (and teaching) requires a substantial change in skills, knowledge, attitudes, and behavior. Not surprisingly, practitioners and academics often respond with anxiety to the degree of change that would be required to meet these expectations (Dubouloz, Egan, Vallerand, & von Zweck, 1999). Therefore, it can be helpful to understand the specific barriers to evidence-based practice and how different individuals have attempted to overcome these barriers and initiate programs of evidence-based practice within their settings. When it comes to evidence-based practice, individual professionals and managers who are better informed about change can plan ahead and be proactive instead of reactive (McCluskey & Cusick, 2002).

International Barriers

From an international perspective, Ilott and colleagues (2006) identify four reasons that have prevented occupational therapy from advancing as an evidence-based profession.

First is its characterization as a **research-emergent profession,** or a profession that has lacked a consistent history and infrastructure to support individuals who conduct research.

A second reason involves variation in the profession's stage of development and status around the world (Ilott et al., 2006). Even within the United States, approaches to OT education vary from state to state. These differences are even more pronounced when one compares educational and certification standards in Canada, different parts of Europe, Asia, Australia, South and Central America, the Middle East, and Africa, for example. OT practitioners with fewer years of education and fewer requirements to enter the field may have less knowledge and fewer skills to utilize or conduct research than those who enter the field with a higher level of education. This affects the extent to which different professionals are capable of supporting and contributing to the evidence base of the field.

A third criterion slowing the incorporation of evidence-based practice into occupational therapy involves language barriers (Dopp, Steultjens, & Radel, 2012; Ilott et al., 2006). Without a requirement for all scientific journals to publish articles in a common language and all professional conferences to hold presentations in a common language, it is difficult for a profession to advance. Other professions, such as medicine and psychology, have adopted English as a universal language. It is difficult to share and compare research findings when investigators are not communicating in a common language.

The fourth barrier to international efforts to build evidence-based practice involves limited economic and educational resources, including the grant funding and expertise required to form long-distance research collaborations. Without funding and time to cultivate collaborations, it is impossible to develop an evidence base for a particular profession.

Barriers for Fieldwork Students and New Practitioners

From a practice perspective, barriers to evidence-based practice are highly complex (Morrison & Robertson, 2011). These barriers affect new graduates as much as they affect highly experienced long-term practitioners. This section focuses on the barriers affecting student practitioners doing fieldwork and recent graduates.

Recently, a number of regulatory professional bodies have required educational curricula to include an emphasis on evidence-based practice. As a result, recent graduates of entry-level OT programs in many regions throughout the world report feeling confident about their knowledge of evidence-based practice (Stronge & Cahill, 2012). Two studies of students from entry-level OT programs in Ireland and New Zealand indicate that final-year students have clear understanding of evidence-based practice and report a willingness to practice it in the future (Stronge & Cahill, 2012). However, they describe the process of actually implementing evidence-based practice during their fieldwork placements as very challenging (Morrison & Robertson, 2011; Stronge & Cahill, 2012).

For example, students from New Zealand reported finding it difficult to link specific research findings to their daily decision-making. Additionally, they reported not having time during their placements to conduct literature searches and critically appraise study designs and findings on their own. They still felt they needed supervision to ensure they were conducting the reviews appropriately (Morrison & Robertson, 2011). Although most surveyed students from Ireland reported accessing the literature weekly or more often, more than one-half reported difficulty locating the articles they needed. Nearly one-third identified lack of support from fieldwork supervisors and lack of time as primary barriers (Stronge & Cahill, 2012).

Once students graduate and enter the profession, it is often difficult for them to incorporate what they learned about evidence-based practice into their daily work behaviors as practitioners (Morrison & Robertson, 2011). An exception to this situation involves a minority of students who may remain professionally active and need information for in-service presentations (58%), professional meetings (39%), involvement in research projects (19%), or grant applications (8%) (Gilman, 2011).

The primary barrier reported by newer occupational therapists for not using research in practice is a perceived lack of time for accessing, reading, appraising, and interpreting research (Morrison & Robertson, 2011). Additionally, many practitioners report that the cultural atmosphere within their settings and attitudes of their supervisors do not support the time and resource requirements necessary to access, appraise, and implement new and evolving evidence into practice (Stube & Jedlicka, 2007).

Barriers for Experienced Practitioners

More experienced practitioners report a lack of skill in conducting literature searches, critically appraising the literature, and linking the literature findings to their everyday practice situations (Dopp et al., 2012; McCluskey, 2003). For example, some practitioners report not knowing how to conduct a literature search or make a critical appraisal of the literature (Metcalfe et al., 2001; Pollock, Legg, Langhorne, & Sellars, 2000). Others report that they do not know how to identify a "good" study from a poorly conducted one, nor do they know how to interpret statistics in the results section of a paper (Metcalfe et al., 2001; Pollock, Legg, Langhorne, & Sellars, 2000). Characteristics of the work setting, such as heavy caseloads and workplace culture, have also been cited as significant barriers (Dopp et al., 2012). It would make sense that therapists who were not as well educated about evidence-based practice when they entered the profession would report deficits in skills and knowledge (Dubouloz et al., 1999). Moreover, experience may have taught some of the therapists what they do not know, whereas students may have a tendency to not yet know what they do not know.

Results of two surveys focusing on these and other barriers are presented in Tables 6.1 and 6.2. These surveys were conducted with occupational therapists in Australia (McCluskey, 2003, 2004). Findings from the first survey, presented in Table 6.1, list the top 10 barriers identified by a convenience sample of 64 occupational therapists. They completed the survey before attending a workshop on evidence-based practice. Consistent with other studies of this topic, most respondents identified lack of time and a large workload or caseload as the major barriers to adopting evidence-based practice, followed by limited searching skills and limited critical appraisal skills.

Table 6.1 Perceived Barriers to Adopting Evidence-Based Practice as Reported by Australian Occupational Therapists (n = 64)

Top 10 Barriers Reported	n	%
Lack of time	56	(87.5)
Large caseload	43	(67.2)
Limited searching skills	32	(50.0)
Limited critical appraisal skills	28	(43.7)
Difficulty accessing journals	28	(43.7)
Lack of evidence to support what occupational therapists do	26	(40.6)
Professional isolation	22	(34.4)
Limited resources and funding to support change to evidence-based practice	20	(31.2)
Difficulty accessing computer	18	(28.1)
The large volume of published research	16	(25.0)

Note: Participants were asked to choose as many barriers as they wished from the list; therefore, the numbers do not add up to 100%.

Adapted with permission from McCluskey, A. (2003). Occupational therapists report a low level of knowledge, skill and involvement in evidence-based practice. *Australian Occupational Therapy Journal, 50*(8), 3–12, table 3.

The second survey was conducted with a different group of Australian occupational therapists who were self-motivated to attend a 2-day workshop on evidence-based practice and complete an assignment that required them to critically appraise a topic.

A **critically appraised topic** is a short summary of evidence on a topic of interest, usually focused around a clinical question. It is essentially a less rigorous version of a systematic review, summarizing and appraising the best research on a topic and typically including more than one study. When a single study is appraised as the "best" available evidence, the outcome is referred to as a **critically appraised paper.** Both of these exercises represent methods of collating and disseminating appraisals to colleagues, and they are increasingly being used as university assignments to assess students' skills in searching the literature and appraising research. (You can obtain a free template for such exercises at http://www.otcats.com.)

Prior to completing the workshop and the critically appraised topic assignment, barriers for the Australian sample included lack of time, a large caseload, limited searching skills, and limited

Table 6.2   Perceived Barriers to Adopting Evidence-Based Practice as Reported by Australian Occupational Therapists (*n* = 114)

Top 10 Barriers Reported	Pre-workshop *n* = 114	Post-workshop *n* = 106	Follow-up *n* = 51
	n (%)	*n (%)*	*n (%)*
Lack of time	86 (75%)	100 (94%)	45 (88%)
Large workload/caseload	76 (67%)	79 (75%)	31 (61%)
Limited searching skills	69 (61%)	56 (53%)	12 (24%)
Limited critical appraisal skills	68 (60%)	69 (65%)	21 (41%)
Difficulty accessing journals	51 (45%)	45 (43%)	18 (35%)
The large volume of published research	33 (29%)	34 (32%)	7 (14%)
Lack of evidence to support what occupational therapists do	31 (27%)	34 (32%)	18 (35%)
Professional isolation	24 (21%)	28 (26%)	7 (14%)
Limited resources and funding to support change to evidence-based practice	23 (20%)	13 (12%)	4 (8%)
Difficulty accessing a computer	19 (17%)	15 (14%)	6 (12%)

Note: Participants were asked to choose as many barriers as they wished from the list; therefore, the numbers do not add up to 100%. Adapted with permission from McCluskey, A. (2004). *Increasing the use of research evidence by occupational therapists* [Final report]. Penrith South, Australia: School of Exercise and Health Sciences, University of Western Sydney, Table 4.1, p. 15. Full copy available in PDF format from http://www.otcats.com (under "Project Summary").

critical appraisal skills. These are presented in the first column of Table 6.2.

Immediately after the 2-day workshop, these therapists were surveyed again (see Table 6.2, middle column). More listed lack of time as a barrier than at the pre-workshop time point. By that time, therapists were more aware of the work involved in being an evidence-based practitioner, particularly the work required to complete a critically appraised topic.

Similarly, more respondents identified limited critical appraisal skills as a barrier than at pre-workshop. Although therapists had learned about and practiced critical appraisal during the workshop, they had become even more aware of skills they still had to learn. For example, they knew they would need to learn about different research designs and statistical analyses to be able to make sense of research articles. Searching skills were seen as less of a barrier than before the workshop, with respondents feeling more confident about searching databases on their own.

Table 6.2 (right column) also indicates that, over time and with practice, a greater percentage of therapists improved their skills. Ten months later, fewer therapists felt their searching and appraisal skills were a barrier to being an evidence-based practitioner. Interestingly, the majority of respondents still identified lack of time as the primary barrier. Nonetheless, many of these therapists had completed a critically appraised topic and developed their skills. As discussed later in this chapter, it was the way in which these therapists managed and reprioritized their time that was critical to adopting evidence-based practice.

Managing Barriers to Evidence-Based Practice

The barriers to adopting evidence-based practice are remarkably consistent across groups of occupational therapists, across professions (Humphris, Littlejohns, Victor, O'Halloran, & Peacock, 2000; Ilott et al., 2006; Mctcalfe et al., 2001), and across countries. Lack of time, a large workload, and limited search and appraisal skills are perceived to be the main problems. Yet little has been done to date to address these barriers or problems. Furthermore, some barriers, such as a perceived lack of time, are unlikely to disappear. Therapists are unlikely to be given, or to find, more time in the day. Instead, they need to reprioritize their time.

One of the most important aspects of being an evidence-based practitioner is anticipating and planning for new challenges. Du Toit, Wilkinson, and Adam (2010) initiated an effort in South Africa to change the way in which OT students are acculturated into the process of practicing according to an evidence-based practice perspective. The faculty and students were charged with developing an OT program on a dementia care ward that was informed by an evidence-based practice perspective. Individual student projects ranged from assembling activity profiles for individual residents to developing multisensory environments (Du Toit et al., 2010).

The educators concluded that by formalizing assignment requirements and evaluation criteria according to an evidence-based practice framework, they were able to enhance program quality for the nursing home residents and improve the educational experience for the students (Du Toit et al., 2010). They referred to this process as *action learning, action research* and explained how the students, educators, and nursing home residents all benefitted from the application of research to program development (Du Toit et al., 2010). This project is perhaps one of the most vivid examples of true integration of an evidence-based practice perspective into fieldwork education.

Another integrated research-training effort (McCluskey, 2004) involved recruiting occupational therapists to participate in a workshop with the primary aim of increasing their skills and knowledge for evidence-based practice. They were asked to identify their stage of readiness to change their practice approach and to discuss their attitudes toward evidence-based practice. Next, they found a "buddy" or peer to work with to promote taking action to initiate and maintain evidence-based practice behavior. They also learned about common barriers to implementing evidence-based practice and developed a plan of action to address their personal barriers. By explicitly thinking about the change process, they planned ahead, anticipated problems, and put strategies in place to manage these barriers.

As noted, some of the occupational therapists in the Australian study successfully managed the barriers and began to adopt evidence-based practice (McCluskey, 2004). During the post-workshop period, their use of research evidence was monitored. They were asked how often they conducted a search or engaged in appraisal. Further, their level of knowledge about evidence-based practice and their skills were measured objectively. These data were used to select a purposive sample. After 18 months, 10 of the most proactive, knowledgeable, and skilled therapists were interviewed to ascertain what factors accounted for their success (McCluskey, 2004). The results of this study are presented in Table 6.3 and discussed in the next section.

Table 6.3	Strategies for Adopting Evidence-Based Practice	
Strategies	**Subcategories**
Finding time for evidence-based practice	• Prioritizing activities • Planning ahead
Developing skills and knowledge	• Using evidence • Teaching evidence-based practice to others • Seeking help
Staying focused	• Making a commitment • Being persistent • Being motivated

Adapted with permission from McCluskey, A. (2004). *Increasing the use of research evidence by occupational therapists* [Final report]. Penrith South, Australia: School of Exercise and Health Sciences, University of Western Sydney, Table 5.2, p. 33. Full copy available in PDF format from http://www.otcats.com (under "Project Summary").

Strategies for Adopting Evidence-Based Practice

Given typical workloads, most therapists need encouragement to spend time searching, reading, and appraising research. Working in pairs, small groups, or with a mentor may help to maintain motivation (Conroy, 1997; Morrison & Robertson, 2011). Presenting the findings of a search to other staff members may also act as an incentive.

The occupational therapists interviewed in the Australian study (McCluskey, 2004) were more successful than others at managing the primary barriers, lack of time and lack of skills. Three main strategies, presented in Table 6.3, were used by these therapists to overcome barriers and adopt evidence-based practice:

• Finding time for evidence-based practice
• Developing skills and knowledge
• Staying focused

First, participants proactively made time by prioritizing the use of research ahead of other tasks for part of their week and by planning ahead. Second, they proactively developed their skills and knowledge upon return to work by teaching others what they had learned and getting help when this was needed. Third, they stayed focused and committed to evidence-based practice and found ways to maintain their motivation.

These therapists reported, and quantitative data confirmed, that new skills and knowledge were acquired relatively quickly as a result of attending the workshop. However, finding time to further develop their skills and changing policy and practice in line with new research was much more difficult. Implementation took longer—more than 12 months—and not all of the therapists interviewed had yet reached this stage. Their strategies for success are described in more detail in the following section.

Finding Time for Evidence-Based Practice

The first strategy involved prioritizing activities and planning ahead. Time was the major barrier to engaging in evidence-based practice for all participants, as indicated by one of the therapists:

> I'm sure everyone finds time a big issue. It is very difficult. Clinically, with just seeing the clients here, it's very busy. And then there are always loads of additional projects that we're working on, meetings and supervision. So, definitely it is very difficult to find the time.

To find time, successful therapists had to make research utilization a priority. They set time aside, both at work and after hours, for these activities. Less successful therapists complained about lack of time and did not prioritize work and personal time for evidence-based practice. Some were not persistent in maintaining their commitment, partly because they and their organizations did not place a high value on activities such as searching, reading, and appraisal.

Searching, reading, and critical appraisal were not always considered an essential part of the occupational therapist's work in some organizations. When these activities were less valued than clinical "hands-on" work, therapists felt guilty engaging in them at work, as one therapist noted:

> I found that every month I had to book over that time for clinical appointments to meet the caseload demands . . . so that was interesting in itself, my own attitude . . . rather than protecting that time and doing evidence-based work, I kept putting it off.

In some cases, therapists had to spend time outside work hours engaged in searching and appraisal. Private practitioners prioritized billable work hours ahead of searching and appraisal because these activities affected their income. They typically completed their activities outside of work hours. Several participants felt that evidence-based practice had to become part of their routine work for it to be sustainable, with a certain number of hours being allocated per week or month. As one therapist noted,

> We've got to change our cultures and job descriptions . . . to include the time . . . rather than it being something you can tack on when you've got a free moment.

Supportive policies were already in place for some participants. Successful therapists planned ahead by booking blocks of time in their schedule.

In summary, finding time for evidence-based practice was difficult for all participants. Lack of time was the major barrier to adopting evidence-based practice. Most struggled to prioritize and plan. Successful therapists managed their time by prioritizing research-related work ahead of other tasks at certain times, by scheduling time in advance in their schedules, and by devoting some time outside work hours. Effective time management was a characteristic of therapists in this study who started to use research in practice.

Developing Skills and Knowledge

Successful therapists developed skills and knowledge by proactively using evidence, teaching evidence-based practice to others, and seeking help when faced with difficulties.

Lack of skills and knowledge was a barrier to using evidence for 9 of the 10 participants. They all struggled with critical appraisal and understanding statistics in research articles. However, successful therapists overcame these difficulties by persisting, practicing, and seeking help. The following is one participant's report of the importance of practice and using newly acquired skills:

> Makes sense doesn't it? If you allow yourself time to do something, you'll get better at it. . . . with more practice [my skills and knowledge had increased].

Five of the 10 therapists were actively involved in journal clubs or similar research-focused activities at work, requiring them to regularly use their skills and knowledge.

Therapists who were successful were more likely to be involved in a journal club, partly because of organizational expectations and partly because of routine questioning at their work. These therapists were keen to find and use research to provide best practice to their clients. Although most therapists hoped to change their practice in response to research evidence, none was yet using this routinely in practice.

Teaching evidence-based practice to others helped therapists to consolidate and practice their new skills and develop confidence in their ability to use evidence. The more successful and active therapists were expected to educate others in the organization about searching and appraisal. Other therapists who were less active did not encounter the same expectations and were less likely to feel they had the skills to educate others.

The role of local opinion leader was one that successful therapists adopted upon their return to work. For instance, one therapist commented that she had been nominated to be the "evidence-based champion." These therapists provided in-services at work for other staff and established journal clubs.

The third way in which successful therapists developed their skills and knowledge was by actively seeking help from others, in person or by phone and e-mail. This help sometimes involved a demonstration of searching techniques or seeking expert advice about statistics. Librarians were a common source of help and support. Work could be delegated to a librarian in some organizations.

Therapists found it helpful to have a "buddy," someone who worked with them on their critically appraised topic. A buddy helped sustain motivation, shared the work, and sometimes supplied journal articles; this was underscored by one therapist who observed the following:

> I think the buddy system . . . worked really well, with everyone being motivated . . . to share out the jobs a little bit, bounce ideas off each other and motivate each other. . . . I think that's a great system, and it helps you to network a little bit too.

Successful therapists, with and without buddies, located and used experts such as librarians and the project outreach support person, who conducted support visits, answered e-mail questions, and helped with searching over the telephone.

In summary, successful therapists in this study developed skills and knowledge by using evidence in practice regularly, by teaching evidence-based practice to others, and by seeking help during times of difficulty.

Staying Focused

The more successful occupational therapists in the study used the strategy of staying focused, which involved making a commitment to evidence-based practice, being persistent when barriers were encountered, and being motivated about evidence-based practice.

They changed their work habits and maintained the changes in spite of many distractions. Their activities were not constant; rather, successful therapists had periods of intense activity followed by periods of inactivity. Despite periods of inactivity and barriers encountered along the way, they did not lose sight of their goals. The first step was making a commitment.

Making a commitment meant holding oneself accountable for completing activities, such as searching and appraisal. One factor that cemented commitment was personal or organizational expectations that a critically appraised topic would be completed. Making a commitment also implied that using evidence was valued.

Being persistent involved hard work and continuing in the endeavor, despite failures and obstacles. It was easier for therapists to persist if they were motivated, were committed to using evidence, and had organizational support. Being motivated meant having the desire and drive to finish the critically appraised topic. All had been motivated initially to participate in the study and the workshop; for example, one participant noted: "I did the 2-day workshop and came back very motivated and very keen . . . and did quite a lot of work into my question." However, as time progressed and deadlines advanced, motivation diminished for some of the participants interviewed. Lack of motivation was characterized by long periods of inactivity and limited time spent searching or appraising evidence and, therefore, limited time spent developing or practicing skills.

The more successful therapists interviewed were motivated to continue using evidence because of comments made by work colleagues, friends, and managers and e-mails sent by the outreach support person. They were also motivated by meeting deadlines for the project, such as completing and then presenting their critically appraised topics to others. One therapist stayed focused because her manager showed interest and asked for e-mail updates on her critically appraised topic. In summary, successful therapists stayed focused on becoming an evidence-based practitioner by making a commitment, being persistent, and being motivated.

Factors and Conditions That Help Occupational Therapists Change

In the Australian study, qualitative analysis identified four factors or conditions that helped therapists change and adopt evidence-based practice or, conversely, that limited their progress and

Table 6.4 Conditions That Promoted Change to Evidence-Based Practice

Conditions	Description
Readiness for change	Time ready, intellectually ready, resource ready, or skill ready. Readiness to change work habits and allocate time to activities such as searching and appraisal.
Personal and organizational expectations	Personal expectations of achievement. Use of evidence encouraged and expected by individuals and their organizations. Managers and supervisors were inquiring and interested and expected new knowledge to be applied and shared with others in the organization.
Presence of deadlines	Intrinsic or extrinsic, negotiable or nonnegotiable, urgent or nonurgent. The presence of deadlines helped initiate and stimulate further activity levels and provided direction and focus for participants.
Availability of support	Encouragement, physical resources (Internet, journals, computer databases), financial assistance, and work concessions. Support from managers, organizations, buddies, and peers.

Adapted with permission from McCluskey, A. (2004). *Increasing the use of research evidence by occupational therapists* [Final report]. Penrith South, Australia: School of Exercise and Health Sciences, University of Western Sydney, Table 5.3, p. 37. Full copy available in PDF format from http://www.otcats.com (under "Project Summary").

presented additional barriers. These four factors or conditions (Table 6.4) are as follows:

- A personal readiness for change
- Personal and organizational expectations that they would apply the skills learned and teach others
- Self-determined deadlines that pushed them along
- Support within the organization, such as computers and journals, as well as encouragement from colleagues and managers

If these conditions were present and positive, participants were more likely to progress. If these conditions were absent or negative, they acted as additional barriers to change, and progress was slower.

Summary

This chapter identifies barriers that limit the use of research by occupational therapists and interfere with the change from "experience-based" practice to "evidence-based" practice. The chapter focuses on factors that allow therapists to overcome some of these barriers. The research presented found that occupational therapists who successfully engaged in evidence-based practice integrated it into their daily work requirements (Du Toit et al., 2010; McCluskey, 2004). They reprioritized their time, proactively developed their skills and knowledge, and stayed focused on answering one or more clinical questions (McCluskey, 2004). They were in control of the change process. They stopped talking about barriers, and instead they changed how they worked. They acknowledged that they

were intellectually ready to change work habits, acquire new skills and knowledge, and prioritize their time differently.

In addition to change on an individual level, the culture of OT practice needs to fully incorporate evidence-based practice into the daily work of most practitioners. Evidence-based practice needs to be mentioned in business plans, annual reports, orientation program documentation, and performance appraisals (McCluskey & Cusick, 2002). It needs to be visible, and it should be considered an important criterion for accreditation of health-care organizations. In the end, organizational culture and the ways in which attitudes and values are espoused by others, particularly managers, appear to enhance or inhibit the adoption of evidence-based practice.

Acknowledgment

Sally Home and Lauren Thompson contributed to qualitative data collection and analysis of the original Australian study as part of their occupational therapy undergraduate honors project in 2003 at the University of Western Sydney, Australia. Categories (strategies and conditions) have been further developed and refined for this chapter.

Review Questions

1. What are four potential explanations for the lack of advancement of evidence-based practice from an international perspective?
2. According to research, what are three primary barriers to implementing evidence-based practice for students and new graduates?

3. According to research, what are three primary barriers to implementing evidence-based practice for experienced practitioners?
4. How would you manage barriers to evidence-based practice as the manager of a large OT practice?

REFERENCES

College of Occupational Therapists. (2003). *Professional standards for occupational therapy practice.* London, England: Author.

College of Occupational Therapists. (2005). *College of Occupational Therapists: Code of ethics and professional conduct.* London, England: Author.

Conroy, M. (1997). "Why are you doing that?" A project to look for evidence of efficacy within occupational therapy. *British Journal of Occupational Therapy, 60,* 487–490.

Coster, W. (2005). The Foundation international conference on evidence-based practice: A collaborative effort of the American Occupational Therapy Association, the American Occupational Therapy Foundation, and the Agency of Healthcare Research and Quality. *American Journal of Occupational Therapy, 59*(3), 356–358.

Coster, W., Gillette, N., Law, M., Lieberman, D., & Scheer, J. (2004). *AHRQ grant final progress report.* Retrieved from http://www.aotf.org/pdf/ahrq_grant.pdf

Dopp, C. M. E., Steultjens, E. M. J., & Radel, J. (2012). A survey of evidence-based practise among Dutch occupational therapists. *Occupational Therapy International, 19*(1), 17–27.

Du Toit, S. H. J., Wilkinson, A. C., & Adam, K. (2010). Role of research in occupational therapy clinical practice: Applying action learning and action research in pursuit of evidence-based practice. *Australian Occupational Therapy Journal, 57,* 318–330.

Dubouloz, C., Egan, M., Vallerand, J., & von Zweck, C. (1999). Occupational therapists' perceptions of evidence-based practice. *American Journal of Occupational Therapy, 53,* 445–453.

Garner, P., Meremikwu, M., Volmink, J., Xu, Q., & Smith, H. (2004). Putting evidence into practice: How middle and low income countries "get it together." *British Medical Journal, 329,* 1036–1039. Retrieved from http://bmj.bmjjournals.com

Gilman, I. P. (2011). Evidence-based information-seeking behaviors of occupational therapists: A survey of recent graduates. *Journal of the Medical Library Association, 99,* 307–310.

Health Professions Council. (2003). *Standards of proficiency: Occupational therapists.* London, England: Author.

Hocking, C., & Ness, N. E. (2002). *Revised minimum standards for the education of occupational therapists.* Perth, Australia: World Federation of Occupational Therapists.

Humphris, D., Littlejohns, P., Victor, C., O'Halloran, P., & Peacock, J. (2000). Implementing evidence-based practice: Factors that influence the use of research evidence by occupational therapists. *British Journal of Occupational Therapy, 63,* 516–522.

Ilott, I., Taylor, M. C., & Bolanos, C. (2006). Evidence-based occupational therapy: It's time to take a global approach. *British Journal of Occupational Therapy, 69,* 38–41.

McCluskey, A. (2003). Occupational therapists report a low level of knowledge, skill and involvement in evidence-based practice. *Australian Occupational Therapy Journal, 50*(1), 3–12.

McCluskey, A. (2004). *Increasing the use of research evidence by occupational therapists* [Final report]. Penrith South, Australia: School of Exercise and Health Sciences, University of Western Sydney. Retrieved from http://www.otcats.com

McCluskey, A., & Cusick, A. (2002). Strategies for introducing evidence-based practice and changing clinician behaviour: A manager's toolbox. *Australian Occupational Therapy Journal, 49,* 63–70.

McKenna, K., Bennett, S., Hoffmann, T., McCluskey, A., Strong, J., & Tooth, L. (2004). OTseeker: Facilitating evidence-based practice in occupational therapy. *Australian Occupational Therapy Journal, 51*(2), 102–105.

Metcalfe, C., Lewin, R., Wisher, S., Perry, S., Bannigan, K., & Moffett, J. (2001). Barriers to implementing the evidence base in four NHS therapies. *Physiotherapy, 87,* 433–441.

Morrison, T., & Robertson, L. (2011). The influences on new graduates' ability to implement evidence-based practice: A review of the literature. *New Zealand Journal of Occupational Therapy, 58*(2), 37–40.

Pollock, A. S., Legg, L., Langhorne, P., & Sellars, C. (2000). Barriers to achieving evidence-based stroke rehabilitation. *Clinical Rehabilitation, 14,* 611–617.

Pollock, N., & Rochon, S. (2002). Becoming an evidence-based practitioner. In M. Law (Ed.), *Evidence-based rehabilitation: A guide to practice* (pp. 31–46). Thorofare, NJ: Slack.

Redmond, A. (1997). Evidence-based medicine: A blueprint for effective practice or the emperor's new clothes? *Podiatry Management, 11,* 123–126.

Sackett, D. L., Straus, S. E., Richardson, W. S., Rosenberg, W., & Haynes, R. B. (2000). *Evidence-based medicine: How to practice and teach EBP* (2nd ed.). Edinburgh, Scotland: Churchill Livingstone.

Stronge, M., & Cahill, M. (2012). Self-reported knowledge, attitudes, and behaviour towards evidence-based practice of occupational therapy students in Ireland. *Occupational Therapy International, 19,* 7–16.

Stube, J. E., & Jedlicka, J. S. (2007). The acquisition and integration of evidence-based practice concepts by occupational therapy students. *American Journal of Occupational Therapy, 61*(1), 53–61.

Taylor, M. C. (2000). *Evidence-based practice for occupational therapists.* Oxford, England: Blackwell Science.

Van Bruggen, H., Renton, L., Ferreira, M. A., le Granse, M., & Morel. M-C. (2000). Occupational therapy education in Europe: An exploration. Amsterdam: European Network of Occupational Therapy in Higher Education.

von Zweck, C. (1999). The promotion of evidence-based occupational therapy practice in Canada. *Canadian Journal of Occupational Therapy, 66,* 208–213.

CHAPTER 7

Professional Responsibility and Roles in Research

Anne Cusick • Gary Kielhofner • Renée R. Taylor

Learning Outcomes

- List the responsibilities of occupational therapy professionals as they pertain to research.
- Describe different roles that occupational therapy professionals may assume when engaging with research.
- Identify reasons why an occupational therapist might decide to become involved with research.
- State examples of ways in which an occupational therapy professional can enter the field of research.
- List the knowledge and skills that are required to participate in research.

Introduction

This chapter explores professional responsibility and roles in conducting and consuming research. It examines ways in which occupational therapists might view research and make choices about research roles in professional life, describes knowledge and skills central to various research roles, and examines strategies that can be used to develop them.

The occupational therapy (OT) student and mentor in the following Case Example are at different stages in terms of their orientation toward OT research. Both are confronted with choices about whether and how to support, use, and produce research to enhance OT practice. Both have the opportunity to network with other professionals to advise them about resources and pathways for learning. These choices and judgments have an impact on their professional and personal lives. Moreover, their decisions about creating and consuming research evidence affect the profession as a whole.

Responsibility, Uncertainty, and Research

Being a professional brings with it responsibilities, and ethical practice is one of them. Evidence from research can be used to inform practice decisions, guide therapeutic processes, and provide tools for interpreting outcomes of service (Cusick, 2001c). When therapists use research evidence in their clinical decisions, they can better know what to do, with whom, when, why, and how best to do it. They can also be more accountable, because they are aware of potential and actual outcomes of their service (Cusick, 2001d). Occupational therapists, thus, have an **ethical responsibility** to be aware of research and to engage with it because staying up to date with practice developments and innovations that are supported by careful and systematic research ensures that clients receive the appropriate level of care.

Occupational therapists also have a **professional responsibility** to use research to help enhance the quality of their clinical decisions. If problems addressed by therapists in practice were straightforward, and if issues and answers were certain, solutions could be provided by simply following protocols. There would be no need for training, responsibility, discretion, expertise, and professional autonomy. Professionals operate within uncertainty in the many complex and high-impact decisions they make every day; therefore, they must find ways to negotiate the uncertainty that comes with practice.

In the past, professional authority or expertise was considered sufficient (Basmajian, 1975). However, in the 21st century, decision-making in professional practice needs to be backed by rigorous and transparent evidence. In recognition of this demand for evidence, OT research productivity has steadily increased (Majnemer et al., 2001; Paul, Liu, & Ottenbacher, 2002).

CASE EXAMPLE

Dr. Starboard, a professor of occupational therapy at a local university, smiles to the audience as she accepts a lifetime achievement award for her contributions to OT practice and research (Fig. 7.1). Over a 40-year career, her achievements include five published books and more than 100 peer-reviewed journal articles funded by large competitive grants.

Hannah, a student in an entry-level OT program, watches Dr. Starboard with simultaneous feelings of admiration and curiosity. She had read one of Dr. Starboard's textbooks during her first semester that year and had deep respect for her ideas about OT practice. About to enter the second year of her program, Hannah recently completed final examinations and is feeling somewhat exhausted and overwhelmed. She wonders how Dr. Starboard got started in research and accomplished all that she did as an OT professional. Moreover, she wonders if Dr. Starboard ever felt equally apprehensive about her career. At the reception that follows the award ceremony, Hannah introduces herself to Dr. Starboard, congratulates her on her award, and proceeds to ask her a few of these questions.

To Hannah's relief, Dr. Starboard admits that she had similar feelings of apprehension as an entry-level student. She describes a career pathway characterized by a lot of self-discipline, networking, and the ability to recognize and seize certain opportunities along the way. She recalls the beginning of her career, when every Wednesday she scrambled across town from her part-time clinical job to volunteer in a colleague's research laboratory and network with other OT faculty members doing research there. She recalls spending hours going through piles of data and background articles, critically reviewing research papers, and preparing a presentation for therapist peers in which practice changes were recommended. She also recalls that her peers could not figure out why she was dedicating all of her free time to these activities when she could be working full-time as an OT practitioner, with better hours and a better salary.

However, in return for all of her work, Dr. Starboard recalls the momentous event of seeing her name appear as fifth author on her first journal article, which was based on that pivotal conference presentation she made with her mentor. At that point, Dr. Starboard decided that she wanted to pursue a research career in occupational therapy, so she enrolled as a full-time PhD student under the supervision of her mentor.

The university in which she enrolled provided a full tuition waiver to attend classes and some very modest living expenses in return for working in her mentor's laboratory as a research assistant for 20 hours per week. Dr. Starboard recalls being anxious about giving up her part-time clinical job at first, but soon her anxiety was replaced by feelings of accomplishment as she continued to gain knowledge, skill, and independence as a PhD program graduate, postdoctoral research professional, and, ultimately, a university professor.

Hannah thanked Dr. Starboard for all of her advice and told her of her deep admiration and respect. Dr. Starboard then gave Hannah her card and offered to have Hannah visit her laboratory if she had an interest in autism. Hannah still did not know the level at which she would be motivated and able to engage in a research career. What she did know was that the brief interaction with Dr. Starboard had gone so well and had made such an impact on Hannah that she went online that evening to begin to look at OTD and PhD programs that she might enter following completion of her entry-level degree, including the one that Dr. Starboard directed.

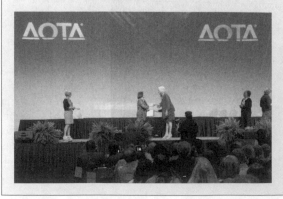

Figure 7.1 A female professor receiving an award on a stage.

Developments in evidence-based practice have provided further opportunities for scientific knowledge to be integrated with expert opinion in forming professional judgments. When used intelligently, evidence-based approaches systematically use a variety of sources of information, including researcher, therapist, and client opinion, to make meaningful and relevant decisions (Bury & Mead, 1998; Dawes et al., 1999; Taylor, 2000). This approach means therapists can responsibly exercise professional discretion in practice within the known limits of their information base.

Therapists need to be discerning about practice priorities, and research information can help in this endeavor. When resources are scarce, difficult decisions must be made about how best to use them. A research orientation to practice helps therapists deal with the interprofessional competition, budget cuts, insurance denials, and other challenges that can emanate from limited resources. Further, when professionals have a research orientation, they can respond to challenges about one's knowledge or service values as opportunities to rationally examine evidence rather than interpreting criticism as a personal affront.

Research Roles

Individual therapists can engage with research in a variety of ways: They can perform original research, collaborate in studies, and engage in reading and critiquing research with peers. Therapists can take on one or more of the following roles (summarized in Table 7.1):

- Research producers
- Research collaborators
- Research consumers
- Research advocates

Each of these research roles makes valuable contributions to the profession. Without research producers, there is no original knowledge base. Without collaborators, clinical studies cannot be implemented. Without supporters, resources needed for research or research dissemination and uptake are not available. Without therapists to advocate for research and guide research questions and priorities, research will not be relevant. Without therapists to use or consume research in their service for the public, the quality of practice suffers. All therapists can help support inquiry based practice in some way. Not everyone will conduct research;

Table 7.1   Research Roles and Related Training, Education, Expertise, and Activities

Role	Typical Education/ Training	Activities
Research producers	Doctorate Postdoctoral training	• Identify original research questions and design methods for answering them. • Secure funding for research. • Supervise/oversee the implementation of research. • Work with interdisciplinary collaborators, statistical consultants, and others with specific research expertise. • Prepare research reports for presentation or publication.
Research collaborators	Professional training Specialized training related to study involvement	• Serve as subjects/participants. • Refer and screen potential subjects. • Collect data. • Implement services that are being tested. • Provide clinical advice/expertise. • Help negotiate the politics and administrative processes. • Help identify a research question and interpret results.
Research consumers	Professional training Training in critical appraisal skills	• Read research and use findings to guide practice. • Identify practice knowledge gaps. • Complete and present/publish critical appraisals.
Research advocates	Appreciation of the value of research that can accrue from training and/or experience	• Serve in professional associations that fund/support research. • Lobby policymakers and legislators. • Ask employers for resources. • Donate money and encourage/support colleagues involved in research. • Comment on research priorities or goals.

however, everyone can contribute to occupational therapy becoming an evidence-based profession.

The following is a detailed description of each of these important research roles.

Research Producers

Research producers can be academics, practitioner researchers, and students who actively engage in research in university, clinical, and community settings. Research producers develop high levels of research expertise. They design and lead investigations, develop teams of dedicated staff, and bring together research resources to produce new knowledge. Research producers generate published papers, conference presentations, books, and multimedia or creative works. These resource products are widely disseminated and critically reviewed prior to and after release.

Some research producers choose this role early in their careers, whereas others take a different route. Occupational therapists who select research-producer roles must commit themselves to the highest level of precision and rigor. For this, they must complete specialized research training at the doctoral and, ideally, at the postdoctoral level (Paul, 2001). Doctoral training emphasizes advanced knowledge and skills in both theoretical and methodological domains. It culminates in the production of a dissertation that requires conception, implementation, and documentation of a major study or study series.

Dissertation research is completed under the supervision of a committee of seasoned researchers who guide doctoral candidates in their research and ultimately judge whether or not the research is sufficiently rigorous and important. Often, the doctoral dissertation process culminates with a "defense," in which the doctoral candidate presents his or her work, answers critical questions, and responds to probing comments about the research from supervisory committees and sometimes a public audience. The defense reflects the very public nature of the research enterprise and serves as a way to evaluate the individual's readiness to engage in the public process of science.

Although the doctoral degree is increasingly common in occupational therapy, postdoctoral training is still growing as an expectation. In mature research fields, postdoctoral training is required before one enters into a fully independent research role. Postdoctoral trainees work alongside accomplished researchers and/or within a research team/laboratory. They are advanced "apprentices" who learn more sophisticated analytical techniques and develop specific expertise in an area of study, a theoretical domain, or a specialized kind of inquiry. They also typically gain experience in grant writing and publication during postdoctoral training.

Research Collaborators

A **research collaborator** is an individual who works in a supportive role to contribute to the production of research. Collaboration can occur in a range of ways, and although a working knowledge of research is always required, not all collaboration needs to be at the level of a research producer. Examples of collaborative activities that do not involve leading research include:

- Being subjects/participants in a study by answering surveys or participating in focus groups
- Referring and screening clients for studies
- Collecting data for an investigation
- Implementing services that are being tested in an intervention study
- Serving on the advisory board of a funded research grant
- Helping investigators negotiate the politics and administrative processes of research in a clinical site
- Identifying a research question and helping interpret the results of a study of practice

Collaboration is a common research role for therapists in clinical settings. Without therapists who are willing to train for study requirements, implement protocols, volunteer time, and maintain quality records, many clinical studies could not be completed. Research collaboration is critical for the field.

Effective collaboration requires careful negotiation, planning, good communication, and relationships of trust. Among other elements, expectations relating to requirements, authorship, and intellectual property need to be negotiated and clearly articulated. Depending on the intellectual contribution made to the design, interpretation, and writing of the study, collaborators may or may not be considered "co-investigators" or "co-authors."

The preparation and expertise required for research collaboration vary widely depending on the nature of the research endeavor. In many cases, the professional education and experience of occupational therapists is all that is needed to be a valuable collaborator. In other cases, therapists may bring skills they learned in a thesis project or research courses taken as part of professional or post-professional education. Sometimes therapists will receive specialized training that enables them to implement an intervention being studied or collect data in a reliable and valid manner. Often this training is provided in preparation for or as part of therapists' involvement in a particular study. Thus, therapists who collaborate learn important skills and knowledge through the research process itself.

Research Consumers

A **research consumer** is an individual who utilizes research to solve problems and/or inform decisions. All therapists should use research to inform their practice.

The preparation for the research consumer role varies. Most professional programs in occupational therapy provide at least the basic knowledge required to intelligently read a research report. Critical appraisal (such as that discussed in Chapter 4) requires more advanced skills. These include, but are not limited to, evaluating the rigor of the research design, ascertaining procedures for data collection, and being able to interpret basic statistics that are used in systematic reviews, for example. Critical appraisal skills are taught in many OT programs and are often available through continuing education. Although all therapists are expected to consume, use, and apply research evidence to inform practice, some will take their role as critical consumers one step further. They will publicize knowledge gaps in practice and identify the information they find that fills those gaps via conference papers, letters to editors, discussion papers, and critically appraised topics. This form of critical consumerism is important both because it stimulates debate and further investigation and because it contributes knowledge to others. The proliferation of OT resources such as critically appraised topics in journals, on Internet sites, and on discussion boards are examples of the importance of this type of research-consumer role and contribution.

Research Advocates

Some therapists support research by identifying knowledge gaps, generating relevant questions, identifying research priorities, and lobbying professional leaders to "do something" to help therapists working on practice problems. They work as **research advocates** by providing the momentum and support for research, even though they do not produce it themselves. The following are some examples of research advocacy:

- Being involved in a local or national professional association that funds or otherwise supports research
- Lobbying policymakers/legislators to improve access to research databases, funds, and professional development for occupational therapists

- Asking employers to provide Internet access to therapists at work so they can consult easily accessible databases for "just-in-time" information
- Donating money to various causes and projects or to organizations that fund OT research
- Encouraging colleagues involved in research through emotional support, praise, and recognition to create research-supportive cultures
- Responding to agency invitations to comment on research priorities or goals

Individuals who advocate for research often have no specialized training or background in research. Their primary qualification is that they appreciate the importance of research to the vitality of the profession.

Deciding to Become Involved in Research

Although individual research role development is important, no one can be successful in a research role when functioning only as an individual. Research roles emerge only in relation to others; that is, research involvement of any form is an intensely social process. Whether serving as a leader or member of a research team, joining a journal club, serving on an editorial board, having one's grant reviewed by a panel, or presenting a paper at a conference, individuals involved in research are always engaged with others. Even the process of publishing a research paper, which can take weeks of private writing time, ends up in a highly public process.

At one time, research was viewed as a solo enterprise; the ideal of the independent investigator was viewed as the epitome of science. Today, however, the best research is created by teams that include diverse members who bring their different expertise and perspectives to the research enterprise. Participatory methods (described in Chapter 30) typically bring researchers together with practitioners, consumers, and community members, all of whom function as integral partners in the research process. Research is also becoming increasingly interdisciplinary in nature. This means that occupational therapists must be prepared to extend their research involvement to those beyond the profession.

Most investigation and discussion of research role development has occurred in relation to research producers, but the processes of role development can be equally applied to other research roles. It starts with the particular stance a therapist takes toward research. That stance is predisposed by personal biography and context (Cusick, 2000, 2001a, 2001b).

An occupational therapist's research standpoint may be:

- Sparked by an event such as meeting someone or experiencing a difficult situation (e.g., deciding to become more involved in research because of funding cuts or insurance denials that referenced a lack of evidence about occupational therapy)
- Incidental to daily obligations (e.g., when charged to develop and justify new services, a therapist becomes engaged with evidence about service outcomes)
- Inspired by meeting an investigator (e.g., at a conference or university)
- Fueled by personal desires (e.g., enriching one's work experience, becoming more credible and able to justify decisions with high-quality information, or achieving the autonomy and flexibility that research roles can bring with them)
- Based on a drive to achieve enhanced status and participate in higher-status groups where one can have an influence on important issues in occupational therapy (e.g., gaining national research grants that provide resources to study therapy, influencing policy decisions, developing advanced educational opportunities for occupational therapists, and creating new services for an underserved population)
- Based on a sense of obligation to contribute to research as part of professional identity
- Fueled by a sense of generosity and gratitude toward the profession coupled with a desire to "give something back"
- As a strategic response to opportunities for professional advancement, or for the advancement of one's interests, or for those of one's organization

Most therapists in research-related roles will identify that a combination of these factors sparked their interest and then influenced their own research role taking.

Where to Begin: Ways to Get Involved in Research

A research standpoint or outlook is only the beginning. Therapists need to then identify, reflect on, and construct research roles that suit them and their life/work context. Beginning one's own research role requires:

- Exposure to role models and role alternatives
- Opportunities to reflect on and try out role behaviors
- Opportunities to obtain feedback
- Opportunities to evaluate new standpoints and experiences

Exposure provides opportunities to see what particular research roles look like. It can happen through encounters in OT education programs, at conferences, on the job, and socially. Strategies for enhancing one's firsthand role exposure include:

- Attending colloquia by visiting speakers
- Joining journal clubs
- Attending professional association meetings
- Seeking supervision or fieldwork placements where research is taking place
- Volunteering to participate in a research project
- Being employed as a research assistant

One can also gain exposure through written profiles, biographies, seminars, and other media that describe not only the technical aspects of research roles, but also the social dimensions and personal processes. This type of information is useful to consider the kinds of attributes required for various research roles and for learning how people balance home and work responsibilities and negotiate the obligations, demands, and politics of research involvement. It is also important to learn about the impact one can have through research involvement and the personal satisfaction that can accrue from it.

Taking on a research role is an important and conscious decision, so opportunities to figuratively "try on" research roles are useful. Therapists need to be able to not only think about a particular research role "out there," but also envision themselves in relation to the role. Conversations with trusted mentors, supervisors, managers, friends, and colleagues permit thinking out loud and provide different views of what is required for various roles. Such conversations can offer realistic feedback on one's capacity, encourage different scenario planning, identify practical constraints and implications of particular role choices, and provide a "reality check."

Knowledge and Skills Required to Participate in Research

Once particular research roles are selected, occupational therapists need opportunities to try out different research role behaviors and to acquire knowledge and technical skills for their preferred roles. Depending on the role, technical knowledge and skills may range from reading research in an informed way, to developing research questions and preparing designs and protocols, to collecting and analyzing data, to deciding how to apply published findings to practice.

Depending on the role one chooses, the necessary skills may be readily learned or may take years of training. For example, many of the technical research skills required for research-consumer roles such as evidence-based practice are taught in professional entry-level courses or continuing education. On the other hand, learning to be a research producer requires earning a doctoral degree and gaining postdoctoral training and/or experience. The fundamental skills required to become a research producer include, but are not limited to, those presented in Box 7.1.

Research-specific and general inquiry skills are facilitated through training opportunities that provide realistic and respectful feedback and couple clear expectations for performance with high degrees of autonomy. This type of training and feedback often begins with the student role, wherein students learn whether or not their literature review, critically appraised topic, or research methods assignment met standards and expectations. It will assuredly continue for the developing researcher when submitting conference papers, journal articles, grants, or requests for release time to be involved in research. Over time, these repeated experiences are opportunities for learning, role feedback, and, if positive, research role validation.

Therapists therefore don't just "do" research; they "become" research producers, consumers, advocates, or collaborators through a reflective and social process (Cusick, 2001a, 2001b; Young, 2004). They think about desired roles, select and practice research role behaviors, obtain feedback on their relative role attainment, and consider whether or not the role feels worthwhile. This self-reflective process involves a continual internal dialogue with oneself about the emerging and changing research role. That dialogue is more meaningful when conversations with trusted friends, mentors, and colleagues provide opportunities to "think out loud" and, in doing so, further refine one's research standpoint, role-taking choices, and views about the worth of the research enterprise in one's life.

Resistance to Research

As covered in detail in Chapter 6, there are individuals in the field who are not particularly

---

BOX 7.1   Skills Required to Produce Independent Research

- Social networking skills
- Willingness to work collaboratively as a member of a research team
- Literature searching skills
- Ability to critically review the literature and identify contradictions or gaps in knowledge
- Ability to identify research topics of professional significance or impact
- Ability to complete an application for human subjects approval
- Ability to generate research questions and/or formulate hypotheses
- Knowledge of how to design a research study to address those questions or hypotheses
- Ability to match a research design to the practicalities of a sample and a setting
- Ability to identify inclusion and exclusion criteria for a sample
- Ability to manage and supervise others working on your team
- Ability to collect data
- Knowledge of measures or other technologies, equipment, or instruments utilized in the research

- Knowledge of statistical or other analytical methods
- Ability to interpret findings from the statistical (or other) analyses
- Ability to synthesize findings in light of the overall study questions/hypotheses and in the context of the literature
- Understanding of the limitations of one's study and of the conclusions that can be drawn from study findings
- Public speaking and writing skills
- Ability to accept responsibility and maximize one's own autonomy
- Ability to clearly articulate the values that underpin the work
- Ability to engage in forward planning by setting priorities, deadlines, and goals
- Ability to integrate and carefully schedule various activities
- Understanding of the system in which one works and manages colleagues, gatekeepers, and people of influence to get resources

supportive of research. There may be a number of reasons to explain this position, including lack of exposure to research, concerns about lack of time for research, and/or anxiety about the perceived or actual lack of skills or knowledge to conduct research. Such individuals may have clinical skills and knowledge that are based on experience, but no way to ensure that their knowledge and skills are not limited or based on outdated information. They may also be primarily guided by personal frames of reference and worldviews outside professional approaches (Cusick, 2001a). They may be research resistant because they actively devalue research or, by default, because they have chosen to do nothing. Research resistance is not consistent with professional responsibility.

Individuals who are resistant to research may be concerned that their experience and expertise are being devalued by the increasing attention being given to research information. However, scientific knowledge is viewed as complementary to knowledge gained through experience, and the latter is valued in the context of evidence-based practice (Richardson, 2001; Titchen & Ersser, 2001). Ironically, individuals who resist using research information place themselves at risk of having their hard-earned expertise dismissed by interdisciplinary colleagues, administrators, and others.

Sometimes people feel intimidated by research because their own professional training did not include research or treated it in a cursory manner. However, even those who have limited research training or understanding have choices. For example:

- One may choose to use research-based clinical guidelines that are presented in practical, user-friendly ways.
- One may adopt service recommendations of managers or supervisors who use research information.
- One may be open to new ideas that students or colleagues bring that might be founded in research and may ask questions to further understanding.

Other ways of addressing and managing barriers to evidence-based research on a wide scale and at the individual level are addressed in Chapter 6.

Summary

This chapter emphasizes the fact that research involvement is a professional responsibility. Occupational therapists make conscious choices about research roles, which can include those of

advocate, consumer, collaborator, or producer of research. Strategies of research role development are also discussed.

Research roles and responsibilities are key features of professional life. In addition to the broad endeavor of contributing to the development of the profession, research underpins ethical practice, provides ways to enhance practice quality, and keeps therapists accountable. Research involvement is part of a community of effort in which people collaborate to advocate for, create, critique, and make use of research evidence for the betterment of the profession and the people we service in practice. The Case Example describes Dr. Starboard, who had a particular approach to her practice and a demonstrable impact on the profession. The entry-level student, Hannah, was poised to develop her own research standpoint and story concerning her future research role. What will your story be?

Review Questions

1. What is a primary responsibility of an OT professional as it pertains to research?
2. What are the possible roles that OT professionals can play with respect to research?
3. Why might a person decide to become involved with research?
4. How can you begin establishing a role as a researcher?
5. What are five skills necessary to produce independent research?
6. What is one negative consequence of not engaging in or supporting OT research?

REFERENCES

Basmajian, J. V. (1975). Research or retrench: The rehabilitation professions challenged. *Physical Therapy, 55,* 607–610.

Bury, T., & Mead, J. (Eds.). (1998). *Evidence-based health care: A practical guide for therapists.* Oxford, England: Butterworth-Heinemann.

Cusick, A. (2000). Practitioner-researchers in occupational therapy. *Australian Occupational Therapy Journal, 47,* 11–27.

Cusick, A. (2001a). Personal frames of reference in professional practice. In J. Higgs & A. Titchen (Eds.), *Practice knowledge and expertise in the health professions* (pp. 91–95). Oxford, England: Butterworth-Heineman.

Cusick, A. (2001b). The experience of practitioner-researchers in occupational therapy. *American Journal of Occupational Therapy, 55,* 9–18.

Cusick, A. (2001c). The research sensitive practitioner. In J. Higgs & A. Titchen (Eds.), *Professional practice in health, education and the creative arts* (pp. 125–135). Oxford, England: Blackwell Science.

Cusick, A. (2001d). 2001 Sylvia Docker Lecture: OZ OT EBP 21C: Australian occupational therapy, evidence-based practice and the 21st century. *Australian Occupational Therapy Journal, 48,* 102–117.

Dawes, M., Davies, P., Gray., A., Mant, K., Seers, K., & Snowball, R. (1999). *Evidence-based practice: A primer for health care professionals.* Edinburgh, Scotland: Churchill Livingstone.

Majnemer, A., Desrosiers, J., Gauthier, J., Dutil, E., Robichaud, L., Rousseau, J., & Herbert, L. (2001). Involvement of occupational therapy departments in research: A provincial survey. *Canadian Journal of Occupational Therapy, 68,* 272–279.

Paul, S. (2001). Postdoctoral training for new doctoral graduates: Taking a step beyond a doctorate. *American Journal of Occupational Therapy, 55,* 227–229.

Paul, S., Liu, Y., & Ottenbacher, K. J. (2002). Research productivity among occupational therapy faculty members in the United States. *American Journal of Occupational Therapy, 56,* 331–334.

Richardson, B. (2001). Professionalisation and professional craft knowledge. In J. Higgs & A. Titchen (Eds.), *Practice knowledge and expertise in the health professions* (pp. 42–47). Oxford. England: Butterworth-Heineman.

Taylor, M. C. (2000). *Evidence-based practice for occupational therapists.* Oxford, England: Blackwell Science.

Titchen, A., & Ersser, S. J. (2001). The nature of professional craft knowledge. In J. Higgs & A. Titchen (Eds.), *Practice knowledge and expertise in the health professions* (pp. 35–41). Oxford, England: Butterworth-Hcineman.

Young, A. F. (2004). Becoming a practitioner-researcher: A personal journey. *British Journal of Occupational Therapy, 67,* 369–371.

CHAPTER 8

The Role of Theory in Occupational Therapy

Renée R. Taylor

Learning Outcomes

- Explicate the components of a theory.
- Understand the difference between theoretical concepts and theoretical application.
- Explain the advantages of grounding one's research within a theory as they relate to research and in terms of evidence-based practice.
- Delineate the rationale for selecting assessments that correspond with a theory.
- Generate examples of theory-based research in occupational therapy.

Introduction

Whether clearly articulated or unspoken, any well-conceived and successful intervention in practice is typically grounded in a theory. A **theory** is a network of explanations; it provides concepts that label and describe phenomena and postulates that specify relationships between concepts (Kielhofner, 2008). **Concepts** describe, define, and provide a specific way of seeing and thinking about some entity, quality, or process. For example, the concept of "strength" refers to a characteristic of muscles (i.e., their ability to produce tension for maintaining postural control and for moving body parts). Exercise is a concept that refers to a process (i.e., the use of muscles to produce force against resistance).

Postulates posit relationships between concepts, asserting how the characteristics or processes to which concepts refer are organized or put together. An example of such a postulate is: Exercise increases the ability of muscles to produce force. When several concepts and postulates are linked together, they constitute a whole network of explanations that make up a given theory (Fig. 8.1).

In occupational therapy, a theory is a set of concepts and postulates that explain how an occupation is performed, an occupational problem, or a particular dynamic or interaction occurring between client and therapist during the course of therapy (Kielhofner, 2008). Research that is grounded in theory seeks to understand and measure a therapist's actions and to show how a theoretical idea is borne out through that action. This chapter defines and discusses the role of theory in research, examining how an occupational therapist might develop a research idea that is informed by theory. It also provides examples of how occupational therapists have applied theoretical concepts when planning and executing research studies.

The following Case Example demonstrates the role of theory in responding to an important question emerging out of occupational therapy practice. This chapter considers the reasons why it is important to link theory to research questions and provides guidance on and examples of how to do so.

The Role of Theory in Occupational Therapy

When an occupational therapist selects a therapeutic activity that emphasizes a client's strengths, rather than revealing the client's areas of weakness, the selection process is driven by a theoretical idea about what is best for that client at that moment. One theoretical idea that is consistent with a strengths-based choice is the concept of **volition,** which is an aspect of a larger theory known as the Model of Human Occupation (MOHO) (Kielhofner, 2009). According to Kielhofner (2009), volition drives occupational performance and participation and is comprised of three elements: the client's interests (the sense of preference toward an occupation), personal causation (the sense of ability to perform an occupation), and values (the sense of personal and societal importance of the occupation). Occupational therapists

CASE EXAMPLE

Kris works as an occupational therapy practitioner in a large outpatient clinic in a rural hospital in Purcell, Oklahoma. She was trained to use the Person-Environment-Occupation-Performance (PEOP) model (Christiansen & Baum, 2005; Christiansen, Baum, & Bass, 2011) as a theoretical frame of reference for practice and research. The PEOP model describes human performance and participation as based on four interactive concepts: person, environment, occupation, and performance. The concept of person refers to a client's intrinsic qualities that are psychological, cognitive, physiological, spiritual, and neurobehavioral in nature. The concept of environment refers to extrinsic variables, such as the client's social support system, built environment and technology, economic systems, and culture. The concept of occupation refers to valued roles, tasks, and activities that are of personal significance. And the concept of performance refers to the ability to perform those activities, tasks, and roles in a holistic sense. According to the PEOP model, these concepts work synchronously to promote or inhibit occupational engagement (Christiansen & Baum, 2005; Christiansen et al., 2011).

Kris is intrigued by the application of the PEOP model to clients participating in hand therapy. Because hand injuries tend to be painful and, depending on the condition, rehabilitation can be lengthy, Kris reasons that the PEOP model may lead to sustained outcomes in occupational performance and participation over time. Kris reasons that this would occur naturally through the transfer of this occupation-based approach to therapy to the clients' everyday activities within their own environments. Kris plans to explore this application through a qualitative study of six clients who completed hand therapy that was grounded in the PEOP model. She begins by interviewing each client using four central questions, each based on a PEOP concept. She begins with the occupation concept by asking each client to identify the valued roles, tasks, and activities that required use of the affected hand. Then she asks them whether and how their experience in occupational therapy impeded or facilitated their performance of these activities. Kris then asks each client about his or her personal characteristics, outlooks, and worldviews; whether and how these were addressed during hand therapy; and how any conversation or intervention in this area facilitated or impeded the desired outcome of therapy. This was followed by similar questions about each client's environment and, ultimately, his or her performance of the desired activities, tasks, and roles.

Kris then conducts a series of layered analyses within and across clients in which subthemes and themes are extracted from the transcribed interview content. Each process involvs ongoing member checks in which Kris confirms or rejects subthemes and themes drawn from the interviews with the clients by checking on the clients' perceptions of the subthemes and themes she extracted. Ultimately, Kris's study provids support for the role of the PEOP model in sustaining rehabilitation outcomes over time in clients participating in hand therapy.

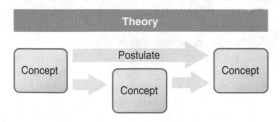

Figure 8.1 A theory is a network of explanations; it provides concepts that label and describe phenomena and postulates that specify relationships between concepts.

emphasizing volition in treatment would choose an activity that is consistent with the client's interests, what he or she feels capable of doing, and what he or she feels is important to do. In the absence of the application of this theoretical concept in treatment, an occupational therapist would likely choose an activity based on a different set of criteria. For example, a therapist might perform joint compressions on a client based on the therapist's view that the client has a sensory or biomechanical need for this manual intervention. Another therapist reasoning from a different theoretical perspective might find a need to pay closer attention to dynamics within the therapeutic relationship as a result of a client's difficult interpersonal behavior. This therapist might decide that it is best for a particular client to take as much time as he or she needs to simply talk about his or her impairment and subsequently make recommendations to the therapist about what needs to be done. The decision to relinquish all control over the goals and process of therapy to the client might be made for a particular client because the therapist knows that, based on past observations of the client, he needs to exert a high level of control within the therapeutic relationship. The therapist knows that the client has this need because the client has resisted any suggestions that the therapist attempts to make based on his own perceived expertise on his condition. In choosing to shift control to the client, the therapist is applying the **collaborating mode** (Taylor, 2008). This mode of action by the therapist is based on the theoretical concept of **collaboration,** which is defined by Taylor (2008) as shifting all control over the therapy process to the client. The term *collaboration* is used to reflect the idea that the only way to truly be collaborative involves willingness on the part of the therapist to relinquish his or her sense of expertise and shift control of the process to the client (Taylor, 2008). Only then may the power between client and therapist truly exist as a shared process (Taylor, 2008). According to the Intentional Relationship Model (IRM; Taylor, 2008), the therapist uses his or her interpersonal reasoning to apply this mode based on the postulate that giving control to a client who appears to need control will facilitate occupational engagement.

In occupational therapy, a theory is a set of concepts and postulates that explain:

- How an occupation is performed
- An occupational problem
- A particular dynamic or interaction occurring between client and therapist during the course of therapy (Kielhofner, 2008)

Why Ground Research in Theory?

Why does occupational therapy need theory? And what would be the consequence if the field did not support the continued development of theory? Theory is particularly important in occupational therapy for educational, technical, scientific, and interdisciplinary reasons.

Occupational therapy education relies on theory to provide a conceptual rationale for why a proposed therapeutic effort is in fact presumed to be therapeutic (Kielhofner, 2008). Theory supports the technical practice of occupational therapy by guiding the nature and sequence of its methods, measures, and adaptations. Theory is important to science as a means of being defined by and defining the concepts and postulates of research. Finally, theory is fundamental in communicating professionally within the field and with other disciplines. Theory defines the boundaries and overlaps between the concepts and corresponding practices of occupational therapy and those of other fields, such as physical therapy, social work, and nursing.

It is important to differentiate between a theory or theoretical concept and the actual application of that concept in a practice situation. This distinction is relevant to occupational therapy practice (Kielhofner, 2005a). It is optimal when the application of a theory or theoretical concept plays out in practice as intended. For example, application of the collaborating mode within the IRM (Taylor, 2008) is based on the theoretical concept of collaboration. But the two are not one and the same. To apply the theoretical concept of collaboration through the use of the collaborating mode, one must use interpersonal reasoning to choose this mode over and above other modes available within the IRM (e.g., advocating mode, encouraging mode, empathizing mode, instructing mode, or problem-solving mode; Taylor, 2008).

It is not always the case that one who embraces a certain theoretical concept is able to enact it through research or practice application. Let's begin with some simple examples from economics and athletics. An economist may present a certain theory about how to lift a country out of a recession while not knowing exactly how that theory would be applied and embraced successfully in a practical sense. Similarly, a soccer coach might have an excellent grasp of the concepts that drive game strategy, but, on a given day, she may lack the ability to actually instruct or motivate her players to carry out her vision on the field.

In occupational therapy, an activity that is not informed by a theory or theoretical concept is not likely to be therapeutic. This is because a theory or theoretical concept is typically applied when a therapist engages in therapeutic reasoning to explain how and why an activity or other therapeutic action is thought to be therapeutic (Kielhofner, 2008). In the absence of theory and the incorporation of theory into therapeutic reasoning, any chosen intervention has no foundation or rationale for its application to a particular client. Conversely, a theoretical explanation for why an activity is likely to be therapeutic is not helpful unless the activity is executed appropriately by the therapist and found to be therapeutic for a given client in a given environment (Forsyth, Summerfield Mann, & Kielhofner, 2005).

With so many new ideas about how therapy should be conducted continually emerging and evolving within the field of occupational therapy, it is important to ensure that they are all appropriately grounded in practice (Kielhofner, 2005b). It is equally important to ensure that new devices, techniques, and activities are sufficiently informed by concepts, plans, and hypotheses about why they are likely to be effective. For example, an occupational therapist might have a concept and a plan about a device that could be designed to help a large-equipment operator return to work. The therapist might collaborate with an engineering company to produce this device. However, if the developers do not inform the design of the device by the body movements of the client, the exact configuration of the equipment that the client will be driving, and the terrain and slope of the land on which the equipment is driven, the device is likely to fail.

In occupational therapy, there is a history of literature that has considered the role of theory in practice (e.g., Costa-Black, Cheng, Li, & Loisel, 2011; Hagedorn, 1997; Kielhofner, 2005a, 2005b). Additionally, our literature has considered the theory–practice gap extensively (Christiansen, 1999; Dobson, 2001; Fisher, 1998; Kielhofner, 2005b; Walker, Drummond, Gatt, & Sackley, 2000; Wood, 1998). The **theory–practice gap** refers to a known gap in communication and collaboration between scholars whose work focuses on the ideas that ground occupational therapy (theory) and the observed actions of therapists whose work focuses on the actual implementation of practice (practice) (Kielhofner, 2005b). Scholars in our field have proposed approaches to address this gap. One of the most widely cited examples is the scholarship of practice (Forsyth et al., 2005; Hammel, Finlayson, Kielhofner, Helfrich, & Peterson, 2001; Kielhofner, 2001, 2005b; Taylor, 2011).

The **scholarship of practice** defines a dynamic and flexible dialectic between empirical and theoretical knowledge (Taylor, 2011). This theoretical perspective distinguishes itself from other approaches to knowledge generation based in **technical rationality** (i.e., Schon's [1983] idea that practical activity is derived seamlessly from basic knowledge). Conversely, the scholarship of practice holds that theoretical knowledge must be derived from the practical problems encountered in therapy (Kielhofner, 2005a). The scholarship of practice calls for an approach to research that contemplates questions raised in practice and

contributes to their answers; characterizes egalitarian partnerships with practitioners; and creates synergies between the needs of scholars, researchers, and practitioners (Hammel et al., 2001). Certainly, there are other approaches to knowledge generation within occupational therapy (Taylor, Braveman, & Forsyth, 2002). However, the scholarship of practice allows for the flexible application of a wide range of theoretical approaches in the field of occupational therapy and serves as a guide for collaboration between educators and practitioners (Crist et al., 2005; Crist, 2010).

Choosing and Applying a Single Theory

In occupational therapy research, the most focused and successful studies are usually grounded in a cohesive theory. Choosing a theory before planning your study is critically important because the approach you choose is a reflection of your knowledge base, practice preferences, and/or ideology about how clients should be served. Choosing a theory may come naturally to a researcher, particularly if she or he has studied or practiced according to the theory in the past.

In planning a study, you should choose a theory that is supported by an ample level of scholarship and prior research. This will allow you to build upon questions and findings contributed by other researchers who have examined or applied the theory with other populations, in other settings, or in other circumstances.

Because many theories share similar concepts or practice approaches, choosing a single theory allows a researcher to link various aspects of that study to the concepts, interventions, and/or interrelationships characterized by the theory. For example, choosing a single theory allows a researcher to select a research question or hypothesis that is consistent with or derives from the theory. Moreover, choosing a single theory allows the researcher to choose an assessment rooted in the concepts of the theory and interpret findings in an integrative and cohesive manner.

For example, a practitioner wants to collaborate with colleagues in electronic visualization, computer sciences, and engineering to develop a new treatment approach for high-functioning postsurgical clients on a neurorehabilitation unit. The treatment approach involves requiring clients to engage in an interactive video game that visually simulates a physical activity and allows for motor input, feedback, and correction of errors. One choice for a client who has enjoyed surfing could be a simulation of someone surfing on a wave using a balance board and a visual image on a computer screen. Given her understanding of motor control theory (Wise & Shadmehr, 2002), the therapist is convinced that the new technology will improve outcomes and is therefore worth purchasing. The administrator of the hospital, an advocate of basic biomechanical approaches, is not as convinced.

To test this question, the therapist forms a research hypothesis that the game-based balance board will lead to better outcomes for high-functioning, post-surgical clients than will usual rehabilitative care. Thus, the underlying theory driving this question is motor control.

In summary, choosing a single theory allows a researcher to:

- Frame the research questions and hypotheses in a focused way, using concepts and relationships outlined by the theory
- Select assessments that capture data that are based on the theory's concepts and relationships
- Interpret findings from an analysis of the data in a way that confirms or weakens a particular exploration or application of concepts and relationships in the theory

In the next sections, these three points are explored in greater detail.

Framing Research Questions and Hypotheses

One of the first steps in planning a research study is to develop research questions and hypotheses. This section is not intended to describe in detail the steps involved in forming research questions and hypotheses (see Chapter 11); rather, it describes the larger picture of how to link research questions and hypotheses to a theory.

Once you have identified a theory, you need to consider that theory when determining your research questions and hypotheses. Unless the purpose of the research is to develop theory by exploring and describing phenomena, research questions and hypotheses in both qualitative and quantitative studies should be grounded in theory. Again, with the exception of research aimed to develop or expand theory, research questions and hypotheses that are not grounded in theory are problematic in three ways. First, a research question or hypothesis that is not linked to theory runs the risk of lacking broader significance, impact, or application. Second, an ungrounded research question or hypothesis leaves the reader wondering

which theory might underlie the research. In the absence of clarity, the reader may come to his or her own conclusions about which theory underlies the research or assume that numerous theories have informed the research. In the absence of clarity within the paper, the reader's assumptions may or may not be correct. Third, when a researcher poses a research question or hypothesis that is not grounded in theory, the remaining methodological and conceptual requirements for conducting the study are more difficult to organize and link together.

Let's look at an example: A researcher wishes to explore whether rural-dwelling women undergoing breast cancer treatment who develop reactive stress disorders will recover from treatment more quickly and report decreased fatigue and distress when an occupational therapy intervention is provided. In this case, the research question is: Will the women who receive the intervention recover from treatment-related fatigue more quickly and report less distress than those who do not? The corresponding hypothesis is: The women who receive the intervention will recover in a significantly fewer number of weeks and report significantly lower levels of distress than those who do not.

Based on this example, one may ask oneself: What is the underlying theory that explains why and how the women will make this important recovery? Without this knowledge, one knows little about what kind of occupational therapy intervention will be provided. One has no means of measuring whether the therapists providing the treatment for the study will do so with fidelity and adherence to the principles of the treatment approach because there is no description of an underlying theory. One does not know how to select from numerous assessments of fatigue or how to select an assessment of distress. This is because both fatigue and distress have multiple meanings depending upon the theoretical basis for understanding them.

Finally, once findings from the study are collected, how does the researcher integrate and make sense of them in light of the profession and current approaches to practice? Without describing those findings in light of the theory that formed the foundation of the study, it is not only difficult, but it limits the impact and interpretability of the work.

This example highlights the reasons why a theory should drive development of research questions and hypotheses. A later section in this chapter provides an example of how a theory can be applied to the same study idea (linking rural women undergoing treatment for breast cancer to an occupational therapy intervention).

Choosing Corresponding Assessments

The previous section explained the importance of linking theory to research questions and hypotheses. It is also important to choose measures that are consistent with that theory. If the theory is well established and widely cited, it is likely that its concepts and postulates have been tested by one or more measures or assessments. In any research study, it is important that the measurement approaches selected to answer the study questions conform to the theory underlying the study. If this does not happen, findings from the assessment cannot be easily interpreted in light of the underlying theory.

Consider, for example, **biomechanical theory,** which describes a client's capacity to engage in movement that is functional. There are numerous measures of movement capacity associated with this theory, ranging from force sensors used to measure directional force in robotics-assisted rehabilitation research (Abdullah, Tarry, Datta, Mittal, & Abderrahim, 2007) to basic goniometers that measure range of motion. If a researcher plans a study of a biomechanical concept with a biomechanical goal, such as increasing range of motion and directional force, the corresponding measures of such concepts are likely to offer the most sensitive and specific means of measuring outcomes associated with this goal.

Another example is sensory integration (Ayres, 1989), which is accompanied by a growing range of assessments, from self-report measures for caregivers such as the Sensory Profiles (Dunn, 1999), to mixed-method assessment batteries such as the Sensory Integration and Praxis Tests (Ayres, 1989). **Sensory integration** describes how sensations are received and organized neurologically to produce human behavior. If one plans a study involving sensory integration, measures that capture concepts of sensation and praxis offer the best means of measuring concepts emerging from this theory.

Another example of a theory on which numerous occupational therapy assessments are based is the Model of Human Occupation (Kielhofner, 2008). The **Model of Human Occupation** (MOHO; Kielhofner, 2008) describes how occupations are motivated, supported by habits and roles, and performed within social and physical environments. This theoretical approach is accompanied by 21 assessments, each of which measures a different aspect of the theory or uses a different approach to assessment. Among them, the Model of Human Occupation Screening Tool (MOHOST;

Parkinson, Forsyth, & Kielhofner, 2006) is a comprehensive assessment of the various aspects of the MOHO that converge to reflect a summary of a client's occupational functioning. It measures a client's volition, habits, and roles; motor skills, process skills, and interaction skills; and functioning within the social and physical environments. Studies drawing upon concepts from the MOHO may benefit from the flexibility and breadth of this approach because one may study a wide range of concepts using a wide range of assessments, including the 21 MOHO-based assessments.

Example of Theory-Driven Research

Let's return to the example of a study that sought to test an occupational therapy intervention for rural women with breast cancer. In that example, the study was not grounded in theory. The following revised example will apply a volitional intervention based on the MOHO. In this revised example, the researcher seeks to test whether women who reengage in an occupation of interest for at least 5 hours per week during radiation therapy are more likely to show motivation to participate in a wider range of their pretreatment occupations and more likely to establish habit patterns reflective of that participation. These outcomes can be measured by an activity diary based on MOHO (Gerber & Furst, 2005) and the MOHOST instrument (Parkinson et al., 2006).

Instead of measuring whether the intervention reduced fatigue and distress, factors that are likely to be less sensitive to change during the study period, the study will measure immediate outcomes that are more closely tied to the theory on which the intervention was based. MOHO-based outcomes include those associated with occupational participation, including increases in volition, the establishment of habit patterns around participation, and the corresponding increases in motor, process, and interaction skills. Applying a theory to the same study illustrates how the clarity, methodological approach, and impact of the study can change dramatically as a result of introducing theoretical concepts and corresponding measures into the process.

Summary

This chapter emphasizes the importance of incorporating theoretical concepts into a research study, including tangible reasons why it is important to begin any research study with a theory. First, a theory allows one to frame the research questions and hypotheses in a focused way, using concepts and relationships outlined by the theory. Second, a theory drives the selection of measures that capture data that are based on the theory's concepts and relationships. Third, a theory facilitates the interpretation of study findings in a way that confirms or weakens a particular exploration or application of concepts and relationships in the theory. It is important to remember that other approaches to research are designed to build or extend theory. These include descriptive and exploratory studies that are qualitative or quantitative in nature. Additionally, the scholarship of practice is introduced as one means of ensuring that research is grounded in a theory. The scholarship of practice illustrates a mutual cycle of how research is informed by practice and theory. Theories in occupational therapy should be flexible enough to account for changes that are informed by occupational therapy practice and by the research that defines the field.

Review Questions

1. What is the definition of a theory?
2. What are two examples of theory-driven research that are not discussed in this chapter?
3. What is the rationale for grounding one's research in theory, including the advantages?
4. Is there a situation or research approach in which one would not ground one's research in theory?
5. What is the rationale for selecting research and clinical assessments that correspond with a theory?
6. What role can the scholarship of practice play in guiding the decision to base research in theory?

REFERENCES

Abdullah, H. A., Tarry, C., Datta, R., Mittal, G. S., & Abderrahim, M. (2007). Dynamic biomechanical model for assessing and monitoring robot-assisted upper-limb therapy. *Journal of Rehabilitation Research & Development, 44,* 43–62.

Ayres, A. J. (1989). *Sensory Integration and Praxis Tests manual.* Los Angeles, CA: Western Psychological Services.

Christiansen, C. (1999). Defining lives: Occupation as identity: An essay on competence, coherence and the creation of meaning. *American Journal of Occupational Therapy, 53,* 547–558.

Christiansen, C. H., & Baum, C. M. (2005). *Occupational therapy: Performance, participation, and well-being.* Thorofare, NJ: Slack.

Christiansen, C. H., Baum, M. C., & Bass, J. D. (2011). The Person–Environment–Occupational Performance model. In E. A. S. Duncan (Ed.), *Foundations for practice in occupational therapy* (5th ed., pp 84–104). London, England: Churchill-Livingstone.

Costa-Black, K. M., Cheng, A. S. K., Li, M., & Loisel, P. (2011). The practical application of theory and research for preventing work disability: A new paradigm for occupational rehabilitation services in China. *Journal of Occupational Rehabilitation, 21,* S15–S27.

Crist, P., Fairman, A., Munoz, J. P., Witchger-Hansen, A. M., Sciulli, J., & Eggers, M. (2005). Education and practice collaborations: A pilot case study between university faculty and county jail practitioners. *Occupational Therapy in Health Care, 19,* 193–210.

Crist, P. A. (2010). Adapting research instruction to support the scholarship of practice: Practice-scholar partnerships. *Occupational Therapy in Health Care, 24,* 39–55.

Dobson, E. (2001). *Occupational therapy intervention with older people who have issues with falls* [Unpublished BS dissertation]. Edinburgh, Scotland: Queen Margaret University College.

Dunn, W. (1999). *The Sensory Profile manual.* San Antonio, TX: Psychological Corporation.

Fisher, A. G. (1998). Uniting practice and theory in an occupational framework. *American Journal of Occupational Therapy, 54,* 509–521.

Forsyth, K., Summerfield Mann, L., & Kielhofner, G. (2005). Scholarship of practice: Making occupation-focused, theory-driven, evidence-based practice a reality. *British Journal of Occupational Therapy, 68,* 260–268.

Gerber, L. H., & Furst, G. P. (2005). Validation of the NIH activity record. A quantitative measure of life activities. *Arthritis & Rheumatism, 5,* 81–86.

Hagedorn, R. (1997). *Foundations for practice in occupational therapy.* Edinburgh, Scotland: Churchill Livingstone.

Hammel, J., Finlayson, M., Kielhofner, G., Helfrich, C. A., & Peterson, E. (2001). Educating scholars of practice: An approach to preparing tomorrow's researchers. *Occupational Therapy in Health Care, 15,* 157–176.

Kielhofner, G. (2001). *A scholarship of practice.* Paper presented at the American Occupational Therapy Foundation Colloquium and Tea at the American Occupational Therapy Association Conference, Philadelphia, PA.

Kielhofner, G. (2005a). A scholarship of practice: Creating discourse between theory, research, and practice. *Occupational Therapy in Health Care, 19,* 7–16.

Kielhofner, G. (2005b). Scholarship and practice: Bridging the divide. *American Journal of Occupational Therapy, 59,* 231–239.

Kielhofner, G. (2008). *Conceptual foundations of occupational therapy* (4th ed.). Philadelphia, PA: F.A. Davis.

Kielhofner, G. (2009). *Model of Human Occupation: Theory and methods in action* (4th ed.). New York, NY: Lippincott Williams & Wilkins.

Parkinson, S., Forsyth, K., & Kielhofner, G. (2006). *The Model of Human Occupation Screening Tool (MOHOST), version 2.0.* Chicago, IL: University of Illinois at Chicago, Model of Human Occupation Clearinghouse.

Schon, D. A. (1983). *The reflective practitioner: How professionals think in action.* New York, NY: Basic Books.

Taylor, R. R. (2008). *The Intentional Relationship Model: Occupational therapy and use of self.* Philadelphia, PA: F.A. Davis.

Taylor, R. R. (2011). Scholarship of practice: Reflections on Gary Kielhofner's legendary vision for occupational therapy. *Occupational Therapy in Health Care, 25,* 3–6.

Taylor, R. R., Braveman, B., & Forsyth, K. (2002). Occupational science and the scholarship of practice:

Implications for practitioners. *New Zealand Journal of Occupational Therapy, 49,* 37–40.

Walker, M. E., Drummond, A. E. R., Gatt, J., & Sackley, C. M. (2000). Occupational therapy for stroke patients: A survey of current practice. *British Journal of Occupational Therapy, 63,* 367–372.

Wise, S. P., & Shadmehr, R. (2002). Motor control. *Encyclopedia of the Human Brain,* 137–157.

Wood, W. (1998). It is jump time for occupational therapy. *American Journal of Occupational Therapy, 52,* 403–411.

SECTION 2
Laying the Groundwork for Evidence-Based Practice:
The Steps of the Research Process

CHAPTER 9

Steps in the Research Process and Characteristics of Sound Research

Renée R. Taylor • Gary Kielhofner • Hector W. H. Tsang • Marian Arbesman

Learning Outcomes

■ Describe each of the key steps in planning and accomplishing a research study.
■ Understand the basic aspects of selecting a methodological approach.
■ Identify the characteristics of sound research.
■ Grasp the differences and the relationships among the research problem, research question, specific aims, and research hypothesis.
■ Define logical reasoning and its role in increasing the rigor, verifiability, and replicability of research.

Introduction

Despite their varying methods, designs, and purposes, all research studies share some common features, procedures, and steps in the process. This chapter provides an overview of those elements that are common to most research studies. It begins by outlining the steps in the research process, identifying the activities that are typically involved from the time a study is planned until its completion. The chapter then describes and examines the accepted characteristics of sound inquiry, or good research. Subsequent chapters in this unit describe the steps of the research process in more detail.

Recognizing a Research Need

Occupational therapists see a wide range of clients with a diverse array of symptoms and impairments. Specialists may work in neonatal intensive care,

or they may work in an outpatient clinic with children and adolescents with developmental disabilities and sensory impairments. Others may work in a school setting with children with motor impairments, neuromuscular disease, and learning disabilities. There is an entirely different group of occupational therapists working in generalist settings, seeing clients of all ages, from infants and toddlers with feeding problems to older adults recovering from stroke. Further, there are geriatric specialists working in skilled nursing facilities, assisted care facilities, home health, mental health settings, and in community-based settings treating problems ranging from Alzheimer's disease, to depression, to fears of falling, to hip replacement.

Given the breadth of our practice, there is no dearth of problems to address when conducting our science. It is important to note that a research problem may emanate out of practice, but it must be further honed and understood in terms of science. Any problem observed in a practice context is only one example of one situation with one particular client. Science encourages us to observe the same problem in multiple settings as it manifests with multiple clients. Furthermore, science demands that we pay respect to all of the previous attempts made to address the problem by other practitioners and scientists. Knowing the historical attempts to identify, analyze, and treat the problem will force new innovations in discovery and treatment. Also, science requires that research problems carry a certain practical and social significance, thereby having an impact on health-care practice and society at large. To summarize, a research problem must:

• Be considerate of prior attempts to address the problem within the practice community

CASE EXAMPLE

Donna recently resigned from her job as a pharmaceutical salesperson to pursue a degree in occupational therapy. Ultimately, she intends to earn a doctoral degree and conduct research that will contribute to practice. Knowing her ultimate goal, her academic advisor suggests that she begin to volunteer for Dr. Kramner, a faculty member with an active research program. Fortunately, Dr. Kramner is at the beginning stage of planning a new study that focuses on the effectiveness of animal-assisted therapy on clients' mobility in an inpatient orthopedic rehabilitation unit (Fig. 9.1).

Donna notes that there are very few studies of the use of a therapy dog on an inpatient rehabilitation unit. The most relevant research was a feasibility study conducted at the Rehabilitation Institute of Chicago (Bode, Costa, & Frey, 2007). These researchers studied the effects of walking with a therapy dog on time spent walking, distance walking, and speed of walking for 23 clients with neurological conditions. Findings were not significant, but the study did demonstrate that it is feasible to examine this question on an inpatient rehabilitation unit.

Donna brings this study to the research team meeting and suggests that the team build on it to identify their research question, aim, and hypothesis. Dr. Kramner appreciates Donna's idea but wonders if there might be other variables that would show stronger treatment effects, leading to an increased likelihood of statistical significance. Namely, Dr. Kramner cites a recent meta-analysis (Munoz, Ferriero, Brigatti, Valero, & Franchignoni, 2011) that found that the use of therapy dogs in rehabilitation has important psychosocial effects, such as enhancing socialization and reducing stress, loneliness, anxiety, and isolation. Moreover, Dr. Kramner wonders if the provision of a dog during therapy might show more significant results with an orthopedic population, rather than a neurologically impaired population, given prior findings.

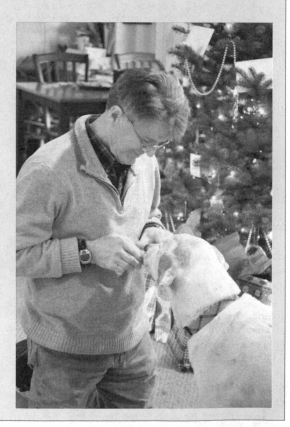

Figure 9.1 An older adult spending time with his dog.

(case example continues on page 88)

Subsequently, the team decides on the following research questions:

1. Does the introduction of a therapy dog to clients on an inpatient orthopedic unit facilitate enhanced mobility?
2. Does it facilitate improved mood and decreased stress?

From these questions, the team establishes the central aims and hypotheses shown in Table 9.1.

By the end of the meeting, the team feels satisfied with the established aims and hypotheses. In subsequent meetings the team selects the research methods, begins to write the research plan and proposal, and applies for ethical review and approval. After the study is ethically approved, the team secures access to the inpatient orthopedic unit at their hospital and begins to enroll subjects according to established inclusion/exclusion criteria. Once the subjects are enrolled and assigned to a condition, data collection begins. At the same time, the team organizes a method for logging completed cases and entering all data into a statistical program for later analysis of results and dissemination of findings.

Table 9.1 Case Example Research Aims and Hypotheses

Number	Aims	Hypotheses
I	To compare a standard walking protocol with a standard walking protocol accompanied by a trained Labrador Retriever on walking distance, speed, and duration among postoperative knee-replacement clients	Clients exposed to a therapy dog during the walking protocol will demonstrate significantly greater walking distance, speed, and duration than controls on all walk attempts during the treatment period.
II	To compare a standard walking protocol with a standard walking protocol accompanied by a trained Labrador Retriever on self-ratings of mood and stress among postoperative knee-replacement clients	Clients exposed to a therapy dog during the walking protocol will demonstrate significantly lower scores on self-ratings of depressed mood, anxious mood, and stress following all walk attempts during the treatment period.

- Have knowledge of and respect for the existing scientific literature related to the problem
- Be innovative so that a new understanding or approach to the problem may be achieved
- Have a practical impact and social significance

For example, Geri decided to study volitional neglect among therapists practicing in orthopedic settings. She arrived at this topic through an integration of practice and science. Aptly, she chose client satisfaction and compliance with the treatment process as being issues of relevance and impact for occupational therapy practice. First, she recalled a personal experience in a practice setting, where she witnessed her grandfather's lack of engagement in rehabilitation following shoulder replacement surgery. Geri recalled his constant feedback that none of the exercises was interesting or relevant to his life or his work. She imagined that other clients must be feeling similarly when going through rehabilitation.

Second, she searched the literature, which revealed a dilemma. There was only one research study on the topic, which found that motivation toward occupation (volition) played a role in compliance with upper extremity rehabilitation in the home setting. Geri observed that the literature did not answer the question as to why therapists did not attend to issues of volition more often when performing upper extremity rehabilitation in an inpatient setting. This led Geri to characterize her research problem as being "a lack of information about volitional neglect among therapists in inpatient orthopedic rehabilitation."

Defining a research problem and reviewing the literature that already exists concerning that problem are two of the initial steps in the research process. The following sections overview these and the remaining steps in the research process.

Steps in the Research Process

When planning and conducting a research study, what steps are required? Research involves the key activities shown in Figure 9.2:

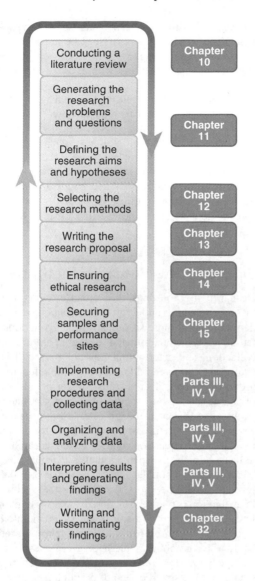

Conducting a literature review	Chapter 10
Generating the research problems and questions	Chapter 11
Defining the research aims and hypotheses	
Selecting the research methods	Chapter 12
Writing the research proposal	Chapter 13
Ensuring ethical research	Chapter 14
Securing samples and performance sites	Chapter 15
Implementing research procedures and collecting data	Parts III, IV, V
Organizing and analyzing data	Parts III, IV, V
Interpreting results and generating findings	Parts III, IV, V
Writing and disseminating findings	Chapter 32

Figure 9.2   Steps in the research process.

- Conducting a literature review
- Generating the research problems and questions
- Defining the research aims and hypotheses
- Selecting the research methods
- Writing the research proposal
- Ensuring ethical research
- Securing samples and performance sites
- Implementing research procedures and collecting data
- Organizing and analyzing data
- Interpreting results and generating findings
- Writing and disseminating findings

These activities are listed in the sequence that investigators generally follow when planning and implementing a study. However, it is typical for an investigator to move back and forth among these activities; that is, they are not necessarily linear. For example, all research begins with a review of the literature. Nonetheless, at the end of a study, when the findings are being prepared for dissemination, researchers should return to the literature to determine whether anything new has been published in the interim.

In the following sections, each of these activities is briefly examined to provide a general orientation to the research process. Subsequent chapters significantly expand on these topics.

Conducting a Literature Review

A **literature review** involves searching relevant electronic databases using key words and synthesizing the findings that are most relevant to the general topic of the research. The aim of reviewing the literature is to identify, evaluate, and understand the existing published theory and research on a given topic. By doing a thorough literature review, investigators learn what information has been generated on the topic and what kind(s) of research methods investigators have used to generate that information.

Thus, the literature review serves to justify or provide a rationale for the research because it allows the investigator to decide what knowledge is lacking and how to best go about generating it.

Literature searches are accomplished through a variety of means, the most common of which uses web-based searching and search engines that retrieve publications based on key words. Another common method is a manual search to examine the references of existing publications to determine what publications previous investigators have considered important.

Once a researcher has exhaustively identified and obtained the relevant literature, it is necessary to analyze it. When analyzing the literature, an investigator asks the following types of questions:

- What is known about this topic?
- What theories are used to explain it?
- What methods are used to generate this knowledge?
- What are the strengths and weaknesses of these methods?
- What gaps exist in knowledge about this topic?

By applying such questions to the existing literature as a whole, the investigator arrives at judgments that allow him or her to identify the research questions and select the methods. A well-done literature review makes it clear why the study is important and needed and provides important information concerning how it should be undertaken. Literature reviews are described in more detail in Chapter 31.

Generating the Research Problems and Questions

After a research need has been recognized and a literature review has been conducted, investigators proceed to clarify a **research problem,** which is a gap or contradiction in current knowledge within a specific topic area, identified by conducting the literature search. The research problem is a statement of the specific knowledge that is being sought in the study. Generating this question is the most important step of the entire research process. The research question informs the study design, the methods for data collection, and the interpretation of findings. Once the research problem is identified, it provides the groundwork for defining specific research questions that can be answered in the research study. Unlike research problems, which are broadly defined gaps in knowledge, a **research question** defines a very specific clinical or scientific problem that the research aims to resolve or a very narrow gap or contradiction in clinical or scientific knowledge that the research aims to address. A key step in any study is deciding what question(s) the research will seek to answer.

Researchers often formulate research questions by beginning with broad questions and then narrowing them. Reading the literature is key to developing research questions. Once a clinical dilemma is defined, reading pertinent studies may help to identify gaps in knowledge that will lead to a research question. For example, reviewing a study involving a specific population or context may trigger the question as to whether a described approach can be applied to different types of clients or in another setting. Or, one may recognize inconsistencies of findings across several studies that point out the need for further research efforts to account for these inconsistencies. In addition to reviewing the literature, investigators generally consult with other researchers in the area to make sure the questions they are developing are warranted and useful.

The topic of identifying research problems and questions is explored in greater detail in Chapter 11.

Defining the Research Aims and Hypotheses

After delineating the research questions, the researcher clarifies the purpose of the research, or the **research aims** of the study, also known as **specific aims.** The statement of specific aims should be precise and concise. It describes what the study will accomplish and what exactly its value will be.

The next step is to define the research hypothesis (or hypotheses). A **research hypothesis** states the expected results of a quantitative study. However, not all quantitative studies will have stated hypotheses. Most commonly, hypotheses are stated when the analysis will involve inferential statistics or when the study compares a dependent variable across two or more groups. The topic of defining specific aims and hypotheses is described in detail in Chapter 10.

Selecting the Research Methods

Research methodology is a broad category that includes selecting and applying a research design, defining one or more **samples** from a given population, applying an approach to assessment or data collection, and determining how the data will be analyzed to produce findings. (A sample refers to a group of people selected from a larger population of people sharing one or more characteristics under study.) The **research design** refers to the specific strategies that the investigator will use to answer the question or questions that guide the research or to test a hypothesis when a hypothesis is included.

Decisions about the design begin on a broad level and become more detailed as the specific investigation is planned. Generally, an investigator first decides whether a study will be quantitative or qualitative or whether it will be a **triangulated** study (i.e., combining methods from these two approaches). Then the investigator makes a decision about the specific type of research design. As described in Chapter 2, examples of study designs include:

* Survey study: A descriptive study reporting findings from a mailed survey to a national sample
* Naturalistic observation: A participant observational study of a specific behavior or other aspect of a specific setting
* Single-subject design: Pre- and posttest data are collected at multiple time points before and following an intervention, replicated across three clients
* Field study: A series of focus groups with providers and consumers of service in a type of setting
* Experimental study: A randomized clinical trial in which subjects are randomly assigned to one of two different intervention approaches

Once the broad decision about research design is made, additional decisions must also be made to refine the study design. For example, in an experimental study, the investigator will need to decide whether random assignment is feasible. The investigator must also determine what different conditions will be compared. In a survey study, the investigator must decide whether subjects will participate in the study only once or whether they will be contacted multiple times over a longer period. In a qualitative study, the investigator will need to decide, for instance, whether it will be an extended participant observation or a brief series of key informant interviews. In designing any given study, investigators will often consider a number of possibilities. It is not uncommon to redesign a study several times while planning. All of these design decisions affect the rigor of the study as well as the resources that will be needed to carry it out.

The investigator must also decide who will participate in the study. This decision involves what characteristics the subjects will have (e.g., age, how they will be recruited and chosen, how many will be included, and what participants will be asked to do in the study). This aspect is referred to as the **sampling approach.**

The final aspect of deciding the research methods is determining how data will be collected and analyzed, or the **data collection approach.** The answers to the study questions depend on the quality of data collected and how they are analyzed. Once again, the choices may range widely. For example, data may be collected with open-ended methods that evolve over the course of the research, or they may be collected through the use of highly standardized procedures and assessments that are valid and reliable and therefore stable among subjects and over time.

Additional information on determining the appropriate research methodology is included in Chapter 11.

Writing the Research Proposal

A **research proposal** is a written plan that organizes the research process in terms of a literature review, the research questions, and the research methodology that will be applied. A research proposal is a document that:

* Details the background literature supporting the need and rationale for the research question
* Describes the anticipated methods that will be used to address the research question
* Describes the anticipated logistics and necessary resources for conducting the research

The proposal serves first to organize the research plan in the investigator's mind and as a blueprint for later implementation of the research. A proposal is also typically used to secure approval, for example, administrative approval or supervisory approval when the investigator is in training.

In other cases, the proposal is used to request funding for the research, in which case it is referred to as a **grant proposal.** These kinds of proposals often include a **management plan,** or description of the major tasks necessary to complete the project, who will perform them, and when they will be done. Included in the management plan is consideration of the necessary resources for conducting the research, such as space and equipment, personnel, and supplies. A budget is also typically prepared for a grant proposal because it forms the rationale for the funds that are being requested. The budget covers the necessary costs of the research for such things as personnel to help carry out the research and supplies necessary for the research.

In addition to these avenues, it is becoming increasingly important in university settings and other organizations to find funding for research. Local, state, and national organizations (for occupational therapy and other fields) develop strategic plans that may incorporate short- and long-term research goals. Agencies that fund research also publish funding priorities. By examining goals, policy statements, and funding priorities, a researcher may discover an approach that can lead to a viable research problem and question.

Chapter 13 provides additional information on writing a research proposal, and Chapter 33 gives more detail on that topic.

Ensuring Ethical Research

Studies involving human beings or animals as subjects undergo **ethical review,** which is a process designed to:

* Protect subjects from harm
* Ensure that subjects' efforts and any risks involved are warranted by the study's importance
* Ensure subjects freely give informed consent to participate

Individuals who are not directly involved in the research conduct a review of the proposed study to make sure it meets these ethical standards. Institutions in which research is routinely conducted maintain ethics boards (sometimes referred to as an **institutional review board**), whose purpose is to review and approve research. Obtaining ethical approval is ordinarily the last step before beginning implementation of a study.

Chapter 14 provides additional information about this step in the research process.

Securing Samples and Performance Sites

A research study cannot be conducted without samples and performance sites. In securing a sample, one must first define the population of interest. One example of a population of interest in occupational therapy research is older adults with Alzheimer's dementia. If one wishes to compare the older adults to themselves before and after a standardized occupational therapy intervention, then the unit of analysis would focus on the individual. To access the older adults and provide them with the intervention, one would need the collaboration and commitment of a performance site, such as a skilled nursing facility. Furthermore, it would be important to develop a sampling plan articulating the sample size, method of recruitment and selection, and inclusion and exclusion criteria. Finally, it is important to implement the sampling process and to begin to obtain consent and enroll subjects. Chapter 15 further explicates the actions necessary to ensure accurate identification of research samples.

Implementing Research Procedures and Collecting Data

Implementation of a study can vary dramatically with the nature of the research. For example, implementing a qualitative field study may involve months of participation with subjects in their natural context, during which time the investigator takes field notes, records interviews, and collects documents. On the other hand, implementing a controlled study comparing two groups of people receiving different therapy approaches may involve assigning subjects randomly to the two intervention conditions, collecting baseline data (i.e., the first measurement takes place before any time passes or intervention occurs), providing the interventions, documenting participant conformity to the intervention protocol, and collecting post-intervention (i.e., posttest) data. Implementing a survey study may require obtaining a random sample of subjects with addresses, mailing the survey instrument, and doing follow-up mailings to ensure the highest possible response rate.

Psychometric studies, or research designed to develop assessments, may involve a series of sequential steps (Benson & Schell, 1997). For example, the investigator may begin with collecting qualitative information (i.e., written observations representing data to be analyzed, such as focus group or interview findings) from clients and/or therapists to ascertain what kind of information should be included in the assessment. Then, once a prototype is designed, a pilot study may be conducted to obtain systematic feedback from individuals who used or experienced the assessment. A pilot study is an initial, often small-scale, version of the larger planned study in which an aspect of the larger study is examined in depth and altered as necessary according to feedback. Following this, the assessment may be revised, and then data will be collected and analyzed to examine whether it has the properties of a sound assessment. Next, revision of the assessment may be followed by further data collection and analysis to determine whether it has improved psychometrically.

A pivotal aspect of implementing any study is recruiting and retaining the participants or subjects necessary for the study. Subjects can be recruited with a variety of approaches, such as presentations that invite participation, fliers or brochures, and mailings. Once subjects have indicated an interest, the investigator must adequately inform the potential participants about the study and obtain and document **informed consent,** a process in which potential subjects learn about the purpose of the study, identify what is being asked of them as participants, and subsequently decide whether or not to participate. More information about informed consent is covered in detail in Chapter 14.

When the research involves a single point of contact with subjects, as in a survey, consent and data collection may occur at the same time. However, many studies require participants to be involved over a period of time and thus require careful attention to subject retention. Once again, a number of strategies, such as subject reimbursement, ongoing contact, and messages to thank and remind, are used to maintain interest in and involvement with the study.

An important consideration in all research is to make sure that the necessary data are collected. Once again, concerns about data collection will depend on the design of the research. In qualitative research, the investigator is concerned that each topic has been saturated, that is, that enough data have been collected from enough different circumstances to ensure that a particular topic is fully informed. In survey research, as noted previously, the researcher is concerned with getting responses from as many persons as possible from the sample chosen. In experimental research, the investigator will be careful to avoid missing data from the pre- and postgroup conditions.

Implementing research procedures and collecting data are covered in detail in Chapters 16 through 19 for qualitative studies and Chapters 20 through 25 for quantitative studies.

Organizing and Analyzing Data

After data are collected, managing, storing, and analyzing the data is the next important step. Typically, but not always, this process follows the original data analysis plan referenced previously. During this step, it is important to monitor data collection to make sure it is being carried out as planned and that the accumulated data are comprehensive. Thus, **data management** refers to the routine monitoring, logging, and/or entry of data into a database as it is collected.

Next, data must be prepared for the analytic process; that is, transformed into a format appropriate to either qualitative and/or quantitative analysis. For qualitative analysis, data are typically in the form of text or narrative, and it is usually entered into a qualitative software package. Quantitative data are typically entered into a computer spreadsheet or other organized format and analyzed according to the available methods offered by the software being used for the statistical analysis.

Another important aspect of data management is to ensure that data are secured so that they will not be accidentally destroyed and so that only members of the research team have access to the data to protect the confidentiality of the study subjects.

Data analysis involves manipulating the data to answer the research question. As noted earlier, qualitative data analysis typically involves coding and sorting the data to identify key themes that will make up the findings, whereas quantitative data analysis involves computing descriptive and inferential statistics. Data analysis is a complex process, and there are a large number of qualitative and quantitative approaches to analyzing data, as discussed in detail in later text chapters, including Chapter 17, Chapter 18, Chapter 22, Chapter 23, and Chapter 24.

Interpreting Results and Generating Findings

A critical and exciting aspect of any research study is the process of making sense of patterns in the data and transforming them into a coherent set of findings to be shared with other members of the scientific community. As with other aspects of the research process, the way in which a researcher interprets the data collected and generates the findings is variable and depends on the type of research and the topic of inquiry.

In some research the process is quite formal. For example, in an experiment in which hypotheses have been postulated, the major task will be to decide whether the data analysis supports the hypothesis or requires the researcher to reject its veracity. In qualitative research, the investigator must ponder the themes and patterns in the data to generate insights into their meaning (Hammell, Carpenter, & Dyck, 2000). This can be a highly creative process in which the investigator's theoretical background and knowledge of the subjects and their life contexts comes into play.

In addition to the major work of generating an understanding of or assigning meaning to the patterns in the data, the process of interpreting results also requires the investigator to analyze the data in light of findings from pilot studies and findings presented by other investigators within the existing literature that formed the background to the study. Additionally, one must skeptically examine the data for alternative explanations to the ones being pursued and ensure there are no problems in the data set (e.g., missing or incomplete data, or an unexpected pattern in the data that affects how it can be statistically analyzed) that need to be considered or corrected. Finally, the investigator must carefully consider the degree of confidence that should be assigned to the findings. This aspect involves several considerations, including how persuasive the data patterns are in supporting the conclusions being drawn and the limitations of the research methods used to generate the findings (Fig. 9.3).

Increasingly, investigators conduct this aspect of the research in public. For example, they may present preliminary findings and seek feedback from peers. They may ask consultants with specialized expertise in the analytical methods (e.g., statistics) to give their opinions about the data and their meaning. They may share their findings with other persons doing research in the same area to gain their insights.

Chapter 18 and Chapter 24 provide additional information on the topics of interpreting results and generating study findings.

Writing and Disseminating Findings

No study is complete until it has been formally shared with other members of the scientific

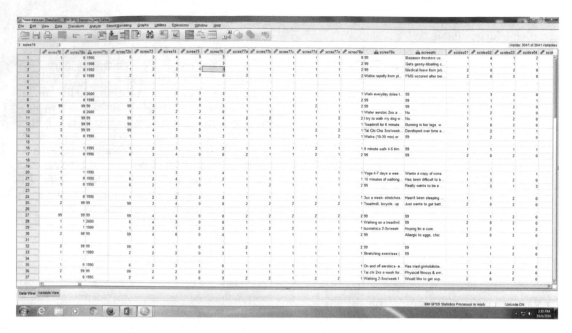

Figure 9.3   Screenshot of an SPSS database.

community and other interested individuals. **Dissemination** defines the manner by which research findings are shared with others. As noted in Chapter 3, investigators typically disseminate their findings through refereed presentations, posters, and published papers. In some cases, the investigator writes a book to disseminate the findings.

The purpose of disseminating research findings in the scientific/scholarly community is twofold. First, one is sharing the information generated through the research with others, thus contributing to what is known about the phenomena under study. Second, and equally important, is that by making the research public, other scientists/scholars can examine the work to determine its rigor and therefore form opinions about how dependable the findings are.

It has become increasingly important to share research results with nonscientific groups that are affected by the research (e.g., individuals whose situations or conditions were studied in the research). In the current information age, consumers are increasingly accessing information generated by research to make informed judgments. For this reason, many investigators also seek to disseminate their findings in formats that are more user-friendly to those outside of the scientific/scholarly community, such as nonscientific articles, books, websites, videos, and brochures.

At the point at which research findings are disseminated, the research process has come full circle. Each investigation begins as an examination of the literature to determine what is known about a topic and how such knowledge was generated. Once published, the research becomes part of that body of literature. By culminating the research process with publication, investigators link their work back to the community of scientists/scholars working in a particular area. Without publication, the research, for all practical purposes, does not exist in the eyes of anyone except the investigators who initiated it. Chapter 32 provides detailed information about successfully publishing research findings.

Characteristics of Sound Research

Considering the potential impact of research dissemination, a research study is not likely to be published in a broadly consumed journal or otherwise shared with a large-scale audience if it is not scientifically sound. The following characteristics are hallmarks of sound research (Crotty, 1998; Polgar & Thomas, 2000; Polit & Hungler, 1999; Stein & Cutler, 1996):

* Rigor
* A scientific attitude of skepticism and empiricism

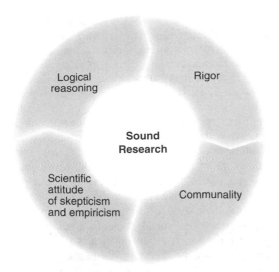

Figure 9.4   Characteristics of sound research.

* Logical reasoning
* Communality

Each of these is interrelated with the others, and high-quality research exhibits all of these characteristics (Fig. 9.4).

Rigor in Research

Research is distinguished from ordinary searching for knowledge by its degree of rigor. The concept of **rigor** means that investigators carefully follow rules, procedures, and techniques that have been developed and agreed upon by the scientific community (Neuman, 1994; Thompson, 2001).

The rules, procedures, and techniques that make up rigorous research are varied and specific to the research questions, the methods and design of the research, and the topic or phenomena under investigation. Following are three examples of how investigators achieve rigor in research.

In experimental research, investigators use standardized research designs that provide control over factors that could bias or confound the results. In a classic text, Campbell and Stanley (1963) outlined the threats to validity in experimental research and detailed a series of experimental and quasi-experimental designs that to various extents controlled for these threats. Today, when investigators use one of these experimental or quasi-experimental designs, members of the research community readily recognize the logic of their design and the extent of rigor it provided in the experiment. The confidence that is placed in the findings corresponds to the rigor of the design used.

In survey research, investigators are concerned that the sample accurately represents the population of interest (Rea & Parker, 1997). To ensure representativeness, investigators must identify the population and sample from it to ensure that the individuals invited to participate in the study characterize the total population. Then, the investigator must engage in a series of steps to ensure that as many of the individuals who are asked to participate actually do. Finally, the investigator must ask whether there is any evidence that survey respondents are systematically different from those who did not respond.

In qualitative research, investigators follow rigorous procedures to ensure that the perspectives, experiences, and actions of the research participants are accurately represented. Because these procedures cannot be prestandardized, as in experimental and survey research, investigators maintain a record of the natural history of the study that documents how insights and new questions arose from the data, how decisions were made to gather new information, how the participants in the study were selected, how the data were coded, and what procedures were used to extract themes and meaning from the data. When researchers have formulated their findings, they return to those they have studied and share these findings to verify that they have authentically captured their experience.

These are only a few examples of the many approaches and procedures that investigators use to ensure rigor in research. In each of these cases, the rules and procedures that the investigators follow have been worked out over time by communities of investigators who sought to improve the soundness of their research. The formal rules and procedures for rigorous research can be found in methodological texts, but the specific processes that are used in a given area of investigation are often shared through various forms of communication, including published reports of research, scientific presentations, and direct communication among investigators in a particular area. These rules and procedures have been shared, scrutinized, discussed, and debated in the scientific community. Eventually prevailing standards have been developed by which investigators execute research and by which their completed research is evaluated for rigor and application.

Research is meticulous, detailed, and reflective. Investigators strive to achieve the highest degree of rigor possible in a given study to optimize the confidence that can be placed in the information generated. Finally, researchers are obligated to honestly document their procedures, any problems encountered, and what limitations of rigor are inherent in the study. With this information, research consumers know how much confidence to place in the findings.

The Scientific/Scholarly Attitude: Skepticism and Empiricism

All research is characterized by a scientific or scholarly attitude that incorporates two elements: skepticism and empiricism (Polit & Hungler, 1999).

Skepticism is the concept that any assertion of knowledge should be open to doubt, further analysis, and criticism. Skepticism is important because it prevents prematurely accepting information as being accurate. Continual questioning of proposed knowledge allows the scientific community to ensure that claims to knowledge are not considered accurate unless they survive constant scrutiny over time (Thompson, 2001).

The scientific or scholarly attitude also demands proof rather than opinion. **Empiricism** means that scientific knowledge emerges from and is tested by observation and experience. Thus, all research involves generating data. Data are information about the world gathered through observation, listening, asking, and other forms of acquiring or extracting information from a situation, event, or person.

Data are valued over opinion because the latter is prone to error and personal bias. Additionally, whether in qualitative or quantitative research, it is important to gather data systematically so that the influence of error and bias are minimized. Moreover, it is common that more than a single opinion will be held about any topic. Consequently, the most systematic way of deciding among differing perspectives is by considering how well they hold up under scrutiny. Empiricism, then, includes the notion that scientists can refine what we know by consistently checking it against what is observed in the world.

Logical Reasoning

Another cornerstone of research is logical reasoning. Importantly, **logical reasoning** is used to systematically link knowledge to the phenomenon being explained through a process of induction and deduction. The logic of inductive and deductive

reasoning has been a topic of constant dialogue, debate, and refinement in the scientific community.

Inductive reasoning, or induction, involves making generalizations from specific observations. For example, suppose that over the course of a week, an occupational therapy investigator observes on several occasions clients who suddenly become aware of another client or a therapist observing them. The researcher also notices that on these occasions, clients appear to increase their efforts. From these observations, the investigator might arrive at the general assertion that clients feel socially obligated to make the most of therapy and that their sense of obligation is strengthened when clients feel socially visible. Creating such a generalization is an example of the process of induction. As the example illustrates, induction involves synthesizing information to generate a theory or an explanation about observed patterns. Induction makes sense of observations by identifying them as belonging to a larger class of phenomena that exhibit an underlying pattern or meaning. Such a generalization is plausible, but, of course, it is not yet tested or verified.

To test it, an investigator would need to use deductive reasoning—that is, to logically derive from this generalization statements that reference observable phenomena. **Deductive reasoning** involves having a general idea in mind and then trying to find evidence to support that idea. The following are some examples:

* Clients are more likely to adhere to therapy tasks if they trust in the therapist's knowledge and experience.
* Clients with lower self-esteem are less likely to adhere to therapy tasks when they are highly challenging.

Each of these statements offers a general idea that would need to be tested through a series of smaller observations.

Induction and deduction allow an investigator to go back and forth between explanations and observations. Different research approaches emphasize either the inductive or the deductive phase. For example, in experimental research, hypotheses deduced from theories are tested. This deductive-empirical approach is typical of quantitative research. On the other hand, qualitative research tends to emphasize the inductive phase. Rich data gathered from participation, observation, and interviews are used to generate new insights, concepts, or theories. Although different research traditions may emphasize one or another aspect of the data–induction–generalization–deduction–data cycle, all research ultimately makes use of both elements.

Communality

Communality describes the context in which research occurs. This context involves a community of scientists who consider how research in a given area should be conducted, scrutinize individual studies, and collectively arrive at judgments about what conclusions should be drawn about a body of research findings (Crotty,1998; Polgar & Thomas, 2000; Polit & Hungler, 1999; Stein & Cutler, 1996). Every study is submitted to a public process in which both the knowledge acquired and the means of acquiring that knowledge are laid bare for others to scrutinize, criticize, and replicate. A review process (typically performed by anonymous peers) ensures that the study to be presented or published meets a basic threshold of rigor.

Once a study has been presented and/or published, others in the scientific community have the opportunity to scrutinize and criticize it. Criticism of existing studies is also a public process that can occur in presentations and publications. In fact, a very typical prelude to presenting the findings of any study is to point out both the findings and limitations of previous investigations, arguing how the current study both builds and improves upon them.

Finally, it is common practice for scientists to replicate a published study (often improving on some aspect of it or conducting it under different conditions) to determine whether they achieve the same results. For this reason, when a study is offered to the scientific community, it is important that it is explained sufficiently so that others can understand exactly what was done and how the conclusions of the study were generated (**verifiability**) and so that others can repeat the study to see if the same results are obtained (**replicability**).

Researchers build upon and place new knowledge in the context of existing knowledge generated by the scientific community. All research is informed by what has gone before. This is why the report of a study always begins with a review of existing literature, which situates the study in the context of what the scientific community already knows. Importantly, researchers not only learn from one another the findings generated by research, but they also learn from others' mistakes and inventions. Innovations in research methods generated by one investigator are routinely used by other investigators to improve their own research. In this way, the scientific community tends to

advance together, with each investigator learning from the experiences of others.

Summary

This chapter outlines the major steps in the research process and the elements of research that define its soundness. It aims to give the reader a broad sense of the activities involved in research. Understanding research and, in particular, being able to conduct research both require detailed knowledge of all the elements that were only touched on in this chapter. Subsequent chapters provide more detail about the essential elements of the research process.

Review Questions

1. What is the sequence and nature of each of the steps of the research process?
2. Imagine that you are assigned to conduct a research study. How would you approach the selection of an overall methodological approach?
3. What are the differences between the research problem, research question, specific aims, and research hypothesis?
4. What are the four major requirements of sound research?
5. What is the role of logical reasoning in research, and how does it help to increase the rigor, verifiability, and replicability of research?

REFERENCES

Benson, J., & Schell, B. A. (1997). Measurement theory: Application to occupational and physical therapy. In J. Van Deusen & D. Brunt (Eds.), *Assessment in occupational therapy and physical therapy* (pp. 3–24). Philadelphia, PA: W.B. Saunders.

Bode, R. K., Costa, B. R., & Frey, J. B. (2007). The impact of animal-assisted therapy on patient ambulation: A feasibility study. *American Journal of Recreational Therapy, 6*(3), 7–19.

Campbell, D. T., & Stanley, J. C. (1963). *Experimental and quasi-experimental designs for research.* Chicago, IL: McNally & Co.

Crotty, M. (1998). *The foundations of social research: Meaning and perspective in the research process.* Crows Nest, Australia: Allen & Unwin.

Hammell, K. W., Carpenter, C., & Dyck, I. (2000). *Using qualitative research: A practical introduction for occupational and physical therapists.* Edinburgh, Scotland: Churchill Livingston.

Munoz, L. S., Ferriero, G., Brigatti, E., Valero, R., & Franchignoni, F. (2011). Animal-assisted interventions in internal rehabilitation medicine: A review of the recent literature. *Panminerva Medic, 53*(2), 129–136.

Neuman, W. L. (1994). *Social research methods: Qualitative and quantitative approaches.* Needham Heights, MA: Allyn & Bacon.

Polgar, S., & Thomas, S. A. (2000). *Introduction to research in the health sciences*. Edinburgh, Scotland: Churchill Livingston.

Polit, D. F., & Hungler, B. P. (1999). *Nursing research: Principles and methods*. Philadelphia, PA: Lippincott.

Rea, L., & Parker, R. (1997). *Designing and conducting survey research: A comprehensive guide*. San Francisco, CA: Jossey-Bass.

Stein, F., & Cutler, S. (1996). *Clinical research in allied health and special education*. San Diego, CA: Singular Press.

Thompson, N. (2001). *Theory and practice in human services*. Maidenhead, England: Open University Press.

CHAPTER 10

Conducting a Literature Review

M. G. Dieter • Gary Kielhofner • Renée R. Taylor

Learning Outcomes

- Distinguish between the two main approaches to searching for information: ready-reference searching and subject searching.
- Differentiate the search strategies of browsing and querying.
- Compare and contrast OPACs, bibliographic citation databases, and the World Wide Web.
- Outline the four steps that comprise the general framework for literature research.
- Describe how keywords and controlled language are used as search terms.
- Explain how Boolean logic is used in search queries.
- Identify generic search syntax functions and commands that are common to many online information-retrieval resources.
- Compare and contrast Web search engines, metasearch engines, and Web directories and list examples of each.
- Identify information sources relevant to occupational therapy.
- Describe search query logic.

Introduction

Possessing an in-depth knowledge of a specific topic area is vital to the success of any research endeavor. One of the best ways to become proficient in a topic area is to conduct a thorough and comprehensive review of the literature. Knowing how to access, summarize, and integrate available information relevant to the topic is essential to conducting and being a consumer of research.

In occupational therapy, the ability to conduct a literature review will serve a wide range of functions. These vary from teaching, to making professional presentations, to grant writing, to publishing articles for professional journals, to writing books and book chapters, to writing the background for a thesis or dissertation. This chapter explains how to locate, summarize, and integrate the evidence resulting from a literature search in order to conduct a thorough and integrative literature review that allows you to respond to an array of professional demands.

Locating Literature on a Topic: Where to Begin

Chapter 4 explains how to appraise the occupational therapy (OT) literature critically, from the perspective of a consumer. This chapter takes that skill further, explaining how to appraise the literature in greater detail. (Note that Chapter 31 in Part 6 covers writing a literature review, which is a separate, but related, task.) The first step in this process involves locating the literature on a topic.

All information-retrieval activities are driven by a need for information. Occupational therapists need information for purposes such as problem-solving, research planning, finding evidence to guide practice, and personal knowledge development. Searching approaches are based on type of need. Approaches generally fall into two categories:

- Ready-reference searching
- Subject searching

Ready-Reference Searching

Ready-reference searching is typically very specific and usually resolved through a closed-ended search process. For example, an occupational therapist may wish to know the following kinds of things about a particular disease: its prevalence, etiology, prognosis, functional implications, and so on. In this case, the information-retrieval task is to identify an appropriate information resource and to access the information (e.g., a text, website, and/or recent review article that contains all of this kind of information about the disease). Ready-reference searching tends to be relatively straightforward and general in terms of level of detail.

Subject Searching

Subject searching is an iterative and ongoing information-seeking process that involves successive steps to arrive at information that is a

CASE EXAMPLE

Jake is a hand therapist at a rehabilitation clinic associated with a university teaching hospital. Involvement in research for 1 day per week is one of Jake's job duties. He has an opportunity to work with a senior hand surgeon on staff on an innovative idea for a grant proposal. In collaboration with scientists, the team has developed an injectable liquid that is hypothesized to significantly speed recovery time following surgery for flexor tendon repair. The substance has been tested in a preliminary pilot study and was found to be safe and effective. The proposed study will extend the number of patients tested, establish safety with a larger sample, and establish optimal dosing. There is also a plan to investigate whether adherence to usual care rehabilitation (recommended exercises), in conjunction with the injection, has an added impact on recovery time.

Jake's role in developing the grant proposal is to ensure that the "usual care" post-surgical exercises that he recommends are updated and reflect best practice as defined by current research. Once he confirms that the exercises are the best ones to use, his next task is to recommend a protocol that will ensure that subjects in the study will adhere to these exercises, in the clinic and at home. Although Jake is effective in his role as a clinician, he cannot be certain that the exercises he currently uses with his clients truly represent the state of the science. He decides to turn to the literature as he develops this aspect of the study protocol.

Jake goes to the webpage for the library that is associated with the university teaching hospital for which he works. He selects two search-engine databases within which he will search for scholarly articles on post-surgical exercises: MEDLINE and the Cumulative Index to Nursing and Allied Health Literature (CINAHL) (see Figs. 10.1 and 10.2). He enters the terms "flexor tendon" and "rehabilitation." He finds 250 articles. Many of them are not relevant to his question because he elected to conduct the most inclusive search possible and did not limit where the terms "flexor tendon" and "rehabilitation" might appear in the articles searched. Once he narrows the field down to truly relevant articles, he finds a number of limitations to the evidence. Most studies do not have a control group, and most advocate for a specific approach. There is controversy regarding the findings for passive versus active flexion and extension exercises that are recommended. Moreover, more information is needed regarding post-surgical time frames and when to introduce unrestricted activity, for example (Matarrese & Hammert, 2012).

Overwhelmed by the evidence, Jake decides to look for rehabilitation approaches that combine best practices. He is particularly intrigued by an article by Groth (2004). This article describes a case-study model in which eight progressively loaded rehabilitation exercises are tested in a specific

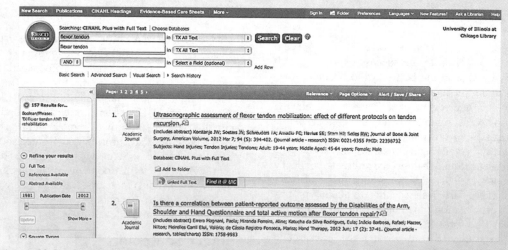

Figure 10.1   CINAHL search for "flexor tendon" and "rehabilitation." *(Copyright CINAHL.)*

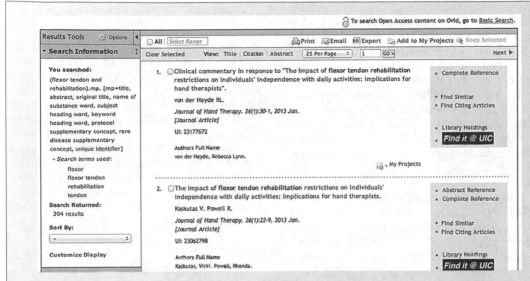

Figure 10.2   MEDLINE search for "flexor tendon" and "rehabilitation." *(Copyright MEDLINE®.)*

sequence, following surgical repair of a zone 2 flexor tendon injury. A 3-point clinical adhesion-grading system is used to rate outcomes. In the case study presented, recovery of active motion was 112%, warranting time for an additional, larger-scale study. The safety and slowness inherent in graded exercise makes sense to Jake in light of his experience.

Based on findings from this article, he decides to contact the author. Jake obtains the protocol and proposes testing it further in the upcoming study.

close-as-possible match to the information being sought. Subject searches use a querying method to transform concepts about which you are seeking information into text search queries. **Information queries** are words or phrases that are entered into the interface of online information-retrieval tools, such as a bibliographic citation database search engine like PubMed/MEDLINE, CINAHL, PsycINFO, or a more general Web search engine such as Google. For example, if you are planning a study of cardiovascular correlates of post-cancer-treatment fatigue, you might enter the following terms into the PubMed/MEDLINE search engine: "cardiovascular" and "cancer fatigue."

The resulting information retrieval is a set of information items ("hits") that have been identified by the search query and organized or prioritized in some fashion. Often, the "hits" or information comes in the form of a citation (e.g., of a published journal article, doctoral dissertation, or book chapter), an abstract (e.g., of a published journal article, doctoral dissertation, or book chapter), or an actual published journal article, depending on the search engine used.

Importantly, when analyzing the retrieved set items, it is common to discover the need to refine

the subject, which necessitates additional search queries. Consequently, searching is essentially a sifting or filtering process intended to produce a core set of information items that are identified by a succession of specific search queries.

As you search using the various search engines, you will notice that searching and scanning the titles and abstracts of the articles/chapters allows you to process and transform the information into knowledge. The purpose of this kind of search is to exhaustively identify all of the information relevant to a topic. In some cases, you may wish to place certain parameters on the kind of information you wish to retrieve in your search. The nature of the evidence you wish to include in your literature review should be guided by the level of evidence (or scientific rigor) that you wish to cover. As explained in Chapter 5, the highest levels of evidence include systematic reviews and randomized trials. Nonrandomized controlled studies and case-series studies are also considered in the levels-of-evidence hierarchy.

Discussed in Section 1, Chapter 4, well-designed and rigorously executed studies reflecting these kinds of levels of evidence will find their way into a **peer-reviewed journal** (i.e., a professional journal in which submitted articles are rigorously evaluated by members of an editorial board who have expertise in research methods and in the topic area under study). **Peer-reviewed journal articles** are published research studies, review articles, and other commentaries that have met with sufficient approval from the members of the editorial review board of a journal to be included in the journal publication. Generally, doctoral dissertations that have not made their way into peer-reviewed journals and book chapters have not undergone the same level of review and evaluation as peer-reviewed journal articles.

For example, if you are searching for a moderately high level of evidence about a historically known topic (e.g., Epstein–Barr virus, the cause of mononucleosis) and need to include information about early discoveries as well as cutting-edge discoveries, you may wish to limit the information source to published journal articles (as opposed to including other sources such as book chapters and doctoral dissertations). At the same time, you may not wish to limit the search to a certain time frame because you need to include early discoveries to show your awareness of the classical studies that formed the foundation of knowledge about this topic.

In another situation, you may be studying a topic that is relatively new to the scientific community, such as Asperger's syndrome. Within the area of Asperger's, you may be studying a particular novel treatment approach that builds upon recent developments within the research community. In this case, you may wish to not only limit the search to published journal articles that include systematic reviews, randomized trials, and controlled studies, but also to studies of treatment approaches published within the past 10-year period (and no earlier studies).

The Process of Information Retrieval

Most information retrieval involves a combination of two broad search strategies: browsing and querying (Taylor, 2004). **Browsing** can be structured or serendipitous and involves entering terms into the search engine, according to either a preplanned approach or an inductive, evolving approach. **Querying** involves seeking matches to a particular text phrase or keyword.

Browsing

Within the category of browsing, there are basically two browsing methods (Taylor, 2004):

* A structured approach
* A serendipitous approach

Structured browsing involves a preplanned organization of a list of topics. These lists often take the form of a hierarchy in which there is a more general list of topics. Then, within each of these topics, there exists a sublist of more specific topics. This approach follows a directed path to the information sought.

Serendipitous browsing is a more random process. In this approach, the searcher travels a nonlinear path to information, for example, randomly following an unfolding series of hyperlinks on the World Wide Web and picking up useful information along the way.

Querying

Querying involves text-phrase matching or keyword matching (Taylor, 2004). **Phrase matching** specifies a particular string of text that is used to reduce the quantity of retrieved items by increasing specificity. For example, an occupational therapist seeking to find appropriate assessments to use in a pediatric setting may begin with the phrase "occupational therapy assessment," proceed to "occupational therapy pediatric assessment," and then to "pediatric occupational therapy observational assessment." **Keyword searching** generally involves using one or more words to retrieve information. Importantly, keywords can be logically combined and uniquely related to one another in search queries.

Online Access to Published Information

There are a number of possible ways to access a variety of information resources available online. One important source of access is through institutions that have access to online information resources, such as Web portals that are supported by a university and/or hospital-based library. An alternative is Web access through local public or community college libraries. Generally, there are three channels to online information retrieval that provide access to published information resources:

* Online public access catalogs
* Bibliographic citation databases
* World Wide Web (WWW or Web)

The following sections focus mainly on strategies for subject query searching involving bibliographic citation databases because these are the major sources for finding research publications used in evidence-based practice and in the literature-review step of the research process.

Online Public Access Catalogs

Individual libraries and networks of libraries rely upon electronic databases of their contents. These are commonly known as online public access catalogs (OPACs). Consortia of OPACs may be networked to provide a wider range of information-locating possibilities. Although OPACs usually have subject-searching functionality, OPAC searches tend to be more closed-ended, seeking known items at a particular site, for example, a book by a specific author or a title. OPAC records include bibliographic descriptions of physical items such as books, pamphlets, and periodicals, as well as electronically formatted materials.

Bibliographic Citation Databases

Bibliographic citation databases allow online access to bibliographic records. Much of the content represented by bibliographic citation databases has undergone some kind of review process that ensures its accuracy, originality, authority, and rigor.

Similar to OPACs, electronic citation databases group information content in certain ways, including by general subject. One example is the PubMed/MEDLINE bibliographic citation databases, which offer access to predominantly biomedical information content. Unlike OPACs, the information items constituting a bibliographic citation database are not limited to resources that are located at a particular site or repository. Instead, bibliographic citation databases such as Medline, CINAHL, and the Cochrane Database of Systematic Reviews index research reports, practice guidelines, literature reviews, editorial comments, letters from subscribers, and other information into content groupings. They include peer-reviewed journal articles, book chapters, and dissertation abstracts from a wide range of sources. These sources include published professional peer-reviewed trade journals, authoritative academic textbooks, and doctoral dissertations made available by various universities throughout the developed world. Among these sources, institutions typically represented include book/journal publishing companies and the universities, medical centers, and other private and public institutions in which academics and researchers work.

What database you use and what is available in the database depend on where you are searching (e.g., through a university or a public library). Each institution has particular subscription arrangements that may provide access to citations only or access to the full text of the publications. Increasingly, however, certain journal articles are being made available online through open access and the use of general search engines on the World Wide Web.

World Wide Web

The World Wide Web, or Web, has made possible a wide variety of electronic publications. Unlike bibliographic citation databases, the Web currently lacks standardized indexing. Although it streamlines the processes of publication and dissemination, the Web also bypasses traditional processes for evaluating the quality of the information included. Web search engines, along with Web directories (e.g., Google or Yahoo) that categorize Web information content, are a means of retrieving a wide variety of content published on the Web.

Subject-Search Considerations for Bibliographic Citation Databases

Selecting an online subject-searching strategy depends on many factors, including:

* Scope and depth of information needs
* Availability of information resources
* Characteristics of the information resources
* Individual's information-retrieval skills
* Available time
* Resources to cover costs

For subject querying of bibliographic citation bases, there are two kinds of search processes: concept expansion and concept contraction. These are often combined in tandem as complementary iterative processes.

Concept expansion refers to broadening a search topic to include all its relevant dimensions. Concept expansion often originates from a specific item of information or a small set of such items. For example, you might receive a few specific research papers from a colleague or find a previously completed literature review on a topic of interest. Alternatively, you might find a key source by browsing the Web and finding a website with a number of bibliographic references on a topic. In each of these instances, these resources are the initial context for conceptual expansion.

The goal of the complementary process, **concept contraction,** is to focus the retrieval into a more conceptually consistent, relevant, and manageable set of information. As noted earlier, a researcher frequently alternates expansion and contraction techniques to modify the developing search concept, resulting in a search process that is dynamic and iterative. You may use expansion and contraction strategies to help identify just how specific the existing knowledge is and to identify the right "pool" of articles and other resources to help develop knowledge of a given topic.

Many online bibliographic citation database search engines and search interfaces have intrinsic search features and syntaxes. It is useful to read all Help screens and judiciously print them out for future reference. The terms and concepts introduced in this chapter are found generally in most advanced search tools and can save much time in defining a search.

Conducting Online Searches in Bibliographic Citation Databases

The following search engines contain citations, abstracts, and links to peer-reviewed journal articles and other sources such as book chapters relevant to a range of scientific and professional disciplines. This is not an all-inclusive list; rather, it includes the premier search engines within the three major disciplines of nursing and allied health, behavioral health, and medicine.

* **CINAHL:** Bibliographic database containing citations, abstracts, and links for peer-reviewed journal articles on topics related to nursing and rehabilitation from around the world. CINAHL may be found through one's local medical library at https://www.ebscohost.com/nursing/products/cinahl-databases/cinahl-complete.
* **MEDLINE:** The U.S. National Library of Medicine's premier database containing citations, abstracts, and links for more than 19 million journal articles from 1946 to present, with some older articles. It is the primary component of PubMed. Topics focus on public health, biomedicine, life sciences, behavioral sciences, chemical sciences, and bioengineering. MEDLINE may be found through the website of the U.S. National Library of Medicine, National Institutes of Health, at http://www.nlm.nih.gov/bsd/pmresources.html.
* **PubMed:** Contains more than 21 million citations, abstracts, and links for biomedical literature from MEDLINE and also includes references to online books and other sources. It allows for free access to MEDLINE. PubMed may be found through the website of the U.S. National Library of Medicine, National Institutes of Health, at http://www.nlm.nih.gov/bsd/pmresources.html.

* **PsycINFO:** A bibliographic database of the psychological literature dating back to the 1800s and continuing to the present. It contains citations, abstracts, and links to peer-reviewed journal articles about a wide range of topics concerning mental and behavioral health. This database may be found through one's local medical library at http://search.proquest.com/psycinfo/advanced/.
* **CIRRIE** (Center for International Rehabilitation Research Information & Exchange): An international database containing citations, abstracts, and full text of research published in the United States and in other countries. A database of workshops and conferences is also available. The link address is http://cirrie.buffalo.edu/monographs/index.php.

This section offers a general framework for subject querying. The overall method involves making choices and decisions that lead to a manageable number of resources that can be examined, evaluated, retained or discarded, and used. An effective search strategy first requires the researcher to:

* Transform concepts (topics) into words that will be used to search
* Logically connect these words by specifying relationships between them
* Format them into search syntax appropriate for the bibliographic citation database being searched

Subject querying involves entering search queries into a database search-engine interface to retrieve sets of information items. Then, you evaluate the information retrieved to ascertain if it is sufficiently relevant, detailed, and focused to the topic. The process is repeated to refine the search until the retrieved information items meet your needs.

The overall search process can be guided by four key questions (Fig. 10.3):

1. *What* (am I looking for)?
2. *Where* (can I find it)?
3. *How* (do I access and retrieve it)?
4. *How well* (does it satisfy my information requirements)?

Step 1: What?

The first step is to identify the information needs. Among other factors, this typically includes consideration of:

* Why the information is necessary
* For whom/what it is intended

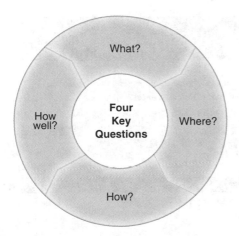

Figure 10.3 The four key questions that guide the search process.

* The format required (e.g., refereed journal articles)
* The time frame

This first step is crucial and not as simple as it may appear. How one initially chooses to define a subject influences later search decisions, the selection of which information items to include (e.g., articles, books, reports), and examination and analysis of the information one retrieves (Rieh, 2002). The ultimate goal of this step is to be clear about what one needs to retrieve so that it can be translated into search terms.

Step 2: Where?

Searching would be greatly simplified if there were a single comprehensive information resource that could be searched. Unfortunately, this is not yet reality. Bates (1989) originally described the process of an information-seeking strategy as "berrypicking" because searchers typically go from resource to resource in search of relevant information items.

An effective search process is characterized by making sound predictions of where relevant information will be and using retrieved information to further define and articulate the search concept and translate it into further search strategies. When making decisions about information resources, it is wise to seek advice from knowledgeable peers, professors, mentors, colleagues, and reference librarians. General knowledge sources, such as dictionaries, encyclopedias, textbooks, and the references sections of relevant journal articles, also are valuable as points of entry into unfamiliar

subject areas. Frequently, universities have created Web information portals where information resources are organized alphabetically or by subject grouping lists, often with appropriate thumbnail descriptions of the scope of each resource's information content. Figure 10.4 shows a page of the Web information portal found on the website of the University of Illinois at Chicago (UIC).

In addition to providing access points to bibliographic citation databases, some Web information portals will also suggest websites that may have useful information content.

Some institutions use metasearch engines that allow **federated searching** of multiple information resources. For example, Figure 10.5 shows the UIC Library's EasySearch. It allows the user to input a single set of search terms into the search interface that will be sent to many different information sources (mainly bibliographic citation databases) to retrieve a set of appropriate information items from each of them. **Search terms** are items used in search queries that connect the intended topic to text in information items that are retrieved. These multiple sets can be combined, ordered, and sorted in a number of ways.

In general, selecting the appropriate information source depends on the topic being researched. This makes it difficult to apply a general rule for selecting an appropriate information source or sources. For the purposes of this chapter, the range of choices has been limited to several bibliographic citation databases that are clearly relevant to occupational therapy. For example, the Cochrane, PubMed/MEDLINE, PsycINFO, and CINAHL bibliographic citation databases are most relevant to OT research. These are not the only citation databases that an occupational therapist might wish to use, but they are generally the most direct and rigorous route to the information you will need.

Once you select a bibliographic citation database, you will need to make a series of search queries to retrieve citations (e.g., the author, title, date of publishing, journal, etc.) of relevant information items. The citation may or may not be linked to an abstract or to the full text of the information item itself.

Citation Searching

Bibliographic citation analysis is another approach to subject searching. **Citation searching** involves looking at the bibliographic citations or references at the end of articles. It offers another way to expand a search from a single article, chapter, book, or Web resource, or from a few such resources. Such

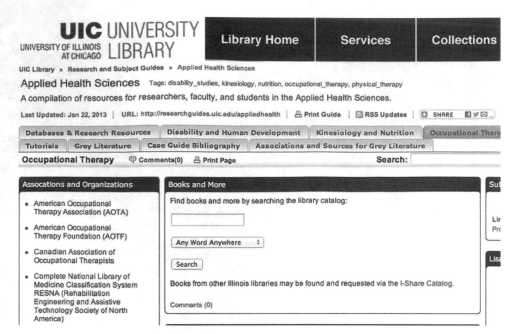

Figure 10.4   UIC Library Subject Page for Occupational Therapy Databases. *(Copyright © 2015 The Board of Trustees of the University of Illinois.)*

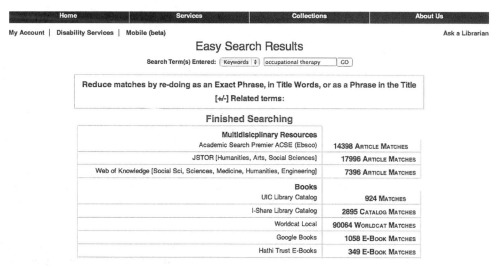

Figure 10.5   UIC's EasySearch metasearch engine results for "occupational therapy." *(Copyright © 2015 The Board of Trustees of the University of Illinois.)*

references represent the author's or Web resource creator's efforts to identify important writings from the work of earlier authors. A searcher can then ready-reference search these cited resources.

A prospective (forward-looking) form of citation searching requires access to a bibliographic citation index database, such as the Thompson Corporation's Institute for Scientific Information (ISI) Web of Knowledge. Using this tool, one can look forward from the original item to identify publications that have subsequently cited it in their own references.

Step 3: How?

Initially, the decisions that searchers make during this stage are guided by the following steps:

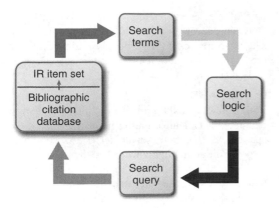

Figure 10.6   Search-query formulation.

1. Articulate and expand the topic into appropriate *search terms* using synonyms.
2. Generate a *search query* defining logical relationships between the search terms.
3. Apply appropriate *search syntax* to the search query as needed to expand and contract search retrieval in terms of precision and recall.
4. Analyze information content to evaluate how well it corresponds to one's intended topic.

As shown in Figure 10.6, these activities are repeated in a cyclical process to refine the search process.

Search Terms

The process of selecting search terms involves a series of steps in which the researcher uses information uncovered from the search to derive new search terms that yield the intended information (Dalrymple & Smith, 2011). As mentioned previously, search terms are items used in search queries that connect the intended topic to text in information items that are retrieved. Researchers continuously identify new search terms to use to expand or contract the retrieval, improving recall and precision, respectively. For example, using synonyms for search terms is a common way to expand a search and, thus, maximize recall. When this results in irrelevant information being retrieved, you will subsequently use contraction strategies to improve precision. The most common search terms used are keywords and controlled language.

Keywords

Some bibliographic citation database search engines allow the user to enter **keyword** search terms by providing a text box with a drop-down label specifying each text entry as belonging to one or more of the database's fields. These keywords are used to find information items in one of two ways. First, bibliographic citation databases sometimes index information items by selecting several key terms that describe the general scope of its content. In this instance, articles and other information items that have been assigned those keywords are retrieved. Second, keywords may be used to identify articles or other information items for which the keyword occurred in the title, author, subject, abstract fields, or full text.

Controlled Language

Some databases have features that allow the user to retrieve specific kinds of information items. For example, the contents in a database may be organized according to a structured classification system. In this case, the user can use controlled language terms to specify a more direct pathway to the information items one wants to retrieve. A **controlled-language term** is a term that matches language that has been preprogrammed into the database. However, effective use of controlled-language search terms requires the user to understand how an information resource's content has been organized. Controlled-language searches result in increased precision when the correct subject headings are used.

In some databases content is already organized (precoordinated) into controlled-language classification systems that use subject headings, thesauri, and ontologies as means of classifying and locating content. In addition, controlled-language systems provide cross-references and links between related terms to assist one in finding the appropriate subject heading.

The National Library of Medicine's MEDLINE Medical Subject Headings system (MeSH) and the CINAHL Subject Headings are examples of controlled languages that are relevant for occupational therapists' information needs. Both are hierarchical arrangements of subject headings. MEDLINE's content is predominantly biomedical and clinical medicine, whereas CINAHL's is related to nursing and allied health. Both systems provide scope notes that explain the use of each subject heading, its position in the hierarchy, and the history of its use. Some bibliographic citation database search interfaces, such as Ovid, map natural-language terms to the correct subject headings or present a list of near matches from which searchers can select a subject heading.

The Search Query

Skill in specifying logical relationships between search terms enhances the user's ability to use expansion or contraction strategies that maximize either the recall or the precision. Both kinds of strategies can be incorporated into a single search query through the use of nesting, a concept that is described in the following section on Boolean logic. A researcher's competence in postcoordinating the logic of information-retrieval processes will enhance the meaning and relevance of the information retrieved.

Search-query logic is arguably the most effective means of applying expansion and contraction search strategies to maximize retrieval recall and precision. When you configure precoordinated controlled-language search terms using postcoordinated search logic, you increase the likelihood of retrieving exactly the information you need. This process is known as set searching.

Boolean Logic

The search logic that is commonly used in bibliographic citation databases is called Boolean logic, after 19th-century English mathematician George Boole (Kluegel, 2011). Boolean logic is a form of algebra in which all values are determined as either true or false. Using Boolean logic, a researcher can connect search terms, allowing more control over the information retrieved than when using individual search terms. Although it may seem intimidating at first, it is well worth learning to increase the precision of searching.

Following the four-step search process described in this chapter, the user enters search queries using syntax appropriate to the bibliographic citation database that is being used. The search engine then retrieves a set of information items that fits the requirements specified in the search query.

Boolean relationships specify the inclusion or exclusion of content that matches the text of search terms in search queries, as illustrated graphically in Figure 10.7. Each circle represents an information-retrieval set that matches a text search term; each

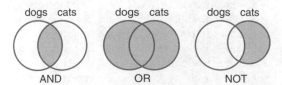

Figure 10.7   A Venn diagram of Boolean search logic.

pair of circles represents the use of a different Boolean search operator to logically relate two search terms, changing what is retrieved. There are three main Boolean operators: AND, OR, and NOT.

Boolean AND

The Boolean AND logical condition creates an exclusive set of information items that match the specific text of both search terms. As shown in the left diagram in Figure 10.7, the relationship between "dogs AND cats" defines a retrieval set that includes only articles that are about both dogs and cats. By specifying dogs AND cats, the user would not retrieve articles that are only about dogs or only about cats. As shown in Figure 10.7, the shaded area representing the intersection of the two sets defines a set of articles mentioning both dogs and cats in their information content. As this example illustrates, the Boolean AND operator can be used in contraction search strategies to increase the precision in retrieval sets.

Boolean OR

The Boolean OR logical condition creates a set of all information items that match the specific text of either of the search terms. As shown in the middle diagram in Figure 10.7, by specifying "dogs OR cats" the user will retrieve articles about dogs, articles about cats, and articles about both dogs and cats. In the diagram, the shaded area represents the union of the two sets, a set of articles mentioning dogs, cats, and both dogs and cats. As this example illustrates, the Boolean OR operator can be used in expansion search strategies to increase recall.

Boolean NOT

The Boolean NOT logical condition creates an exclusive set of all information items that match only the specific text of one of the search terms. As shown in the right diagram in Figure 10.7, specifying "cats NOT dogs" defines a retrieval set that includes articles about cats only. In this instance, any articles about cats that also contain information about dogs would be eliminated from the search set. In this case, the shaded area represents elimination of the dog set from the cat set; that is, articles about dogs and articles about both cats and dogs are eliminated, leaving articles about cats only. The Boolean NOT operator can be used in contraction search strategies to increase precision.

Nesting

Nesting allows Boolean search-term relationships to be combined with one another in a search query to improve control over the set of retrieval items. Parentheses are used to separate the search-term relationships. For example, a nested statement would be "((cats OR dogs) AND pets) AND health." This search query would result in the retrieval of items about the health of cats and/or dogs that are pets. It is important to remember that leading and closing parentheses must enclose each logical set. You can readily see how much more precision is achieved by using this kind of search logic than simply searching for the key terms "cats, dogs, pets, and health." Among many other kinds of articles irrelevant to the intended topic would be those about pets that are not cats or dogs and those about the health of humans.

The Search Syntax

In general, each bibliographic citation database search interface has its own syntax or format rules specifying operations on search terms and queries. Researchers can use printouts of Help screens to become familiar with the commands. However, some generic syntax functions and commands that are common to many online information retrieval resources can be used to expand or contract retrieval, including case sensitivity, truncation, phrases, and proximity.

Case Sensitivity

In general, most bibliographic citation database search engines are not case sensitive. The default condition is typically lowercase, and the retrieval includes lowercase and uppercase occurrences of the search term(s).

Truncation

Truncation refers to inserting a character, instead of a letter, into a word in order to expand the word's reach during the search process. This is a useful search operator for expanding retrieval to account for multiple forms of a term, or when the exact spelling of the term is uncertain. The most frequent types of truncation functionality are termed "right-hand" and "left-hand"; most search engines offer right-hand (the end of the term) truncation. The specific operator varies, but often the "?," "#," or "*" character is used for truncation. An example of right-hand truncation is the search term "librar*." The retrieval would include items with "library," "libraries," "library's," "librarian," "librarians," and "librarianship." Left-hand truncation is situated at the leading end of a search term, and it is used infrequently. Middle truncation functionality is less commonly available than right-hand truncation, but more so than left-

hand truncation, for example, "wom#n" used for "woman" or "women."

Phrases

Some bibliographic citation databases allow phrase searching. Phrase searching searches for an exact string of text. This increases precision and reduces retrieval. For example, a search for "reduce tactile defensiveness" or "increase range of motion" would retrieve only information items in which those specific phrases occurred.

Proximity

Proximity searching (also called adjacency or positional searching) is a useful tool for specifying the relationship of terms by their nearness to one another in the text of the information item. For example, the user might search for items about health-care workers, and could search using the phrase "health-care workers." This strategy might eliminate a number of useful information items that do not use the exact phrase "health-care workers," such as "workers in health care" or "workers employed by health-care providers." A proximity search operator allows one to expand the search, increasing the recall to include terms that are near one another in an article or other information item. Some bibliographic citation database search engines use "adj," "n," or "w" to specify proximity. The order of the search terms often specifies the order of occurrence in the text. More powerful search engines can specify the number of words that may occur between the terms in the item, or their order of occurrence. Proximity can be used as an expansion or contraction strategy.

Analyzing Information Content

When new information items are retrieved, the user must evaluate them in terms of their relevancy to the topic being searched. Also, the retrieved information may be used as feedback that can lead to broadening or narrowing of the intended topic. This reflects the fact that the search process is iterative, with each step informing the next.

Sample Query

Prior to searching online, a good way to begin is by diagramming the terms you intend to use along with their logical relationships in a matrix. By doing this, you are constructing a nested search query from search terms that best represent the topic for which you are searching.

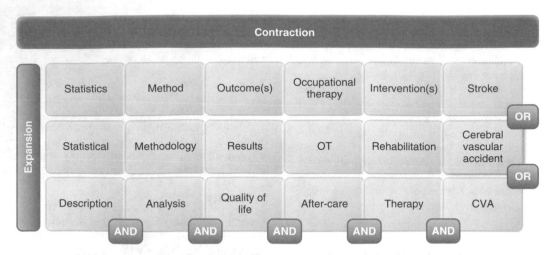

Figure 10.8   Initial topic expansion and contraction using Boolean relationships of search terms for the research question: "What statistical methods might be used to describe the outcomes of occupational therapy interventions for persons with stroke?"

Figure 10.8 shows how a searcher might begin the process on paper with a search matrix for the research question: "What statistical methods might be used to describe the outcomes of occupational therapy interventions for persons with stroke?" The matrix rows show search terms related with the Boolean AND, which would contract the search, facilitating precision. The columns relate terms with the Boolean OR, which would expand the concept, facilitating recall.

Ideally users employ an information resource that allows set searching, allowing one to use search terms related by Boolean logic. For the purpose of demonstration, Figure 10.9 illustrates and explains an example of a single search query that combines the matrix search terms according to the specified Boolean logic, using a generic syntax.

Note that in the examples in Figure 10.9, lowercase and truncation functionalities are used to expand the terms further. In addition, positional syntax is substituted for phrase matching as a means of fine-tuning contraction. Truncation also reduces the number of search terms required for entry by accounting for variants of several terms (e.g., "rehab*" for "rehabilitation," "rehabilitate"). In bibliographic citation databases such as CINAHL, which use controlled language, there is precoordination of terms such as "occupational therapy," which eliminates the need for positional syntax. Many variations of the query shown in Figure 10.9 are possible for querying the research question, as is true for all online subject-search queries.

Note: Assume that "*" is used as a right-hand truncation symbol for 0 to *n* characters, and "**w**" is a proximity operator, where an optional number can be used to specify positional distance in number of words, for example, the use of "w2" to specify the positional arrangement as shown in the example below. A logical representation of the relationships in the matrix could apear as below. In this case each "AND" separates text representing a column of the matrix.

(statistic* OR (descript* OR describe*)) AND (method* OR analy*) AND (outcome* OR result* OR (quality* w2 life)) AND ((occupational w therapy) OR OT OR (aftercare OR (after w care)) AND (intervent* OR rehab* OR therap*).

- (statistic* OR (descript* OR describe*)) Inclusive expansion of column 1 of the matrix
- AND Used to contract the retreival
- (method* OR analy*) Inclusive expansion

Figure 10.9   A sample search query derived from Figure 10.8.

Post-Qualification and Limiting

At any point in the retrieval process, searchers can choose to further focus a retrieval set by limiting the retrieval to a certain time period, type of publication, language, or source. Typically, this is done near the final steps of the process. Searchers can also post-qualify terms by specifying occurrence in a particular database field, such as the title, which reduces the amount of retrieval.

Step 4: How Well? How Reliable?

There are two levels of analysis at this stage; they concern:

* How well the information retrieved fulfills one's needs
* The reliability of the information items

Although published literature often undergoes some form of a prepublication review process (e.g., peer review), it is important for searchers to develop their criteria for evaluating evidence. For example, you may establish the criteria that all the articles you want must employ random sampling of subjects or that they have a minimum sample size.

Critical evaluation requires that researchers select, weigh, and apply appropriate criteria to the information retrieved. For purposes of critically evaluating reports of research, the various discussions of methodological rigor in this text are a useful source of criteria. In the end, the criteria used will vary by the purpose for which the information was retrieved. For example, in conducting a general literature review to refine a research question, you may include a wide range of studies that employ different research methods. A meta-analysis, however, is a more rigorous and statistically systematic way of summarizing the literature. For a meta-analysis you may have very strict criteria related to sampling, the nature of the independent variable, presence of a control group, and so forth.

Searching the World Wide Web

Searching the World Wide Web (WWW) for scientific information may be used cautiously if one understands the topic area and the state of the science well enough to be able to determine the quality and rigor of the information being retrieved. The following section covers specific search approaches and strategies that may be used.

Web Search Engines

Web search engines must comb a vast information space that grows larger every day. Unlike comparatively small, well-organized, and well-structured bibliographic citation databases, the WWW lacks a systematic schema of organization. Therefore, search engines used for searching the WWW have several distinguishing characteristics. Kluegel (2011) has suggested that Web search engines are in reality comprised of three parts:

* The crawler
* The index
* The search engine itself

The search engine crawler is a software tool that continually traverses the WWW looking for new information content and for information content changes. Information that the crawler locates is stored in an index. The search engine searches the index for query matches to terms that one enters. The way in which specific Web search engines identify, select, and prioritize information content for retrieval display is commonly proprietary knowledge, often patented by software designers. The most important thing to remember is that no one Web search tool has yet indexed or catalogued the entire WWW. An example of a Web search engine is Google (http://www.google.com/), one of the most extensively used search engines.

As with searching bibliographic databases, it is important to apply logical strategies for searching the Web. Box 10.1 lists general considerations for using Web search engines to search the WWW.

BOX 10.1 Web Search Tips

* Utilize the Help function to identify search functionality and proper syntax.
* Use topic-appropriate keywords.
* Add more search terms to reduce retrieval.
* Check spelling; although some Web search tools may prompt for spelling errors, not all search engines have this function (this tip applies generally to all search queries).
* Look for an Advanced interface that gives more control to the searcher.
* Use phase searching to increase specificity and reduce retrieval size.
* Check for Boolean and nesting functionality; when entering multiple search terms, the default connector is usually "AND." Check if "+" and "-" can be used to force inclusion or exclusion of terms, respectively.
* Look for word stemming or truncation functionality to increase recall.
* Use the text search function in your browser to find text in the pages you select for examination; hit Ctrl-F to open the search text box.

Metasearch Engines

Metasearch engines provide a single search interface for a cluster of individual search engines. The search terms the researcher enters are transmitted to each of the component search engines. The resultant retrieval is usually categorized according to the component search tool. Additional processing of the information retrieval may eliminate multiple occurrences and organize the content in some fashion. Because individual search engines index only portions of the WWW, metasearch tools are a way to expand the scope of information retrieval, effectively improving the search recall. Examples of metasearch engines are Vivisimo (http://vivisimo.com/), metacrawler (http://metacrawler.com/), and DogPile (http://www.DogPile.com/).

Web Directories

Web directories are organized lists of WWW information content. The typical organizational structure is hierarchical. Unlike Web search engines, Web directories do not use crawlers to seek out or refresh information content, relying instead on Web authors to register their webpages or websites with the directory. Most use a search engine to find a suitable subject point of access for searchers to subsequently browse from by clicking links. An example of a Web directory is Yahoo (http://www.yahoo.com/), a well-known Web information portal that provides links to many different kinds of information and many commercial sites.

Information Resources Relevant to Occupational Therapy

Ultimately, there is a wide range of resources potentially relevant to occupational therapy. Box 10.2 lists some of the journals and websites devoted to occupational therapy. This section describes some of those most frequently used by occupational therapists. As explained earlier, publicly available databases accessible through most university libraries include, but are not limited to, PubMed/MEDLINE, CINAHL, and the Cochrane Library search engines. Other relevant sources include OT SEARCH, gray literature, and specific content websites.

OT SEARCH

OT SEARCH is a bibliographic database that includes literature pertinent to occupational therapy

---

BOX 10.2 Occupational Therapy Journals and Websites

Journals and Periodicals

- *ADVANCE for Occupational Therapy Practitioners*
- *American Journal of Occupational Therapy*
- *Australian Occupational Therapy Journal*
- *British Journal of Occupational Therapy*
- *Canadian Journal of Occupational Therapy*
- *International Journal of Rehabilitation Research*
- *Irish Journal of Occupational Therapy*
- *Occupational Therapy in Health Care*
- *Occupational Therapy in Mental Health*
- *Occupational Therapy International*
- *Occupational Therapy Journal of Research*
- *Occupational Therapy Now*
- *Occupational Therapy Practice*
- *Physical and Occupational Therapy in Geriatrics*
- *Physical and Occupational Therapy in Pediatrics*
- *Scandinavian Journal of Occupational Therapy*
- *South African Journal of Occupational Therapy*
- *Therapy Weekly*

Websites

- American Occupational Therapy Association (AOTA) ■ http://www.aota.org/
- American Occupational Therapy Foundation (AOTF) ■ http://www.aotf.org/
- Canadian Association of Occupational Therapists ■ http://www.caot.ca/
- Illinois Occupational Therapy Association ■ http://www.ilota.org/
- National Board for Certification in Occupational Therapy (NBCOT) ■ http://www.nbcot.org/
- British Association of Occupational Therapists / College of Occupational Therapists ■ http://www.cot.co.uk/
- OTseeker ■ http://www.otseeker.com/

---

and related subjects. It includes monographs, proceedings, reports, doctoral dissertations, master's theses, and most international OT journals (published in English), as well as journals related to the field. This database includes only bibliographic information and the abstract when there is one. The Wilma L. West (WLW) Library, which is part of the American Occupational Therapy Foundation (AOTA), owns a copy of all the material indexed in OT SEARCH. If you are unable to otherwise locate material found through OT SEARCH, you can contact the WLW library to arrange for an interlibrary loan or to receive a photocopy (for a nominal charge) when copyright restrictions do not prohibit it. OT SEARCH is available on a subscription basis only. More information on the database can be found at http://www.aotf.org.

Gray Literature Relevant to Occupational Therapy

Gray literature refers to information that is not published or available in usual formats such as journals. Examples of gray literature are abstracts of conference papers, dissertations or unpublished theses, and unpublished reports—all literature that may contain vital and specific information. Some organizations, such as the United Kingdom College of Occupational Therapists, London (http://www.cot.co.uk), have developed specialist libraries of gray literature that are available to review on request. The Internet significantly augmented the availability of gray literature. However, not all of this type of information is electronically available. Additionally, not all gray literature has been peer reviewed, and so it must be evaluated carefully in terms of its quality and rigor.

Specific Content Websites

Numerous websites are available that can provide access to various sources of information (including publications) related to a specific topic. One example is the website for the National Multiple Sclerosis Society (http://www.nationalmssociety.org/), a nonprofit organization dedicated to providing information about the diagnosis and treatment of multiple sclerosis. The website lists publications relevant to multiple sclerosis and provides a number of other resources. Another example is the Model of Human Occupation (MOHO) Clearinghouse website (http://www.cade.uic.edu/moho/). It not only maintains an up-to-date bibliography of publications related to the model, but also has a search engine that can be used to identify published materials related to specific topics, such as MOHO-based assessments and interventions in specific practice areas.

Summary

Skill in online searching is fundamental to information literacy and is a valuable asset for professional development and practice. Occupational therapists seeking to improve information literacy skills should begin by identifying a core set of useful OT information resources, and then concentrate on mastering the intricacies of the search tools and interfaces required to access information. Ultimately, the only way to improve online searching skills is by continuing to actively perform and refine searches and to evaluate information retrieval.

Review Questions

1. What are the four key questions that guide the literature-search process?
2. How does a researcher use search-query logic?
3. What are two bibliographic citation databases relevant to occupational therapy, and how do you find them?
4. What is meant by "browsing," and how is it different from querying?
5. What is gray literature, and can it be useful to a researcher?

REFERENCES

Bates, M. J. (1989). *The design of browsing and berrypicking techniques.* Retrieved from https://pages.gseis.ucla.edu/faculty/bates/berrypicking.html.

Dalrymple, P. W., & Smith, L.C. (2011). Organization of information and search strategies. In R. E. Bopp & L. C. Smith (Eds.), *Reference and information services: An introduction* (4th ed., pp. 95–96). Englewood, CO: Libraries Unlimited.

Groth, G. N. (2004). Pyramid of progressive force exercises to the injured flexor tendon. *Journal of Hand Therapy, 17*(1), 31–42.

Kluegel, K. M. (2011). Electronic resources for reference. In R. E. Bopp & L. C. Smith (Eds.), *Reference and information services: An introduction* (4th ed., pp. 121–122). Englewood, CO: Libraries Unlimited.

Matarrese, M. R., & Hammert, W. C. (2012). Flexor tendon rehabilitation. *Journal of Hand Surgery, 37*(11), 2386–2388.

Rieh, S. Y. (2002). Judgment of information quality and cognitive authority in the web. *Journal of the American Society for Information Science and Technology, 53*(2), 145–161.

Taylor, A. G. (2004). *The organization of information* (2nd ed.). Library and Information Science Text Series. Westport, CT: Libraries Unlimited.

Generating Research Questions and Defining Specific Aims and Hypotheses

Renée R. Taylor • Hector W. H. Tsang • Marian Arbesman

Learning Outcomes

- Outline the process of generating a research question.
- Differentiate between a research question, a specific aim, and a hypothesis.
- Explain the impact of theoretical frameworks on research questions.
- Identify sources from which research questions may ultimately be derived.

Introduction

Research questions, specific aims, and study hypotheses articulate the central meaning and impact of a study and are closely associated with one another. Together, they offer different perspectives on how a particular study will advance and/or shed more light on a problem or topic of concern, such as a particular impairment or community-based concern. The **research question** probes specific knowledge that is being sought in a research study. The **specific aims** summarize the ways in which the investigators will approach knowledge discovery within the study. The study **hypotheses** serve as direct predictions that point to the anticipated findings or outcomes of the study.

Research questions uncover deeper aspects of a problem or act as a launching pad for treatments aimed to solve a problem. Generating the research question serves as a critical step in the entire research process because it reveals the impact or importance of a problem and directs the course of the subsequent study, particularly the topic, design, and methods of the investigation (Bordage & Dawson, 2003). Not surprisingly, generating this question, along with determining the specific aims and hypotheses, is also one of the most challenging aspects of the research process. This chapter examines key aspects of this process and describes the role of creativity in developing sound research questions, specific aims, and hypotheses.

Generating Research Questions, Specific Aims, and Research Hypotheses

Investigators usually begin the research process by identifying their main area of interest. After this, they proceed to clarify a **research problem,** which is a gap in current knowledge and/or an absence of a needed treatment within a specific topic area. The best research problems are:

- Succinctly stated,
- Derived from practice,
- Informed by the existing scientific literature,
- Innovative, and
- Of high potential impact.

Once the research problem is identified, it provides the groundwork for defining specific research questions that can be answered in the research study. Often, but not always, researchers choose problems based on a topic of personal interest, meaning, or importance.

Whereas research problems are broadly defined gaps in knowledge, **research questions** are narrow, focused, and specific questions intended to generate knowledge to help close the gap within the scientific literature. After delineating the research questions, the investigator clarifies the **specific aims.** As stated previously, the specific aims derive from the research questions and are similarly precise and concise. They describe how the study will approach the research questions. Implicit in the statement of specific aims lies the ultimate value and impact of the study (Fig. 11.1). Finally, the **research hypotheses** restate the research questions and offer a definitive prediction of study findings or outcomes.

Where to Begin?

Research problems and questions are initially derived from a number of sources. In the field

CASE EXAMPLE

Leigh is a first-year occupational therapy (OT) student taking a research methods course. She has been assigned to identify a high-impact problem facing OT practice, and based on that problem, identify corresponding research questions, aims, and hypotheses. Having been born and raised in a small Wyoming town, Leigh is particularly concerned with reaching people living in remote rural areas who return home from a hospital or skilled nursing facility without access to local home health care or outpatient care. After graduating from OT school, Leigh has definite plans to work at a medical center in a remote rural area. Based on the experience she and many of her family members have had, she knows that it will be difficult to serve all of the patients in the broad catchment area of a given medical center.

At a recent American Occupational Therapy Association (AOTA) conference, Leigh learned a little bit about the use of tele-rehabilitation as a means of reaching people in remote rural areas from a vendor in the exhibit hall. However, the sessions presenting research evidence on this topic did not fit her schedule. Leigh remains curious about the feasibility and effectiveness of the use of different approaches to tele-rehabilitation with different types of client populations.

For this reason, she decided to focus her thesis project on the following research questions:

1. Is tele-rehabilitation as effective or more effective than in-person approaches to delivering rehabilitation services to improve motor function?
2. Are there specific populations for which tele-rehabilitation is as effective or more effective in terms of improving motor function?

From these questions, Leigh established the specific aims and hypotheses shown in Table 11.1. In the next phase of her work, Leigh will select the research methods, begin to write the research plan, and apply for ethical review and approval.

Table 11.1 Case Example Specific Aims and Hypotheses

Number	Aims	Hypotheses
I	To compare motor outcomes from a usual-care outpatient rehabilitation protocol with the same protocol delivered online via teleconferencing	There will be no significant differences in motor outcomes for clients exposed to the tele-rehabilitation protocol versus those receiving usual outpatient care.
II	To test whether motor outcomes in the tele-rehabilitation condition differ according to the following primary diagnoses: neurological event, cardiovascular event, multiple sclerosis exacerbation, and total knee arthroplasty	Clients with less complicated diagnoses involving motor impairment (i.e., cardiovascular event and total knee arthroplasty) will show significantly greater improvements in motor functioning as compared with those with more complicated diagnoses (i.e., neurological event and multiple sclerosis exacerbation).

of occupational therapy, research problems and questions often originate from clinical experience. For example, therapists often encounter problems, such as not having an assessment for a specific purpose or not knowing which services will best help a given client group. Therapists routinely raise questions about clinical phenomena, such as:

• Is this assessment reliable or valid?
• Is this treatment approach or modality effective?
• What explains the different treatment outcomes within a defined population?

• Are there ways to improve the treatment outcome for a particular group?

Clinical dilemmas such as these may be tremendously helpful in identifying relevant research questions. Developing a research question should be a public process that benefits from the input of people who know something about the problem from a research and/or practical perspective, such as OT practitioners, managers, policymakers, and clients. Consulting with such people enhances the likelihood that the study will address an important

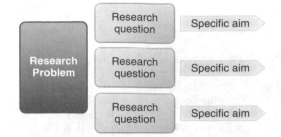

Figure 11.1   The relationship among research problems, research questions, and specific aims. Research problems describe gaps in current knowledge. Research questions are narrow, focused, specific questions intended to help close the gap. Specific aims are the precise and concise ways that investigators approach knowledge discovery.

and relevant question. Participatory approaches to research stress the importance of involving stakeholders such as these who will be influenced by or who would be expected to be consumers of the research.

Carefully deciding on the research question is worth all of the effort and time researchers can give it because it influences all subsequent decisions and procedures and ultimately shapes the worth of the study. Taking time to consider information from the literature and from others' perspectives is a wise investment for any research project.

All research sets out to generate new knowledge that fills a current gap. Such questions may have their origins in clinical experience. They might emerge from the literature. Or, they may have their origins in the findings of previous research. Articulating and refining the research question involves identifying what it is that is not currently known and what the investigation will address.

Formulating Research Questions

How the research question is formulated determines much of the rest of the study. In particular, the question shapes the selection of the research methodology. For example, if an investigator formulates a question about motivation that asks what factors influence motivation, then the design of the study will be largely descriptive and could involve either qualitative or quantitative approaches. On the other hand, if an investigator wants to know whether an intervention improves motivation, then a quantitative design such as a control group study or a single-subject study will be required. If an investigator wants to identify unique factors

that motivate individuals in a particular context, a qualitative field study is likely to be the design of choice. Finally, if an investigator wants to determine whether different factors motivate individuals of different ages, a quantitative survey is needed.

Research questions may start out broad and become narrowed upon revision. An investigator might begin with the following types of questions:

- Why do so many individuals who are hospitalized with serious mental illness tend to be rehospitalized?
- What kinds of characteristics predict which individuals will be more successful following rehabilitation?
- What is the personal experience of individuals following a cerebrovascular accident?
- What differentiates clients who tend to be motivated to get the most out of therapy and those who lack motivation?

The process of formulating a research question involves going from such broad formulations of research problems to research questions that are much more specific and addressable in a single study. For example, the first research problem noted in the previous list (i.e., Why do so many individuals who are hospitalized with serious mental illness tend to be rehospitalized?) could be narrowed into one of the following research questions:

- Is functional level related to the frequency of hospitalizations over a 3-year period?
- Do individuals who have family support have a lower rate of hospitalization in 1 year than those without family support?

As these examples illustrate, choosing a research question requires the researcher to select an aspect of the broader problem being studied that is manageable. Every research question has costs in terms of resources and time needed to generate an answer. Thus, research questions should be formulated with an eye toward what will be feasible in the study being planned.

Formulating a research question usually involves the following steps:

- Reviewing the literature (as discussed previously) to determine what is already known about the topic, what type of questions have been asked in previous research on the topic, and how people have gone about asking those questions.
- Consulting with others about the relevance, significance, and timeliness of the research question/topic. Depending on the objectives and scope of the study, this may involve:

- Talking to people who have done research in the area to receive their input about how to best formulate the problem. This can include getting direct supervision or consultation from expert researchers in the topic area.
- Discussing the topic with practitioners or consumers to ensure the question has relevance and significance to contemporary practice.
- Obtaining information from public policy-makers and potential grant-funding agencies regarding their perspective on the significance, relevance, and timeliness of a given research question. Within the field of occupational therapy, these may include members of public advisory boards, clinical organizations, hospital administrators, self-help or advocacy-based organizations, and governmental agencies that provide funding for research and/or services.
- Presenting an early version of the question to get feedback from others.

The Role of Theoretical Frameworks

As explained previously in this text, a number of theoretical frameworks have been developed in occupational therapy. Theory often serves as the basis for developing research questions, specific aims, and hypotheses. Theories explain phenomena and predict what will happen, given certain circumstances. Researchers can use theories to logically deduce expected observations and to make predictions.

Research questions, aims, and hypotheses derived in this manner can be used to guide studies that test OT theory. Consider, for example, an investigator who wants to examine the broad area of what factors increase clients' motivation to participate in therapy. To formulate a question, the investigator needs to begin with a theoretical idea about what constitutes motivation. This process can be fairly straightforward if there is a single, well-formulated theory that characterizes the particular research topic; in this case, the Model of Human Occupation (MOHO; Kielhofner, 2008) could be used to define the aspects of motivation that are pertinent to participation in occupational therapy. According to MOHO, these include a client's interests, personal causation (perceived ability to do something), and values. Subsequently, these constructs that drive a client's motivation might be utilized to examine participation during therapy.

In other cases, there may be competing theories, so the researcher must select from among them. In still other cases, there may be no clear theoretical

approach, so the researcher must identify a theoretical approach that might be appropriate to the topic. Even if an investigator does not specify a theory, certain assumptions and concepts will be implicit in how any question is posed. Thus, research is more logical and transparent when the theory underlying it is made explicit.

Defining Specific Aims

Specific aims and hypotheses should be derived from the research questions that were originally built upon the research problem. They should be stated clearly in any research paper or proposal. Similar to a research question, the aims and hypotheses should be clear and succinct. A **specific aim** (also called a *research aim*) describes the purpose of the study and/or how it intends to accomplish what it intends to accomplish. Any statement of the research aim should begin with a phrase such as "The central aim of this study is to...." or "The main objective of this research is to...."

Examples of research aims from the field of occupational therapy include:

- "To test the effects of an intervention that helps families manage distressing behaviors in family members with dementia" (Gitlin, Winter, Dennis, Hodgson, & Hauck, 2010, p. 1465);
- "To investigate the effects of a token economy—a behavior therapy technique for controlling drooling in children with cerebral palsy and mild intellectual disability" (Sethy, Mokashi, & Hong, 2011);
- "To follow the rehabilitation outcomes of war fighters who sustained combat amputations in Operation Enduring Freedom or Operation Iraqi Freedom" (Melcer, Walker, Galarneau, Belnap, & Konoske, 2010); and
- "To provide a description of the experiences of dinnertime and bedtime routines and rituals in Australian families with a young child with an Autism Spectrum Disorder (ASD), as well as common challenges experienced" (Marquenie, Rodger, Mangohig, & Cronin, 2011).

As evident in these examples, research aims may involve a qualitative phenomenon, such as describing an experience, or they may involve something quantitative, such as testing the measurable effects of a behavioral intervention. In other cases, they may be both descriptive and quantitative, such as following rehabilitation outcomes for combat veterans. In all of these cases, the aims identified by the researchers were clear, succinct, and at the focal point of the research problem.

Writing the Research Hypothesis

A **research hypothesis** is a carefully written phrase that definitively describes the expected outcomes of a quantitative study. Not all quantitative studies will have stated hypotheses. For example, an exploratory or descriptive study may stop at the level of a research question: "What is the incidence of chronic fatigue syndrome following mononucleosis in adolescents?" Typically, hypotheses are stated when the analysis will involve inferential statistics or when the study is comparing a dependent variable across two or more groups.

If a study includes more than one hypothesis, the hypotheses should be labeled and numbered (e.g., Hypothesis I, Hypothesis II, etc.). Alternatively, a hypothesis may be introduced with a phrase: "It is hypothesized that...." or "We hypothesize that...." Some examples of hypotheses from the OT literature include:

- "It was hypothesized that caregiver-patient dyads in Advancing Caregiver Training would experience the targeted problem behavior and associated caregiver upset less frequently than a no-treatment control group...." (Gitlin et al., 2010, p. 1466); and
- Hypothesis I: There will be a significant decrease in the frequency of drooling in the experimental group as compared with the control group (Sethy et al., 2011).

In reviewing the OT literature, you will notice that a number of studies do not contain stated hypotheses. Qualitative studies, such as descriptive or exploratory studies, may include an exploratory hypothesis or no hypothesis at all. For example, an exploratory hypothesis might read as follows:

- Hypothesis I (exploratory): Rehabilitation outcomes of war fighters who sustained combat amputations will be explored in terms of physical, cognitive, and mental health functional outcomes.

As stated previously, hypotheses are generally included in quantitative (and some qualitative) studies that involve testing groups before and after an intervention or comparing groups on an important characteristic or outcome.

Summary

For OT practice to have a true impact within health care and on policies relevant to public well-being,

the importance of a research problem (and its corresponding questions, aims, and hypotheses) cannot be emphasized enough. Studies that make a difference will pose research questions that are up to date, relevant, and innovative. They will build upon existing knowledge and, ideally, stretch the boundaries within what is currently being practiced in rehabilitation clinics throughout the world in order to improve the lives of clients served.

Review Questions

1. What is the role of the research problem in shaping a subsequent study? Where does one begin in attempting to define such a problem?
2. What is the process by which a research question is defined? How are gaps in the existing knowledge discovered?
3. How does a specific aim differ from a research question? Provide an example of a specific aim.
4. When is a statement of a research hypothesis required in a research study? Under what circumstances would a hypothesis not be required?
5. Why is it important that a research question be grounded in a theoretical framework?

REFERENCES

Bordage, G., & Dawson, B. (2003). Experimental study design and grant writing in eight steps and 28 questions. *Medical Education, 37*(4), 376–385.

Gitlin, L., Winter, L., Dennis, M., Hodgson, N., & Hauck, W. (2010). Targeting and managing behavioral symptoms in individuals with dementia: A randomized trial of a nonpharmacological intervention. *Journal of the American Geriatrics Society, 58*(8), 1465–1474.

Kielhofner, G. (2008). *Model of Human Occupation: Theory and application* (4th ed.). Philadelphia, PA: Wolters-Kluwer.

Marquenie, K., Rodger, S., Mangohig, K., & Cronin, A. (2011). Dinnertime and bedtime routines and rituals in families with a young child with an autism spectrum disorder. *Australian Occupational Therapy Journal, 58*(3), 145–154.

Melcer, T., Walker, G., Galarneau, M., Belnap, B., & Konoske, P. (2010). Midterm health and personnel outcomes of recent combat amputees. *Military Medicine, 175*(3), 147–154.

Sethy, D., Mokashi, S., & Hong, C. S. (2011). Effect of a token economy behaviour therapy on drooling in children with cerebral palsy...including commentary by Hong CW. *International Journal of Therapy & Rehabilitation, 18*(9), 494–499.

CHAPTER 12

Selecting the Research Method

Renée R. Taylor • Ellie Fossey • Gary Kielhofner

Learning Outcomes

- Provide examples of validity in research.
- List the quantitative research designs that are commonly used in occupational therapy research, and outline their strengths and limitations.
- Differentiate between experimental and quasi-experimental research designs.
- Describe the threats to validity that accompany the use of quasi-experimental designs.
- Identify the qualitative research designs that are commonly used in occupational therapy research, and outline their strengths and limitations.
- Explain how validity is defined differently in qualitative versus quantitative research.
- Explain the major considerations in selecting an appropriate design to address a given research question.

Introduction

In Chapter 2, quantitative research is defined as an objective approach in which reports and observations are converted into numerical data that are then analyzed using statistical approaches. In contrast, qualitative research is an approach that explains individuals' subjective experiences, actions, interactions, and social contexts through various approaches involving interviewing, note taking of events and actions, examining written and visual documents, and making audio and video recordings. Within the field of occupational therapy, these overarching approaches are considered equally valid and practical, depending on the research topic, question, and resources at hand.

Within the broader frameworks of quantitative and qualitative research, a **research design** refers to the specific procedures and guidelines that a researcher uses to answer a research question and/or test a research hypothesis. This chapter reviews the specific types of quantitative and qualitative research designs that are most commonly recognized in occupational therapy (OT) research and explains the steps involved in choosing an appropriate design for a given research project. It would not be practical to describe each of the numerous and sometimes complex research designs that are used in research, so this chapter focuses on the most basic types.

In addition to becoming familiar with commonly utilized design choices, it is important to understand the concept of validity and its importance in research. Chapter 2 contrasts experimental designs with quasi-experimental designs and identifies other descriptive, psychometric, and case-study approaches to research. Before reading this chapter, it may be helpful to review the contents of Chapter 2. The concept of validity and the design choices most commonly utilized in quantitative and qualitative research are further explained in this chapter.

Validity and Its Threats

Validity refers to the degree to which a research experiment offers the best evidence available to be able to approximate the truthfulness of a proposition or an inference about cause (Shadish, Cook, & Campbell, 2002). In the case of OT research, validity most commonly refers to the degree to which the effectiveness of an intervention may be estimated.

Types of Validity

There are four general types of validity:

1. Statistical conclusion validity
2. Internal validity
3. Construct validity
4. External validity

CASE EXAMPLE

Sandie is a school-based occupational therapist working at an elementary school in an underserved urban neighborhood. One aspect of her practice involves an obesity prevention and wellness program in which developing healthy activity patterns, along with healthy eating habits and knowledge of nutritionally balanced foods, are emphasized. She has just returned from a state conference, during which she became aware of a grant-funding opportunity that would allow her to expand her program and develop a research study to evaluate its outcomes.

In developing the grant proposal, Sandie is clear about her research topic and question. Her topic is obesity in children, which is a problem of national significance and a funding priority in her state. Specifically, she aims to study the effectiveness of a school-based obesity prevention and wellness program in pre-adolescent children (grades 3 and 4) in an underserved urban area. Sandie's desired program would target three levels of change: the child, family, and school system.

At the level of the child, Sandie plans to host nutritional education sessions with the students during science class. She will educate the children about healthy activity patterns and food groups, and teach personal decision-making skills to influence eating and activity choices. At the level of the family, Sandie plans to host monthly after-school potluck dinner parties, in which parents and siblings are invited to bring a healthy meal to the school and socialize while sharing and discussing healthy eating and activity choices. At the level of the school system, Sandie is working hard with the school district to ensure healthy activity schedules for school children, to change the food choices served at lunchtime, and to ensure that there are neither vending machines nor other vending carts offering unhealthy foods on school property.

If she can time the implementation of these changes so that the changes occur simultaneously with the student nutritional education sessions and the family potlucks, Sandie may be able to coordinate a fairly systematic intervention plan and utilize a quantitative approach with a single-group pretest–posttest design. This design, illustrated in Figure 12.1, would allow her to analyze the program outcomes and draw tentative conclusions about the role of the intervention in affecting the children's eating habits and activity patterns.

In this design, the pretest observation (A_1) would include measuring the body mass index of the child, followed by a test of nutritional knowledge given to the child and his or her family member and a 30-day food and activity diary to measure the child's daily eating habits at home and at school. The intervention or treatment (TX) is a three-level program consisting of child nutritional education, family potlucks, and the elimination of unhealthy food options at school. The posttest observation (A_2) would include the same measurements as in the pretest observation (child's body mass index, child interview, and family interview).

However, if Sandie cannot coordinate the timing of the three levels of intervention, she may need to consider another design. For example, in planning her project, Sandie may discover from preliminary focus-group interviews and informal inquiries with family members that many parents are working at least one job, if not two; will be unlikely to supervise their children in filling out a 30-day food and activity diary; and unlikely to be able to attend the family potluck dinners. Or she may discover that it will take approximately 1 year to get approval for the removal of the vending machines and for a change in the food choices served at the school cafeteria. In these instances, Sandie might have to shift her research design and measurement outcomes.

Instead of a quantitative approach, it may be more practical for Sandie to utilize a qualitative approach, in which she will use semistructured interviews and observational methods to learn more about the children's activity choices, as well as attitudes and preferences toward food, and to collect more detailed information about the children's home lives, activity patterns, and family attitudes and preferences toward food. Qualitative designs are useful in terms of providing information about unique circumstances that are either poorly understood, or faced by groups

A_1 TX A_2

A_1 = Pretest assessment
A_2 = Posttest assessment
TX = The treatment

Figure 12.1 Single-group pretest–posttest design.

of people who are perhaps misunderstood. For example, an ethnographic approach using interactive interviewing and field observations of families within the school district would yield narratively based data that could then be classified and summarized in terms of specific themes or meanings extracted from the interviews and observations. Before Sandie develops a program to promote healthy eating and activity patterns, she would be able to benefit from the knowledge gained from this type of approach.

Clearly, Sandie has a choice to make in terms of what kind of research design and approach she will take as she writes her grant proposal. Knowledge of her community, the feasibility of carrying out her intended intervention, and the information she would need for the project will help her make this important decision.

Statistical Conclusion Validity

Statistical conclusion validity is relevant to research studies and designs that rely on statistics to test hypotheses about cause and effect. **Statistical conclusion validity** defines the extent to which an independent variable and dependent variable are related (or covary). Measures of effect size, statistical power, and statistical significance are collectively relevant when examining statistical conclusion validity (Shadish et al., 2002). Threats to statistical conclusion validity, particularly from an inferential perspective, include:

- Low statistical power (i.e., not a large enough sample size to accommodate the study design and number of variables under investigation)
- Improper use of statistical tests, thus violating certain statistical assumptions or "ground rules"
- The extent to which a researcher studies multiple variables in an attempt to fish for findings (sometimes referred to as "exploratory research" or "data mining")
- Limits to the reliability of measures used in the study
- Limits to the reliability of the manner in which the treatment was carried out
- Variations in the setting in which the study is conducted
- Unanticipated variations among participants in the study

Internal Validity

Internal validity is defined as the extent to which we may infer that (a) an explanation for a particular phenomenon is true or (b) a specific action or intervention has caused an effect (Shadish et al., 2002). In OT outcomes research, another way of defining internal validity is estimation of the extent to which the relationship between the independent (causal) variable and dependent (outcome) variable is causal (as opposed to merely associative or correlational). Two variables may be related, but it may not be possible to determine that an action by one variable had an effect on the second. Internal validity represents the extent to which one may estimate that such a relationship between variables is causal.

Common threats to internal validity include history, maturation, practice effects, regression to the mean, selection bias, attrition, measurement approach, contamination effects, and ethical and social confounds related to inequities between treatment groups. These threats are summarized in Table 12.1.

The degree of internal validity is most often used as the standard against which the rigor of many research studies is determined by one's professional peers. The selection of a research design weighs heavily on the degree to which one can maximize the extent of internal validity and minimize any threats thereof.

Construct Validity

Construct validity is defined as the extent to which a researcher may make a generalization about a particular concept or phenomenon based on what the researcher observes in an actual research study. Taking an example from psychometric research, imagine that a researcher develops a set of questions that she thinks will measure the use of empathy in occupational therapy. Indicators of construct validity will help her estimate the degree to which the questions have accurately captured this concept. In an outcomes experiment, construct validity also measures the extent to which the implied cause-and-effect relationship between

Table 12.1 Threats to Internal Validity

Threat	Definition
History	Events in the natural course of history may have an unanticipated influence on outcomes. For example, if a researcher was studying the effects of a public education campaign on building accessibility and, during the course of the study, the county passed a law that all doorways must be modified to be a certain width, history has clearly played a role in study outcomes.
Maturation	Maturation occurs when participants in a study change over time, and that change affects their measurements on study outcomes. Participants may change in terms of age, physical size or strength, impairment status, cognitive or psychological capacity, experience, and/or other features. Maturity is considered a threat when participants systematically change in a way that might affect study outcomes.
Practice effects	Practice effects may occur when a subject receives the same assessment more than once and recalls his or her previous responses or behaviors during the assessment. If what is being measured is influenced by practice (e.g., knowledge of pop culture), then a threat to validity exists.
Regression to the mean	Regression to the mean refers to the degree to which an initial observation or score contains error. For example, if a recent graduate from occupational therapy school scores very high on the National Board Certification Exam for Occupational Therapy (NBCOT), it is likely that she will score lower the next time she takes the examination. In this case, the lower score will have less to do with the graduate's ability and more to do with error (e.g., it is possible that she was not feeling well during the second examination session, did not get enough sleep the night before, or that there was a distracting noise outside of the room). Regression to the mean can explain some differences between pretest and posttest scores that are attributable to error.
Selection bias	Selection bias refers to another type of error that occurs when there are natural differences between the groups under study. For example, selection bias occurs when there are different kinds of people in the treatment group as compared with the control group. Error attributable to selection is more likely in quasi-experimental research designs because one cannot rely on random assignment to groups to minimize existing differences between groups.
Attrition	Participants discontinue participation in studies for a variety of reasons. They may no longer have time to participate or may no longer perceive that their participation is valuable. Attrition is a threat to internal validity because when a subject drops out or dies during a study, it differentially affects who remains in the treatment and control groups. If, for example, in a study of a fatigue intervention, more participants drop out of the treatment group than in the control group, it is likely to bias outcomes about the effects of the treatment on fatigue, particularly if the participants dropped out because they found participation to be too fatiguing.
Measurement approach	Any change in the assessments or measurement approach used at pretest versus posttest can introduce error into the study. For this reason, it is typically important to use the same measures and the same measurement intervals at every assessment time point.
Contamination effects	Also referred to as "bleed" effects, contamination effects occur when an intervention becomes available to others under study who are not in the treatment group (such as members of the control group). Contamination effects occur when an intervention is widely available or when it occurs in a single institution, such as a hospital, group home, or school, but not all participants receive it. Examples of studies that are subject to bias from contamination include studies involving public education campaigns, life skills training, and other occupationally focused intervention groups that occur in a single institution or close-knit area.
Ethical and social confounds	When a treatment or therapy has positive effects, it becomes desirable to all participants in the study. In studies that have no-treatment controls, placebos, or delayed-treatment control groups, concerns about the ethicality of denying certain groups the treatment or therapy become relevant.

the intervention and the outcome is explained by the intervention (as opposed to some other unanticipated action or event). These unanticipated actions and events are referred to as **confounding variables,** and they represent the primary threats to construct validity. Other threats to construct validity include expectancy effects (i.e., when the researcher or participants expect a certain outcome and therefore behave in a biased way), interaction effects (i.e., in cases in which participants receive more than one type of therapy or treatment), and testing anxiety (i.e., when participants' fears of the testing or assessment procedures bias the findings).

External Validity

External validity is defined as the extent to which we can generalize an inference to different persons, settings, and times (Shadish et al., 2002). Even positive findings from a study can be limited when one cannot reproduce them with a different group of participants, in a different setting, or at a different time point. Outcomes may not be easily replicated if participants in one group are particularly enthusiastic about the study topic, whereas those in the other group are not (i.e., interaction of selection and treatment). Similarly, if one laboratory prepares and processes a genetically based finding according to specific procedures, but those procedures are not replicable in another setting or there is an environmental variable that has an unanticipated effect (e.g., laboratory room temperature), the same genetically based finding may not be observed in another laboratory.

Finally, history may affect external validity. For example, if a social skills intervention occurs on a unique day (e.g., the day of the Boston Marathon bombing), and this event causes a unique level of concern and sharing among research participants, the same outcomes may not be reached with another group of participants on a different day, when no such event has occurred.

Importance of Validity in Design Choice

Quantitative research offers many types of design choices, each with its own practical strengths, feasibility, rigor, and limitations, including threats to validity. The more rigorous the design, the fewer the limitations and threats to validity. However, no matter how rigorous the design, it is always important to speak about one's conclusions in a qualified or considered manner. One of the most important points to keep in mind about validity

is that in any type of discussion or write-up about a research study, it is never acceptable to make a direct inference about cause and effect. When making any inference that an intervention led to a specific outcome, a skillful researcher should avoid using the word "truth" and discussing a research finding in black-and-white terms. From your reading of abstracts and research articles, you may have already noticed that conclusions are typically qualified as "tentative," "limited," "estimated," "approximated," "preliminary," or "speculative."

Moreover, a researcher is responsible for describing all of the limitations to the truthfulness of whatever is being postulated or concluded, including the threats to the validity of the study. The following section examines the three major design classifications in quantitative research, from the most rigorous (and typically least feasible) to the least rigorous (and typically most feasible).

Designs Used in Quantitative Research

Quantitative research incorporates three major design classifications: experimental, quasi-experimental, and nonexperimental designs. In occupational therapy, all studies seeking to determine the effects of a given treatment approach involve the following: (a) a treatment, (b) at least one outcome measure, (c) categories or conditions to which participants are assigned or classified into groups, and (d) at least one point of comparison from which a change or outcome may be inferred and attributed to the treatment (Shadish et al., 2002).

Experimental Designs

The earmark of an **experimental design** is that it involves random assignment of participants to treatment versus control groups. Random assignment differs from random selection in that **random assignment** is conducted without participants' knowledge of the group (or treatment condition) to which they are being assigned. In **random selection,** participants are aware of the condition to which they are being selected. Because knowledge that you are receiving a particular treatment may introduce a **placebo effect** (i.e., the perception or experience that a treatment has been successful even if no treatment or a placebo treatment is being applied), random assignment is a more rigorous approach.

Random assignment forces a degree of equivalence between the groups, both in terms of raw numbers of participants assigned to each group and in the degree to which the groups naturally differ on variables that are extraneous to the research question but nonetheless may create differences that have the potential to influence outcomes. For example, if body mass index is an extraneous variable that could affect the degree of movement in post-stroke hemiparetic adults, then random assignment would reduce this potential confound. It is presumed that randomly assigning participants to comparison groups would greatly reduce the chances of an uneven number of individuals with high body mass ending up in one group and those with lower body mass index ending up in the other group. Controlling for these types of extraneous variables through random assignment maximizes the likelihood of inferring that a given intervention led to a discovered outcome.

Types of Experimental Designs

There are two basic experimental designs found in the literature: the two-group posttest-only randomized experiment and the two-group pretest–posttest randomized experiment.

The **two-group posttest-only randomized experiment** is the most basic experimental design in which participants are randomly assigned to either a treatment group or the no-treatment control group. The treatment group receives the treatment, and both groups are assessed following the treatment to see if they differ on the desired outcome. There is no pretest assessment in this design because the random assignment to groups renders the groups **probabilistically equivalent** (i.e., although the two groups are not equal in terms of all variables, any differences between the two groups are likely to be based on chance rather than on some systematic pattern of variation). A depiction of this design is presented in Figure 12.2.

The **two-group pretest–posttest randomized experiment** is nearly identical to the two-group posttest-only randomized experiment; the only difference is the addition of a pretest before the treatment is offered (Fig. 12.3). The addition of a pretest introduces greater control within the experiment in that it allows for the measurement of change within the two groups of participants and between the two groups of participants. The ability to measure change within the two groups of participants further demonstrates that any observed difference between groups did not occur independently without the treatment and was not attributable to error, such as an unanticipated difference between participants in the two conditions.

Blinding of Participants

In true experimental designs, it is important that participants do not know whether they are receiving a treatment, which is referred to as **blinding.** The primary way of maintaining blinding is to offer participants who are assigned to the no-treatment condition a **placebo treatment.** In pharmacotherapy, this treatment is generally a pill that is administered in capsule form and filled with a substance that is not likely to have an effect on the subject (e.g., a sugar pill). In rehabilitation, a placebo treatment may involve instruction or coaching to engage in a particular task that occupies the client and leads the client to believe he or she is receiving treatment but is unlikely to have any effect on the desired outcome (e.g., a guided relaxation placebo as a control group in a study of a systematic stress management intervention that incorporates cognitive reframing to facilitate physical activity).

Types of Control Groups

There are four common types of control groups used in research studies. In experimental studies

R_T TX A
R_C ---- A

R_T = Random assignment to
          the treatment group
R_C = Random assignment to
          the control group
TX = The treatment
A   = Assessment

Figure 12.2 Two-group posttest-only randomized experiment.

R_T A_1 TX A_2
R_C A_1 A_2

R_T = Random assignment to
          the treatment group
R_C = Random assignment to
          the control group
TX = The treatment
A_1 = Pretest assessment
A_2 = Posttest assessment

Figure 12.3 Two-group pretest–posttest randomized experiment.

with true random assignment, placebo control groups are generally utilized because they enhance subject blindness to condition. **Placebo control groups** include individuals who are led to believe they are receiving a treatment of significant benefit, when in fact the treatment that is actually given has been found to have no significant benefit. In contrast, in **usual-care control groups,** the participants simply continue to receive what is considered to be the usual standard of care for their particular impairment.

Another type of control group is the **delayed-treatment control group,** in which participants are put on a wait list (and sometimes receive periodic pretest assessments while waiting) and then receive the treatment a period of time after the treatment group has already received the treatment. A third circumstance is the **no-treatment control group,** in which participants are either naïve to any treatment for their particular impairment or have independently withdrawn from or have been deliberately withdrawn from treatment for purposes of the study (the latter of which is likely to pose ethical issues, particularly if treatment is necessary to manage or ameliorate the impairment).

Usual-care, delayed-treatment, and no-treatment control conditions are often utilized in quasi-experimental designs, in which control groups still exist, but participants are not randomly assigned to a condition and so are more likely to be aware that they are not receiving the experimental treatment.

Other Experimental Designs

More sophisticated experimental designs that incorporate multiple levels of analysis exist. Among these are factorial designs, randomized block designs, covariance designs, and hybrid experimental designs. Further discussion of these designs is beyond the scope of this chapter, and readers seeking advanced knowledge are encouraged to consult other resources (e.g., Shadish et al., 2002).

Quasi-Experimental Designs

In OT research, experimental designs requiring true random assignment to groups can be practically challenging and sometimes ethically controversial. Imagine you are proposing a major randomized clinical trial examining the effects of portable, robotically assisted movement therapy on range of motion and movement recovery time for upper extremity paralysis immediately following neurosurgical treatment of cerebellar brain tumor

and for 12 months thereafter. You are comparing the effects of two experimental conditions on the postsurgical clients: Group 1 is usual-care rehabilitation plus robotically assisted movement therapy, and Group 2 is usual-care rehabilitation alone. Your preliminary pilot study research and your clinical experience both suggest that the robotically assisted movement therapy is likely to decrease recovery time by at least one-third compared with usual care. These recovery gains are sustained up to 1 year postsurgery, compared with the usual care group, which tends to level off and regress in terms of range of motion and movement.

Based on these preliminary findings, if you were to conduct a formal study with true random assignment using a usual-care placebo control, this would mean that you would have to recruit participants while knowing that some of them will be assigned to a condition in which they think they are receiving a beneficial treatment (usual care) but the treatment may actually be of less benefit to them. Is this ethical? On one side of the debate, an argument might be made that usual care represents the standard of care, and so it is ethical because the clients are not being denied any care. On the other side of the debate, one could argue that knowingly denying care following surgery that is thought to be superior and not telling clients is not ethical.

Imagine that, instead, you decide to employ a **quasi-experimental design** that relies upon random selection using a delayed-treatment control group. You decide to deny care to the controls for the first 3 weeks after surgery and bring them back as outpatients to learn how to utilize the robotics machine at home. Those who agree to be in the delayed-treatment control group understand the risks of not being included in the experimental group, but they know they might still be able to benefit from the experimental treatment, even if it is administered at a later time point. Given the results of your pilot study, it is highly likely that the control participants on the waiting list for treatment will not benefit as much as those in the experimental group who receive the treatment immediately following surgery. Is this ethical? One could argue that it is more ethical than denying them the opportunity to utilize the treatment, but it still poses a dilemma if the critical window for treatment efficacy lies in the immediate 3 weeks following surgery.

Quasi-experimental designs utilize random selection or other methods of nonrandom assignment to groups based on **convenience sampling,** in which participants may be fully aware of the group to which they are being assigned, and researchers estimate that the groups are equivalent in terms of key features, but they cannot be as sure as if the groups were determined by random assignment. Quasi-experimental designs allow for ethical issues and concerns about feasibility of implementation to be addressed. However, these designs are limited in that they do not permit reasonable causal inferences (Shadish et al., 2002). Instead, one may only suggest that a treatment is associated with a hypothesized outcome, citing all of the limitations that constrain such a possibility.

Nevertheless, quasi-experimental designs are the most commonly employed designs in rehabilitation research because of their flexibility and relative rigor. The four quasi-experimental designs that are most commonly utilized in occupational therapy research are:

• One-group posttest-only design
• Two-group posttest-only design
• One-group pretest–posttest design
• Two-group pretest–posttest design

The following sections describe each of these designs, providing examples of their use in OT research. Other variations on these designs that incorporate more than two groups or more than two levels of analysis are also utilized, but they are beyond the scope of this chapter.

One-Group Posttest-Only Design

In the **one-group posttest-only design,** a single group of participants receives an OT treatment, and then a posttest is given to determine whether the treatment was successful. This design is presented in Figure 12.4.

This design is not rigorous, and it is limited in the amount of information it provides. First, it does not include a pretest assessment of the participants before treatment is received. Second, it does not include a control group wherein any posttest differences might reveal themselves when comparing controls, for example, who did not receive a sensory-based classroom intervention with participants who did. Information provided by a one-group posttest-only design would only be useful if a researcher was able to make educated guesses about the participants prior to having received the intervention or if the researcher could retroactively

collect information via interview or from other historical records that might be available.

Imagine a school-based occupational therapist recommends that an entire integrated kindergarten classroom of 12 children with and without developmental disabilities receive sensory-based toys and play equipment and supervised interaction during recess breaks. Imagine that this new approach to sensory-based recess breaks and equipment is continued within the school for a period of 6 months. After 6 months, very few interpersonal and behavioral problems are observed. If the therapist has no prior knowledge about the behavior of the children prior to the introduction of the sensory intervention, then the fact that few behavioral issues are observed is meaningless. However, if the therapist knows that more than one-half of the children in the classroom had chronic and ongoing behavioral problems prior to the 6-month intervention period, a cautious inference that the intervention was effective might be made. The validity of this inference might be strengthened by a retroactive interview of the teacher and of the children's parents about the interpersonal and behavioral status of the classroom before and after the 6-month intervention period.

A second circumstance in which a one-group posttest-only design might reveal useful information is one in which an intervention is characterized by a signature cause that is so unique that it would be impossible to link the outcome to any other explanations. For example, if an occupational therapist on an outpatient neurorehabilitation unit requires that all persons recovering from cerebrovascular accident with speech impairment attempt to sing the vowels of the alphabet in tune with the song "Row, Row, Row Your Boat," and most of her clients are able to accomplish this task spontaneously and without practice within a certain time frame, it is clear that the rote practice of a signature intervention led to the clients' ability to spontaneously sing the vowels. However, if one wanted to link the incidence of brain tumors to radiation from cell phone use, one would have a much more difficult time weeding out the effects of all of the other sources of radiation in daily life, let alone all of the other causes of brain tumors.

Two-Group Posttest-Only Design

The **two-group posttest-only design** offers slightly more rigor than the one-group posttest-only design. It allows the researcher to test whether a certain therapy or other action led to a desired outcome by allowing for a direct comparison between a group of participants receiving the therapy and one

---

TG   A

TG = Treatment group
A   = Posttest assessment

Figure 12.4 One-group posttest-only design.

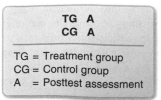

Figure 12.5   Two-group posttest-only design.

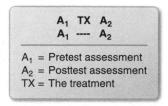

Figure 12.7   Two-group pretest–posttest design.

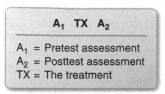

Figure 12.6   One-group pretest–posttest design.

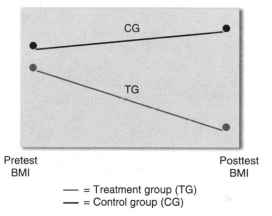

Figure 12.8   The effects of a cardiovascular fitness program on body mass index (BMI) for adolescents with Down's syndrome.

not receiving the therapy. However, because this design only offers one assessment, it is difficult to determine whether history, maturation, or other confounds related to the passage of time affected findings. This design is presented in Figure 12.5.

One-Group Pretest–Posttest Design

The one-group pretest–posttest design is a commonly utilized design in OT research. Other names for this design include the within-participants pretest–posttest design or the within-groups pretest–posttest design. According to this design, one group of participants is administered a pretest before the intervention occurs. This group then receives the intervention, and a posttest is administered thereafter (refer to Fig. 12.6).

This design is superior to the one-group posttest-only design in that findings from the pretest assessment (comprised of the same measure or set of measures administered in the posttest assessment) can be directly compared with findings from the posttest assessment.

Two-Group Pretest–Posttest Design

The two-group pretest–posttest design, presented in Figure 12.7, is more rigorous than the two-group posttest-only design because it offers two types of comparison in terms of outcomes—one comparison between groups of participants and another comparison within each group of participants over time. To some degree, this reduces some, but not all, of the threats to validity.

Consider Amy, an OT student who is interested in studying the effects of a cardiovascular fitness program on the physical health and activity

levels of adolescents with Down's syndrome. With parental consent, she recruits participants from two local community-based centers serving individuals with developmental disabilities. Participants from the first center receive the therapy, and participants from the second center receive a placebo intervention consisting of guided relaxation training. Pretest and posttest assessments of body mass index, muscle strength, peak oxygen uptake (VO_2 max), and activity level measured with a pedometer over 24 hours/7 days are taken from both groups of participants, and the outcomes are observed after 1 year. Participants from the first center improved significantly on all three measures. Visual depictions of these findings are shown in Figures 12.8, 12.9, and 12.10.

Despite the promising look of these findings, there are several threats to validity when using a single-group pretest–posttest design. In writing up her findings, Amy must consider a number of threats. First, she must consider history in the sense that a different set of events could have occurred at the control group center as compared with the therapy group center. For example, it is possible that the control group center hosted a significantly greater number of fundraising parties during which rich foods and desserts were served,

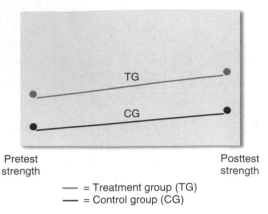

Pretest
strength

Posttest
strength

—— = Treatment group (TG)
—— = Control group (CG)

Figure 12.9   The effects of a cardiovascular
fitness program on muscle strength for
adolescents with Down's syndrome.

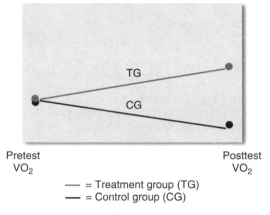

Pretest
VO$_2$

Posttest
VO$_2$

—— = Treatment group (TG)
—— = Control group (CG)

Figure 12.10   The effects of a cardiovascular
fitness program on peak oxygen uptake (VO$_2$
max) for adolescents with Down's syndrome.

or significantly less regular physical activities
may be organized for people attending the control
group center. This could have negatively affected
the body mass index and overall fitness of participants in the control group. This could explain
why the controls were slightly heavier during the
pretest phase.

Selection bias (i.e., participants self-selecting
into a study or condition out of self-interest or a
researcher's bias in assigning certain participants
to a specific condition) and **experimenter expectancy** (i.e., the researchers expecting that participants from the therapy group center would do
better) might also explain differences. The control
group center might not have placed a high value on
a cardiovascular training program or might regularly serve highly calorific meals. These variables
may have been directly or indirectly evident to

the researchers, thus influencing the designation
of that particular center as the center from which
control group participants would be derived. From
the data presented in Figure 12.8, it appears that
something must have affected the fact that individuals in the control group were heavier at pretest
than those in the therapy group.

Another threat to validity is maturation. As a
group, adolescent participants at one center may
have been slightly younger than those at the other
center. The effects of the timing of puberty in the
older participants may have led to weight gain and
increased muscle strength in one group as compared with the other. Regression to the mean represents an additional threat to validity, particularly
when examining pretest and posttest performance
on the muscle strength and VO$_2$ max testing.

As evident from the figures, the treatment and
control groups are not equivalent on the variables
of interest from the time of the pretest. This nonequivalence reduces the rigor that true random
assignment offers because true random assignment typically accounts for many of the issues
of nonequivalence that arise in quasi-experimental
designs.

Nonexperimental Designs

Nonexperimental designs represent the final
category of quantitative research. These designs
include studies that are purely descriptive or observational in which variables that are thought to be
associated with one another are analyzed statistically (Shadish et al., 2002). Another term used to
describe these types of designs is *correlational*
because the central question concerns an association between variables that may not be causal or
ordered in a specific way. The design typically
lacks manipulation of an independent variable and
only relies on measurement for information.

These designs are employed when the researcher
wishes to quantitatively explore people's behavior
as it naturally occurs, in the absence of any upfront
assignment to treatment or control groups, and in
the absence of any planned therapy or intervention.
These designs include data that may only be interpreted in terms of the strength of their relationship
to one another. In these designs, it is typically not
possible to predict whether one variable preceded
or directly led to another variable—particularly
if the sample taken was cross-sectional in nature,
meaning it was taken at only one point in time.

For example, Pete serves as the Director of
Graduate Studies at a large OT school. He is
interested in student success and would like to
know whether passing the National Board for

Certification in Occupational Therapy (NBCOT) examination is associated with students' final grade-point averages (GPAs) upon graduation. He conducts a cross-sectional study of the class of 2014 and, with the written consent of the graduated students, gathers NBCOT scores and compares them to the GPAs. He finds that the data on the two variables reveal a significant association. However, because the sample is cross-sectional and the study is merely descriptive, he is not able to discern whether higher GPA predicted or caused better NBCOT performance. Too many threats to validity exist.

Designs Used in Qualitative Research

In contrast to designs used in quantitative research, the perspectives and methods of qualitative research originally grew out of the challenges of studying groups of people who were dramatically different from the investigator. Because qualitative researchers encountered foreign languages, perspectives, and practices, they recognized that behavior reflected rules specific to the social and cultural context (Denzin & Lincoln, 1994).

Qualitative methods were developed in response to the recognition that the everyday world that people experience is a valid focus of inquiry (Neuman, 2003). Thus, qualitative research traditions generate a unique set of assumptions about, and approaches to, investigating the phenomena studied.

Because qualitative researchers seek to understand the actions of people, they must know the everyday meaning and contexts that inform and shape those actions (Corbin & Strauss, 2008). Qualitative researchers are concerned with accurately capturing research participants' subjective meanings, actions, and perceptions of their social contexts (Popay, Rogers, & Williams, 1998). Consequently, qualitative researchers use methods to actively engage their study participants in dialogue, and participate with them in the activities under study, to achieve an insider (or **emic**) understanding.

Unlike quantitative researchers, who strive to maintain an objective stance on the phenomena under study, qualitative researchers aim to immerse themselves in the subjective reality of the persons whom they study. Qualitative researchers also reflect on their own personal reactions in the research setting to gain better access to how study participants experience their reality. The greatest threat to rigor in qualitative research is that researchers may erroneously substitute their own meaning for the meanings of the individuals whose experiences they are studying, creating fictitious and, thus, invalid findings.

The focus of qualitative research is on authenticity and groundedness. Qualitative researchers aim to "illuminate the subjective meaning, actions and context of those being researched" (Popay et al., 1998, p. 345). Thus, central to the quality of qualitative research is:

- "Whether participants' perspectives have been genuinely represented in the research (authenticity)
- Whether the findings are coherent in the sense that they 'fit' the data and social context from which they were derived." (Fossey, Harvey, McDermott, & Davidson, 2002, p. 723)

Qualitative researchers ordinarily begin their inquiry, like quantitative researchers, with guiding theoretical concepts and questions. However, they formulate broader questions, rather than narrowly defined questions or specific hypotheses. As data are gathered and inform these broad questions, they are refined, leading to more focused sampling and information gathering. Thus, qualitative research is flexible, emergent, and responsive to the study setting, data, and data analysis. The participants and their social context shape the kinds of information gathered and the themes and explanations that emerge in the study.

This means that in qualitative research, the resulting abstractions, or theory developed, are grounded in the participants' experiences and social context. Valid representation centers on the transformation of the meanings, perspectives, and behaviors of those studied into theoretical abstractions. These abstractions must authentically represent how those studied experience and organize their world (Rice & Ezzy, 1999).

Data collection in qualitative research focuses on gaining understanding of the phenomena under study as they are experienced by the participants. This means that researchers strive to preserve the ways in which participants characterize their experiences and actions. Digitally recorded interviews that allow for extensive quotation of participants' own words, detailed notes that describe events and actions, written and visual documents, and recordings are typical data. These data provide a rich source for the qualitative investigator, but they also pose a challenge to coherently and concisely present findings.

Qualitative findings are represented as textual descriptions or narratives. Consequently, analysis involves translating a wealth of detailed qualitative information into a textual account. Importantly, this account or narrative must authentically describe the phenomena being studied. That is, it must preserve for the reader some essence of what was studied.

Qualitative data analysis requires the researcher to explore the meanings, patterns, or connections among data. This process involves the researcher's own thought, reflection, and intuition. There are many different qualitative procedures and tools for analyzing qualitative data. They share the common feature of progressively exploring the data and comparing and contrasting different parts of the data to evolve a more sophisticated understanding (Tesch, 1990).

Often data gathering and data analysis occur iteratively, with each influencing the other. Because the researcher seeks to generate findings that are clearly grounded in participants' viewpoints, various safeguards are built into the analytic process. For example, qualitative research requires adequate sampling of information sources (i.e., people, places, events, types of data) so as to develop a full description of the phenomenon being studied (Rice & Ezzy, 1999). In addition, qualitative researchers typically return to the participants to seek their feedback as to whether the findings generated truly characterize their experiences.

Presentations of findings must enable the reader to appreciate the phenomena studied and to gain insights into how they are experienced by the participants. One way of accomplishing this is through "thick description" (Geertz, 1973). Thick description refers to a sufficiently detailed depiction, drawn from the raw data, of people's experiences, actions, and situations to convey the layers of personal and contextual meanings that inform them (Denzin, 1971). For this reason, qualitative findings are generally presented with substantial quotes, verbatim field notes, and other data that help point to the essence of the phenomena that the researcher is attempting to characterize.

Types of Qualitative Research Designs

There are four general types of qualitative research designs: case-study, grounded-theory, phenomenology, and ethnographic designs.

Case-Study Designs

In **case-study** designs, researchers obtain and reveal information about a phenomenon from a single subject under study by gathering in-depth information about that phenomenon from that subject. The "case" may represent an individual client of occupational therapy, an event, a group, or an institution. Consider an occupational therapist who works in a prison setting and wants to better understand the occupational hazards of female gang membership in Chicago. Because it could be impractical or dangerous to immerse herself in an actual observational study of real-time gang life, she invites a highly capable female inmate with extensive experience of gang membership to participate in an in-depth interview, so as to learn more about the phenomenon, and then analyzes the findings in terms of emergent themes. To authenticate her findings, she invites this same inmate to also write a biographical account of her life with the gang, following which these two sources of information can be analyzed together by the research team and the emerging themes reviewed with the participant herself to check how well they represent her gang experience. Additional information about case-study research is presented in Chapter 26. It should be noted that case-study research may also be approached using quantitative methods.

Grounded-Theory Designs

Researchers employing grounded-theory designs strive to create a theoretical understanding of a phenomenon by extracting meaning from social interactions (Miller & Fredericks, 1999). In a **grounded-theory** approach, data are typically gathered using emic (insider) approaches and then read, reread, and coded to discover or label variables and their interrelationships. Through constant comparison, concepts emerge from the data, and those data are used to establish a hypothesis involving relationships between certain phenomena (Glaser, 1965). For example, a researcher interested in systematically understanding how individuals with disabilities become engaged in advocacy-related social action may begin by accessing social networks and recording interactions among persons with disabilities within those networks that concern advocacy-related topics. The digital data would then be downloaded and coded by multiple individuals to ensure accuracy. After concepts are labeled, the researcher would check them with members of these same social networks to ensure the accuracy of the coding and labeling. Then, associations would be drawn between the concepts to form a theoretical understanding of advocacy network formation among individuals with disabilities. It should be noted that grounded-theory research may also use mixed methods, drawing on quantitative and qualitative data.

Phenomenology

Researchers employing **phenomenology** strive to explain the ways in which individuals experience their lives from their viewpoint, placing emphasis on understanding the subjective meaning of experiences and situations for individuals themselves without reference to theory or knowledge from other discipline perspectives. This approach relies on personal knowledge and subjective experience, and its main means of data collection include interactive interviewing, focus groups, and the analysis of the personal writing of participants. Additional information about phenomenological research is presented in Chapter 16.

Ethnographic Designs

Ethnographic designs are derived from sociology and focus on the social definitions and meanings of behavior or other phenomena. Ethnographic researchers generally work in community-based settings and study entire groups of people. Specifically, ethnography seeks to define and describe the characteristics, actions, and behaviors of a cultural group from an insider perspective, according to the perspectives of members of that group (Neuman, 2003), with the aim of developing an account of how a particular societal, cultural, or organizational context shapes meaning and behavior. Hence, ethnographic studies typically use interview and observational methods suited to investigating naturally occurring interactions and practices of people in social settings.

Deciding on the Appropriate Design for Your Study

There are many avenues from which an investigator may approach the selection of a research design. Developing criteria for selecting the appropriate design is helpful when making this consequential decision. The criteria outlined in Table 12.2 are important to consider.

Knowledge

As evident in the Case Example at the beginning of this chapter, it is important to have intimate knowledge of and experience with the population before embarking on a research study. Having knowledge of a potential research population has different meanings depending on the type of research.

In basic science laboratory research, there is often little contact with human participants outside of the consent procedures. Initial knowledge about the characteristics of a subject population is often derived from the literature and immediate clinical experiences with patients. For example, if an OT researcher seeks to improve range-of-motion recovery in post-mastectomy clients under the age of 45, he or she will look to personal experience treating these types of clients. Additionally, he or she is likely to turn to the literature on this topic to achieve knowledge about the types of pain

Table 12.2 Criteria for Selecting a Research Design

Criteria	Description
Knowledge	The extent of knowledge of the participants and problem under study
Impact	The anticipated value, impact, and sustainability of the research question, hypothesis, or proposed outcome
Feasibility	The practicality and feasibility of locating and retaining participants in the study
Environment	The available environment(s) for research
Resources	The available resources (money, staff, and time) for research
Mentor approval	The importance of adequate support from mentors, collaborators, and institutions involved
Time frame	The acceptability of the expected time frame for completion of the study (to the participants, the researchers, the mentors/collaborators/involved institutions, and the funding agencies)
Safety and ethics	Assurance that the design will support a safe and ethical process for those involved

medications used to facilitate movement following surgery and other movement-related recommendations that facilitate mobility of the associated muscles, joints, and other involved tissues, so as to enable activity participation.

In laboratory research, investigators are generally analyzing human tissue, blood, radiographic images, biomechanical parameters, and other data retrieved while a client is already undergoing treatment. Participants are often, but not always, recruited because they are existing clients within a medical or rehabilitation facility. Participants may be available for this type of research because they have an existing disability or medical problem, and they may be interested in the topic under study because they perceive it may be of benefit to them and others in the long term. In laboratory research, knowledge of the research population will be characterized narrowly in terms of sociodemographic and physical characteristics (e.g., age, ethnicity, sex, height, weight) and in terms of health or disease status. Intimate knowledge of the social customs and resources available within the community in which the patient lives are typically less relevant to the research question.

Given these realities, quantitative research approaches are often applied in basic laboratory research. If it is possible to eliminate or control external and confounding variables (i.e., unwanted variables that may influence and confuse the study findings), it is likely to be quite feasible to conduct controlled and experimental studies when conducting basic laboratory research.

By contrast, applied research (i.e., research conducted in a clinic or in a setting where findings can be easily translatable to practice or some other type of productive action) requires broader knowledge of the participants and a willingness to be flexible to accommodate cultural traditions, work hours, parenting requirements, and other aspects of life that accompany people when they consent to participate in a research study. For example, instead of studying a particular pain medication or type of movement found to facilitate post-mastectomy recovery in clients under the age of 45, imagine you are studying the effects of attending a daily tai chi group on post-mastectomy recovery. Your occupational therapist, who is also a tai chi instructor, is only available to host the group session on Wednesday afternoons. If the majority of your participants have child-care responsibilities or lack transportation to the group sessions, a traditional experimental or quasi-experimental study will fail. In this situation, it would be better to follow a qualitative case-study design, in which tai chi sessions could be conducted in a small number of participants' homes during times that are most convenient to the participants. Knowledge of these and other unique characteristics of your study population is paramount in terms of selecting a research design that is actually possible to execute.

Impact

Most rigorous quantitative research studies involve retaining groups of participants that are large enough (e.g., $N > 15$ to 20 participants per group) to allow for statistical comparison. Typically, studies this large require some type of funding to support activities such as the creation and distribution of consent forms and assessments, implementation of the given treatment, purchase of supplies needed for the treatment, and any reimbursement to the participants for their time and travel. To garner a sufficient amount of grant funding and enthusiasm among participants to participate in the research, the study topic and expected outcome must have sufficient impact and value. Studies that anticipate obvious outcomes or those with little value to participants are not likely to generate the degree of participation that is required for comparison studies. Studies designed to reveal a new innovation, adaptation, or remedy for a significant problem are ones that are considered to have value and impact.

There are circumstances, however, in which a research study is still necessary, even if the anticipated outcome does not have wide-ranging impact or is not perceived as being of any value to the participants. For example, a researcher might need to learn something specific about the participants before designing or applying a treatment or other intervention. In these cases, survey study designs, observational studies, or qualitative (interactive) interviewing may be appropriate design choices.

Participant Feasibility and Preferences

Another important consideration in design choice involves the degree of practicality and feasibility of carrying out the study with the available participants. The easier it is for individuals to participate in your study, the more likely they are to enroll and sustain participation over time. Variables that make it easier for individuals to participate in research include, but are not limited to, the location of the study, the degree of discomfort they may experience during study assessments or procedures, the time required to participate, side effects of any therapies or treatments, and any additional personal risks that may be assumed during or after their participation. Increasing feasibility of participation reduces selection bias and other limitations caused by attrition. Therefore, choosing designs that allow participants to self-select into conditions honors participants' preferences to participate in a certain treatment condition. This will also affect participation and retention rates. If you design a study in which participants are free to self-select into groups, you may bias the findings in terms of selection and nonequivalence of groups, but you may also reduce biases and other feasibility and completion issues introduced by attrition.

Environment

The environment that is available to conduct one's research study may play a significant role in terms of design choice. If you do not have an adequate environment in which to introduce the level of research control necessary in a basic laboratory study, then it is best not to conduct this type of study. Similarly, if you do not have access to the type of community-based environment that would allow participants to share an insider understanding of a certain cultural group, then trying to approximate that environment is not recommended.

Resources

Available resources, such as money, staff, and time, will affect the type of research design you select. Money, staff, and time are all determinants of variables such as:

- How long you may spend with each participant (e.g., 1 day, several weeks, several months, years)?
- How many participants you are able to include in your study?
- How many times you may assess the participants?
- The rigor with which you are able to approach assessment.
- The type, dosage, and length of any intervention you provide.

Mentor Approval

Adequate approval and support from mentors, collaborators, and institutions involved in your research is paramount and must be treated as a first priority in planning any type of study design. If you do not have these approvals and supports, progress of even the best study proposal will be seriously hampered.

Time Frame

Studies range in length, and data collection may take place during a single day, week, month, year, or years. The expected time frame for completion of your study must be acceptable to you, your participants, your mentors and other study collaborators, the sponsoring institution (e.g., your OT department), and the agencies that are funding the research. For example, a study design that involves a lengthy intervention period or multiple measurements over time may not be the best choice for your capstone project, master's thesis, or doctoral project or dissertation. However, if you have been awarded multiple years of funding to conduct a study involving multiple variables, multiple treatment groups, and multiple time points, then you will be expected to work efficiently and quickly within the time that has been provided by your funding agency.

Safety and Ethics

Above all, any design choice must provide for a safe and ethical process for those people involved as participants (as well as for everyone involved in the research). Certain designs may pose unexpected safety or ethical constraints for participants. For example, if a study design involving a no-treatment control group requires participants to undergo a wash-out period in which any current therapy that is being received is discontinued, one must be careful that discontinuing a current therapy is safe and ethical for those involved. Similarly, if, during a study, a treatment is found to be highly successful for the experimental participants and, due to the nature of the design, it is being denied to the control participants, provisions should be made to make the treatment available to all members of the study. The timing of these provisions may need to be immediate if, for example, a treatment is found to be life-saving or extremely vital in preserving functioning, or it may be delayed so that control comparisons can be made before administering the treatment to everyone. Institutional ethics boards approving and overseeing your research will be able to assist you in your decision-making in situations such as these.

Summary

This chapter describes the importance of design choice in research and reviews the major types of designs utilized in quantitative and qualitative research. Additionally, it presents information about the role of validity in selecting a design approach, and it defines four of the most relevant types of validity in quantitative research: statistical conclusion validity, construct validity, internal validity, and external validity (or generalizability). Within the quantitative tradition, true experimental designs that involve random assignment to groups, blinding participants and experimenters to the condition to which participants are assigned, and placebo controls offer the highest level of rigor and minimize threats to validity. However, quasi-experimental designs (in which participants may be randomly selected from an available pool or convenience sample) and nonexperimental designs (that measure associations between existing variables in a data set) may be more feasible, practical, and ethical for many researchers. Qualitative designs, such as case studies, grounded-theory research, phenomenological studies, and ethnographic research, define validity in terms of accuracy of understanding of the subjective experience, values, behaviors, ideology, and other characteristics of participants. Qualitative approaches are typically applied to smaller samples and require in-depth and repeated data collection approaches with multiple reviews and extensive analytic procedures. Choosing the appropriate design for your study ultimately relies on a number of variables, including extent of knowledge of the population, anticipated impact of your study, feasibility, environment, resources, approvals, time frames, and, most importantly, safety and ethics.

Review Questions

1. What are the main considerations in choosing an appropriate design for a given study question?
2. What is an example of a quantitative research design that appropriately balances experimental rigor with feasibility and ethics?
3. What are two additional quantitative research designs that are commonly used in OT

research, and what are their strengths and limits?
4. What are the four types of validity to consider when choosing a research design?
5. How is validity defined differently in qualitative research?
6. What are three threats to validity that accompany the use of quasi-experimental designs?

REFERENCES

Corbin, J., & Strauss, A. (2008). *Basics of qualitative research: Techniques and procedures for developing grounded theory* (3rd ed.). Thousand Oaks, CA: Sage.

Denzin, N.K. (1971). The logic of naturalistic inquiry. *Social Forces, 50,* 166–182.

Denzin, N. K., & Lincoln, Y. S. (1994). Introduction: Entering the field of qualitative research. In N. K. Denzin & Y. S. Lincoln (Eds.). *Handbook of qualitative research* (2nd ed., pp. 163–188). Thousand Oaks, CA: Sage.

Fossey, E., Harvey, C., McDermott, F., & Davidson, L. (2002). Understanding and evaluating qualitative research. *Australian and New Zealand Journal of Psychiatry, 36*(6), 717–732.

Geertz, C. (1973). Thick description: Toward an interpretive theory of culture. In C. Geertz (Ed.), *The interpretation of cultures: Selected essays* (pp. 3–30). New York, NY: Basic Books.

Glaser, B. G. (1965). The constant comparative method of qualitative analysis. *Social Problems, 12*(4), 436–445.

Miller, S., & Fredericks, M. (1999). How does grounded theory explain? *Qualitative Inquiry, 9,* 538–551.

Neuman, W. L. (2003). *Social research methods* (5th ed.). Upper Saddle River, NJ: Prentice Hall.

Popay, J., Rogers, A., & Williams, G. (1998). Rationale and standards for the systematic review of qualitative literature in health services research. *Qualitative Health Research, 8*(3), 341–351.

Rice, P., & Ezzy, D. (1999). *Qualitative research methods: A health focus.* Melbourne, Australia: Oxford University Press.

Shadish, W. R., Cook, T. D., & Campbell, D. T. (2002). *Experimental and quasi-experimental designs for generalized causal inference* (2nd ed.). Stamford, CT: Wadsworth Publishing.

Tesch, R. (1990). *Qualitative research: Analysis types and software tools* (Vol. 337). New York, NY: Falmer Press.

CHAPTER 13

Writing the Research Proposal

Renée R. Taylor

Learning Outcomes

- Identify the uses for a research proposal in occupational therapy.
- Describe the eight major elements of a research proposal.
- Understand the necessity of impact as it relates to a study's background and significance.
- Define a methodological approach that will best accomplish the aims of a study.
- Understand approaches to data analysis.
- Recognize the necessity of a timeline.
- Consider approaches to identifying key personnel in a study.
- Acknowledge the processes and limits involved in defining a study budget.

Introduction

As noted in the previous chapter, a research problem and any corresponding research questions must satisfy two criteria. They must identify any gaps or contradictions in knowledge about a given issue, and they must be of high importance or impact, which is often illustrated in an introductory section addressing the study's background and significance. In occupational therapy, research problems often address issues facing the practice community, such as a particular impairment that is escalating in prevalence or a new treatment method that warrants evaluation. A **research proposal** is a written document that organizes and describes a planned process of research to address the research problem or answer a question. Writing a research proposal is one of the most important skills that an occupational therapy (OT) researcher will develop. Proposals offer blueprints for executing research studies and are often used to secure funding for such studies. As demonstrated in the following Case Example, researchers build their proposals around a specific research problem, which leads to one or more questions of high impact. A clear sense of the research problem and corresponding

questions will facilitate development of a research proposal that is cohesive and easy to follow.

This chapter explains how to incorporate statements of the research problem and question into a comprehensive research proposal, and it outlines the other essential content of a proposal.

Why Write a Research Proposal?

Beyond the fact that students may be required to write a research proposal as part of their coursework in research methods or grant writing, knowing how to write a research proposal opens doors to a wide range of professional opportunities. Outside of formal coursework, many students have their first experience writing a research proposal as part of their master's thesis or doctoral dissertation. During that experience, students quickly learn the importance of writing an effective proposal because the proposal shapes the remainder of their work toward completing the research study or studies that will earn them a degree.

For practicing occupational therapists, the ability to write a research proposal is extremely important in many careers, particularly in industry or government, for OT managers, for those working in not-for-profit or community-based organizations, and for professors in academic settings. OT managers may have the opportunity to write research proposals that have the potential to bring new practice knowledge or equipment into their treatment settings. Occupational therapists working in industry or government may be invited to compete internally within the organization to write a research proposal that, for example, introduces or tests a new assistive technology or device under development. Working for a not-for-profit or community-based organization presents opportunities to write grant proposals to fund applied research and program evaluation research that examines whether the programs offered to clients are needed and effective. For professors in an academic setting, the ability to compete for

CASE EXAMPLE

Geri, an OT doctoral student, just received an assignment to write a research proposal about a topic of relevance to practice. At first, she panics because she does not know where to begin. Her professor encourages her to think critically about a practice situation or a personally relevant experience in health care that made her question something or wish something had been different. Geri thinks for a while, and then she remembers a time when her grandfather underwent shoulder replacement surgery. She recalls that her grandfather was moody from the anesthesia and interpersonally difficult with the occupational therapist who saw him at the time. She considered her grandfather's feedback to the therapist harsh but truthful. He continued to insist that the exercises were uninteresting and had no relevance to his life or his work. Although Geri recalls having been a little unnerved by her grandfather's behavior, she recalls having been more concerned about the occupational therapist, who kept insisting that her grandfather engage in meaningless, repetitive exercises that only caused him pain and aggravation. Geri wondered to herself, "Is this all there is to occupational therapy?" and began to think twice about her career choice.

Once in OT school, Geri discovered different conceptual practice models, one of which is Kielhofner's (2008) Model of Human Occupation (MOHO), which describes how occupational engagement in rehabilitation activities is shaped by the client's interests, perceived self-efficacy, and values (i.e., volition) (Fig. 13.1). Immediately, she accesses her college library from her computer portal and uses various search engines and databases, including the Cumulative Index of Nursing and Allied Health Literature (CINAHL), to search for evidence about the use of MOHO to advance outcomes related to upper extremity rehabilitation in older adults. She is surprised to discover two things: First, she is not the only person who has thought about studying this particular topic. An article by Chen, Neufeld, Feely, and Skinner (1999) found that volition as defined by MOHO (Kielhofner, 2008) was associated with client cooperation and satisfaction with an upper extremity home exercise program. Second, Geri is surprised to find that there have been no extensions of that study or additional publications on this topic since 1999.

Geri faces a choice: (a) She can replicate and extend the Chen et al. (1999) study by studying the role of volition in compliance and satisfaction with inpatient treatment, or (b) she can study the reasons behind therapists' neglect of volition in inpatient orthopedic care. Geri reasons that because it has already been shown that tailoring therapy to a client's volition makes a difference in terms of compliance and satisfaction, she will choose to define the research problem as being a lack of scientific information about the reasons behind therapists' neglect of volition in orthopedic rehabilitation settings. She is now ready to write a proposal for a research study that focuses on this problem of volitional neglect among therapists.

Geri begins by defining three central questions for her study, which are exploratory and descriptive in nature: (1) What proportion of occupational therapists practicing in orthopedic settings formally assess and address elements of a client's volition as a central aspect of treatment? (2) What variables explain a therapist's choice to attend to volition or not to attend to volition in the treatment of a given client? (3) Do treatment approaches incorporating volition lead to

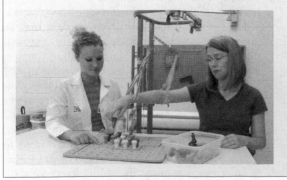

Figure 13.1 MOHO posits that therapeutic interventions are less effective if they do not harness a patient's volition.

improved short- and long-term orthopedic outcomes as compared with those not incorporating volition?

Following definition of the research questions, Geri then reviews the literature in more depth to define the background and significance of these questions. In her review, she looks for studies that illustrate the prevalence and functional and occupational consequences of orthopedic injuries within the general population. It is important for readers to know that orthopedic problems have a significant negative impact on the personal and professional lives of patients and their families, as well as on work productivity and output, leading to larger social and economic consequences. This literature will form the preliminary background to the general problem at hand (orthopedic injury). Next, Geri searches for studies that describe positive outcomes associated with the use of MOHO (Kielhofner, 2008) in practice, seeking to isolate findings that point to a particular emphasis on a client's volition during rehabilitation. Together, the argument that orthopedic injuries are a significant personal and societal problem, and that treatment approaches that incorporate MOHO's volition as an element of treatment, are successful form the background and significance of the proposed study.

grant funding from a range of local, private, and federal funding sources will be determined by how well they are able to write a research proposal.

In sum, learning how to write an effective research proposal affords a range of opportunities, both as a student and as an OT professional. The next section explains how to write each of the components of a clear and effective research proposal.

Elements of a Research Proposal

After conducting a literature review, generating research questions, defining specific aims and hypotheses, and selecting the research methods, the next step is writing the research proposal. A research proposal should contain the following eight components (Fig. 13.2):

1. Statement of the research problem and questions
2. Statement of the research aim and hypothesis
3. Background and significance
4. Methodological approach
5. Data analysis approach
6. Timeline
7. Key personnel
8. Budget

The following sections describe what should be included within each of these components.

1. Statement of the Research Problem and Questions

As covered in Chapter 11, the research problem is a concise phrase or sentence that characterizes

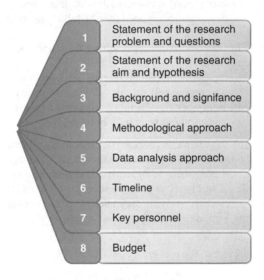

Figure 13.2   The eight elements of a research proposal.

the topic of study. The research question is a similarly concise and detailed question that reflects the knowledge sought in the study. Recall from the Case Example that Geri's research problem was "a lack of information about volitional neglect among occupational therapists working in inpatient orthopedic settings." Some additional examples of research problems and their corresponding research questions include:

- "Lack of parental follow-through on recommended sensory activities at home"
  - What variables explain a complete lack of parental follow-through?
  - What variables explain a partial lack of parental follow through?

- What role does parent education play in rates of parental follow-through?
- "Insufficient knowledge about the role of ergonomic handles in preventing fatigue and injury in a factory setting"
  - Do rates of injury and fatigue decrease significantly when ergonomic handles are installed in a factory setting?
  - What types of ergonomic handles are more effective in preventing fatigue and injury than others?
- "Fear of falling among community-dwelling older adults with cardiovascular illnesses"
  - Are adults who have lost consciousness during a cardiovascular event more likely to report a fear of falling than adults who have not lost consciousness?
  - Are the number and severity of prior cardiovascular events associated with the number of times adults report a fear of falling using a mobile monitoring device?
- "Fine motor difficulties resulting from traumatic brain injury"
  - Compared with usual OT care, will wearing a newly engineered robotics device for at least 12 hours per day facilitate greater fine motor gains following traumatic brain injury?

If you are unable to state your research problem and corresponding question(s) succinctly, you may need to revise them to ensure that the ideas possess the level of clarity and focus necessary for building a research study. It may take several attempts before you are satisfied with the result.

2. Statement of the Research Aim and Hypothesis

As described in Chapter 11, research aims and hypotheses should be built on the research question. Similar to your statement of the research question, your aim and hypothesis should be stated in clear and succinct language. A research aim describes the purpose of the study or what it intends to accomplish. Any statement of the research aim should begin with a phrase such as "The central aim of this study is to...." or "The main objective of this research is to...." Aims should be stated toward the beginning of the first paragraph of the introduction of the research proposal, rather than after several paragraphs or pages. Refer to Chapter 11 for more information and examples.

In quantitative research proposals, the research hypothesis describes the expected outcomes of the study. If there is more than one hypothesis for a study, the hypotheses should be labeled and numbered (e.g., Hypothesis I, Hypothesis II, etc.). Alternatively, a hypothesis may be introduced with the phrase "It is hypothesized that...." or "We hypothesize that...." Refer to Chapter 11 for more information and examples.

3. Background and Significance

The intent of the background and significance section is to accomplish two highly important tasks:

1. Demonstrate your knowledge of the topic area through a focused, comprehensive, and up-to-date review of the literature.
2. Make an argument that your topic is of imminent importance and that your study will have an important impact in terms of increasing knowledge and/or altering outcomes related to the problem.

The ability to demonstrate a keen depth of knowledge and expertise in the topic under study and to link this display of knowledge to the specific aim and study hypothesis is critically important to an effective research proposal. The only way to accomplish this is to know and study the surrounding scientific literature in depth, including any literature and studies that test relevant theoretical concepts that may be referenced in the study. In addition, the planned research must carry the promise of impact. Some people refer to this as the "so what?" question. If your research topic does not leave an individual with the feeling that the world would be a better place for having the knowledge or outcome intended by the study, the time, effort, and money necessary to invest in the research might be better spent studying something else.

The topic must not only carry the promise of impact, you must also be able to effectively convey that potential in writing, as early in the proposal as possible. The fact is, some individuals may not continue reading the proposal beyond the first page, particularly if there are competing proposals to read and time is at a minimum.

To demonstrate that you know enough about the research problem to justify the study, it is important to demonstrate two areas of knowledge:

1. A broad knowledge of the topic area (e.g., traumatic brain injury).
2. A focused knowledge of the research that pertains specifically to your particular aim (e.g., to test an intervention for mild traumatic brain injury resulting from blast concussion sustained by combat veterans).

This kind of expertise is achieved by conducting a comprehensive literature review and doing an extensive amount of reading, then summarizing both areas (the broad and the focused). When conducting the literature review, it is often helpful to organize the articles in terms of categories.

In the example of research on traumatic brain injury, the researcher might categorize one set of studies as "general articles on the prevalence and functional impact of traumatic brain injury" and another set of studies as "interventions for mild traumatic brain injury." If the planned study covers a controversial topic or is a comparative effectiveness study of two interventions that both have a track record of success, the researcher may create two additional categories: one for articles supporting "Intervention A" (e.g., customized video games for improving cognition in mild traumatic brain injury) and one for articles supporting "Intervention B" (e.g., assistive technologies for improving cognitive functioning in mild traumatic brain injury).

The background and significance section of the proposal is where the researcher tells a historical, scientific "story" about the topic and explains why the research could make a difference in people's lives.

4. Methodological Approach

The next important section of the research proposal is the **methods section,** which encompasses the following elements:

- Research design
- Sample, population, and sampling approach
- Subject retention plan
- Assessments or measures
- Procedures
- Ethical review and approval

Research Design

The research design section specifies the overarching methodological tradition (qualitative or quantitative) and the manner in which the sample or sample groups will be compared or otherwise analyzed over time. Examples of research designs covered in this text include, but are not limited to, the following:

- Experimental (randomly assigning subjects to groups and comparing the effects of an intervention on one group against the effects of a placebo or usual-care condition on another group).
- Quasi-experimental (nonrandomly assigning subjects to groups and comparing the effects of

an intervention on one group against the effects of a placebo or usual-care condition on another group).

It is important that the research proposal contains a clear statement about which design is being followed and how that design will be used to address the research questions and hypotheses.

Sample, Population, and Sampling Approach

After determining the most appropriate study design, the researcher decides how to select the research subjects. This involves first identifying the population from which the sample will be drawn, or the **sampling population.** For example, if you want to study the effects of guided meditation on bone pain in end-stage prostate cancer, the sampling population could be identified as men with end-stage prostate cancer who are patients at one of six regional urology clinics in the area. You will then need to determine how to recruit the men into the study, which is referred to as the **recruitment approach.** Ethical review boards are appropriately cautious about what researchers are and are not allowed to do when inviting people to participate in research studies. The main consideration is that people do not feel pressured or coerced to participate. Continuing the example, a brochure about the study distributed at the urology clinics that describes the study and provides a preaddressed, postage-paid form that subjects may mail back to the investigators if interested in participating represents an acceptable means of recruiting subjects into the study.

Next, the researcher chooses the characteristics that the subjects who are actually participating in the study will have (e.g., age, inclusion and exclusion criteria, and what interventions they might be eligible to receive in the study). How the characteristics of the subjects being selected are determined is referred to as the **sampling approach.** The group of subjects who are ultimately eligible to participate in the study defines the **sample.**

Taking the example of men with end-stage prostate cancer, it is known that certain centrally acting medications, such as antidepressants, sleep medications, antianxiety medications, and pain medications, can affect pain perception. Thus, in determining inclusion and exclusion criteria, because you know that medication has the potential to affect the outcomes for men who would be assigned to the guided meditation intervention, you will need to be cognizant of medication usage when recruiting the sample of men from the six urology clinics. Because most men with end-stage cancer experience significant pain and are likely to be taking one or more of these medications, it would not be practical to exclude subjects from participating in the study based on medication usage. However, to measure the effects of medication in a more controlled way, you may decide to exclude subjects taking more than one centrally acting medication and those taking particularly high dosages. All of this information pertaining to your sample is important to include in a research proposal so that readers know that you understand your sampling population well and you have considered and adjusted all of the potential confounds that might interfere with the validity of study findings.

Subject Retention Plan

Proposals that describe **follow-up studies** (i.e., studies examining the long-term effects of an intervention) and descriptive **longitudinal studies** (in which subjects are tracked over time) include retention plans. A **retention plan** specifies how the researcher plans to maintain participation from the subjects in the study over time. Typically, longitudinal and follow-up studies include more than one data collection time point. For example, an epidemiological study is a study of the development and course of an illness over time and the variables that might be associated with that particular illness. A researcher designing an epidemiological study to determine the **incidence** (i.e., rate of new cases of illness) of chronic fatigue syndrome following mononucleosis infection would want to contact prospective participants at the time of initial infection (time 1) and then follow up at 6 months (time 2), 12 months (time 3), and 24 months (time 4) after the infection. This would allow the researcher to determine which subjects do or do not develop fatigue over a 2-year period. Given that most subjects are likely to recover from the infection in the first few weeks or months, it is likely that many would lose interest in participating over time or drop out of the study for other reasons, such as lack of time or other priorities. Moreover, some subjects are likely to move, and they may forget to inform the researchers of their new addresses. Additionally, some subjects may be lost to other forms of attrition, such as death.

For these reasons, a strong retention plan provides a means for researchers to remain in regular contact with subjects between data collection time points. For example, the researchers might contact subjects on their birthdays to wish them a happy birthday, and/or they might conduct monthly outreach calls to thank the individuals for participating in the study and remind them of the importance of their sustained participation. Another retention strategy is to obtain tracking information for each subject at the time of enrollment, such as information about planned moves, contact information of a close friend or relative, alternative phone numbers, employment information, and social security numbers. All of these details are critical to include when writing an effective research proposal.

Assessments or Measures

Another important aspect of the methods section is the description of **assessments** or **measures.** Measures and assessments are the means used to collect the data for studies. In a qualitative study, open-ended interviews or field observations might be used to collect data. For example, a quantitative study might include:

- A survey questionnaire (mainly comprised of a series of fixed-choice questions, with some open-ended questions, assessing factual information, sociodemographic data, opinions, attitudes, or behaviors to be completed in the absence of researcher influence),
- A validated self-report measure (same as a survey questionnaire, but supported by reliability, validity, and/or normative data),
- An observational assessment (systematic observations of specific behaviors made by a trained professional in a predefined setting),
- A structured interview (a series of specific questions that are supported by reliability, validity, and/or normative data, and therefore must be asked as written, in the order presented), or
- A semistructured interview (an interview that contains at least some questions that can be rephrased or reordered).

Additionally, a quantitative study might use a medical instrument or other piece of equipment to record data. For example, a researcher might use goniometry to measure joint range of motion before or after heat therapy. A study of the cardiovascular effects of exercise in adults over 40 with Down syndrome might record peak oxygen uptake as one of the outcome variables. Another study might employ functional magnetic resonance imaging (fMRI) to track brain changes as subjects with Parkinson disease are asked to perform a cognitively stressful task.

In this section of the research proposal, the type of measure or assessment the researcher plans to use should be identified and described in detail. If a self-report, observational, or interview measure will be used, the title of the measure, the full citation with authors, and a description and citation of any study conducted showing the reliability and/or validity of the measure should be included. Similarly, if a piece of equipment will be used, as much information about the equipment as possible (e.g., the name and location of the manufacturer, version or serial number, calibration information, etc.) should be included in the proposal.

In qualitative studies that do not use standardized measures or assessments, sample questions that will be used for interviewing individuals or groups, or prompts that will be used for journaling, are included in this section.

Procedures

The next important component of the methods section that is essential for inclusion in the proposal is the description of **procedures.** The procedures section outlines what will happen in the study, the order in which it will happen, and the timeline according to which it will happen. In an intervention study, the procedures section typically details the intervention plan and contains any **fidelity measures** that will be used to ensure that the therapists abide by the intended treatment protocol. The procedures section also includes a description of the **data collection approach,** detailing how and where data will be elicited from the subjects. Some study topics may necessitate that you follow highly standardized procedures and utilize assessments that are valid and reliable and therefore stable between subjects and over time. Other topics will allow you to use open-ended methods that evolve over the course of the research. Whichever approach is used, the outcome of your study will depend on the accuracy and quality of the data you collect.

Ethical Review and Approval

The final component of the methods section is a statement of plans to obtain approval or existing documentation of **ethical approval** for the study. This may not be required for an in-class assignment in which you are writing a proposal for a fictitious study or one that has not yet been approved by your advisor. However, when writing a research proposal for an actual study, most universities, major teaching hospitals, governmental agencies, and other major organizations that support the conduct of research will require the researcher to apply for ethical approval. The process for obtaining ethical approval is explained in Chapter 14.

5. Data Analysis Approach

A **data analysis approach** should build on the aims and hypotheses, and it should follow the methods section in the proposal. As introduced in the previous chapter, the data analysis approach describes how the data will be organized and scrutinized to test whether the original aims or hypotheses were accomplished. At the broadest level, the approach to data analysis depends on whether the study is qualitative or quantitative.

If the study is qualitative, the nature of the data collected will shape data analysis. Qualitative data may be collected using an interview, focus group, or observational field approach. Qualitative data are most frequently analyzed using some kind of coding procedure that is based on written transcriptions of interview data, photographs, or other data collected. The process of collecting the data may be inductive, and it may evolve as the study evolves (Hammell, Carpenter, & Dyck, 2000). As data are collected, the researcher may begin to notice themes or commonalities. To analyze qualitative data, the researcher may rely on a range of theoretically guided approaches. These approaches are explained in more detail later in this text, and all of these approaches should be detailed in the proposal.

Quantitative data are typically analyzed using statistical methods. Depending on the design of the study, the researcher may use descriptive statistics, inferential statistics, or a combination. **Descriptive statistics** are often used to describe the social and demographic characteristics of the study sample and are also used in descriptive studies to summarize the data. Data are often summarized using frequency, proportion, and percentage data, as well as measures of central tendency and variation, such as means, standard deviations, medians, ranges, and modes. **Inferential statistics** are used in hypothesis testing because they allow the researcher to test whether two groups of people differ in terms of an important characteristic. For intervention studies, they allow the researcher to test whether the study intervention has had an effect on a desired outcome.

For quantitative studies, the proposal should include a description of the specific statistical test that will be used to analyze each aim and/or hypothesis. Often, but not always, the data analysis section pairs the statistical test with the hypothesis, so that the approach to analysis is better understood. For example, a study of workforce resources on an American Indian reservation may offer the following hypothesis and approach to analysis:

Hypothesis 1: Tribal members will be significantly more likely to seek out traditional healers for assistance with a substance abuse problem as compared with licensed mental health providers.

Analysis 1: For each subject, the average number of minutes spent visiting both types of providers during a 1-year period will be summarized in terms of means and standard deviations and compared using a paired samples t-test.

This is just one example of what a statistical analysis plan might look like for a single-hypothesis study.

6. Timeline

Creating a timeline that includes deadlines by which certain activities for your study must be achieved is very helpful when planning any research study. Often, the time during which a study takes place is limited, either by funding, by time available, or both. For example, when conducting a study to fulfill the requirements of a master's degree or doctoral dissertation, most universities allocate a certain number of years until a student is placed on academic probation or dismissed for failure to complete the research in a timely manner. Funding is another factor. Tuition is high, and many studies cost money. Many students do not have the funds necessary to prolong a research study, and most funding agencies will extend funding for a project for only a limited time period. Timelines can be very simple or highly detailed, depending on the complexity of your study and the number of personnel and performance sites. Figure 13.3 presents an example of a simple study timeline for an OT student aiming to complete her doctoral dissertation during a 2-year period.

7. Key Personnel

Unless you propose a small and highly focused research study, most studies will require assistance along the way. If you are a graduate student, it is not highly likely that you will be conducting independent research without the support of your mentor. Generally, your mentor will facilitate your work in a collaborative study involving other students, faculty, and/or professional research collaborators from other departments or institutions. However, in some cases, graduate students are expected to conduct research independently. In these cases, the students may hire or recruit the help of undergraduate volunteers who are interested in the topic under study. Typically, arrangements are made so that the volunteers receive class credit or some other kind of formalized credit as research volunteers. Undergraduate volunteers may be trained in very basic tasks, such as helping to collate forms and enter, check, and clean data. Particularly talented students may even be trained to collect certain types of basic data.

Whether using a staff of volunteers or a paid staff on a grant, whenever you conduct independent research, it is wise to include a personnel plan in the research proposal. A personnel plan should include a list of the key collaborators in the study, their specific roles in the study, and planned duties and contributions. Next to each person's name, an estimation of percentage of workload effort (or hours per week that the person agrees to dedicate to the project) should be provided. This type of plan clarifies the roles and expectations for participation on both sides (the principal investigator managing the study and the project staff), allowing for a means for a manager to remind staff of their duties and for differences to be resolved should questions arise about performance.

8. Budget

No matter how small, every research study costs money. Many graduate students fund their own research, apply for small fellowships or grants dedicated to graduate student research, or piggyback on the funding provided by their faculty mentors or sponsors. Larger studies are more expensive and require more formal mechanisms of funding, such as external grants or internal sponsorship from the home university or institution. These studies require formal budgets, with different categories for each aspect of the research, such as personnel costs (typically a percentage of each collaborator's salary plus fringe benefits, calculated in terms of the workload effort that the collaborator agrees to put forth in the study), supplies costs (e.g., to purchase assessments, make photocopies, etc.), equipment costs (e.g., to purchase computers and other forms of equipment necessary to conduct the research), and indirect costs. Indirect costs are typically a predetermined percentage of the budget that will be allocated to the home institution of the principal investigator to cover the costs of space, facilities, and in-kind resources and equipment that will be used during the study. Different funding agencies will have different budgetary formats and requirements, and it is important to familiarize yourself with these when the time comes for you to apply for formal means of funding.

Year 1   **Months 1–3:** recruit, consent, and enroll subjects; assemble and collate charts containing forms and assessments; order statistical software licenses and set up database for data entry; train study volunteers on data collection approach and data entry, checking, and cleaning.

Months 4–12: continue to recruit, consent, and enroll subjects; collect data as subjects are enrolled; enter data into the database; begin to check and clean entered data.

Year 2   **Months 1–3:** close study to accrual and discontinue enrollment of subjects; continue to collect data for all subjects enrolled; continue to enter data into the database; continue to check and clean entered data.

Months 4–6: finish data collection on all subjects enrolled; discontinue data collection for all subjects by month 6; continue to enter data into the database; continue to check and clean entered data.

Months 7–10: complete data entry, checking, and cleaning; conduct statistical analyses; prepare dissertation for review; begin to present findings and dissertation chapters to committee members and obtain feedback.

Months 11–12: present drafts of dissertation to committee members; respond to feedback; defend final version of the dissertation.

Figure 13.3   Timeline for completion of doctoral dissertation (assuming initial proposal has been written and approved).

Summary

As health-care professionals, we all strive to make a difference in the lives of our clients. One of the primary ways we can make a difference on a large scale is through scientific research. However, all studies require approval from a human subjects review board and/or other persons, such as one's mentor or representatives from a grant funding agency. In this chapter, we reviewed the essential steps required to write a research proposal. Research proposals generally follow a very standard structure that is the same as, or highly similar to, the one presented in this chapter. If you follow this structure, it will naturally guide you through the writing process, and you will not forget any of the requirements that make up a solid research proposal.

Review Questions

1. How should a researcher approach the definition of impact in a research proposal?

2. What roles do a study timeline and budget play in a research proposal?
3. What are two reasons why an OT student or researcher might need to write a research proposal?
4. What are three of the eight major elements of a research proposal?

REFERENCES

Chen, C., Neufeld, P., Feely, C., & Skinner, C. (1999). Factors influencing compliance with home exercise programs among patients with upper-extremity impairment. *American Journal of Occupational Therapy, 53*(2), 171–180.

Hammell, K.W., Carpenter, C., & Dyck, I. (2000). *Using qualitative research: A practical introduction for occupational and physical therapists.* Edinburgh, Scotland: Churchill Livingston.

Kielhofner, G. (2008). *Model of Human Occupation: Theory and application* (4th ed.). Philadelphia, PA: Wolters-Kluwer.

CHAPTER 14

Ensuring Ethical Research

Don E. Workman • Gary Kielhofner • Renée R. Taylor

Learning Outcomes

■ Critique two historical examples of unethical research practices that prompted the need for the regulation of research.
■ Describe key regulations in place to ensure ethical research.
■ Explain the role of HIPAA in occupational therapy research.
■ Outline the role of an institutional review board in protecting human subjects.
■ Summarize the main features of an application to an institutional review board.
■ Delineate ownership issues related to collected data.
■ Define the three main types of research misconduct.
■ Describe the role of the principal investigator in ensuring ethical research.

Introduction

Occupational therapists conducting research are responsible for doing so ethically and with integrity, whether or not there are specific regulations that pertain to the study. To ensure that there is a reasonably objective review of the ethical issues related to human subjects research, many institutions worldwide require that research plans be reviewed and approved by a committee prior to the initiation of a research study. This requirement is reflected in the national regulations of many countries throughout the world. Examples of regulatory bodies in the United States, Canada, Australia, and the United Kingdom are provided in Table 14.1.

Occupational therapy (OT) research may fall under the jurisdiction of specific federal regulations, or it may not be specifically governed by any regulations, depending on the institution and/or country where the research is conducted. In much of the world today, investigators doing research that involves human subjects come under the jurisdiction of national principles and regulations

that govern the ethical conduct of research. When discussing such governmental regulations, this chapter focuses mainly on the United States. However, because these regulations reflect degrees of international consensus about research ethics, they parallel many aspects of how ethical conduct of research is managed throughout much of the world.

Conducting research in an ethical manner requires that the researcher develop knowledge beyond a commonsense understanding of moral issues. This chapter describes the basic ethical principles that should guide the conduct of research and explains the general requirements of applying to an institutional review board for approval of a study. The structure of this chapter is partly based on an Office of Research Integrity publication entitled *Introduction to the Responsible Conduct of Research* (Steneck, 2013).

It is important to note that the practical application of the general principles of integrity and ethics is a complex matter. There are situations when it is impossible to perform research without impinging upon one or more of the ethical principles, in which case the investigator may need to develop additional safeguards to protect the subjects of the research.

For example, one of the basic principles of research ethics requires that subjects only be enrolled in research when they have provided fully informed consent (this is included under the principle of "respect for persons") (National Commission for the Protection of Human Subjects of Biomedical and Behavioral Research, 1979). However, to answer important questions about clinical interventions, some OT research needs to be performed with individuals whose impairments prevent them from fully understanding the research and who therefore have a limited capacity to give informed consent, as mentioned in the Case Example. In such cases the investigator may be required to obtain permission on behalf of the patient from a spouse or other family member before enrolling the patient as a subject of research. In still other situations, it may simply

Table 14.1 International Regulations Governing Research

Country	Regulations
Australia	The National Statement on Ethical Conduct in Research Involving Humans of the National Health and Medical Research Council (available at https://www.nhmrc.gov.au/guidelines-publications/e35) provides guidelines made in accordance with the National Health and Medical Research Council Act of 1992, to which research involving humans must conform.
Canada	The Tri-Council Policy Statement: Ethical Conduct for Research Involving Humans describes the policies of the Medical Research Council (MRC), the Natural Sciences and Engineering Research Council (NSERC), and the Social Sciences and Humanities Research Council (SSHRC).
United Kingdom	The 2005 Research Governance Framework for Health and Social Care (2nd ed.) establishes the standards, principles and requirements that apply to research as it is conducted within the UK health-care system. The framework is available at https://www.gov.uk/government/publications/research-governance-framework-for-health-and-social-care-second-edition.
United States	All research that is funded through the U.S. Public Health Service (PHS) falls under the jurisdiction of the Office for Research Integrity (http://ori.dhhs.gov/). PHS-funded research must be conducted in compliance with the federal regulations at Title 42 of the Code of Federal Regulations (CFR), Part 50 and Subpart A (http://ori.hhs.gov/reg-sub-part-a). In addition, all human subjects research that is funded through the Department of Health and Human Services (HHS), which is part of the PHS, is subject to the oversight of the Office for Human Research Protections (OHRP) (http://www.hhs.gov/ohrp/). The OHRP is responsible for ensuring that HHS-funded research is conducted in accordance with the federal regulations at Title 45, Part 46 of the CFR. The OHRP is the federal office that provides oversight over the local institutional review boards (IRBs), just as the local IRB provides oversight of the human subjects studies that are under way.

not be ethically permissible to enroll the subjects at all (e.g., when the research represents more than minimal risk).

In the end, ethical research depends on the knowledge and integrity of the investigator. Everyone who undertakes an investigation assumes a moral responsibility to abide by commonly accepted ethical standards. This chapter describes compliance with regulatory principles and procedures that enforce these ethical standards. However, it is important to underscore the fact that ethical conduct in research extends beyond compliance with the letter of the law and, instead, requires behavior that is consistent with a knowledgeable awareness of research ethics and an underlying spirit of integrity.

Protection of Human Subjects in Research

Of all the ethical considerations in research, the most compelling pertain to humans who will be subjects or participants in a study. Unfortunately, the impetus for contemporary ethical standards for the protection of human research subjects is grounded in previous abuses of humans under the guise of research.

Historical Unethical Research Practices

Two of the most well-known cases of unethical research practices are the Nazi Doctors Trials and the Tuskegee Experiments.

Nazi Doctors Trials

In the **Nazi Doctors Trials** investigating war crimes following World War II, the tribunal identified numerous experiments that had been conducted in the "interests" of science, which represent horrific abuses of human beings. For example, concentration camp prisoners were exposed to low atmospheric pressures to simulate what might happen to pilots if they were exposed to atmospheric conditions at high altitudes. Individuals would lapse into coma, and sometimes died, as the Nazi scientists established some of the limits of human endurance. In other experiments, prisoners were placed naked into tubs of icy water to establish limits for hypothermia. They were then often "rescued" using various techniques that sometimes produced scalding burns and even death.

Although these experiments provided the Nazi military with valuable information regarding the length of time human beings can survive in water at various temperatures and information

CASE EXAMPLE

For her doctoral research project, Reina is planning to complete a study on therapeutic empathy in a neurosurgical rehabilitation unit. For her study, she intends to videotape therapy sessions during which occupational therapists interact with clients during standardized (usual-care) rehabilitation activities. One-half of the occupational therapists will have been exposed to Taylor's (2008) Intentional Relationship Model, and one-half will not. Using an observational measure based on the Intentional Relationship Model, she plans to have a panel of three experienced occupational therapists view the digital recordings of the recorded therapy sessions and rate the level of empathy shown by the therapists during the standardized rehabilitation activities. Reina's hypothesis is that occupational therapists who have been exposed to the Intentional Relationship Model will be more likely to show empathy during rehabilitation sessions than those who have not been exposed.

Although this study would likely be classified by an institutional review board (IRB) as involving minimal risk, Reina must consider a number of issues when making her application for human subjects approval. First, she must consider the issue of consent. Because of the effects of medication and/or post-neurosurgical cognitive impairment, many of the subjects in her study may have impaired decision-making ability. This may interfere with their capacity to read the consent form and give informed consent to be observed and videotaped during treatment. Reina would have to build in assurances for consent, such as gathering consent from the client's partner, relative, or attorney who may be serving in a guardianship capacity during the client's recovery period.

Another issue for consideration is the risk-versus-benefit ratio in the study. Clearly, there is no direct benefit to clients for participating in the study. One might argue that videotaping them during treatment will not change the treatment in any significant way, particularly if the therapists being videotaped are blinded to the exact reason that they are being recorded. By contrast, there are some risks to clients, including the intrusiveness and lack of privacy involved in having a person in the treatment room operating the video camera and the risk for loss of confidentiality and Health Insurance Portability and Accountability Act (HIPAA) violations, should the recorded material become lost or otherwise fall into the wrong hands.

In addition to considering these risks, Reina must be sure that all of the personnel assisting her with her study have been trained in ethics, the protection of human subjects, and HIPAA regulations. The confidentiality of participants must be protected to the greatest extent possible. This can be done by separating the consent forms containing subject names and any other assessments containing identifying information from study data (e.g., the digital recordings), keeping the consent forms in a locked cabinet in a separate room from the digital recordings, and redacting the identifying information on the assessment forms.

Moreover, Reina must train the individuals who obtain informed consent from the clients and/or guardians to obtain consultation from a neurosurgeon, neurologist, or neuropsychologist regarding the client's capacity to give consent. Study personnel should also be able to assess this capacity independently as a cross-check measure. Therapists working with the clients and the person operating the video camera should also be trained to respond to the client's questions about the equipment and to provide an explanation of assurances for the protection of confidentiality, when questioned. All of these risks must be identified, and provisions must be explained in Reina's IRB application. Once the study begins, the provisions must be followed as written.

about effective methods for reviving soldiers who were partially frozen, those hapless prisoners were involuntarily exposed to experimental torture and even death.

The experiments by the Nazi doctors were ethically reprehensible because they caused harm without regard for the well-being or for the informed consent of the subjects. They also exposed individuals to unacceptably high levels of risk without regard for their pain and suffering, and in ways in which the risks were not reasonable in light of the benefit that might be gained from the information that was derived from the research.

Tuskegee Experiments

When an agency of the U.S. Public Health Service (PHS) began its study of syphilis in the African

American male in 1932, the researchers selected a rural area in the South (Macon County, Alabama) where there was a high concentration of men who had the disease (Dunn & Chadwick, 2012). They intended to study the natural history of the disease for a period of 6 months, but then considered the research important enough that it was continued for 40 years. They collected spinal fluid through nontherapeutic lumbar punctures, telling the unknowing research subjects that they were being provided with treatment for "bad blood." This research later became known as the **Tuskegee Experiments.**

In 1943, penicillin was recognized as an effective treatment for syphilis. In the eyes of the researchers from the PHS, this made the cohort of patients in the "Tuskegee" experiment even more valuable because they might be one of the last cohorts of individuals with the disease who would be studied longitudinally (over a long period of time). For this reason, the PHS researchers made additional efforts to ensure that their research subjects remained under study. This meant preventing them from knowing they had a disease and from obtaining medical treatment for syphilis. During World War II, the PHS investigators managed to convince the local draft board not to enlist any of the "Tuskegee" subjects into the armed forces because they would have been readily diagnosed and treated.

In retrospect, and from a perspective outside of the investigators, this is easily viewed as a morally repugnant study. Investigators deceived innocent and vulnerable men into thinking they were getting some form of treatment, when they were actually being denied information about a disease they had (and were sharing with others in their community), were not being provided with treatment for their syphilis, and were actively prevented from receiving a newly validated treatment (penicillin). This study was exposed by the media in 1972 and finally halted in 1973. The public outcry led to regulations, the IRB, and federal oversight processes that make up today's human subjects protection programs in the United States (Dunn & Chadwick, 2012).

Nuremberg Code

One of the earliest U.S. codes regarding the ethical conduct of research was written during the Nazi Doctors Trials. Because the trials were conducted in Nuremberg Germany, the 10 principles of ethical human subjects research became known as the **Nuremberg Code.** The full code can be accessed at https://history.nih.gov/research/

downloads/nuremberg.pdf. Box 14.1 gives an abbreviated version.

The Principles of Belmont

In 1979, the U.S. National Commission for the Protection of Human Subjects of Biomedical and Behavioral Research published a document summarizing for the Department of Health, Education and Welfare (later to become the U.S. Department of Health and Human Services, or HHS) the basic ethical principles for human subject research. The paper distinguishes between clinical practice and clinical research and sets out three basic principles that are intended to apply to all research involving humans (U.S. Department of Health and Human Services, 1979). The three **Principles of Belmont** are respect for persons, beneficence, and justice.

Respect for Persons

Respect for persons, the most basic of the three principles, asserts that humans must be respected in terms of their right to self-determination. Key to this principle is the notion of informed consent as a required prerequisite for most kinds of research, especially when the research involves imposing some risks on the subjects.

The Belmont Report's principle of respect for persons emphasizes the importance of the individual to make choices regarding whether or not to participate in a research study as an exercise of free will. Respect for persons assumes that the researcher can provide enough information, in a language the prospective subject can understand, for the individual to provide fully informed consent to be involved in the research. The report states that there are circumstances and populations for which fully informed consent is not possible, and the report requires that additional protections be afforded to these "vulnerable populations." Pregnant women and fetuses are considered to be a vulnerable population, as are prisoners and children.

Beneficence

Beneficence is the principle requiring that human subjects research must minimize risk to the greatest extent possible and maximize the potential for benefits to be gained from the research (either for the individuals participating in the research or from the knowledge that will be gained). Risks must be reasonable in relation to the potential for benefit to be derived from the research. The risks considered include reasonably anticipated physical and mental risks and physical and mental discomforts.

BOX 14.1   Selected Content From the Nuremburg Code

1. The voluntary consent of the human subject is absolutely essential.
2. The experiment should be such as to yield fruitful results for the good of society, unprocurable by other methods or means of study, and not random and unnecessary in nature.
3. The experiment should be so designed and based on the results of animal experimentation and a knowledge of the natural history of the disease or other problem under study, that the anticipated results will justify the performance of the experiment.
4. The experiment should be so conducted as to avoid all unnecessary physical and mental suffering and injury.
5. No experiment should be conducted, where there is an a priori reason to believe that death or disabling injury will occur; except, perhaps, in those experiments where the experimental physicians also serve as subjects.
6. The degree of risk to be taken should never exceed that determined by the humanitarian importance of the problem to be solved by the experiment.
7. Proper preparations should be made and adequate facilities provided to protect the experimental subject against even remote possibilities of injury, disability, or death.
8. The experiment should be conducted only by scientifically qualified persons. The highest degree of skill and care should be required through all stages of the experiment of those who conduct or engage in the experiment.
9. During the course of the experiment, the human subject should be at liberty to bring the experiment to an end, if he has reached the physical or mental state, where continuation of the experiment seemed to him to be impossible.
10. During the course of the experiment, the scientist in charge must be prepared to terminate the experiment at any stage, if he has probable cause to believe, in the exercise of the good faith, superior skill and careful judgement required of him, that a continuation of the experiment is likely to result in injury, disability, or death to the experimental subject.

Source: *Trials of War Criminals Before the Nuremberg Military Tribunals Under Control Council Law No. 10,* Vol. 2, pp. 181-182. Washington, DC: U.S. Government Printing Office, 1949. Retrieved from https://www.loc.gov/rr/frd/Military_Law/NTs_war-criminals.html

Beneficence also requires the use of sound research methodology because no degree of risk is acceptable if the research design is inadequate. That is, there would be little likelihood for benefit from the knowledge to be gained if the study is not sound, and without any anticipated benefits, no risk to subjects is justified.

Finally, beneficence also requires that risks must be minimized. This means that investigators should take every precaution and make every effort to anticipate and prevent or minimize physical or mental discomfort or harm that may accrue from participation in the study.

Justice

The principle of **justice** requires that the research impose the burden of risk and the potential for benefit upon the same groups of people. It is unacceptable from the perspective of the principle of justice for an investigator to take advantage of a vulnerable population (e.g., the poor) in order for others to reap the benefits of the research. Consequently, ensuring justice typically involves examination of the composition of subjects who have been enrolled according to such categories as gender and race/ethnicity.

Declaration of Helsinki

In addition to the Belmont Report, the Declaration of Helsinki sets forth the principles regarding the ethical conduct of human subjects research originally adopted by the World Medical Association in 1964. The current document, adopted in 2000, includes 32 principles and has two subsequent clarifications (World Medical Association, 2015). It is the responsibility of the investigator to determine the applicable rules and procedures for any study being initiated.

Health Insurance Portability and Accountability Act of 1996

Within the United States, the Health Insurance Portability and Accountability Act (HIPAA) was introduced by the U.S. Congress and signed into law by President Bill Clinton in 1996. It may be accessed online through the website of the U.S. Government Printing Office (http://www.gpo.gov/fdsys/pkg/PLAW-104publ191/html/PLAW-104publ191.htm).

Title II of HIPAA provides policies and procedures for ensuring the privacy and security of each person's medical records and other health information. It also provides for protections against fraud and abuse within the health-care system and requires the development of rules aimed to increase efficiency within the health-care system by creating standards for using and disseminating the health-care information of all individuals seeking care.

Maximizing Potential for Benefit

In light of these important reports, declarations, and acts, it is important to maximize the potential that subjects will benefit from participating in a research study. There are numerous ways in which the IRB and the investigator can design the study to maximize potential for benefit, both for the individual subjects and from the potential knowledge that may be gained from the research. For instance, a study might increase the potential for individual subjects to benefit by incorporating a crossover design rather than a placebo control. In the case of the placebo control, those subjects receive no therapy at all, whereas in the crossover design, everyone has a period of time when they are receiving the new treatment. The IRB's insistence on sound research methodology is a way for ensuring that there is a maximum potential for benefit from the research in terms of its provision of generalizable knowledge.

Institutional Review Boards and Ethics Committees

An **institutional review board (IRB)** is a mechanism for regulatory oversight that exists within a university, medical center, or other industry in which one or more committees of informed individuals review research proposals to ensure that the proposed study is safe and ethical for all participants (including any animals and biological materials that may be used in the research).

Most institutions that have research involvement have established committees that oversee issues of ethical conduct in research. In the international context, these bodies are usually referred to

as ethics committees. In the United States, research institutions that receive federal funding for human subject research are required to have an IRB that exercises oversight authority over the research (Steneck, 2013). In such institutions, an individual must be designated to oversee this process; that individual is usually given a title such as research integrity officer.

IRBs are comprised of a group of diverse individuals with both scientific and nonscientific interests. Often, there are requirements for representation from a specific number of scientists from specific disciplinary backgrounds plus representation from a community member who is not a scientist. There may be other requirements, such as the necessity for representation of both men and women and the inclusion of individuals from diverse racial and ethnic backgrounds.

The IRB is responsible for reviewing applications, and each application must include a study protocol. The study protocol may be included within an appended research proposal (such as a grant-funding application or similar proposal) to ensure there are adequate provisions to minimize risk and maximize the potential for benefit from the research (to the subjects or from the knowledge that will be gained). The IRB is also responsible for ensuring that adequate safeguards are in place, including the requirements for informed consent, so that the risks to subjects are minimized to the greatest extent possible.

The IRB process starts with the submission of an application, which is typically completed on a paper or electronic form and submitted in person or via a secure online portal. The application is then reviewed by a board of appointed individuals who read the applications and then meet to deliberate on a specific date (Fig. 14.1). Following

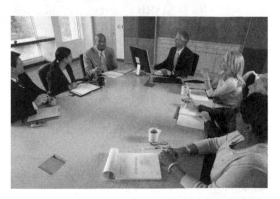

Figure 14.1 An institutional review board (IRB) reviews a research proposal. *(ThinkStock/Digital Vision/Thomas Northcut.)*

review and deliberation, the board may write back to the candidate via a letter containing specific questions, requirements, or concerns for the applicant to address in a subsequent, revised application. Subsequent exchanges between the applicant and review board, which are typically all done in writing, may involve several series of responses to questions and modifications of the research plan, recruitment materials, and informed consent documents before the project is approved. Once a study is approved and started, the IRB will notify the applicant in writing. After this time, continuing review applications will be required from the applicant (typically annually) until study completion, at which time a final report of research activity is required.

The extensiveness of this process varies by institution, but it typically involves furnishing the research application or an abbreviated version of the application. It also requires that the researcher respond in writing to a series of questions about the safety and ethicality of the research. The reviewers will want to know that subjects will not be coerced to participate or remain in the study, that any interventions or assessments will not harm the subjects, that any risk of harm introduced by the study is significantly outweighed by the predicted outcomes of the study, and that subjects are fully consented and informed about all aspects of the research as it unfolds during the study. Additionally, review panels often require researchers to provide samples of the materials used to recruit subjects and examples of the written consent forms (and any other scripted procedures) used to obtain informed consent from subjects.

The specific operations of the IRB and the application of the regulations (laws) vary from one institution to another. They also may vary depending on the source of funding or the nature of the research. For these reasons, it is important to consult your local IRB to obtain the application and follow-up policies and procedures required by the institution for which you are working. IRBs are responsible for making numerous determinations about the level of risk related to participation in the research, the adequacy of the informed consent documents or processes, and the appropriateness of recruitment materials, as well as ensuring there are additional safeguards for protecting vulnerable subjects.

Many institutions provide forms or structured formats for submitting information to the IRB for approval. They generally publish guidelines, procedures, and forms that are used to submit proposed research and research progress reports. Investigators are responsible for identifying and complying with these procedures and completing the necessary documentation. In some institutions, the principal investigator and other members of the research team are required to undergo training in research ethics before submitting research for approval.

If a study receives initial approval and is started, investigators are required to promptly submit to the IRB information related to unanticipated problems involving risks to subjects or others. The IRB then reviews the issue and requires changes or approves any planned modifications to the research before they are implemented. Exceptions are made if changes to the protocol would remove subjects from risk of immediate harm; in this case, investigators immediately make the changes, notify the IRB, and submit an amendment as soon as possible.

If a research study is not approved by the IRB, the IRB is required to inform the investigator what changes to the research would make it approvable. It is then up to the researcher whether she or he will revise the study protocol and application accordingly. If the researcher refuses to revise the study protocol and application as requested by the IRB, then she or he will be prohibited from conducting the research study.

Until the IRB has approved the study, the investigator cannot proceed with the research. As noted earlier, approval sometimes involves several steps in which the IRB responds to the original or previous submission with questions and required changes. Investigators should determine the deadlines for submission of IRB documentation and the schedule of IRB meetings, factoring these into overall deadlines and planning for a research project.

Once the research is under way, the IRB is responsible for substantive re-review of the research no less often than once every 365 days.

Submitting an Application to an IRB

One of the first steps in planning and ensuring the ethical nature of a research study involves submitting an application to your local IRB. As discussed previously, most institutions provide guidelines and forms for investigators to use. Generally, IRB applications require the following major components: informed consent, description of the research protocol, an assessment of the risks and benefits of the study, assurance of adequate representation (by gender, race, age, and ethnicity), consideration of issues related to vulnerable populations, and evidence of the training of key personnel. In the following sections, each of these aspects is reviewed.

Informed Consent

The principle of **informed consent** requires that prospective research subjects be given enough information, before they choose to participate in a research study, that they can make an informed decision as to whether or not they wish to participate. Although circumstances exist in which the requirement of prospective informed consent may be waived or altered, usually research involving human subjects requires that they provide written informed consent (and possibly a HIPAA authorization for research use of protected health information, or PHI) before they participate in the research.

Informed consent usually requires that subjects be prospectively informed that they are being asked to participate in research, that their participation is voluntary, and that they may choose to discontinue their participation at any time. Prospective subjects must also be informed of reasonably anticipated risks and discomforts from participation, as well as any benefits that may be expected to result from their participation or from the knowledge gained from the study. The IRB may waive or alter the required elements of informed consent under some circumstances. For example, if a researcher has access to data that were collected in the past as part of a treatment or educational process, those data do not contain information that would identify the respondents in any way, and the researcher now wants to analyze those data for a research study, the researcher may apply for a waiver of consent. Because it would be impossible to go back to the subjects who originally provided the data (because they are anonymous), an IRB might grant a waiver of consent that would allow the researcher to conduct the requested analyses. This would be particularly likely if the proposed analyses were of low risk and high value to the scientific community and to the public.

The Process of Consent

Two central components of informed consent are a well-written informed consent document and a process for obtaining consent that involves a careful review of the information in the document with ample opportunity for the prospective subject to have any questions answered. The process under which investigators inform prospective subjects about the research is as crucial as the document that the subject signs. The discussion about consent that occurs between the researcher and the subject should reflect the information in the consent document, but it should also include questions to allow the person obtaining consent to be assured that the potential subject understands the information that is being presented.

Consent is not usually a one-time event; rather, it is an ongoing process throughout a subject's participation in research. During a prolonged study, it may be prudent to revisit the consent document, ask about willingness to continue in the research, and offer to answer questions about ongoing participation.

Assent and Surrogate Permission

Because consent refers to the process whereby competent adults give permission for something to be done to their own person or information, one cannot give consent for something to be done to another individual. Therefore, in the case of children and adolescents, the regulations usually require a combination of parental permission and the active assent (not the failure to dissent) of the children and adolescents. In the case of adults who may have cognitive impairments (e.g., psychotic episodes or dementia), the researcher must obtain the assent of such persons to the extent they are able to provide it and the permission of a surrogate. Ideally the surrogate is a legally authorized agent under the local laws. When such laws do not exist, it is important for the investigator who is enrolling adult subjects who are cognitively impaired to consult with legal counsel to ensure that appropriate surrogate consent is being obtained.

Documentation of Consent

The documentation of consent refers to obtaining the appropriate signature on IRB-approved consent or assent document(s). The original documents are very important to keep because any audit of the research study will require the investigator to produce them. Funding agencies require that these original documents be maintained for a number of years after the completion of the study. Investigators are usually required to provide a copy of the consent document to the subjects as an information sheet they can take with them. Under HIPAA, if an investigator is also obtaining an authorization for the research use of PHI, the investigator is required to provide subjects with a copy of the signed consent document.

Informed consent is often a complex process that involves a number of considerations. These include, for instance:

- Making sure the prospective subject understands the study and the risks/benefits involved (this increasingly involves not only ensuring that the study will be explained in lay terms but also indicating how the researcher will ascertain that the subject has understood what was explained).
- Consideration of whether prospective subjects have the ability to give consent and whether others may provide consent on their behalf.
- Balancing any incentives or reimbursement for participation to avoid coercion (e.g., giving financial incentives that would be difficult for some potential subjects to decline).

Ensuring freedom of consent in situations in which other obligations or roles might pressure individuals to consent is important. For example, a charge nurse might feel pressured to participate in a study being conducted by her colleague, who is an OT professor, because she wants to maintain good relations between the college of nursing and the department of occupational therapy. It is important that the investigators consider and make plans to manage these and other considerations that may be unique to a particular study when developing informed consent procedures.

Description of the Research Protocol

When applying for IRB approval, it is important to describe every aspect of the study in lay language. A clear and cross-disciplinary description of the study protocol ensures that all members of the review panel, regardless of their level of knowledge, are able to understand the relative risks and benefits of the study. From reading the protocol, reviewers should understand exactly what will happen to the subjects, both during and after their participation.

Assessment of Risks and Benefits

Every IRB application requires a thorough consideration of all potential risks to the individuals participating in the study. Many basic OT studies do not pose more than minimal risks to subjects. Many of the procedures used within the rehabilitation environment are noninvasive and do not require subjects to take medications, provide biological samples, or endure surgical procedures. Examples of risks to subjects in these types of OT studies include the loss of confidentiality, negative emotional consequences of responding to assessments that tap sensitive content, and falls and other types of physical harm or injury during rehabilitation-related physical activities or exercises. In these kinds of studies, it is not only important to explain and demonstrate how the experimenters will enforce assurances to minimize risk, but it is also important to justify how the expected benefits of the experimental procedures outweigh the risks.

For example, a study of the effects of daily stretching and self-massage on pain levels in otherwise healthy older adults with hypertonic muscles carries the risks of increased pain during stretching of pulled muscles and increased pain related to carrying out the procedures improperly. The benefits, however, are likely to exceed the risks if the stretching and self-massage are performed properly and at a level that the client can tolerate. For an IRB application, the investigator would need to explain that the anticipated reduction in pain far outweighs the risks for increased pain as a result of improper execution of study procedures.

Occupational therapists pursuing more complex, multidisciplinary studies may be involved in procedures that pose more than minimal risks to subjects, such as surgical procedures, higher-risk exposures, and pharmaceutical agents. All invasive procedures are accompanied by the risk for infection, at minimum. Risks when using pharmaceutical agents include negative and/or unknown side effects, withdrawal effects, and interaction effects. In these cases, it becomes particularly important that the potential benefits expected to emerge from the study outweigh the anticipated risks and that all risks are minimized to the greatest extent possible.

Assurance of Adequate Representation of the Sample

Racial, ethnic, and sociocultural diversity characterizes the U.S. population and many other populations around the world. Ensuring that a sample of individuals in a study adequately represents the diversity within the general population of subjects to which your findings may be generalized is not only methodologically indicated, it is also an ethical imperative. If an investigator intends to systematically exclude any group of subjects from a study based on gender, race, ethnicity, age, income level, educational level, national origin, language, or any other variable, he or she needs to have a sound rationale for the exclusion. For example, one might make an argument for the exclusion of men from a study of breast cancer if the group of individuals under study includes women with a sex-linked genetic polymorphism. In this case, it would be impossible for men with breast cancer to have this polymorphism. Unless there are well-justified exceptions that are grounded in science, researchers must ensure that the sample adequately represents the diversity of the population under study.

Consideration of Issues Related to Vulnerable Populations

Vulnerable populations include individuals who do not have the capacity to consent to participate in research or who may be pressured into participating for the wrong reasons. Examples of vulnerable populations include:

- Prisoners (because they represent a captive audience and may fear negative consequences for not participating).
- Pregnant women (because research may pose additional unknown risks to pregnant women and their fetuses).
- Fetuses and neonates (because it is not known how certain research activities would affect fetuses and neonates because these populations are not easily accessible and thus have not been studied extensively).
- Employees and students of the institution out of which the study is being conducted (because these individuals may feel unduly pressured to participate or fear that findings that emerge from participation may negatively affect their status as students or employees).
- Individuals with impaired decision-making capacity (because they are not able to provide consent in a fully informed way).
- Educationally or economically disadvantaged people (because they may be more vulnerable to coercion or pressure to participate out of a need to access health care or for some other gain unrelated to and not guaranteed by the intentions of the study protocol).
- Other individuals who are vulnerable to coercion or undue influence.

When conducting research with these populations, extra protections must be in place to ensure that the subjects are not, by virtue of their vulnerable status, subject to undue risk for harm.

Evidence of the Training of Key Personnel

Another critical aspect of an IRB application is the requirement to show evidence that anyone participating in obtaining consent from subjects, collecting data, administering interventions, analyzing data, and presenting or writing findings has adequate training and knowledge about the protection of human subjects. Depending on your institution, trainings may include face-to-face classroom sessions and/or online courses on human subjects protection, ethics, and HIPAA regulations. Training must then be supplemented by continuing education throughout an investigator's career.

Research Integrity

The Office of Research Integrity (2013) has identified nine core areas that need to be addressed for investigators to know how to conduct research responsibly (DuBois & Dueker, 2009):

1. Data acquisition, management, sharing, and ownership
2. Conflict of interest and commitment
3. Human subjects
4. Animal welfare
5. Research misconduct
6. Publication practices and responsible authorship
7. Mentor/trainee relationships
8. Peer review
9. Collaborative science

The subsequent sections explain the primary issues for consideration within these nine areas.

Data Acquisition, Management, Sharing, and Ownership

In the practice of science, data collection and storage are crucial activities. Given the advent of the personal computer and the proliferation of easy ways to replicate, share, and store electronic copies of data (e.g., laptop computers, handheld storage devices, flash memory cards, e-mail, and cloud-based computing), there are many new mechanisms that can be used to facilitate the acquisition, management, sharing, and ownership of data. Although these mechanisms streamline many aspects of research, they also require additional care to ensure that confidentiality protections and verification agreements are in place regarding how data are stored, managed, shared, and owned.

In conducting research, there may be one or many people who collect the data, but collecting the data does not necessarily infer rights of ownership over that data. There may be important limits to what one can ethically do with the data that are collected. For instance, when research is funded through a grant by the federal government, the research institution (e.g., university or hospital) is assigned ownership rights to the data gathered under that research. In this case, the research institution is accountable for ensuring the integrity of the data that are collected, and neither the individual researcher nor the government has immediate ownership rights to the data—they belong primarily to the research institution that received the award (e.g., grant).

In other cases, the federal or state government may fund research through a contract, in which case the data are usually required to be "delivered" to the government, which then retains ownership interest. In the case of research that is sponsored (funded) by a private corporation, there is usually a contract that specifies the terms of the funding that is provided and clarifies that ownership of data resides with the private corporation, which retains this right in hopes of applying it for commercial use. Philanthropic organizations can also fund research; these organizations may either retain rights or give them away depending on their interests.

Finally, there are student research projects and clinician-initiated studies in which the ownership interests in the data are not clearly articulated or understood. It is important for researchers to understand the nature of the agreements that provide funding for the research as well as any applicable policies in the settings where the research is conducted in order to know whether or not they have the right to publish those data.

Accepted Practices

For the results of research to be of value, it is essential that the data that are gathered are reliable. There is no one way to ensure the reliability of the data, but responsible investigators will use acceptable standards within their fields of research to ensure the careful collection of accurate information. In addition, investigators must understand (or consult with others who understand) statistical methods adequately to ensure that they are using an appropriate strategy for the analysis of the data. Although this point is covered elsewhere in this text as an issue of scientific rigor, it is important to understand that following accepted scientific practice is also an ethical mandate.

Data Collection

Investigators must also understand what levels of authorization might be required in order to collect data. For instance, under HIPAA, individuals who are collecting PHI for research purposes in a setting such as a clinic or hospital are required

to obtain the written authorization of the patient/subject, a data use agreement from the clinic or hospital, or a waiver of authorization from the IRB.

Data Storage

Finally, the investigator must ensure that data are properly protected to ensure the integrity of the data. This often means using appropriate filing strategies, including security measures such as locked file cabinets within locked offices and password-protected files on electronic storage devices. In many circumstances data must be retained for a number of years after they are published or after the funding period is over. Specific data retention policies for the institution where data are gathered and stored should be consulted before data, signed consent documents, and authorizations are destroyed.

Investigators frequently store their raw data on paper documents called case-report forms. This information may subsequently be summarized in computer files for statistical analysis or for creating charts or graphs. The investigator should maintain the "source documents" in a locked file cabinet as well as the appropriately protected and secured electronic files for some time after the results of the research are published or the grant or contract has ended.

Under HIPAA, individuals who collect PHI for research purposes are required to store all electronic protected health information (e-PHI) according to acceptable standards. Each covered entity (e.g., clinic or hospital) is required to develop its own policies and procedures for ensuring the security of e-PHI. When using Internet-based storage, your institution should have a written agreement with a provider that protects your data under HIPAA. Researchers must be sure to comply with the applicable policies for their institutions.

Conflicts of Interest and Commitment

A **conflict of interest** is a situation in which the researcher derives personal benefit from the research at the expense of subjects and/or the institution in which the research is being conducted. There can be numerous conflicts of interest in a research enterprise. One of these conflicts stems from the desire to attain status and gratification from being the one to make new information available to others. It is important in research not to make public statements about the results of the research prematurely. When preliminary results are presented, this practice is usually limited to presentations at scientific meetings where the audience will understand and the presenter can clearly articulate the results as being preliminary and subject to additional analysis and the scrutiny of peer review before being published for more general scientific consumption. Another source of conflict of interest occurs when a researcher is a part owner of a company whose product is being tested.

In addition, there are circumstances in which the research results are not favorable, and thus the reporting of those results could compromise the funding opportunity or career of the researcher. There are times when it would be a clear violation of principles of integrity to hide or suppress unexpected, contrary, or negative results for the sake of self-promotion or interest.

Conflict of commitment refers to issues that may prevent researchers from expending their full energy and effort for their primary employment and, in particular, for discharging research obligations. Examples include hours spent on an outside job or other income-generating activity. Local institutions often develop their own thresholds and definitions of when an activity constitutes a conflict of financial interest or commitment. Both the investigator and the research team members are responsible for complying with the institutional and federal requirements for disclosure and management of conflicts of interest and commitment.

Human Subjects

Whenever a person is invited and consents to participate in any kind of research (i.e., information gathering and sharing), that person is defined as a **human subject.** People are considered to be human subjects at the time they consent and are enrolled in a study. This is true regardless of whether they serve as controls (receiving no intervention) or as experimental subjects receiving assessments and/or interventions. Conflicts of interest and commitment must always be considered when conducting human subjects research.

Animal Welfare

Animal welfare involves protecting the physical and emotional well-being of animals that are being used in research. When animals are used in research, numerous protections must be in place requiring veterinary oversight over any procedures that are conducted. Provisions are made to ensure that animals are properly anesthetized and cared for throughout any study procedures.

Research Misconduct

In the United States, the Office of Research Integrity (ORI; refer to Table 14.1) is responsible for the promotion of the responsible conduct of research (RCR) and resolution of allegations of research misconduct. The criteria for research misconduct are outlined in the U.S. regulations at Title 42 of the Code of Federal Regulations (CFR) 50.102. More information about the Title 42 regulations may be accessed at the website of the U.S. Government Printing Office (http://www.gpo.gov/fdsys/granule/CFR-2000-title42-vol1/CFR-2000-title42-vol1-sec50-102).

To qualify as misconduct, the behavior of the investigator or member of the research team must represent a significant deviation from commonly accepted practices. Moreover, it must be intentional, knowing, or reckless. The ORI has established and follows a number of federal policies for resolving allegations of misconduct. The following is the ORI's definition of misconduct:

> **Misconduct** in Science means fabrication, falsification, plagiarism, or other practices that seriously deviate from those that are commonly accepted within the scientific community for proposing, conducting, or reporting research. It does not include honest error or honest differences in interpretations or judgments of data. (*Cited from 42 CFR 50.102*)

Fabrication, falsification, and plagiarism constitute the primary issues that fall under research misconduct. **Fabrication** is defined as making up data or results and recording or reporting them (42 CFR 93.103[a]). For example, an OT graduate student has been told by his advisor that a minimum of 30 subjects will be needed for a thesis project he is undertaking. The student obtained data on 29 subjects and is facing a deadline that would prevent graduation on time. Under the pressure of time, the student fabricates a 30th subject, entering that subject into the database for analysis.

Falsification is defined as manipulating research materials, equipment, or processes or changing or omitting data or results such that the research is not accurately represented in the research record (42 CFR 93.103[b]). For example, two OT researchers involved in a qualitative study have data providing support for a conceptual argument they have previously published in the literature. They are discussing the data in a research team meeting when a research assistant points out a number of instances in the field notes that call into question their argument. Nonetheless, the investigators decide to complete an article based only on the data that support their argument. They not only ignore the contravening data, but they do not mention the data's existence in the research report. This is an instance of falsification, and it constitutes scientific misconduct.

Plagiarism is the appropriation of another person's ideas, processes, results, or words without giving appropriate credit. For example, an occupational therapist has been working on a paper and discusses it with a colleague from nursing. This colleague points out that an article addressing the issue has been published in the nursing literature and provides a copy. The occupational therapist uses the fundamental ideas of the article and structures the OT paper much the same as the nursing paper. When the OT paper is published, it has no reference to the nursing paper. This would be an example of plagiarism that constitutes scientific misconduct. The ORI considers plagiarism to include outright theft and misappropriation of intellectual property, as well as the substantial unattributed textual copying of another's work. Plagiarism does not include authorship or credit disputes.

In each of the hypothetical instances of scientific misconduct just described, it is likely that the individuals involved will have "good reasons" for their behavior. The student who fabricates a subject may reason that 1 subject out of 30 won't really change the findings. The qualitative investigators are convinced that their conceptual argument is mainly correct, and reason that mentioning contradictory data will only undermine others' confidence in what is basically a sound conceptual argument. The writer of the OT paper argues that because the original work was published in another field, it doesn't matter if the author is not cited. However, in each situation, the reasoning masks the fact that all of these hypothetical persons gained something from their misconduct.

Allegations of misconduct need to be proven by a preponderance of evidence for such a determination to be made. Thus, there are forms of misconduct that clearly breach ethical standards but may not warrant sanctions. Therefore, conduct in research is better guided by a concern for ethics and integrity than a concern for avoiding sanction. An investigator must always be careful to ask whether personal gain is influencing a decision that involves an ethical issue. Moreover, decisions should always be guided by the ethical principles involved and not by personal, logistic, political, or other considerations.

Mechanisms for Resolving Allegations

Research institutions usually develop policies for resolving allegations of misconduct in a timely manner and through a two-step process. Typically, there is an inquiry phase in which the allegation is initially explored to determine whether it meets the institutional and federal definitions of misconduct and whether there seems to be evidence of the alleged misconduct. If the allegation appears meritorious, then the matter is referred to a more comprehensive investigation phase, during which the allegations and the evidence are reviewed by a larger group. During the investigation, the institution seeks to determine whether the allegation of misconduct is true. The institutional policy must also identify a person with authority in the institution to act on the results of the investigation. That person can impose sanctions upon the individual if found guilty of misconduct or vindicate the person if cleared of the allegation. Finally, the institutional policy makes provisions for reporting the findings to the ORI.

The Price of Scientific Misconduct

- Requirements that federal funding be returned (paid back)
- Additional penalties and fines to the individual investigator and the institution for not maintaining regulatory compliance
- Imprisonment for up to 5 years in severe cases (e.g., presenting and publishing fraudulent data in publications and using this data to secure federal research grants)
- Institutional sanctions such as halting of all federal funding of research, or possibly even halting all ongoing human subjects research (regardless of the source of funding), until the institution is "brought into compliance"

When researchers receiving federal funding are investigated and judged to have engaged in research misconduct, they can bring significant penalties and consequences upon themselves and their host institutions.

In addition, there are agencies that "blacklist" investigators so that they are prevented from participating in future research.

Publication Practices and Responsible Authorship

The sharing of the results of research occurs in numerous contexts and can easily be one of the more contentious issues related to research integrity. Early results from experiments are often shared in laboratory meetings, local research meetings and clinical conferences, and scientific meetings. Later analyses of research results are frequently published in scholarly journals and books.

At a minimum, any communication of the results of research must be accurate and honest. Researchers should strive to accurately report their methods, the results obtained, and the conclusions they have drawn from the research. Scientific publication allows for the replication of methods and the generalization of results from the study being reported. In human subjects research, it allows for the generalization of the results from the experimental sample to others from a larger population. The publication of findings allows others to learn from the experiences and data collected during the conduct of the research. Detailed information about writing research findings can be found in Chapter 32.

Assignment of Due Credit

Authorship, or the assignment of names to a publication or presentation, is an important aspect of the responsible conduct of research. Individuals who made substantive contributions to the research should be represented by inclusion in the authorship listing. This ordinarily can include:

- Persons who were instrumental in the initial conception and design of the study
- Persons who were responsible for the collection and interpretation of the data
- Individuals who wrote the results or substantively edited the presentation before publication

Individuals who play more minor roles are often acknowledged in the publication but not given authorship credit. Individuals should not be given "honorary" authorship credit by virtue of their relationship to one or more of the authors, and they should only be included in the author listing if they have made a substantive contribution. Open conversations between the parties conducting the research are essential regarding this topic because it is a frequent area of misunderstanding.

Many organizations in which members engage in research (e.g., a department or college) develop policies that govern authorship. These policies usually reflect:

- Consideration of ethical issues involved
- Protection of less powerful individuals (e.g., students in relation to faculty members)
- Local consensus about issues of fairness and responsibility

Deciding authorship can be a challenging issue when students are involved with research under the supervision of faculty advisors and/or within the faculty member's research projects/teams. In such cases, it is useful to have departmental policies that guide decisions about authorship.

Because policies alone can never cover all contingencies, open and honest communication combined with fair-minded negotiation is also important. This process should begin before the research commences and continue as persons shift responsibilities, contributions, and roles. The website of the American Psychological Association contains guidelines for deciding on authorship in a wide range of situations (http://www.apa.org/research/responsible/publication/index.aspx).

Repetitive and Fragmentary Publication

It is not ethical to publish the same results more than once without clear acknowledgement of the prior presentation or publication because the scientific community and public may be misled into thinking that a given finding has more impact than it actually has, for example. This avoids wasting resources and keeps the research record clear. It is also important for readers to know whether one is reporting the same results again or an independent replication of the previous research (whether it is the same data being presented again or a new set of data). This is also important when researchers conduct meta-analyses because it is essential that the "sample of samples" contains an accurate accounting and that research samples are not inadvertently repeated.

Citations

The appropriate and accurate citation of supporting evidence for one's own research is an important aspect of research integrity. When ideas, data, or conclusions are based on other published work, including prior publications of the author or coauthors, there must be appropriate attributions made through inclusion of a citation. Failing to properly cite someone else's work can be cause for allegations of plagiarism.

Mentor–Trainee Relationships

One of the most important, but least standardized, mechanisms for training professional students in the proper conduct of research is the mentor–trainee relationship. Students are usually required to have a supervisor over their research activities, but the form and quality of the supervision will vary widely from mentor to mentor, and supervision may be different with each trainee.

Mentors are required to invest time and resources in their trainees. Because of their experience base and relative power in the relationship, it is usually helpful for mentors to establish many of the "ground rules" for the mentoring relationship. These might include topics such as:

- How much time will the trainee be required to spend on the mentor's research?
- How much direct time will the mentor spend with the trainee in providing individual or group supervision?
- What criteria will be used to evaluate the performance of the trainee?
- What are the authorship expectations for different research projects?
- What are the standard operating procedures regarding the conduct of the research, including the acquisition and storage of data?
- Who is entitled to access and use the data that are collected by the trainee?
- How will the data be stored, and by whom, after the trainee has completed his or her training?

It is helpful for a research laboratory to consider development of standard operating procedures governing the nature of the mentor–trainee relationship and for standardization of authorship/publication practices. Ensuring that trainees are treated appropriately and not exploited is not only an ethical obligation but also a legal responsibility.

The trainee also has responsibilities in the mentoring relationship, such as conscientious conduct that is consistent with research protocols and other local institutional requirements. In the mentoring relationship, as in other aspects of academic training, trainees are responsible for understanding the nature of their role and seeking out opportunities to learn from their teachers and mentors.

Many institutions or agencies funding research or research training require trainees to undergo formal training in the responsible conduct of research. This requirement has led to the development of a significant number of online resources that are sponsored by research institutions. Individuals who plan to collaborate in research or conduct research would be well advised to take advantage of these educational tools and to consider ways in which they can maximize their benefit from the mentoring relationship.

Peer Review

One of the hallmarks of scholarly publication is the practice of peer review. This process involves a review of the planned publication by other scientists who are neutral in response to the publication and have sufficient expertise to provide a scientific critique and evaluation. Part of their evaluation includes judgments as to the potential value of the research to the current literature.

Peer review, like IRB review of human subjects research, is intended to be an evaluative process through which quality scientific publications are vetted. The role of peer review, then, is one that requires honest appraisal and feedback. Journal and book editors rely on peer reviewers to provide them with expert opinions in regard to potential publication manuscripts. Granting agencies rely on peer review to make decisions about which research proposals should be funded. Therefore, it is important that the peer reviewer adopt a facilitative role. This requires putting aside personal disagreements with others in the discipline or deferring one's own ambitions for the sake of the scientific enterprise. Reviewers must also respect the confidentiality of the information with which they are provided. These are among the most important ethical requirements of peer review.

Peer reviewers are usually selected in confidence by the editors of a journal or book. The reviewers usually are blind to the author of the manuscript under review, and the authors of the manuscript are not informed regarding the identity of the reviewers. Reviewers are not always paid for their time and efforts, but they are expected to provide timely and honest reviews in accordance with the format of feedback desired by the editors. Typically, editors will provide reviewers' comments to the author, who will then revise the manuscript to address the issues raised. The editor may also notify the author that there is not support for the publication of that manuscript in the editor's journal, in which case the author can consider submission of the manuscript to another journal for review. It is important to refrain from submitting a manuscript to more than one journal at a time.

Peer reviewers are obligated to provide honest feedback regarding the grants or manuscripts they are reviewing. It is not acceptable for reviewers to allow someone else to assist them in performing the review because this would be a breach of the confidentiality requirement. They also must not use ideas they find in grants or manuscripts until the information is publicly available. The manuscripts or grant applications that have been reviewed should be returned to the editors/granting agencies after the review is completed, or they should be shredded or otherwise destroyed.

Collaborative Science

Scientific investigation is becoming increasingly interdisciplinary and inter-institutional. This has led to an increase in collaborative efforts between investigators and between scientific disciplines. It has also led to consortium arrangements whereby multiple institutions may share some common scientific resources. The responsible conduct of collaborative science entails attention to establishing clear roles, responsibilities, and written agreements that will satisfy institutional officials at the various institutions. This is an ethical obligation of the senior researcher within the collaborative team.

It is helpful to establish the ground rules for conduct and reporting of the research early in the collaboration. Various co-investigators may share interest in common research aims, and so there should be some discussion of the proposed authorship arrangements in relation to the proposed conduct of and responsibility for the study.

Sharing of Materials and Data With External Collaborators

Contractual agreements may need to be developed, including material transfer agreements that convey ownership rights to intellectual property or materials that will change hands during the course of the study. These agreements are usually negotiated through the grants and contracts office of a larger institution and by corporate counsel at a smaller institution.

Special Concerns Related to HIPAA

Following implementation of the HIPAA privacy rule, and more recently the security rule, it is prudent to consider any HIPAA-related issues early in the research development process to ensure adequate time to accrue the appropriate waivers, agreements, and/or approval for authorization agreements. It is important to remember that the institution where PHI is created has a primary responsibility for ensuring that there are appropriate mechanisms for accessing PHI for research, especially when PHI will be shared with co-investigators outside of the covered entity.

The Role of the Investigator and Research Team

The principal investigator and research team have the most direct responsibility for ensuring that research is conducted ethically, including that human subjects' protections are implemented and maintained as approved by the IRB. The principal investigator is ultimately responsible for ensuring that the required human subjects' protections are followed. He or she may delegate some of the responsibilities for the conduct of the study, but the principal investigator may not delegate ultimate responsibility for the conduct of the research team. In addition, the principal investigator is responsible for reporting any unanticipated problems involving risks to subjects or others and for abiding by the IRB-approved protocol and consent document/process.

Ultimately, it is the principal investigator who is held responsible for the conduct of the research, but each individual member of the research team is also responsible for his or her own conduct. When questions arise regarding research integrity or some aspect of the research conduct in light of regulations, it is the responsibility of the principal investigator and the research team to find a satisfactory answer.

There is often an inherent tension that arises concerning compliance and noncompliance with regulations. It is easy to feel inherently offended when one is told that one has "broken a rule" (consider the average response to a police officer when someone has been pulled over for speeding). Moreover, higher stages of moral development involve guiding one's behavior by ethical principles rather than rules. This allows one, at times, to understand that the morally right thing to do may indeed be inconsistent with an established rule.

In watching *Les Miserables,* for example, one readily identifies with the hero, who has been imprisoned for 20 years because he broke into a house and stole a loaf of bread for his sister's starving child. Nonetheless, one would also concede that laws against stealing are generally "just" and that there should be consequences for individuals who break into houses and steal from others.

The regulations regarding research ethics and research integrity are no different. Knowing the regulations is helpful for understanding the broad parameters for acceptable conduct. Ethical research behavior is usually achieved by being compliant with those regulations. Nonetheless, as already noted, investigators should think beyond regulations to a thorough consideration of ethical issues that inevitably arise in doing research. Moreover, investigators should seek to become as knowledgeable about ethical issues as they are in other aspects of the conduct of research.

Summary

There are many policies that govern the ethical conduct of research. These policies reflect a long history of efforts to correct past abuses of human rights as well as efforts to identify and attain the highest standards of integrity in research. Researchers and students who participate in research are well advised to familiarize themselves with the basic requirements for the responsible conduct of research. This can be accomplished through online browsing of appropriate resources and through continuing education sections at professional meetings and those offered within research institutions. Some useful websites are noted at the end of this chapter in the resources section.

In addition to the federal regulations, researchers need to be familiar with their own local policies and procedures. These local policies will often go into greater detail regarding how the researcher needs to conduct the research and stay in compliance. Many institutions have administrative offices that handle conflicts of interest, outline and enforce guidelines for responsible conduct of research, and coordinate grant and contract applications and/or ethical approval of research. Officials in those offices and their local websites are both likely to be a rich source for additional guidance.

In the end, the best way for investigators to ensure compliance with human subjects' protections is for the investigators to be well informed. Understanding the ethical principles and the regulatory requirements should increase a researcher's motivation to ensure that adequate protections are provided. A commitment to and thorough understanding of the ethical principles and the requirements for the responsible conduct of research are essential to conducting research with integrity.

Review Questions

1. Why are researchers required to submit study proposals to an institutional review board?
2. How did historic ethics violations lead to the regulation of research studies?
3. What is research misconduct, and what are some of its consequences?
4. What are some of the considerations in obtaining informed consent from vulnerable populations?
5. What are the Principles of Belmont, and how have they influenced the contemporary conduct of research throughout the world?

REFERENCES

DuBois, J. M., & Dueker, J. M. (2009). Teaching and assessing the responsible conduct of research: A Delphi Consensus Panel report. *Journal of Research Administration*, 40(1), 49-70.

Dunn, C. M., & Chadwick, G. L. (2012). *Protecting study volunteers in research: A manual for investigative sites* (4th ed.). Boston, MA: Thomson.

National Commission for the Protection of Human Subjects of Biomedical and Behavioral Research. (1979). *The Belmont report*. Retrieved from http://www.hhs.gov/ohrp/regulations-and-policy/belmont-report/

Office of Research Integrity. (2013). RCR objectives: A Delphi study. Retrieved from http://ori.hhs.gov/rcr-objectives-delphi-study

Steneck, N. H. (2013). *ORI introduction to the responsible conduct of research*. Washington, DC: U.S. Department of Health and Human Services. Retrieved from http://ori.hhs.gov/ORI-INTRO

Taylor, R. R. (2008). *The Intentional Relationship: Occupational Therapy and use of self*. FA Davis: Philadelphia.

U.S. Department of Health and Human Services. (1979). *The Belmont Report*. Retrieved from http://www.hhs.gov/ohrp/humansubjects/guidance/belmont.html

World Medication Association. (2015). *WMA Declaration of Helsinki—ethical principles for medical research involving human subjects*. Retrieved from http://www.wma.net/en/30publications/10policies/b3/

RESOURCES

U.S. Federal Research Integrity Policies: There are several U.S. federal research integrity policies posted on the Office of Research Integrity (ORI) website, including those from the Public Health Service and the National Science Foundation (http://ori.dhhs.gov/). The federal regulations regarding the conduct of human subjects research that is funded by the Department of Health and Human Services and guidance and online information resources are readily available at the Office for Human Research Protections (OHRP) website (http://www.hhs.gov/ohrp/) and the U.S. Food and Drug Administration (FDA) website for regulating medical devices (http://www.fda.gov/). Many academic careers have ended with a finding of research misconduct or have been impaired because of noncompliance with other regulations. In addition, institutions have faced very stiff fines or sanctions that have cost millions of dollars. The ORI website contains informative case summaries of closed cases and the sanctions that have been made (http://ori.hhs.gov/). The OHRP website also includes access to determination letters regarding findings of noncompliance (http://www.hhs.gov/ohrp/compliance/letters/index.html). Reviewing these documents can be quite informative for the student and researcher alike as we all try to better understand how to conduct research responsibly.

The Belmont Report: Information about the Belmont Report may be found at http://www.hhs.gov/ohrp/regulations-and-policy/belmont-report/#.

The Declaration of Helsinki: Within the international context, the major document summarizing ethical principles for research is the Declaration of Helsinki. The World Medical Association (WMA) initially adopted this statement of ethical principles in 1964, and the document was last amended in 2000. It is available online at the WMA website: http://www.wma.net/en/30publications/10policies/b3/

Promoting Research Integrity in the Next Generation of Occupational Therapy Researchers: A study course titled "Promoting Research Integrity in the Next Generation of Occupational Therapy Researchers" is available to occupational therapists. It was developed through a contract awarded to the American Occupational Therapy Association (AOTA) and American Occupational Therapy Foundation (AOTF) by the Office of Research Integrity administered by the American Association of Medical Colleges. Information can be found at the AOTA website: http://www.aota.org/.

CHAPTER 15

Securing Samples and Performance Sites

Anne E. Dickerson

Learning Outcomes

■ Discuss the fundamental considerations when identifying a subject pool, including available resources, inclusion/exclusion criteria, and sample representation.
■ Describe each of the five steps involved in sampling.
■ Provide examples of different types of performance sites in occupational therapy research.
■ Differentiate the methodological considerations in quantitative versus qualitative approaches to sampling.
■ Outline three approaches to sampling in quantitative research.
■ Explain the key considerations for sampling in qualitative research.

Introduction

One of the critical steps in the research process is identifying a population of research participants from which the researcher draws the sample. Equally important is identifying a performance site in which to conduct research. An adequate, carefully selected sample and one or more accessible and confidential locations in which to conduct the study are essential to a successful research study. Whether undertaking quantitative or qualitative research, there is a process for defining and selecting the participants in the study and locating where the study will take place.

As is evident in the Case Example, there are times when accessing a sample of participants and locating a performance site go hand-in-hand. If the researcher is not able to gain access to a location that serves, houses, or otherwise attracts people who might be willing to participate in a study, it will take more deliberate advertising and more pronounced efforts to locate prospective participants.

The selection of a research design will also determine **sample size** (i.e., how many participants

will be invited to participate), **sampling approach** (i.e., how participants are selected), and **inclusion criteria** and **exclusion criteria** (i.e., the specific type of participants or criteria by which the study includes or excludes people from participating). Practical issues, such as available student resources and funding for studies, may drive you to make certain design decisions and take certain methodological approaches.

For example, do you conduct a quantitative study with a large number of participants or a qualitative study with only a few? These decisions, as well as the method of developing a sample, are best guided by the step-wise process that is detailed in this chapter.

Sample Fundamentals

Research samples are groups of participants that represent a larger population of individuals with a common phenomenon under study. Selecting a sample determines who is studied. However, it is intimately tied to what is studied. For example, if one intends to study the effects of passive-range robotics therapy on individuals with high-level spinal cord injury that has affected movement according to a very specific pattern, then one needs to select a sample that adequately represents all individuals with the same type of spinal cord injury that has had the same pattern of effects on movement.

Inclusion and Exclusion Criteria

It is important to delimit, or determine the boundaries of, the specified group of individuals who will be studied according to the phenomena or conceptual idea under investigation. For example, if an investigation is examining the use of a training technique for increased mobility in clients who experienced a cerebrovascular accident (CVA), it

CASE EXAMPLE

Professor Johnson has decided to relocate from a large university in the Midwest to a smaller university in the Southwest. The university with which she was affiliated in the Midwest owned a medical school and a large urban medical center. In the Midwest, Professor Johnson had access to multidisciplinary teams of research scientists through her physician colleagues at the medical school and an abundance of doctoral students who needed to engage in research projects in order to graduate. Moreover, as a health sciences professor in the Department of Occupational Therapy, she had unrestricted access to the medical center building, which housed confidential patient databases, high-tech equipment, and laboratories, as a performance site (i.e., a place where the research is actually taking place). Taken together, all of these resources gave Professor Johnson an advantage in terms of securing an ample amount of grant funding to conduct large-scale clinical trials involving large numbers (e.g., $n = 300$) of participants who are clients from the university medical center.

The smaller university in the Southwest does not have its own medical school or hospital, and it trains predominantly bachelor's and master's level students. It is located in a rural town, and the Department of Occupational Therapy relies largely on rural primary care practices, schools, and community-based rehabilitation centers for educational practica and research collaborations. Given the small size of the hospitals, schools, and primary care practices, Professor Johnson will need to conduct quantitative studies that employ quasi-experimental designs and typically involve more than one location as a performance site. Importantly, gaining access to those performance sites will not be easy. A colleague tells her that gaining access to community hospitals and practices for research often depends on one's social connections and on mutual trust with gatekeepers from each site. Such relationships must develop over the course of many visits and following long hours of negotiation and correspondence.

Given these realities, Professor Johnson knows that the nature and pace of her research may need to be modified when she relocates to the Southwest. She may need to consider quantitative research designs that involve smaller sample sizes and low-tech equipment. Additionally, it may be beneficial for her to consider qualitative approaches to research, such as case-study designs and narrative ethnographic research, that involve a fewer number of subjects and in-depth approaches to understanding their experiences.

may be very important to limit the scope of the research to those who had either a right or left CVA because training may differently affect clients depending on the location of the CVA. On the other hand, if the research question involves the effectiveness of the Canadian Occupational Performance Measure (Law, Baptiste, McColl, Polatajko, & Pollock, 1998), it will likely make no difference if CVA clients with both right and left CVA are included. By contrast, persons with expressive aphasia would not be appropriate subjects because they could not participate verbally in the assessment. Inclusion criteria define the characteristics that a person must have in order to participate in a given research study. Exclusion criteria define the characteristics that a person cannot have in order to participate in a given research study. If a researcher wishes to study the effects of a centrally acting medication on fatigue following radiation therapy for breast cancer treatment, then it would

be important that people who are, by necessity, taking any other centrally acting medications not be included in the study.

Defining the Sample

The term **subject pool** refers to those who are identified as eligible to participate in the study. How a subject pool is selected depends on several issues. First, as mentioned earlier, the subject pool clearly depends on the study question. For example, if a study question asks about the efficacy of sensory integrative (SI) therapy for children, the subject pool would be children who have SI problems. If the question pertains to SI effectiveness with children who have tactile defensiveness, then the subject pool would be further narrowed to those children with this particular SI problem. Thus, the specific nature of the research question directly affects the selection of subjects.

The research approach also affects sampling. For example, a quantitative study of the efficacy of sensory integration would compare a group of children randomly assigned to receive sensory integrative treatment to a group randomly assigned to a control group. In this instance, there would be concern to have a sufficiently large sample size in order to achieve statistical significance. By contrast, a qualitative researcher examining efficacy would be likely to select a small number of children who could be interviewed and observed in great depth. In this instance, the researcher might systematically select children who are better able to articulate their experience.

A researcher may address the research question using a single case design. Such an inquiry would require only one subject. Alternatively, a narrative history design could involve an in-depth interview with a child, members of the child's family, and the therapist providing the SI therapy. As these examples illustrate, a third issue that affects sampling is the research design.

Finally, such practical considerations as access to the populations of interest influence the selection of subjects. In many cases, these logistic issues have a major impact on a researcher's sampling plan. For example, if a study focuses on a population that has limited numbers (e.g., people with amyotrophic lateral sclerosis), the sample size will be limited by access. More commonly, the limitations of budget, time, and space lead the researcher to limit the sample size or diversity. Often, sampling limitations undermine the integrity of a study, jeopardizing its usefulness. Unfortunately, many studies are ultimately not published because the sample size or sampling approach was inadequate to provide the necessary rigor. Although practical considerations will influence aspects of a study, a researcher will need to be prepared to explain and defend the sample and sampling strategy at the conclusion of the study. In the end, the researcher has to balance the research question, the approach to inquiry, the research design, and pragmatic considerations to achieve an optimal sample.

Ensuring Representation

Do heart attacks, spinal cord injuries, strokes, or cancers occur only in white men? Given that these events occur in people of all races, sexes, and ethnicities, it is essential to the rigor of your research and an ethical requirement that you ensure that your research sample represents the diversity of people who are affected by the phenomenon under study. Before contemporary ethical regulations and established practices were put in place, large-scale studies funded by national grants primarily focused on white male subjects. The National Institutes of Health (NIH) is now mandated by law to ensure the inclusion of women and minorities in research (see the policy at http://grants.nih.gov/grants/funding/women_min/women_min.htm). This is a positive step toward placing more emphasis on identifying potential differences between men and women and between individuals of diverse racial and ethnic backgrounds in research. It is expected and hoped that all research, regardless of whether it is funded by NIH, will abide by and embrace these important requirements.

As with any research question, it is important to consider whether the factors of sex or race will impact the study. For example, in a study of persons with spinal cord injury, Tzonichaki and Kleftara (2002) found that males had a higher level of self-esteem than females. In a study of persons with stroke, Kizony and Katz (2002) found that significantly more women than men scored above the cutoff point on the process scale of the Assessment of Motor and Process Skills. As these examples illustrate, gender can make a difference in occupational performance and volition and must be taken into consideration when ensuring representation and when interpreting and explaining the findings from a study.

Relevant to occupational therapy, there is evidence that U.S. Latinos and African Americans with disabilities who are also of low income are more likely to receive fewer comprehensive services and less culturally relevant services compared with white families (Wells & Black, 2000). Therefore, as one is designing a study with a representative sample, it is important to conduct a careful assessment of the past treatment history of all participants to ensure that some do not have a head start or advantage in treatment because they have had more access to treatment prior to the study.

Decisions about sampling should always, therefore, give careful consideration to issues of gender and race/ethnicity. Including diverse samples and analyzing data within these subcategories can also have important implications for sample size. This is addressed later in the chapter.

Steps in Sampling

The sampling process involves five critical steps: defining the population of interest, considering the unit of analysis, identifying a performance site, developing a sampling plan, and implementing the sampling procedures (Fig. 15.1).

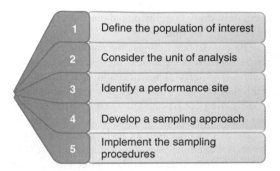

1	Define the population of interest
2	Consider the unit of analysis
3	Identify a performance site
4	Develop a sampling approach
5	Implement the sampling procedures

Figure 15.1   The five critical steps of sampling.

Step 1: Define the Population of Interest

The first step in the sampling process is defining the population of interest. This is ordinarily done through a literature review. A thorough examination of completed research in the area of concern will define the parameters of the population that will be important for a given study. Knowing the population of interest is the first step in defining the sample.

Step 2: Consider the Unit of Analysis

The next step is to consider the **unit of analysis.** What is analyzed in the study will determine the unit. In most occupational therapy (OT) research, the unit of analysis is an individual (e.g., the client). However, the unit of analysis can be settings (e.g., comparing long-term care facilities with rehabilitation centers); families, caregivers, or couples; geographical areas; or other elements. For example, in comparing the efficacy of sensory integration by evaluating performance of children, the unit of analysis would be individual children because each child's scores would be used in the data analysis. However, if the goal is to determine the efficacy of one private pediatric setting using sensory integration against another setting, the unit of analysis would be the settings, which include the groups of clients as a whole. If the goal of the study is to examine the impact of therapy on families with a disabled child, the unit of analysis would be the family.

Step 3: Identify a Performance Site

The performance site is the location in which one ultimately conducts the research study. Having access to one or more performance sites is of paramount importance to the success of a study and therefore must be one of the first steps in the planning process. Common performance sites in OT research include, but are not limited to, university laboratory facilities, inpatient units, outpatient rehabilitation centers, skilled nursing facilities, and community-based organizations. Gaining access to a performance site typically requires that the researcher or a collaborator is employed by the site, that the researcher has close professional ties with the site, or that the researcher has a positive professional reputation and a willingness to work at a collaborative relationship over time.

Step 4: Develop a Sampling Approach

Once the population, unit of analysis, and performance site have been identified, the fourth step is developing a sampling approach. This involves making a plan that outlines how the researcher will select the sample. In quantitative research, researchers should use theoretically defined methods of sampling that are required for making inferences about the population of interest and that are assumed by more powerful parametric, and even some of the nonparametric, statistics. As part of the plan, the researcher determines the sample size or how many individuals are needed for the study. The rigor of a quantitative study depends on well-planned sampling that is strictly followed.

In qualitative studies, sampling is designed to be less rigid, but it is not any less important. A key distinction of the qualitative design is that although the qualitative researcher does outline a sampling plan, the sample can be changed during the study, including the number, type, and description of the subjects to be studied. In some cases it is critical to the study rigor to change the boundaries of the sample.

Step 5: Implement the Sampling Procedures

The last step is to implement the sampling procedures. The next sections elaborate on this and other critical implementation steps for quantitative and qualitative research.

Sampling in Quantitative Research

In quantitative research, the specifications of the subjects are set before the study begins. As noted earlier, defining the population is the starting point in sampling. The population of the study includes all the individuals who share the defined characteristics of interest. Sometimes the population is the key element of the research question. For example, consider a researcher who wants to find out the most appropriate assessment for determining whether the client with a head injury is ready to return to work. The population for the study would be individuals with brain injuries who are of working age.

By contrast, if a researcher wants to validate an assessment, the actual focus or question of the research is the construct validity or the predictive validity of the assessment tool. In this case, the population could be very broad (i.e., all persons who could potentially be assessed with the instrument). Nonetheless, the population is still important because the assessment should be shown to have validity for the entire population for whom it is intended. Depending on the assessment, the population may be defined either broadly (e.g., any disabled clients) or narrowly (e.g., clients with chronic mental illness). Whatever the research question, the researcher must clearly define the characteristics of the population about whom the conclusions will be drawn from the study.

The target population is the population to which the researcher wants to generalize his or her intended findings. For example, if the study's target population is defined as individuals with schizophrenia, it would include all individuals who have this diagnosis. The researcher selects a subset of that target population for the sample. The sample will be the subjects the researcher uses in his or her research study. The degree to which the selected sample represents the target population is the degree to which the results can be generalized to the population.

The researcher wants to ensure that the sample is representative of the population so that the results of the study are valid for the population whom the sample was chosen to represent. For instance, if a researcher wants to investigate an OT intervention for clients who have had a CVA, the sample must represent all clients with CVA who are candidates for occupational therapy. If the study was done in a regional hospital in a specific state, the researcher would need to defend how clients with CVA admitted to this hospital are typical of the population. Just as importantly, the researcher will need to define how the individuals in the study sample were actually selected from this hospital to maximize their representativeness of the target population. The main purpose of sampling in quantitative research is to be able to

accurately draw conclusions about the population by studying the sample.

The researcher defines the parameters of the target population by specifying the inclusion and exclusion criteria. The inclusion criteria are the traits that the researcher has identified as characterizing the population. They serve as the criteria that qualify someone as a subject or participant in the study. For example, an inclusion criterion for the earlier example would be a diagnosis of CVA. The exclusion criteria are the characteristics that will prohibit the subject from being an appropriate candidate for the study. These are typically factors that could potentially confound the results of the study (Portney & Watkins, 2008). In other words, the subject may have characteristics that would interfere with the interpretation of the results of a study, and thus need to be excluded from the study.

For example, if the investigation sought to examine the impact of an intervention on persons with CVA, it might produce different outcomes if the person with CVA also has a major mental illness. In such a case, comorbid mental illness might be an exclusion criterion. In some instances, clients are excluded because they are unable to participate in the study.

The sample pool must possess the inclusion criteria, not possess the exclusion criteria, and be available for selection. Good inclusion and exclusion criteria are specific and clearly identified. For example, Mathiowetz (2003) had the following specific inclusion criteria for his study of the Fatigue Impact Scale for persons with multiple sclerosis:

- A diagnosis of multiple sclerosis
- 18 years of age or older
- Functional literacy
- A Fatigue Severity Scale score of 4 or greater (i.e., moderate to high fatigue severity)
- Living in the community
- Functionally independent in the majority of self-care and daily activities

In this same study participants were excluded if they:

- Did not attend at least five support group and energy conservation sessions
- Had an exacerbation of symptoms
- Changed fatigue medication
- Had other major illnesses, hospitalizations, or rehabilitation during the course of the study

In quantitative research, the specification of the number of persons in the sample is established after the design is determined. For example, if the research study calls for a pretest–posttest control group design, the researcher will know that two groups of subjects are required. The number of subjects necessary will depend on the desired power, as discussed later in the chapter.

External Validity

The purpose of getting a representative sample is to increase the generalizability of the study. A worthwhile study is one whose results can be generalized to a broader population or similar populations. **External validity** relates to this generalizability (i.e., a study whose sample allows generalization to the broader population has greater external validity). Validity refers to the "approximate truth of propositions, inferences, or conclusions," and external validity refers to the "approximate truth of conclusions that involve generalizations" (Trochim & Donnelly, 2007, p. 1).

To make generalizations, the researcher must be able to assume that the characteristics of the sample members will represent those of the target population. Unfortunately, sampling bias occurs when a disproportionate number of individuals are selected who happen to possess (overrepresent) or lack (underrepresent) important characteristics that may produce or interfere with a certain type of finding or outcome in the study. Bias can be deliberate, such as when a researcher purposefully includes certain kinds of subjects. However, even when bias is unplanned, it can jeopardize a study's external validity.

The three major threats to external validity are people, place, and time (Trochim & Donnelly, 2007). A potential criticism of any study is that the study's results occurred because there was an "unusual" group of subjects in the study. For example, if the sample for an intervention study included individuals who volunteered for the study and were highly invested in results, these volunteers may "work" beyond what the nonvolunteer or average individual would choose to do. Thus, their outcome from the intervention may not generalize to all others who might receive the intervention.

Another threat to external validity is the place or location of the study. For example, if an outcomes study occurs in an area of a city where the average income is well above average, affluence may influence the results. Other areas with fewer resources or more environmental stressors linked to poverty may not achieve the same benefits from an intervention because there may not be any follow-through or resources to meet the basic requirements of an intervention (i.e., no resources to pay for assistive devices).

The element of time (i.e., when data are collected from the sample) must also be considered. For example, a study on the incidence of depression could be affected if the study occurs immediately after the holidays, a time when more people report depression. Thus, the researcher must evaluate these factors prior to starting any study to limit threats to external validity with sampling or sampling bias.

Types of Sampling

In quantitative research, there are two types of sampling: probability and nonprobability. Both are described in the following sections. Each approach to probability-based sampling has its strengths and its weaknesses, as does each approach to nonprobability sampling. Selected examples of sampling bias in quantitative studies are presented in Box 15.1, and general examples of quantitative studies using specific types of sampling strategies are presented in Box 15.2.

Probability Sampling and Assignment

Probability, or random, sampling is based on probability theory. **Random sampling** means that each member or element of the population can theoretically have an equal chance of being selected for the sample. For example, consider a study in which the population consists of all the voters in a particular state. If a researcher could obtain a complete voter list, then a sampling design could be developed that ensures that each voter will have an equal chance of being selected for the sample.

Randomization is considered to be the cornerstone of quantitative research. It balances both the measured and unmeasured characteristics that affect the outcomes of a study, allows for masking, and provides a basis for inference (Berger & Bears, 2003). In other words, it is the best method of removing selection bias (Torgerson & Roberts, 1999). Randomization can be used both for subject selection (sampling) and subject assignment (allocation to different experimental groups).

When the population is known, methods of probability sampling can be relatively simple and unbiased. With simple random sampling, all the individuals in a defined target population have an equal and independent chance of being selected for a sample. Simple random sampling is also known as sampling without replacement (Portney & Watkins, 2008); once a person is selected, he or she is out of the pool and has no further chance of being selected again. Often a table of random

BOX 15.1   Examples of Sampling Bias in Quantitative Studies

- The sample was composed of college students in an introductory psychology class who got credit for participation in the study. Although it was possible that there were students with varying degrees of health, the sample was biased toward healthy college students. "The extent to which the participant sample of college students might be representative of other participant samples is unknown. This leaves some uncertainty about the generalizability of the results of the study" (Reich & Williams, 2003, p. 55). Additional research comparing healthy individuals with those of varying degrees of illness would need to be conducted to enhance the validity of this particular study. Reich, J., & Williams, J. (2003). Exploring the properties of habits and routines in daily life. *Occupational Therapy Journal of Research, 23*, 48–55.

- Participants were recruited from the "students, faculty, and staff at the university, friends, and family" (Pohl, Dunn, & Brown, 2003, p. 101). Older adults were recruited from a research registry developed at the university. The participants all lived in the Midwest and most in urban areas. Findings may not be generalized to those who reside in other parts of the country and other settings. Additionally, the sample of older adults was highly educated. "A more diverse representation of education levels in future work is needed" (p. 105). Pohl, P., Dunn, W., & Brown, C. (2003). The role of sensory processing in the everyday lives of older adults. *Occupational Therapy Journal of Research, 23*, 99–106.

- The response rate from the survey was 52%. "This response rate indicates a self-selected sample (volunteers) that may be biased in their views about *AJOT* and the usefulness of research. Consequently, study results may not accurately reflect general leadership views" (Philibert, Snyder, Judd, & Windsor, 2003, p. 457). Philibert, D. B., Snyder, P., Judd, D., & Windsor, M. M. (2003). Practitioners' reading patterns, attitudes, and use of research reported in occupational therapy journals. *American Journal of Occupational Therapy, 57*, 450–458.

- The participants were kindergarten students from one school district. "The participants did not effectively represent a heterogeneous population of kindergarten students as a random sample would have" (Daly, Kelley, & Kraus, 2003, p. 462). Daly, C. J., Kelley, G. T., & Krauss, A. (2003). Brief report: Relationship between visual-motor integration and handwriting skills of children in kindergarten: A modified replication study. *American Journal of Occupational Therapy, 57*, 459–462.

- The participants were kindergarten students from one school district. "Only typically developing students were assessed; thus, the research has no implications for learning disabled students" (Daly et al., 2003, p. 462). Daly, C. J., Kelley, G. T., & Krauss, A. (2003). Brief report: Relationship between visual-motor integration and handwriting skills of children in kindergarten: A modified replication study. *American Journal of Occupational Therapy, 57*, 459–462.

- One hundred and twenty-nine volunteers were recruited. There was no effect for gender on the reaction time to the visual stimulus. "However, it should be remarked that the relatively small number of female participants (28) did not reflect the actual gender distribution of older drivers" (Lee, Lee, & Cammeron, 2003, p. 327). Lee, H. C., Lee, A. H., & Cammeron, D. (2003). Validation of driving simulator by measuring the visual attention skill of older adult drivers. *American Journal of Occupational Therapy, 57*, 324–328.

- One hundred and twenty-nine volunteers were recruited. "The participants who volunteered for this study cannot be taken as representative of the target population because the sample was not randomly selected but only came from some sectors of the community" (Lee et al. 2003, p. 327). Lee, H. C., Lee, A. H., & Cammeron, D. (2003). Validation of driving simulator by measuring the visual attention skill of older adult drivers. *American Journal of Occupational Therapy, 57*, 324–328.

numbers or a computer-generated list of random numbers is used to select the sample from the list of the target population.

In addition to using random sampling to choose a subject pool from a population, researchers who are studying groups of subjects use random assignment to allocate subjects to groups. The principle of random assignment is the same as for sampling. However, instead of eliminating bias that makes the sample unrepresentative of the population, random assignment seeks to eliminate bias resulting from differences in the groups being

BOX 15.2   Examples of Specific Types of Sampling Strategies in Quantitative Studies

Randomly Assigned

- Subjects needing bathing devices were chosen from inpatient and outpatient services from one hospital in Hong Kong (Chiu & Man, 2003). The subjects were randomly assigned to the intervention group or a control group. Chiu, C., & Man, D. (2003). The effect of training older adults with stroke to use home-based assistive devices. *Occupational Therapy Journal of Research, 24,* 113–120.
- Subjects were randomly assigned to test administrators and either of the two treatment groups or control group. "Environments and treatment schedules for both groups were matched" (Shaffer et al., 2001, p. 157). Shaffer, R. J., Jacokes, L. E., Cassily, J. F., Greenspan, S. I., Tuchman, R. F., & Stemmer, P. J. (2001). Effect of interactive metronome training on children with ADHD. *American Journal of Occupational Therapy, 55,* 155–162.

Stratified Random Sampling

- Stratified random sampling was used in order for the total sample to have "... equal numbers of boys (n = 20) and girls (n = 20), 6- and 7-year-olds (n = 20 each), and to allow for equal numbers of right-handed (n = 32) and left-handed (n = 8) children in each group" (Smith-Zuzovsky & Exner, 2004, p. 383). Smith-Zuzovsky, N., & Exner, C. E. (2004). The effect of seated positioning quality on typical 6- and 7-year-old children's object manipulation skills. *American Journal of Occupational Therapy, 58,* 380–388.
- Adolescents of ages 12–18 years were recruited from a target population of 110,000. "The use of a sample stratified by age allowed for exploration of the potential differences to emerge during adolescent development..." (Passmore, 2004, p. 66). Passmore, A. (2004). A measure of perceptions of generalized self-efficacy adapted for adolescents. *Occupational Therapy Journal of Research, 24,* 64–71.
- The researchers selected five states from various parts of the country based on their geographic location and variety of occupational therapy programs (Philibert, Snyder, Judd, & Windsor, 2003). American Occupational Therapy (AOTA) member mailing lists were ordered. Faculty members, students, and occupational therapy assistants were eliminated from the mailing lists. The proportion of AOTA members in each state was determined; based on proportions, the surveys were mailed to randomly selected AOTA members from the five states. Philibert, D. B., Snyder, P., Judd, D., & Windsor, M. M. (2003). Practitioners' reading patterns, attitudes, and use of research reported in occupational therapy journals. *American Journal of Occupational Therapy, 57,* 450–458.

Purposive

- "Participants were identified by their occupational therapist, school psychologist, or special education teacher according to predetermined criteria including having a learning disability as defined by the State of Washington" (Handley-More, Deitz, Billingsley, & Coggins, 2003, p. 141). Handley-More, D., Deitz, J., Billingsley, F. F., & Coggins, T. E. (2003). Facilitating written work using computer word processing and word prediction. *American Journal of Occupational Therapy, 57,* 139–151.
- The sample of low income older adults was purposely selected if they met inclusion criteria of reporting impairments in one or more areas of the Functional Independence Measure motor subscale and indicated a need for environmental modifications to their home to increase performance capacity (Stark, 2004). Stark, S. (2004). Removing environmental barriers in the homes of older adults with disabilities improves occupational performance. *Occupational Therapy Journal of Research, 24,* 32–39.

Convenience

- The sample consisted of 140 participants who were selected from four groups with different levels of neurological impairment and community participation (Goverover & Josman, 2004). There was a limitation in that the levels of education were not equal among the four groups. Education was controlled for as a covariate in the statistical analysis to compensate. Goverover, Y., & Josman, N. (2004). Everyday problem solving among four groups of individuals with cognitive impairments: Examination of the discriminant validity of the Observed Tasks of Daily Living—Revised. *Occupational Therapy Journal of Research, 24,* 103–112.
- Participants were recruited through day programs located in one large metropolitan area and postings at two mental health centers

(Laliberte-Rudman, Hoffman, Scott, & Renwick, 2004). Participants received a small monetary honorarium. Sampling bias may be present since more motivated and socially oriented individuals may have volunteered. Laliberte-Rudman, D., Hoffman, L., Scott, E., & Renwick, R. (2004). Quality of life for individuals with schizophrenia: Validating an assessment that addresses client concerns and occupational issues. *Occupational Therapy Journal of Research, 24*, 13–21.

- Volunteers were recruited by the researcher at the acute psychiatric hospital where she was employed (McNulty & Fisher, 2001). McNulty, M. C., & Fisher, A. G. (2001). Validity of using the Assessment of Motor and Process Skills to estimate overall home safety in persons with psychiatric conditions. *American Journal of Occupational Therapy, 55*, 649–655.

Snowball or Network

- "All were recruited via word-of-mouth" (Niemeyer, Aronow, & Kasman, 2004, p. 589).

Niemeyer, L. O., Aronow, H. U., & Kasman, G. S. (2004.) Brief report: A pilot study to investigate shoulder muscle fatigue during a sustained isometric wheelchair-propulsion effort using surface EMG. *American Journal of Occupational Therapy, 58*, 587–593.

- Posters and brochures were used to recruit subjects. "Word of mouth and personal contacts were also used" (Clemson, Manor, & Fitzgerald, 2003, p. 109). Clemson, L., Manor, D., & Fitzgerald, M. (2003). Behavioral factors contributing to older adults falling in public places. *Occupational Therapy Journal of Research, 23*, 107–117.

- Participants were recruited from several settings, including "a health club, a school employee retirement community, a folk dancing group, a student group, and a military base community" (Dickerson & Fisher, 1997, p. 248). Participants helped recruit other participants within their network. Dickerson, A. E., & Fisher, A. G. (1997). *Psychology and Aging, 12*, 247–254.

compared. Thus, by randomly assigning subjects into the groups that make up a study, a researcher achieves groups that, according to probability theory, are likely to be equivalent.

True randomization is often difficult or prohibitive in OT studies because of the structure of the practice environment. Fortunately, randomization is also considered as referring "to a broad collection of allocation methods" (Berger & Bears, 2003, p. 468). For example, Berger and Bears argue that in studies where groups are compared, strict allocation (assignment) methods can eliminate selection bias as effectively as randomization. If the terms of allocation are identified before identification (or screening) of subjects, selection bias is controlled. However, if terms of allocation are done after the identification of subjects, then direct selection bias is introduced. In other words, if it is determined how subjects will be assigned to particular groups prior to the start of the study, then it can be argued that bias is eliminated (e.g., every other subject will be assigned to the control group). If subjects are identified and *then* assigned to groups, direct selection bias is likely (e.g., the more willing subjects might be assigned to the treatment group).

Bias can also be introduced if the researcher has discretion to approve or deny enrollment

in the study or has advanced knowledge of the groups. Additionally, if alternation of assignment of subjects (e.g., every other identified subject is assigned to a particular group) is used instead of randomly assigning groups, the sequence becomes predictable and problematic (Berger & Bears, 2003).

Stratified Random Sampling
If a study requires that certain groups be represented equally, a stratified random sample may be more appropriate. **Stratified sampling** is similar to a simple random sample, but the selection is from identified subgroups in the population. For example, if a study about the OT profession is being undertaken, the researcher may want to ensure that both the professional and technical levels of the profession are represented. Therefore, stratified random samples of the professional level therapists and the OT assistant population would be separated and the appropriate number from each group selected randomly. It is important to ensure that representation from the stratified categories is proportional to that category's proportion of the whole population. For example, if there were two occupational therapists for every assistant in the profession, then the resulting sample should reflect that proportion.

Systematic Sampling

Systematic sampling is considered equivalent to random sampling as long as there is no reoccurring pattern or order in the listing (Portney & Watkins, 2008). The number of subjects for the sample is known and divided into the number of the population. Then, individuals are selected from the list by taking every "k"th name. For example, if a list of licensed occupational therapists from Pennsylvania includes 1,500 occupational therapists and the researcher has decided to survey 300 therapists, the research would select every 5th individual from the comprehensive list to survey.

Cluster Sampling

Another common probability sampling method is **cluster sampling.** In cluster sampling, individuals are not randomly selected. Rather, groups or programs are selected, and every member of that group or program is invited to participate in the study. For example, cluster sampling may be used to determine the usefulness of an evaluation in outpatient rehabilitation centers. Centers in certain states or counties may be selected, and all therapists in the centers asked to participate.

Nonprobability Sampling Methods

When the parameters of a population are not known or when it is not feasible to do some type of probability sample, nonprobability sampling (nonrandom sampling methods) is used in quantitative research. In this instance, it is very important to try to attain the greatest degree of representation for the sample. When nonprobability sampling is used, the researcher must:

- Clearly define the process of the sampling.
- Acknowledge the limitations of the sampling procedure.
- Justify why the sampling limitations do not jeopardize the research question being answered.

The sample characteristics still need to be defined clearly in terms of inclusion and exclusion criteria.

Convenience Sampling

Convenience sampling is the most problematic, yet widely used, nonprobability method to obtain subjects. Convenience sampling is the use of volunteers or easily available subjects such as a group of students in a program or clientele in a clinic. In a convenience sample, subjects are enrolled as they agree to enter the study, until the desired number is reached. Although a convenience sample is always the weakest sampling method, the degree of appropriateness of using a convenience sample depends on the research question. For example, if

the research question is about normal grip strength for female college students, selecting the women in an OT class, on the face of it, does not appear to enter a large amount of bias. However, if the research question asks about average knowledge of health issues among college students, an OT class might be very biased in terms of such knowledge. In the latter case, using the class as a convenience sample is much less defensible.

Purposive Sampling

Purposive sampling is the deliberate selection of individuals by the researcher based on certain predetermined criteria (usually stated as inclusion and exclusion criteria) (Portney & Watkins, 2008). For example, if a study sought to understand the impact of being involved in a wellness group on health behaviors among women, a researcher might seek subjects from a wellness group at a local women's center.

Snowball or Network Sampling

Snowball or **network sampling** is a method in which initially identified subjects provide names of others who may meet the study criteria. Snowball sampling is used when potential subjects are difficult or impractical to obtain and when the intended subjects are likely to be aware of others who share their characteristics. For example, consider a researcher who wants a sample of mothers of children with spina bifida. If the researcher has some initial contacts, such mothers usually know other members of the same group through support groups and other means. The initial mothers can then be useful in recruiting additional subjects. However, with the snowball method, the sampling pool can become biased, and the researcher has no control over who is nominated for the study.

Quota Sampling

Quota sampling is used when different proportions of subject types are needed so that there is appropriate representation in the sample that may not be attainable with purposive or convenience sampling. For instance, a researcher who wanted to compare male to female occupational therapists might use quota sampling to attain equal numbers of subjects in both groups.

Sampling Error

Sampling error represents the difference between the values obtained by the sample and the actual values that exist in the population. If the population parameters are known, the sampling error can be calculated. However, it is very unusual to have this information. Therefore, calculating the exact sampling error is usually not possible. When this situation occurs, an estimated sampling error can be calculated. Because sampling error represents the degree to which the sample is representative of the population, the larger the sample error, the less representative the sample is to the population and the lower is the external validity.

Sampling error is attributable to random error or systematic error. **Random errors** are those that happen by chance. For example, suppose 50 subjects for a study on normal grip strength were randomly selected in a geographic area. If one of these subjects happened to be an Olympic shot putter, his grip strength will skew the mean higher than the true average because there is not 1 Olympian for every 50 persons in the population. This type of random error is expected, but it cannot be predicted. For this reason, larger numbers of subjects are preferred because they reduce random errors. For example, if 500 subjects had been selected for the study of grip strength, it is highly improbable that another Olympian would have been selected, in which case the effect of the one Olympian on skewing the mean grip strength would be much less.

Systematic error is a serious problem for a study. It represents a flaw in the sampling process, which results in the subjects differing from the population systematically. For example, if the researcher studying grip strength recruited subjects at a men's gym, the resulting sample would include individuals who are likely to have greater grip strength than average.

The major sources of systematic error are:

- Using volunteers (because those who volunteer for any study are likely to be different from those who refuse).
- Using groups that are available and convenient (but likely to share some common characteristic that makes them different than the intended population).

Avoiding these two sources of error often creates a dilemma for researchers. For example, consider an occupational therapist who wants to study the efficacy of sensory integration for children with learning disabilities. If the researcher seeks volunteers from a clinic that evaluates and treats children using sensory integration techniques, which parents are most likely to volunteer? Those who volunteer will tend to be motivated parents who want any kind of information that might help to address their child's issues.

Because the children with the most motivated parents are not "typical" of all children with learning disabilities, systematic error will be introduced into the selection of subjects.

Determining Sample Size

It is important to determine the right sample size (number of participants) in each group for every study. The sample size will influence many factors in the design and implementation of a study, especially the costs and time involved in a study. A general rule of thumb is that one should obtain the largest sample possible. Larger samples make a study more challenging to complete and require more resources. On the other hand, if there are too few subjects, a study is not worth undertaking because any findings would be suspect because of a number of threats to validity and a lack of statistical power, which increases the likelihood of type II error (i.e., not detecting statistical significance when statistical significance is present).

Researchers have agreed on a minimum number of cases needed for specific research designs. For example, in correlational research, it is traditional to use a minimum of 30 subjects (Gall, Borg, & Gall, 2006). Survey research requires a minimum of 100 in each major subgroup and 20 to 50 in each minor subgroup whose responses will be analyzed (Gall et al., 2006). In causal comparative or experimental research, there should be at least 15 subjects in each group. However, within this category, there are variations of appropriate numbers of subjects. For example, in cross-over two-period designs, the same subjects are used in the treatment and control groups. The subjects are their own control, and therefore sample sizes for this group can be substantially smaller than those for the parallel groups (Shaw, Johnson, & Borkowf, 2012).

Statistical Power and Sample Size

It has become good research practice to base decisions about sample size on statistical power. **Statistical power** refers to the likelihood of finding a significant difference between groups or association between variables when one exists (Shaw et al., 2012). The number of subjects is directly related to the statistical power of a study. As discussed in other chapters of this text, researchers can determine before a study is undertaken how many subjects are needed.

To determine the number of subjects necessary to have sufficient statistical power, four interrelated components need to be considered:

1. Sample size
2. Effect size
3. Alpha level or level of significance
4. The power or the odds of observing a treatment effect when it occurs (Trochim & Donnelly, 2007)

If the values of three of these components are known, computation of the fourth factor is possible. Thus, the number of subjects needed can be determined based on reasonable estimates of the other factors. The goal is to balance these components so that maximum level of power is available to detect an effect if one exists given constraints on the other components (Trochim & Donnelly, 2007).

Effect Size

The **effect size** represents a desirable way to describe the findings from a research study because it defines the extent of difference between two means or the size of the relationship between variables in a research study (Stein, Rice, & Cutler, 2012). The smaller the effect size, the more subjects a study will need. For example, consider a study about the changes in handwriting for children who were enrolled in a 6-month-long sensory processing program. Such a study would compare handwriting proficiency in children who received the sensory processing programming to that of a group of children who did not receive the program. The size of the expected difference in handwriting proficiency between the two groups (the effect) would need to be estimated. Several considerations might enter into this estimate. For instance, the researcher might consider the sensitivity of the measure of handwriting used, any pilot data or previous studies that give an indication of how much change could be expected as a result of the intervention, and how much change might occur naturally in the control group as a result of maturation or learning.

Level of Significance

The **level of significance,** or "alpha," is typically set at .05 in OT studies. This means that researchers are willing to accept a 5% chance that they will find an effect by chance when there really is no true effect. This is known as a type I error (we mistakenly accept the alternative hypothesis when the null hypothesis is in fact correct and should be accepted). Decreasing alpha (for example to .01) decreases the chances of making a type I error; however, it also decreases the "power," or the chances of rejecting the null when the alternative hypothesis is true (Shaw et al., 2012).

Calculating Sample Size

Using expected effect size, alpha level, and power, an appropriate sample size can be established. Traditionally, OT studies use .05 as the alpha level and .80 for statistical power. The following are points that need to be considered in calculating a necessary sample size:

- As the sample size increases, the power increases.
- If variation in outcome decreases, the power increases.
- If variation in outcome increases, the sample size needs to increase.
- The power increases as the effect size increases.
- If the effect size decreases, the sample size needs to increase.

Researchers often consult with a statistician to perform analyses that determine the right number of subjects based on a power estimate.

Other Factors Affecting Sample Size

In addition to the statistical power analysis, there are several other factors that affect the determination of sample size, including subgroup analysis, expected attrition, and reliability of measures (Gall et al., 2006). In group comparison studies, there is often a need to compare subgroups after the primary analysis is complete. For example, there may be a need to compare right-handers and left-handers within the experimental and control groups. If the subgroups do not have enough subjects, the analysis may not yield any significant results. Thus, it is important to plan for any subgroup analysis prior to the start of the study in order to plan for enough subjects.

Attrition (or subject dropout) is an issue that needs to be considered. Especially for studies that involve considerable time and effort on the part of the subjects, the projected sample size should take into account the possibility of attrition. Finally, if the measure used has a low reliability, the power of tests of statistical significance is decreased, and an increase in the number of subjects is justified (Gall et al., 2006).

Box 15.3 outlines selected examples of quantitative studies in occupational therapy in which sample size presented a limitation to the study.

Sampling in Qualitative Studies

Morse and Field (1995) identify two principles that guide qualitative sampling: appropriateness and adequacy.

Appropriateness is the identification of participants who will best inform the researcher about the phenomena under inquiry. In qualitative research, although the sample size is often small, the amount of data can be substantial and expensive to collect.

BOX 15.3   Examples of Sample-Size Issues in Quantitative Studies

- "The sample size precluded researchers from conducting a factor analysis to further establish validity" (Laliberte-Rudman, Hoffman, Scott, & Renwick, 2004, p. 20). Laliberte-Rudman, D., Hoffman, L., Scott, E., & Renwick, R. (2004). Quality of life for individuals with schizophrenia: Validating an assessment that addresses client concerns and occupational issues. *Occupational Therapy Journal of Research, 24*, 13–21.
- With this pilot study's small sample size, the study was able to identify one significant difference in self-care performance between the control and experimental groups. However, "... further research, with a greater number of participants over longer duration, is recommended in order to detect other differences that may exist" (Gange & Hoppes, 2003, p. 218). Gange, D. E., & Hoppes, S. (2003). Brief report: The effects of collaborative goal-focused occupational therapy on self-care skills: A pilot study. *American Journal of Occupational Therapy, 57*, 215–219.
- To help determine what sample size was needed for this study, the researcher looked at similar studies and found two in which a sample size of 20 was needed to achieve a power of .91 at .05 with an effect size around 31. However, in this study, the researchers wanted to compare males and females, thus requiring a larger sample. "Therefore, in order to achieve a power of .08 at .05 with an affect size of .68, a sample size of 56 was needed" (Dudek-Shriber, 2004, p. 511). Dudek-Shriber, L. (2004). Parent stress in the neonatal intensive care unit and the influence of parent and infant characteristics. *American Journal of Occupational Therapy, 58*, 509–520.

Therefore, research must be efficient and effective (Meadows, 2003). The researcher must interview participants who are in a position to offer the most information.

Because randomization would not serve this end, random selection is not considered an effective sampling strategy for qualitative research. The researcher theoretically should know who would be the best participant based on the needs of the study. Moreover, the *number* of participants or informants is not as important as their amount of exposure to and knowledge of the phenomena to be studied.

Adequacy of the data means that enough data will be available to provide a rich description of

the phenomena of interest (Meadows, 2003). The goal is saturation, meaning that after continued interviewing and/or observation, no additional information is gained.

Depending on the study, participants may be obtained from the community or formal or informal groups. Frequently, volunteers are sought to participate, and those who usually volunteer tend to be more receptive to the interviewer and readily offer information (Meadows, 2003). However, it is important not to select informants based just on convenience, but on what that person can offer in terms of illuminating a particular concept, experience, or cultural context.

In some organizations or groups, there will be key informants who are in positions or have information that will be more beneficial compared with other individuals in the organization. It is important to identify those key informants and include them as participants. Key informants are selected on the basis of their role, knowledge, or insights and the type of relationship they have with the others involved. However, it can be valuable to also pay attention to the quiet, less verbally expressive individuals (Meadows, 2003). These individuals may have a different perspective and offer insight that would otherwise be ignored.

Douglas (1976) has identified four types of individuals as being useful to the qualitative researcher in any setting:

1. The "social gadflies" are the well-liked and lively individuals who mix with and talk to everyone in the group.
2. The "constant observers" are the individuals who are the longer, well-established members of the group who will freely speak of the details of past events.
3. The "everyday philosophers" are those who think a great deal about the setting and can give insights to what is going on, but they are not as forthcoming with their ideas.
4. The "marginal people" are the individuals who do not feel like they really belong to the group or feel ambivalent about the group. Because they do not have strong loyalty, they will often talk to outsiders and be able to give valuable insights about the group.

Using marginal participants requires caution lest the researcher be seen as aligned with a member whom the others believe to be the least trustworthy.

Most participants can only give part of the picture or have only one perspective on a setting that includes many perspectives. It is therefore critically important to make sure that all perspectives are represented in the collection and verification of the data. Sometimes the researcher does not know who the best participants are. In this case, Morse (1991) recommends that the researcher use secondary selection. This means that the researcher conducts many interviews. If a participant does not have the information that is needed or does not meet the qualities of a good interviewee, the researcher does not use the interview in the analysis. Such data are set aside for possible use in the future if they are found to have some validity.

A necessary factor in acquiring good participants for qualitative research is the amount of rapport and trust established between the participants and researcher. This element is paramount to the success of the study. If the key participants are not receptive to the researcher or the project, they may give shallow or partial information, not disclose their true feelings, or provide invalid information on the topic.

As with all research studies, the sampling methods are determined by the nature of the study. The fluid nature of the qualitative study process is also reflected in how participants are selected. This process is inductive and dynamic and may change as the study evolves. In fact, it is common for new participants to be sought out as a study progresses.

Unit of Analysis

The unit of analysis for qualitative studies tends to be either people focused or structure focused (Patton, 2014). In people-focused studies, the researcher examines individuals and small informal groups, such as friends, families, or gangs. Structure-focused units include projects, programs, organizations, or units within organizations (Patton, 2014).

Some of the most common factors that are considered when determining participants for a qualitative study are:

• Culture
• Geographic or organizational location
• Time or event-related experience
• Personal experience of a unique condition

One of the most common considerations in qualitative research is the culture of the participants. For example, in Bazyk, Stalnaker, Llerena, Ekelman, and Bazyk's 2003 study on the use of play in Mayan children, how culture influenced play was a major concern. Another example is a study of two undocumented immigrants and their child's participation in an early intervention program (Alvarado, 2004). As these two examples illustrate, qualitative studies often focus on individuals who represent unique cultural experiences.

Geographic location or membership in an organizational group can be used to initially define the participants for a study. Ward's (2003) study of the clinical reasoning of occupational therapists working in community mental health is an example of such a study. Other factors leading to sample selection may be related to a specific time or event. For example, qualitative studies often focus on experiences during events such as the Great Depression, 9/11, or the Vietnam War era (Patton, 2014).

Personal experiences are frequently a focus of qualitative studies, particularly phenomenological studies. Neville-Jan's (2003) study of chronic pain and Kinnealey, Oliver, and Wilbarger's (1995) study of the experience of being an adult with sensory defensiveness are both examples of this type of research focus. In such studies, researchers seek out participants who experience the phenomena under study.

Strategies for Selecting Participants

Selection of participants in qualitative research is always purposeful. That is, the researcher strategically determines who would make the best participants. Obviously, the best participants are those who have the knowledge and are willing and able to share their knowledge in enough depth so as to be understandable and useful to the researcher.

Nevertheless, there are specific strategies for selecting informants. One of the most commonly used strategies is maximum variation. Maximum variation involves seeking individuals who have extremely different experiences of the phenomenon being studied. In this strategy, the researcher is seeking to find the broadest range of experiences, information, and/or perspectives possible. For example, a researcher studying the gainful employment of workers over the age of 70 may choose to seek subjects from a wide range of work settings. Homogenous selection is the opposite. In this instance, the researcher seeks informants who have the same experience. The researcher wants to simplify the number of experiences, characteristics, and/or conceptual domains under investigation. This strategy is used for exploring a particular phenomenon in depth, rather than examining all the variations of which it is an instance. For example, a researcher who wishes to learn more about workplace ergonomics for adults with multiple sclerosis would be wise to define the population of individuals with this disease in a very narrow way, ensuring that subjects are as similar as possible in terms of symptoms, fatigue levels, pain levels, and mobility.

Theory-based selection is when the researcher selects only individuals who exemplify a particular theoretical construct for the purpose of expanding the current understanding of a theory. This strategy focuses on a particular concept and seeks to explore its meaning in depth. For instance, a researcher interested in learning more about how to maximize the volition of older adults with dementia may choose to study three groups of individuals, each of whom are able to demonstrate the three levels of volition as defined by the Model of Human Occupation (Kielhofner, 2008). Thus, the researcher would select one group of individuals who demonstrate volition at the exploratory level, another group who demonstrate volition at the competency level, and a third group demonstrating volition at the achievement level.

Yet another strategy involves finding confirming or disconfirming cases. In this instance, the researcher looks purposefully for the informant who will support or challenge an emerging interpretation. This is a useful strategy in the later stages of a qualitative study, when the researcher begins to feel confident that the data are leading the investigation in a specific direction. Finding informants who can confirm or disconfirm that direction is critical for increasing the confidence of the analysis and expanding the understanding of the phenomenon.

Finally, the researcher can select cases on the criteria that they represent an extreme example of a phenomenon or that they represent the average case. In each of these instances, the design or purpose of the study determines what the most useful strategy is.

Determining Sample Size in Qualitative Research

In qualitative research, there are no standards or set rules for determining the "right" number of subjects or informants. In fact, the number of participants is less important than selecting participants who can ensure richness of information and depth of understanding. In some instances, exploring the experiences of a very few subjects in depth may be sufficient to thoroughly exhaust a topic. In other instances, a researcher may need to continue selecting participants to gather necessary information on all elements of the question.

In the end, the quality of the data obtained in relation to the study question drives the sampling process. When the researcher wants to explore a phenomenon, explain diversity, or understand variation, then a larger sample is needed (Patton, 2014). Lincoln and Guba (1985) recommend that

the appropriate sample size be determined by the information gathered. When no new information on the study question is forthcoming from new subjects, then the "right" number of subjects has been achieved. Patton (2014) recommends that the design specify minimum samples based on the expected description of the phenomena. As with all other aspects of qualitative study, the sample size will need to be flexible, fluid, and subject to change.

Depth Versus Breadth

Before and during the data collection process, a qualitative researcher must be acutely aware of the implications of the participant selection choices and be prepared to define why all participants were selected, interviewed, and/or observed. There is generally a tradeoff between breadth and depth. The researcher needs to decide whether to explore specific experiences of a large number of individuals (seeking breadth) or a greater range of experiences from a smaller number of individuals (depth) (Patton, 2014).

Gaining Access

Gaining access is the entry point into a qualitative inquiry and affects the selection of subjects. Frequently the researcher enters the setting through the gatekeeper or the person in charge of the setting or organization. Winning the trust of the gatekeeper through a straightforward approach or through contacts in the organization affects the ability to freely select participants.

Domain Analysis

The researcher makes ongoing judgments about whom to interview and/or observe based on the unfolding research question(s) and how well the questions are being answered. Usually, the researcher starts with broad sampling. As the research progresses, the question (and thus sampling) becomes more focused and narrowed. **Domain analysis** is the critical process of selecting and adding pieces of information through interview and observation and analyzing it for further discovery. The subject selection process is strategically guided by the aim of achieving rich data for discovery.

Similar to the limitations inherent in different approaches to sampling in quantitative studies, qualitative studies also have such limitations. Box 15.4 displays selected examples of qualitative

BOX 15.4   Examples of Types of Sampling in Qualitative Studies

Purposefully Selected Settings

- The study's aim was to investigate the use of occupation with individuals with life-threatening illnesses (Lyons, Orozovic, Davis, & Newman, 2002). A hospice attached to a hospital was selected. Lyons, M., Orozovic, N., Davis, J., & Newman, J. (2002). Doing-being-becoming: Occupational experiences of persons with life-threatening illnesses. *American Journal of Occupational Therapy, 56*, 285–295.
- The study was limited to physical rehabilitation settings because of the variability of occupational therapy settings and physical rehabilitation represents one of the largest areas of practice (Scheirton, Mu, & Lohman, 2003). Scheirton, L., Mu, K., & Lohman, H. (2003). Occupational therapists' responses to practice errors in physical rehabilitation settings. *American Journal of Occupational Therapy, 57*, 307–314.

Purposefully Selected Participants

- Participants were recruited from local Parkinson's disease support groups. The criteria included individuals who would be able to hear and respond verbally in a face-to-face interview (Doyle Lyons & Tickle-Degnen, 2003). "Purposive sampling (Lincoln & Guba, 1985) was used to select four participants from the pool of seven people who indicated interest" (p. 28). Doyle Lyons, K., & Tickle-Degnen, L. (2003). Dramaturgical challenges of Parkinson's disease. *Occupational Therapy Journal of Research, 23*, 27–34.
- "I used purposive sampling to select three children with physical disabilities." (Richardson, 2002, p. 298). Richardson, P. K. (2002). The school as social context: Social interaction patterns of children with physical disabilities. *American Journal of Occupational Therapy, 56*, 296–304.

Purposefully Selected Process

- Participants were adults with acute hand injuries who were receiving outpatient therapy. "Usual treatment protocols are followed because the intent is to document the adaptation process as it naturally occurs" (Chan & Spencer, 2004, p. 129). Chan, J., & Spencer, J. (2004). Adaptation to hand injury: An evolving experience. *American Journal of Occupational Therapy, 58*, 128–139.

Maximum Variation

- Participants interviewed were from many different sites, varied in years of experience, and used the income for a variety of purposes (Dickie, 2003). The participant craft workers used a variety of media processes. Dickie, V. A. (2003). Establishing worker identity: A study of people in craft work. *American Journal of Occupational Therapy, 57*, 250–261.

Homogenous

- All the participants were Caucasian females who graduated from the same occupational therapy program at the same university (Scheerer, 2003). Scheerer, C.R. (2003). Perceptions of effective professional behavior feedback: Occupational therapy student voices. *American Journal of Occupational Therapy, 57*, 205–214.

Convenience

- The participants were recruited through support groups associated with the local chapters of the National Multiple Sclerosis Society (Finlayson, 2004). Interested individuals contacted the study office and were screened to determine eligibility. Finlayson, M. (2004). Concerns about the future among older adults with multiple sclerosis. *American Journal of Occupational Therapy, 58*, 54–63.

Snowball or Network

- Seven participants were selected from known contacts and an additional participant was suggested by one of the original participants (Egan & Swedersky, 2003). Egan, M., & Swedersky, J. (2003). Spirituality as experienced by occupational therapists in practice. *American Journal of Occupational Therapy, 57*, 525–533.
- Participants were chosen based on their reputation as expert occupational therapists in community mental health as well as their ability to communicate and reflect on their practice (Ward, 2003). Ward, J. D. (2003). The nature of clinical reasoning with groups: A phenomenological study of an occupational therapist in community mental health. *American Journal of Occupational Therapy, 57*, 625–634.

studies in occupational therapy that have used specific types of sampling, illustrating some of the limitations discussed in this chapter.

Summary

This chapter provides an overview of the process of securing samples and performance sites to conduct effective research. Issues affecting the selection of subjects include the study question, research approach and design, and pragmatic considerations. The steps to sampling include defining the population through a literature review, considering the unit of analysis, identifying a performance site, developing a sampling plan, and implementing the sampling procedures.

In quantitative research, the main concerns of sampling are whether the sample represents the target population, whether compared groups are equivalent, and whether sample size is large enough to achieve statistically significant results.

In qualitative studies, the researcher seeks participants who will best inform the researcher about the topic under inquiry and purposefully samples until the topic is saturated. The number of participants is not as critical as selecting participants who can ensure richness of information and depth of understanding.

Careful sampling is essential to a rigorous study. Nevertheless, each approach carries its own strengths and limitations, which must be disclosed in every study. Good sampling takes planning, effort, and resources. In the end, it is the foundation for having confidence in the study findings.

Review Questions

1. What are applied examples of the five steps in the sampling process?
2. Why is it important to define inclusion and exclusion criteria for one's research pool before beginning a study?
3. What are the advantages of gaining access to a performance site in the early stages of a study? Portray a scenario in which this did not happen and describe a possible consequence.
4. What are the more common sampling approaches in quantitative research, and what would the corresponding performance sites be?
5. What are common examples of sampling approaches in qualitative research?
6. What are the key methodological considerations in quantitative versus qualitative approaches to sampling?
7. What is a methodological limitation in qualitative sampling approaches?

REFERENCES

Alvarado, M. I. (2004). *Mucho camino*: The experience of two undocumented Mexican mothers participating in their child's early intervention program. *American Journal of Occupational Therapy, 58*, 521–530.

Bazyk, S., Stalnaker, D., Llerena, M., Ekelman, B., & Bazyk, J. (2003). Play in Mayan children. *American Journal of Occupational Therapy, 57*, 273–283.

Berger, V. W., & Bears, J. D. (2003). When can a clinical trial be called "randomized"? *Vaccine, 21*, 468–472.

Chan, J., & Spencer, J. (2004). Adaptation to hand injury: An evolving experience. *American Journal of Occupational Therapy, 58*, 128–139.

Chiu, C., & Man, D. (2003). The effect of training older adults with stroke to use home-based assistive devices. *Occupational Therapy Journal of Research, 24*, 113–120.

Clemson, L., Manor, D., & Fitzgerald, M. (2003). Behavioral factors contributing to older adults falling in public places. *Occupational Therapy Journal of Research, 23*, 107–117.

Daly, C. J., Kelley, G. T., & Krauss, A. (2003). Brief report: Relationship between visual-motor integration and handwriting skills of children in kindergarten: A modified replication study. *American Journal of Occupational Therapy, 57*, 459–462.

Dickerson, A. E., & Fisher, A. G. (1997). *Psychology and Aging, 12*, 247–254.

Dickie, V. A. (2003). Establishing worker identity: A study of people in craft work. *American Journal of Occupational Therapy, 57*, 250–261.

Douglas, J. D. (1976). *Investigative social research: Individual and team research*. London, England: Sage Publications.

Doyle Lyons, K., & Tickle-Degnen, L. (2003). Dramaturgical challenges of Parkinson's disease. *Occupational Therapy Journal of Research, 23*, 27–34.

Dudek-Shriber, L. (2004). Parent stress in the neonatal intensive care unit and the influence of parent and infant characteristics. *American Journal of Occupational Therapy, 58*, 509–520.

Egan, M., & Swedersky, J. (2003). Spirituality as experienced by occupational therapists in practice. *American Journal of Occupational Therapy, 57*, 525–533.

Finlayson, M. (2004). Concerns about the future among older adults with multiple sclerosis. *American Journal of Occupational Therapy, 58*, 54–63.

Gall, M. D., Borg, W. R., & Gall, J. P. (2006). *Educational research* (8th ed.). White Plains, NY: Longman.

Gange, D. E., & Hoppes, S. (2003). Brief report: The effects of collaborative goal-focused occupational therapy on self-care skills: A pilot study. *American Journal of Occupational Therapy, 57*, 215–219.

Goverover, Y., & Josman, N. (2004). Everyday problem solving among four groups of individuals with cognitive impairments: Examination of the discriminant validity of the Observed Tasks of Daily Living—Revised. *Occupational Therapy Journal of Research, 24*, 103–112.

Handley-More, D., Deitz, J., Billingsley, F. F., & Coggins, T. E. (2003). Facilitating written work using computer word processing and word prediction. *American Journal of Occupational Therapy, 57*, 139–151.

Kielhofner, G. (2008). *Model of Human Occupation: Theory and application* (4th ed.). Philadelphia, PA: Wolters-Kluwer.

Kinnealey, M., Oliver, B., & Wilbarger, P. (1995). A phenomenological study of sensory defensiveness in adults.

American Journal of Occupational Therapy, 49, 444–451.

Kizony, R., & Katz, N. (2002). Relationships between cognitive abilities and the process scale and skills of the Assessment of Motor and Process Skills (AMPS) in patients with stroke. *Occupational Therapy Journal of Research, 22,* 82–92.

Laliberte-Rudman, D., Hoffman, L., Scott, E., & Renwick, R. (2004). Quality of life for individuals with schizophrenia: Validating an assessment that addresses client concerns and occupational issues. *Occupational Therapy Journal of Research, 24,* 13–21.

Law, M., Baptiste, S., McColl, M. A., Polatajko, H., & Pollock, N. (1998). *Canadian Occupational Performance Measure* (3rd ed.). Ottawa, Ontario: Canadian Association of Occupational Therapists Publications ACE.

Lee, H. C., Lee, A. H., & Cammeron, D. (2003). Validation of driving simulator by measuring the visual attention skill of older adult drivers. *American Journal of Occupational Therapy, 57,* 324–328.

Lincoln, W. S., & Guba, E. G. (1985). *Naturalistic inquiry.* Beverly Hills, CA: Sage.

Lyons, M., Orozovic, N., Davis, J., & Newman, J. (2002). Doing-being-becoming: Occupational experiences of persons with life-threatening illnesses. *American Journal of Occupational Therapy, 56,* 285–295.

Mathiowetz, V. (2003). Test-retest and convergent validity of the Fatigue Impact Scale for persons with multiple sclerosis. *American Journal of Occupational Therapy, 57,* 463–467.

McNulty, M. C., & Fisher, A. G. (2001). Validity of using the Assessment of Motor and Process Skills to estimate overall home safety in persons with psychiatric conditions. *American Journal of Occupational Therapy, 55,* 649–655.

Meadows, K. A. (2003). So you want to do research? 3: An introduction to qualitative methods. *British Journal of Community Nursing, 8,* 519–526.

Morse, J., & Field, P. (1995). *Qualitative research methods for health professionals.* Thousand Oaks, CA: Sage.

Morse, J. M. (1991). Strategies for sampling. In J. D. Morse (Ed.), *Qualitative nursing research: A contemporary dialogue* (Rev. ed., pp. 127–145). Newbury Park, CA: Sage.

Neville-Jan, A. (2003). Encounters in a world of pain: An autoenthography. *American Journal of Occupational Therapy, 57,* 88–98.

Niemeyer, L. O., Aronow, H. U., & Kasman, G. S. (2004.) Brief report: A pilot study to investigate shoulder muscle fatigue during a sustained isometric wheelchair-propulsion effort using surface EMG. *American Journal of Occupational Therapy, 58,* 587–593.

Passmore, A. (2004). A measure of perceptions of generalized self-efficacy adapted for adolescents. *Occupational Therapy Journal of Research, 24,* 64–71.

Patton, M. Q. (2014). *Qualitative research and evaluation methods: Integrating theory and practice.* Thousand Oaks, CA: Sage.

Philibert, D. B., Snyder, P., Judd, D., & Windsor, M. M. (2003). Practitioners' reading patterns, attitudes, and use of research reported in occupational therapy journals. *American Journal of Occupational Therapy, 57,* 450–458.

Pohl, P., Dunn, W., & Brown, C. (2003). The role of sensory processing in the everyday lives of older adults. *Occupational Therapy Journal of Research, 23,* 99–106.

Portney, L., & Watkins, M. (2008). *Foundations of clinical research: Applications to practice* (3rd ed.). Upper Saddle River, NJ: Prentice Hall Health.

Reich, J., & Williams, J. (2003). Exploring the properties of habits and routines in daily life. *Occupational Therapy Journal of Research, 23,* 48–55.

Richardson, P. K. (2002). The school as social context: Social interaction patterns of children with physical disabilities. *American Journal of Occupational Therapy, 56,* 296–304.

Scheerer, C. R. (2003). Perceptions of effective professional behavior feedback: Occupational therapy student voices. *American Journal of Occupational Therapy, 57,* 205–214.

Scheirton, L., Mu, K., & Lohman, H. (2003). Occupational therapists' responses to practice errors in physical rehabilitation settings. *American Journal of Occupational Therapy, 57,* 307–314.

Shaffer, R. J., Jacokes, L. E., Cassily, J. F., Greenspan, S. I., Tuchman, R. F., & Stemmer, P. J. (2001). Effect of interactive metronome training on children with ADHD. *American Journal of Occupational Therapy, 55,* 155–162

Shaw, P. A., Johnson, L. L., & Borkowf, C. B. (2012). Issues in randomization. In J. I. Galli & F. P. Ognibene (Eds.), *Principles and practice of clinical research* (3rd ed., pp. 243–255). San Diego, CA: Academic Press.

Smith-Zuzovsky, N., & Exner, C. E. (2004). The effect of seated positioning quality on typical 6- and 7-year-old children's object manipulation skills. *American Journal of Occupational Therapy, 58,* 380–388.

Stark, S. (2004). Removing environmental barriers in the homes of older adults with disabilities improves occupational performance. *Occupational Therapy Journal of Research, 24,* 32–39.

Stein, F., Rice, M., & Cutler, S. K. (2012). *Clinical research in occupational therapy* (5th ed.). Clifton Park, NY: Delmar Cengage Learning.

Torgerson, D. J., & Roberts, C. (1999). Randomization methods: Concealment. *British Medical Journal, 319,* 375–376.

Trochim, W. M. K., & Donnelly, J. P. (2007). *The research methods knowledge base* (3rd ed.). Mason, OH: Atomic Dog.

Tzonichaki, I., & Kleftara, G. (2002). Paraplegia from spinal cord injury: Self-esteem, loneliness, and life satisfaction. *OTJR: Occupation, Participation, and Health, 22,* 96–103.

Ward, J. D. (2003). The nature of clinical reasoning with groups: A phenomenological study of an occupational therapist in community mental health. *American Journal of Occupational Therapy, 57,* 625–634.

Wells, S. A., & Black, R. M. (2000). *Cultural competency for health professionals.* Bethesda, MD: American Occupational Therapy Association.

CHAPTER 16

Design Considerations in Qualitative Research

Mark R. Luborsky • Cathy Lysack

Learning Outcomes

- Understand the role that social interactions play across all qualitative research designs.
- Explain the importance and necessity of qualitative study methods.
- Outline the unique aims of qualitative research.
- Define epistemology, and describe its role in qualitative research.
- Outline the five major epistemological traditions (or designs) in qualitative research.
- Evaluate the various traditions (or designs) in terms of their utility in different research contexts.
- Provide an example of a unique contribution of qualitative research in occupational therapy.

Introduction

Because research in the behavioral sciences and health care was historically dominated by quantitative methods, for many decades qualitative research was misunderstood and viewed as less rigorous. Fortunately, this circumstance has changed in most sectors of science. In many fields of knowledge there is a complementary and interdependent relationship between quantitative and qualitative approaches. In occupational therapy, as in other fields, scholars are increasingly trained in both qualitative and quantitative traditions, although they may specialize in one or the other.

There is growing recognition that rigorous criteria for qualitative data exist. These criteria are recognized increasingly in top-tier medical journals (e.g., *British Medical Journal;* Mays &

Pope, 1995a, 1995b, 1995c, 2000) and by research funding agencies (National Institutes of Health, 2001; Ragin, Nagel, & White, 2004). There has also been a rapid expansion of specialty journals and book series attending to qualitative research. It has been estimated that upwards of several hundred journals exist across disciplines that publish qualitative work (Wark, 1992).

Although it would be tidy if the phrase "qualitative research" denoted one single methodological approach, this is not the case. There are many different forms of qualitative research, depending on the discipline and its assumptions about what constitutes knowledge and how it is generated. Probably the best-known approaches in the qualitative tradition arise from anthropology and sociology. These disciplines have provided a wide array of tools and approaches with which to gather qualitative data, including ethnography, life histories, narrative analysis, symbolic interactionism, content analysis, discourse analysis, critical theory, semiotics, and action research, among others.

Each of these qualitative approaches is different with respect to the type of research designs commonly used, the methods used to gather data, data analysis approaches, and the form in which study findings are disseminated. In spite of their differences, there are some common characteristics and procedures for the conduct of qualitative research, and several philosophical assumptions that are shared among them. Most basically, all qualitative researchers are intrigued with the complexity of social interactions as expressed in daily life. This interest takes them into natural settings as opposed to laboratories. For this reason, qualitative research is sometimes referred to as naturalistic inquiry.

In its broadest sense, **qualitative research** must be understood as the systematic study of social phenomena. Irrespective of its particular

CASE EXAMPLE

Melissa is a doctoral student in occupational therapy taking a course on qualitative research methods. Her assignment is to conduct a brief literature review to demonstrate how qualitative research methods may further inform answers to questions whose answers are limited by the methods of quantitative research. For the assignment, Melissa is permitted to select any topic provided that it relates to occupational therapy. Melissa decides to select the topic of health appraisals and their relationship to mortality.

In her exploration, Melissa first uncovers quantitative research showing that individuals' appraisals of their own health are among the most powerful predictors of disability and death. She encounters a range of studies demonstrating that persons who rate their health as fair or poor have a three times greater likelihood of death than those who rate it as good or excellent. These findings emerged from the analyses of many large-scale secondary data sets on health services utilization. Yet, after extensive replication in multiple international studies, these studies revealed little about what people have in mind or how they go about reasoning on their way to such self-labels for their health.

Melissa then locates some studies that have employed qualitative methods. Epidemiologists use a variety of qualitative interview methods to learn firsthand what was in the minds of individuals as they provided these self-ratings, and qualitative findings can shed light on this issue. For example, Idler and Benyamini (1997) reported that persons making self-rated health judgments are influenced not only by factors associated with the physical body and its maladies, but also by social aspects of the impact of their illnesses and disabilities. McMullen and Luborsky (2006) have found that self-appraisals and interpretations of health include complex belief systems related to the perceived moral consequences associated with labeling yourself as "good or bad." The social fall-out associated with functional independence, and the meaning associated with participation in roles, activities, and settings, exerts an overwhelmingly powerful influence on how individuals rate their health, well-being, and overall life quality.

What Melissa discovers is that none of these evaluations is or ever can be predicted by blood values, medical diagnoses, or the severity of one's illness or injury. Similarly, research has shown that injury severity is not a useful predictor of either long-term physical functioning or social participation and community integration (Dijkers, 1997, 1998; Lysack, Zafonte, Neufeld, & Dijkers, 2001; Mossey & Shapiro, 1982).

For her assignment, Melissa concludes that qualitative research allowed the scholarship in the area of health appraisals and mortality to advance. Qualitative studies demonstrated that one's social desire to appear useful and moral to others and to participate in a wide range of roles and environments are important missing pieces of the puzzle in terms of understanding the issues of health appraisals and mortality.

disciplinary roots, qualitative studies ask questions that are rarely specifiable as conventional hypotheses, as is the case in quantitative research. The ultimate goal of qualitative research is to go beyond the *what* of research to explain the *why* and *how*. This empirical pursuit requires concepts and tools that yield such information and approaches.

The aim of this chapter is to provide a broad overview of qualitative research. It considers the nature and uses of qualitative research, discussing its place and importance in health care in general and occupational therapy in particular. This chapter also introduces the major epistemologies, or traditions, of thought within qualitative research, and it describes the primary design considerations of this research methodology.

The Nature and Necessity of Qualitative Research

Research is, simply, asking informed questions. The hallmark of all research is curiosity about the nature and functioning of the world, including its people, and working to develop some generalizations about this world. In this quest for understanding, investigators make use of existing concepts and knowledge, including wisdom received from others while growing up as human beings and from professional training (**deductive processes**). Investigators also keep their eyes open to see in new ways and build up new ideas (**inductive processes**).

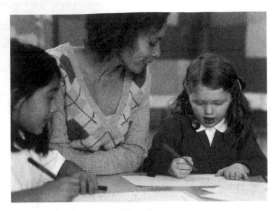

Figure 16.1 A school-based occupational therapist keeps her eyes open to see in new ways and build up new ideas. *(ThinkStock/Photodisc/Katy McDonnell.)*

Both approaches are needed. Scholars continually move between studying things in terms of what is already known to be true about the world and studying things from a fresh point of view. The latter is especially important when previous knowledge seems not to apply to a new situation or cannot explain why things go poorly in certain circumstances (Fig. 16.1).

The Nature of Qualitative Research

Qualitative study methods are needed when researchers ask certain kinds of questions. Qualitative research is a broad term for approaches to developing new knowledge that have as their main goal the naturalistic discovery, identification, and description of basic features of the worlds people live in and their experiences of those worlds. Qualitative methods are used when it's important to learn more about the kinds of features that are present in those worlds and the salient contents and meanings of a given phenomenon. Simply stated, qualitative methods are well suited to the task of discovering what needs to be measured or described and how to measure it.

Questions Addressed by Qualitative Research

Occupational therapy contributes outstanding questions to the wider scientific research enterprise. These include, for example, questions about the impact of disability on occupation, meaningful activities, and habits. As a relatively young field, its scholars are continuing to develop the tools for answering these questions. Qualitative research is an important tool for answering many of the questions generated in the field.

First, qualitative methods enable discovery of the basic form of salient things to measure in situations in which there is insufficient prior work. In this case, qualitative research is often the first step for investigating a particular phenomenon. In addition, it is often the case that certain phenomena, experiences, or processes are inadequately captured by the preconceived concepts and predefined tools. This is the second major reason for qualitative research.

Many phenomena in occupational therapy are best studied with qualitative methods. For example, an investigator who wishes to learn about the evolution of occupational therapists' acquisition of professional competencies could count words or behaviors or collect data on constructs such as independence, judgment, reasoning, and control. Although such a strategy would answer certain questions, it would likely not capture the dynamic range of issues, dilemmas, and struggles that real occupational therapists grapple with as they seek to design and implement therapies and interventions to facilitate the recovery and well-being of their clients. A qualitative, narrative approach would be required to discover these aspects of professional development. Narratives discovered in qualitative research reflect the lived experience of therapists. They reveal layers of intention, emotion, and meaning, including complex contradictions that fixed questions may miss. The following are some additional examples of questions that require qualitative research.

Consider the question of what factors affect adherence to adaptive device use. Research shows that the answers to this question reside in the interface between the device and the person, the social settings of device use, and even within the person's ideals and expectations with respect to the perceived benefits afforded by the device. Research also shows that adaptation of environments can dramatically alter the need for assistive devices. Conducting qualitative research in naturalistic settings, such as people's homes and communities, has been essential to discovering these factors (Fig. 16.2) (Gitlin, Luborsky, & Schemm, 1998; Luborsky, 1997).

Consider the question of what factors affect outcomes in stroke rehabilitation. In a series of studies, researchers have shown that rehabilitation after stroke is sometimes devalued by health-care professionals, in contrast to the views of stroke patients (Becker & Kaufman, 1995; Kaufman & Becker, 1986). For patients, rehabilitation

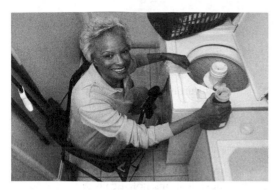

Figure 16.2 Conducting qualitative research in people's homes and communities has been essential to discovering the factors that affect adherence to using adaptive devices. *(ThinkStock/ moodboard.)*

represented a hopeful opportunity for recovery if they worked hard enough, which resulted in feeling let down when recovery did not occur. On the other hand, professionals' views were dominated by the idea that the potential to influence the illness trajectory is quite limited. As a result, rehabilitation professionals in stroke settings tended to divide patients into two categories: rehabilitation candidates and geriatric care patients. This practice was found to be based on culturally based assumptions about aging and notions of appropriate rehabilitation for older people that ultimately served to limit costs.

Tham and Kielhofner (2003) studied older women with stroke, focusing on unilateral neglect. They found that how the women experienced neglect differed from professional conceptions of neglect. Professionals generally conceive of neglect as an inability to recognize one side of the body as a result of paralysis. By contrast, clients experience the neglected side of their bodies more as an estranged part of the body that is at once a nuisance and an aspect that requires ongoing care and supervision. Consequently, the strategies that were most helpful in assisting these women to manage daily life were not those that emanated from professional conceptions of neglect treatment. Rather, as the women's experience of neglect changed over time, an evolving set of strategies helped them reclaim and occupy the neglected half of the world. Tham and Kielhofner concluded that occupational therapy (OT) interventions for persons with neglect as a consequence of stroke could become more effective by systematically incorporating the kinds of strategies identified in this study.

Consider the question of what it is like for clients and families to live every day with the

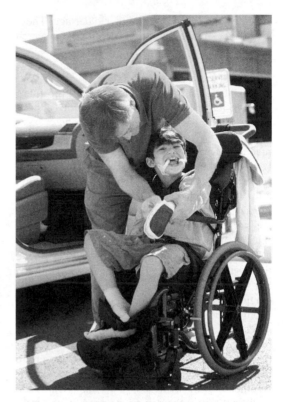

Figure 16.3 Consider the physical and social challenges that this father and son face every day. *(ThinkStock/iStock/jarenwicklund.)*

physical and social consequences of chronic illness and disability (Fig. 16.3). Understanding what that is like from their perspectives can provide invaluable insights. Examples of qualitative research studies that provide such understanding are abundant. For example, some research has centered on observations of a particular person or group, such as persons with cancer, autism, and mental retardation (e.g., Langness & Levine, 1986). In other instances, the researcher is simultaneously the author and the subject of the study, as in the case of Murphy's (1987) classic *The Body Silent,* which powerfully illustrates living with a disabling and terminal disease.

Edgerton's (1967, 1993) *Cloak of Competence* reports research that showed how the stigma of mental retardation pushed individuals to hide and even deny their cognitive handicap in attempts to pass as normal in society and thus escape the social inspection and surveillance that accompanied their disability. Edgerton also revealed the unexpected skills, resources, and insights of his study participants, dispelling myths about the public's sense of their incompetence. Finlayson's (2004) qualitative research illuminated the perspective of adults with multiple sclerosis, describing the challenges they encounter and fear as they enter older age. These are only a few examples of qualitative research that provided an insider's viewpoint on illness and disability. Such research offers important insights that can shape and improve OT practice.

Qualitative research aspires to learn the entire range of features characterizing a patient's experience, "paint" a picture, and evaluate how existing trait systems (such as those used in clinical practice) are useful, when they miss important phenomena, and even when they do harm. Medical and rehabilitation classifications are powerful and enable the control or management of impairment, the treatment of serious injuries, and the prevention of disease. Nonetheless, medical science and discovery require methods and tools to better address patients' continuing lives within the social fabric of daily life in the community. For example, current qualitative research on the diagnosis of depression focuses on asking patients about the presence, duration, and effect of feelings of sadness and despair. To extend this knowledge base, qualitative research must also be undertaken to seek to learn about individual and group concepts of depression. Such research would ask whether the way laypersons understand depression is different from the definitions used by researchers and professionals. It would seek to understand laypersons' beliefs about the nature, causes, and natural course of depression. It would ask about their views of what should be done about depression. No doubt such research will yield unexpected insights. These insights will likely have direct, and perhaps dramatic, practice implications.

Occupational therapists have already recognized that the approach to classifying disease and dysfunction inherited from medicine and rehabilitation is too limiting. Recognition of the limitations of a narrow biomedical focus led Reilly (1962), Kielhofner (2008), and others (Zemke & Clark, 1996) to attempt to develop a more integrative conceptual framework for the profession that more properly included human occupations, meaningful activities, and personal values. Occupational therapists increasingly are examining the embodied experiences of patients as social beings (not only physically functioning beings) and as intending and feeling persons. The notion of embodiment has, at its core, the idea that substance and spirit are inseparable (Csordas, 1994; Kielhofner, 1995).

The Features of Qualitative Research

All qualitative research is characterized by several features. It seeks to discover:

- The insider's (emic) view and compare it with the observer's (etic) view
- Meanings, symbols, beliefs, and values in the language of the participants
- The multiple perspectives of persons, groups, and organizations across the spectrum of positions in a social setting or culture, including those at the margins of society, not just the center
- Features of the worlds of everyday lived experience

Additionally, qualitative research seeks to capture these features holistically within naturalistic settings as information emerges and evolves within the unique context of the research environment (Rossman & Rallis, 1998). Another critical feature of qualitative research is that it acknowledges that the information provided through applying the scientific methods that characterize this approach is fundamentally interpretive and subject to the influence of the presence of the investigators within the study context and vulnerable to the unique interpretations of the investigators and subjects involved in a given study. Although these features are common to all forms of qualitative inquiry, there are different epistemologies, or traditions of thought, within qualitative research. These are considered next.

Major Epistemologies in Qualitative Research

Epistemology refers to the broad arena of philosophy concerned with the nature and scope of knowledge. Epistemology asks such questions as: What does it mean to know the truth, and what is the nature of truth? What kinds of things can be known? Can we believe in knowledge about what goes beyond the evidence of our senses, such as the lived experiences of others or events of the past? What are the limits of self-knowledge?

Today in qualitative research, major epistemological traditions include:

- Participatory action research
- Ethnography
- Grounded theory
- Critical theory
- Phenomenology

Terms such as *philosophical traditions* and *epistemology* may seem abstract and unrelated to daily life. Yet everyone has a philosophy and uses philosophy when thinking about and addressing questions about life, meaning, society, and morality. Philosophies, usually subconsciously, form the foundations of everyone's approaches to thinking and acting.

Qualitative research is an inherently social process, and qualitative research traditions are somewhat akin to social traditions. They are gestalt ways of seeing the world. Qualitative methods integrate pieces of social interpretation and social interaction to define events, practices, activities, ideals, and goals of the groups under study. Just as deeply held cultural values and beliefs shape the expression of individuals' lives, the perspectives of qualitative research traditions shape how researchers within those traditions see and act on the world in their studies.

Each epistemological approach presents a particular philosophical stance that directs investigators to certain questions and ideas about what counts as answers. Each stance involves contrasting ideas not only about how to go down the path to new knowledge, but also about the destination. The rules of each epistemological tradition directly shape the type and style of research questions asked and the specific procedures used.

This section provides an appreciation of each stance and describes its basic principles, definition, and procedures. OT researchers can benefit from learning the different stances that have shaped qualitative research epistemologies. Investigators who adopt one stance are led to investigate particular problems that can be answered within the perspective of that stance, whereas those who adopt a different stance will be directed to other problems.

Participatory Action Research

Participatory action research (PAR) is an approach to research used to confront pressing social problems. Although PAR can be combined with quantitative designs (Taylor, Braveman, & Hammel, 2004), it most often employs qualitative research strategies. Moreover, because PAR involves important ideals and principles about how knowledge should be generated and used, it is viewed by many qualitative researchers as a particular epistemological tradition.

PAR combines both research efforts and active intervention within a single project. PAR is unique in how the research goal is formulated and pursued: it involves multiple stakeholders, including research participants, institutional representatives (e.g., teachers, physicians, service providers), and researchers, as equal partners. In addition to concerns for research rigor, PAR adds concern with creating community trust and a sense of ownership of the project and findings. The people who conduct the study, the procedures and forms of the

findings, and methods of dissemination are collaboratively planned and conducted to ensure that the results both represent all the stakeholders and that they are able to trust the processes by which it was developed.

Taylor et al. (2004) describe a study based on the principles of PAR. The central aim was to determine whether a chronic illness self-management program utilizing a PAR approach led to higher perceptions of quality of life and psychosocial resources compared with usual care. Participants in the PAR study defined and led the very rehabilitation program in which they participated. They decided what topics were important to cover, and they delivered these topics to their peers. The role of the researcher was limited to providing an appropriate and accessible setting for the participants to meet, coordinating meeting times, and facilitating meetings and resource sharing. The advantages to this approach included active participation and engagement in the program by all participants, and positive outcomes.

Conducting a PAR Project

The aphorism "Look, think, act" (Stringer, 2014) sums up the main features of PAR and highlights its socially engaged stance. When looking, investigators collect information to discover, define, and describe a phenomenon or setting. When thinking, they explore by interpreting, analyzing, and explaining. Finally, when acting, investigators develop, implement, and evaluate a purposeful plan formulated to meet a local need or change something in the context. These three steps provide PAR collaborators with a script of explicit orientations and goals. They serve as an iterative process so that looking, thinking, and acting can be repeated throughout the research process as new information, agendas, and questions emerge from the input and shared experiences of all the PAR partners.

Overall, the structure of PAR proceeds in the following steps:

1. A project begins with the initial identification of a problem by the researchers or the participants, or both together.
2. Collaborative discussions and negotiations among all stakeholders serve to refine the sense of the problem.
3. The research partners review what is already known and published about the issue and/or attempt to address a problem.
4. Researchers work to redefine the problem more clearly and formulate an agenda for change.

5. Methods for research and evaluation are selected.
6. Research partners implement the change and collect and analyze data to evaluate their efforts.
7. The results are prepared, including recommendations, and disseminated for wider audiences.

Generally, the investigators return to refining the problem, goals, and procedures as they make use of the emerging knowledge and experiences, including evaluation of the changes.

In the United States, the federal Agency for Healthcare Research and Quality (AHQR) has published the results of a consensus conference and literature meta-analyses; it confirmed the positive outcomes of PAR and summarized key design criteria (Viswanathan et al., 2004). The AHQR also issued a fact sheet on participatory research (see http://www.ahrq.gov/research/findings/factsheets/minority/cbprbrief/). PAR has been vital to the success of projects spanning from patient-centered mental health and substance abuse treatment to community-based health and in many primary health-care and international development projects, including the community-based rehabilitation movement (Lysack & Kaufert, 1994) around the world. Excellent studies using the PAR approach include those featured in the *American Journal of Public Health* (2003 August, 2003 September), those by Hart and Bond (1996) and Stringer (2014), a report commissioned by the AHRQ (Viswanathan et al., 2004), and that by Minkler, Blackwell, Thompson, and Tamir (2003). One of the most comprehensive reviews of the history, development, and international uses of PAR is given by De Koning and Martin (1996). An excellent text published by the American Psychological Association with OT contributors discusses the use of PAR in community contexts (Jason et al., 2004). Finally, an OT text by Crist and Kielhofner (2005) illustrates the use of PAR in advancing practice.

Contributions of Participatory Action Research

Interest in PAR has grown rapidly. In part, this is because the collaborative design incorporates core progressive social ideals. PAR seeks to ensure that the interests of all the partners are on an equal footing; it is often described as "democratic" (Gitlin, Lyons, & Kolodner, 1994). It is also popular because the results of PAR are more likely to be trusted by consumers and professionals and are more likely to be used because they are transparent and personally, politically, economically,

and/or socially relevant to consumer participants. Thus, the end result of PAR is not only new knowledge, but also changes in practices, in organizations, and in governmental, legal, economic, and social rules. It is also socially progressive because it is designed to enhance the life of individuals and communities. Although PAR is still developing within the field of occupational therapy, a number of projects using this approach have demonstrated how services can be improved and how therapists and clients can be empowered to achieve desired ends (Forsyth, Summerfield-Mann, & Kielhofner, 2005; Taylor et al., 2004).

Ethnography

Ethnography is a research approach that aims to discover and describe the point of view of a people or social scene. Ethnography is a dynamic tradition with a long history. From its early days in the late 1800s, it was defined by a fieldwork tradition. Investigators, such as Franz Boas (1966), who first studied the Eskimo (Inuit), or Malinowski, who studied the natives in the South Pacific Islands, lived among the people they studied and immersed themselves in the settings and events being studied. These investigators systematically learned and spoke the local language, and they described the material lives, activities, structures of social life, relationships, and cultural beliefs that they observed. By conducting such fieldwork to learn directly from the natives about their viewpoints, these early ethnographers developed a method of firsthand discovery.

Ethnography continues to evolve. For example, ethnographers now see researchers as instruments; their experiences and reactions are part of the process of gaining insight into the people and settings studied. What distinguishes ethnographic fieldwork from other methods conducted in field settings is a quest for the naturally occurring language, insider's viewpoint and values, and cultural patterns.

The term *ethnography* embraces a wide range of approaches that share an interest in learning:

• The patterns in how a people define and view the world
• Habitual patterns and ways of life
• Categories of thought
• Symbols and meanings
• Kinds of social relationships
• Systems of moral goals, values, and social structures

Ethnographers strive to gain an insider's view of the social scene (Spradley 1979, 1980). Geertz

(1973) summed up the ethnographic task as figuring out what those under study think they are up to. This aim contrasts with trying to force fit a description of those under study into the language categories and values held by the researcher.

Ethnography is distinctive in several ways. Among these are its aims to:

• Describe the insider's view, categories of language, thought, rules for behavior and relationships, and symbols.
• Conduct studies in the natural settings of informants' lives by immersion and participation.
• Regard participants as informants who help to direct and interpret the topic of study and verify or refute conclusions.
• Focus on exploring the particulars of the specific setting in time (historical, life course, developmental), people, and place (physical and culturally constructed).

Ethnography also aims to build, validate, and refute generalizations about human society. Although ethnography focuses on the detailed case of a particular culture or setting, it does so with an eye to proposing larger patterns of human life by using what has already been learned about the beliefs and structures of other societies. Generalizations grow from the accruing record of each society, which reveals recurrent patterns of similarity and difference across systems of cultural values, relationships, and symbols. General theories about the sociocultural lives of humans are built and constantly case tested by the ethnographic veto, a term for the use of the rich record of empirical ethnographic studies of societies to provide counter-examples to a theory or prevent oversimplification. For example, to provide a newer model of stigma (the social labeling of a person as undesirably different), researchers used a comparative global perspective to reveal institutional practices that covertly perpetuate stigma (Das, 2001; Link & Phelan, 2001).

Ethnography's insider view also helps to dispel myths. For example, economic development experts engaged to help subsistence peasant farmers living high in the Andes Mountains believed their poverty was attributable to idleness and underemployment. These experts wanted to get more of the "lazy" peasants working because they saw that few were laboring to dig or work the fields, tasks associated with busy productivity in the economists' industrial models. Ethnographers used time allocation cultural methods (Gross, 1984) to observe and ask peasants what they did, when, and why. Their findings showed that the crops required seasonal effort, not constant intense work. Moreover, of equal importance was that people must be posted to stand watch over the fields to protect the grain harvests from predation by birds and animals. Thus, crop watching was a very important economic routine. When understood and counted as productive activity (not idleness), the employment rate was 98% (Brush, 1977).

Conducting Ethnographic Research

Ethnographic research is conducted in a series of basic phases:

• Preparation and entry
• Immersion using participation and observation
• Exit
• Writing up

Study participants are properly called "informants," because they inform and teach about their lives and communities; they are not "subjects" controlled by the researcher.

The start of immersion can take several forms, from preparation by reading in an archive or publications, to entry into the field site. As an outside participant, the ethnographer begins to learn the language and folk categories; how to ask and answer questions; the history, kinds, and structure of relationships; behavioral expectations; social and life values; and life as defined by the participants. Next, with continued immersion and increasing insider knowledge, the questions reach into deeper realms of cultural values and philosophy; they explore diversities in beliefs and individual and group histories. Comparisons between observed actions and events and the informants' expressed beliefs and social rules become possible with extended time in the field. An ongoing field journal is used to monitor accruing insights and highlight gaps and questions. In the final stage, ethnographers exit the setting to begin summarizing and interpreting their field data, but now at a distance. The distance allows them to mentally compare insider and outsider viewpoints to explore and analyze the fieldwork data.

The data collection toolkit for ethnography features direct interview and observation of people, events, and artifacts; personal participation in the ongoing routine and special events of social life; and interpretation of the stories, symbols, and objects in the field site. The traditional handwritten journal notebooks and maps for collecting data are now being replaced by a range of technology, including digital audio or video recordings, global positioning system (GPS) mapping, and computer software for taking field notes, indexing, and analyzing observations and interpretations.

Contributions of Ethnographic Research

Because ethnography can provide systematic data on people's own perceptions, meanings, expectations, needs, and structures for action, it is a powerful tool for the health and social service fields. Ethnography is used to study topics that range from the social structure and value systems in hospitals and rehabilitation facilities to patterns of practitioner–patient interactions. Such research has provided important insights to problems and practices. For example, ethnographic studies of the culture of nursing homes have shown that disruptive behavior by residents on a Alzheimer's care unit may be tied to the timing of nursing shift changes (e.g., during meals) (Stafford, 2003); incontinence is defined and managed by nursing home staff as a wetness problem requiring diapers instead of a potentially reversible medical condition that can be treated (Schnelle et al., 1989); and malnutrition is a major problem in American nursing homes (Kayser-Jones et al., 2003). Without such sustained ethnographic field research, these important health issues would never have been identified.

The ethnographic tradition shares with occupational therapy the desire to work to learn, not predefine, individuals' own meaningful desired habits, values, and actual life settings as well as perceived challenges and resources. Perhaps this is why occupational therapists have looked to and welcomed ethnographic insights offered by anthropology researchers, and reciprocally, anthropologists have benefited from the insights of OT clinicians to guide and frame their own work on disability and rehabilitation (e.g., Mattingly, 1998).

Grounded Theory

Grounded theory is an inductive method designed to construct theory from qualitative data (Glaser & Strauss, 1967). It does so by following a defined set of procedures for data collection, but without direction from existing constructs or theory about the phenomena. The term *grounded* refers to the aim to have the theory emerge from, or be grounded in, the data. The grounded theory approach seeks to ensure that the theory derives from the experiences of the individuals on whom the study is focused. In this instance, the theory is a generalization about the empirical data. That is, the investigator seeks to explain the data from the specific study, not to propose a conceptual or philosophical model. Imagine that a researcher aims to develop a theoretical concept that defines suboptimal therapeutic responses to client resistance. Instead of imposing the concept onto a situation and then testing whether the concept holds during a standardized client–therapist interaction, a grounded theorist would observe numerous client–therapist interactions within their naturalistic environments, extract the ones that involve client resistance, and then derive theoretical concepts that link the resistance to the therapist's suboptimal responding.

Conducting a Grounded Theory Study

The procedures for conducting a grounded theory study can be described individually, but they are undertaken concurrently during the project rather than in a sequence. Researchers use data collection methods such as narratives, focused interviews, informal discussion, participant observation, and field notes. Sample sizes often are not large, usually in the range of 20 to 50 participants at the most.

What distinguishes the grounded theory method from other qualitative methods is the structured formalized process for data collection and theory development. It specifies a continuous interplay between data collection and interpretation, leading to a generalization that is project-specific for that data (Corbin & Strauss, 2014). The work of evolving a theory from the data is one of constant comparison by which each new piece of information (a belief, explanation for an event, experience, symbol, or relationship) is compared to each other piece of data as it is gathered.

Investigators code the conditions, actions, strategies for interactions, and outcomes observed. Should the information be similar to other already existing information, it is assigned to that category and labeled, or coded, with the descriptive word or phrase for that group. On the other hand, if the idea or phenomenon does not fit a category already created, then a new one is created.

Over time, a set of categories emerges that is refined and confirmed, and the resulting set of categories is used to make a more abstract generalization (i.e., the grounded theory) to explain the phenomenon. The published reports from grounded theory studies follow a similar design; they usually would not contain a detailed literature review (preexisting theory and data). The report is a descriptive discussion of the structured procedures followed and the findings.

Contributions of Grounded Theory Research

Grounded theory studies have the potential to offer important understanding of how people live with the challenges of illness and disability. For example, the goal of a grounded theory study by Clements, Copeland, and Loftus (1990) was to learn how parents coped with the adversity of living and caring for a child with a chronic illness. This study included focused interviews with 30 families who attended a clinic where the children were treated. They found heightened challenges and resource needs at the critical changes in the child's condition. A grounded theory developed by the researchers focused specifically on the phenomena described by participants in that study. The theory they proposed was that the specific ways of coping developed by a family with a chronically ill child attempt to meet the needs of all the family members. A balance or equilibrium is reached if there are resources, but that cannot be maintained if the demands rise or the support changes.

Critical Theory

Critical theory researchers take the stance that knowledge (and theory) is not universal and absolute. Instead, it starts with the basic premise that social reality is embedded and constructed in specific historical times and places and that it is produced and reproduced by people. Simply stated, then, adherents of critical theory see social reality and knowledge as relative to particular people and times. They contend that multiple social realities exist that are distributed across the various segments of society and groups.

Critical theorists contrast starkly with "positivists," who assume that there is but one objective reality that can be captured and measured by instruments that are independent of the observer. Positivist studies generally attempt to test theory, in an attempt to increase the predictive understanding of phenomena. On the other hand, critical theory's purpose is to enlighten people and make them critically aware.

The goal in critical theory research is to bring to light or become aware of the social realities that create barriers or allow for progress rather than passively acting according to the reigning sociopolitical structures and settings that shape ways of thinking. In this context the term *critical* does not mean to demean or ridicule; rather, it means to pose questions. The aim of critical theory is positive social and political transformation, including reducing social injustices. Thus, it focuses on ways of thinking that are taken for granted, insights gathered through heightened awareness of the diversity, and inequalities afflicting many segments of society. More fundamentally, critical theorists view human inaction in the face of social injustices as resulting from domination by the status quo.

Critical theory is reflected in the work of a wide range of scholars, from Marx and Hegel to Foucault and Derrida. One of the best-known proponents of critical theory, Habermas (1988), along with others, argued that scientific and philosophical constructs are enmeshed in and serve to re-create wider social-historical patterns. More general critical theory programs are sometimes also described as critical research (Mishler, 1986) or analytic induction (Corbin & Strauss, 2014). Cogent reviews of the limits of critical theory are also available (Hammersley, 1992; Honneth, 1991). Critical theory is less familiar to occupational therapy than some other qualitative epistemological traditions.

A critically informed OT research study will be reflective about the nature of the research questions it asks, their historical origins, and the forms for answers and solutions it allows. Because occupational therapy is centrally concerned with practices that are "client centered" (Law, 1998; Townsend, Langille, & Ripley, 2003) and morally concerned with clients' social positions in society, occupational therapists must be attentive to the diversity in their clients' desired goals and the methods by which their clients' rehabilitation needs can be met within that broader social context.

One limitation of this approach to research that is particularly relevant to occupational therapy is that in critical theory the individual is not conceptualized as a willful, autonomous person. Instead, individuals are viewed as bound by social rules or norms; they are defined simply as the sum of family, work, and community roles.

Conducting a Critical Theory Study

No formalized procedures exist for critical theory, compared with those for grounded theory. However, a generalized approach can be outlined (Luborsky & Sankar, 1993). The critical theory approach rests on the systematic pursuit of a set of clearly articulated questions.

There are four general components:

1. A clear definition of a key concept or problem is presented.
2. A description of how the construct is currently conceptualized is stated, and that formulation's place in the continuing (past to present) thought on the issue is summarized, often as a literature review.
3. The current definition is critiqued to reveal gaps and limitations in the concept/problem formulation's ability to explain the phenomena on

which it is focused, and other problems that it does not highlight. Notably, one would ask in what ways the problems defined for study are consonant with the wider sociopolitical climate of that time, and in what ways they implicitly embody visions for continued re-creation of the existing social organization and values for human life.

4. The researcher conducts research and presents data that are informed by the analytical and historical critique. The form of results for critical theory research is new data as well as new questions and analytic frames for thought.

The Contributions of Critical Theory Research

Critical theory helps reveal how each culture and group has its own definitions for familiar scientific categories such as health, illness, ethnicity, family, or self. It points out that such familiar categories are not universal. For example, historically unrecognized ethnic and social class differences in how age relates to health, morbidity, and mortality have shaped the scientific portrait of what constitutes normal aging. Although these intertwined social influences have always been present, research allows them to become understood (Dannefer & Sell, 1988). In many respects, this is because it is difficult to be reflective about the times in which one lives. It is only afterward, with the benefit of hindsight, that investigators can see a historical period more clearly. For example, consider how clothing styles and fashions, tastes in music, and design of automobiles evolve over a period of years. The same is true for less visible attributes of a historical period that are limited to a local context or a small and reclusive part of the population. People during different decades hold very different attitudes and values than generations before and after.

A case in point is the public's attitudes toward people with disabilities. These attitudes have changed substantially over the last several decades. For example, disabled persons are no longer systematically segregated in asylums and institutions. Moreover, although the status of persons with disability can still be much improved, there are now disability rights laws, protections against disability discrimination in the workplace, more accessible buildings, and more public visibility and acceptance of disabled persons.

Occupational therapists are in a position to utilize the results of critical theory research to enhance their interventions and positively influence the occupational well-being of their clients.

For example, occupational therapists are more aware of the disproportionate prevalence of disability among economically disadvantaged people (House, Kessler, & Herzog, 1990; Townscnd & Wilcock, 2003) and the exclusion of oppressed persons from opportunities or resources needed to engage in meaningful activity (Kronenberg, Pollard, & Sakellariou, 2010; Whiteford & Wright St. Clair, 2004). The promise of critical theory for occupational therapy is in examining and documenting underlying assumptions that reflect power imbalances and social injustices.

Phenomenology

Phenomenology is both a way of doing research (method) and a way of questioning and conceptualizing thought (philosophy). Like critical theory, phenomenology is a complex and multifaceted philosophy that is not easily characterized. Moustakas (1994) explains, "The understanding of meaningful concrete relations implicit in the original description of experience in the context of a particular situation is the primary target of phenomenological knowledge" (p. 14). Schwandt (1997) reminds us that phenomenology "rejects scientific realism and the accompanying view that the empirical sciences have a privileged position" (p. 114) in identifying and explaining features in our world.

At its most basic level, this approach focuses on the everyday life-world and gives great attention to the careful description of how the ordinary is experienced and expressed in the consciousness of individuals. Phenomenology rests on the assumption that there is a structure and essence to personal experience that can be communicated to others in a systematic way using narratives. The primary question that is asked from this perspective is: What is the meaning of one's experience, and how does one interpret it?

When William James appraised kinds of mental activity in the stream of consciousness (including their embodiment and their dependence on habit), he was practicing a form of phenomenology (as quoted in McDermott, 1967). The discipline of phenomenology as we know it today is largely due to Edmund Husserl, who launched the modern-day movement in 1913 with his seminal work *Logical Investigations* (Husserl, 2001). For Husserl, phenomenology integrates psychology with logic. It is psychological in the sense that it describes and analyzes types of subjective mental activity or experience, and it is logical in the sense that it describes and analyzes the objective contents of consciousness (i.e., experience). Other famous phenomenologists are Heidegger, Sartre, and Merleau-Ponty. Each holds different conceptions of phenomenology, however, and uses different methods to study human experience. The *Encyclopedia of Phenomenology* (Embree, 1997) is an excellent reference that comprehensively details the features of seven separate forms of phenomenology, including those of these prominent theorists.

Phenomenology contrasts with other qualitative research approaches in its stance toward the informant and the researcher. Phenomenological research regards the sense of lived experiences and meanings as fully knowable only by those who share the experience. That is, in ordinary life, people are somewhat limited in their ability to grasp and intuit the meanings of lived experiences of other individuals. This is because the meanings of experience must be transmitted and filtered from the person who has the experience to the other persons who wish to understand that experience (Luborsky, 1994a, 1994b, 1995). Of course, things can be lost in translation.

There are many forms of expressive media beyond words that are used to communicate experience with other people (e.g., body language, art, music, etc.). Nonetheless, it is not easy for one person to comprehend or appreciate another's experience in exactly the same way. Therefore, a critical element in phenomenological studies is the skill of the researcher in identifying an appropriate source of information about the experience to be studied, a topic addressed in the following discussion.

There is a second major contrast with other qualitative approaches worthy of notice: In terms of the researcher, phenomenological research differs from ethnographic and grounded theory. In the latter forms of qualitative research, the meanings emerge through a back-and-forth unfolding exploration between the researcher and the researched, and they are then further interpreted and explained during data analyses. In phenomenology, no structure or framework is imposed on the data by the researcher. Rather, the researcher must find and (re)present the experiences in the form in which they are expressed. This can be very challenging, and considerable investigator effort must be devoted to the choice of sample to ensure that it can provide the fundamental insights into the experience that is the target of the investigation (Luborsky, 1994b; Luborsky & Rubinstein, 1995).

For example, if a phenomenological study is designed to understand the experience of surviving a hip fracture and returning to normal life in the community, then it would be imperative that an informed participant is selected for interview and perhaps even observation. Importantly, qualitative researchers must remember that in a study about the experience of hip fracture, the unit of study would be the individual with this injury, but the focus of research enterprise, or the units of analysis, would be the participant's experience of hip fracture and the experience of reconnecting to a personally meaningful life. The intent of a phenomenological researcher in such a study would be to gain understanding of what it is like to live with an altered body that limits mobility and perhaps makes other people think of one as old. Phenomenological researchers would also want to know how these experiences shape the participant's sense of self as a full adult person (Luborsky, 1994a).

As stated earlier, one's choice of informant is critical in phenomenology. Sampling in this tradition must be purposive and theoretically driven in an effort to maximize the range of experiential phenomenology of people with the experience of interest (Karlsson, 1993). Sampling in this tradition must also build on what is already known (Bertaux, 1981; Glaser & Strauss, 1967; Luborsky & Rubinstein, 1995). If phenomenological research is to be successful in capturing what particular experiences are like, it must gather their data from informed samples with firsthand access to the experience of interest. Only then can the investigation gain access and insight into the informant/participant's experiences.

Conducting a Phenomenological Study

Phenomenological researchers conceptualize the person and the environment as a whole. A central tenet of this perspective is that the only reliable source of information to answer questions about personal experience is the person with the experience. Because each individual has his or her own unique reality, the task of the phenomenologist is to engage in lengthy discussions with participants about their experiences and then to locate and summarize common themes in their expressions of experiences that convey a central essential meaning. To begin to achieve this goal, four or more aspects of human experience need to be explored. These include:

- The lived space (spatiality)
- The lived body (corporeal embodied experience)
- Lived social relationships (relationality)
- Lived time (temporality)

Thus, phenomenology is simultaneously holistic and also relativistic in regard to the particular experiences and situations of each person.

Understanding human experience also requires that the person with the experience must self-interpret these experiences for the researcher, and then the researcher must further interpret the individual's explanation provided by the person. Thus, the method of phenomenology is one of interactive dialogue and exchange as the researcher seeks to know what the experience is like.

Typically, the data in phenomenological studies are collected by in-depth conversations in which the researcher and the subject (informant) are fully interactive. Analysis begins when the first data are collected. This analysis guides decisions related to further data collection. The meanings attached to the data are expressed within phenomenological philosophy. The outcome of analysis is a theoretical statement responding to the research question, and the statement is validated by examples of the data, often direct quotes from the subjects.

The procedures for phenomenological research involve biographical storytelling and informal discussion, with encouragement to reflect on at least the four aspects of experience outlined previously. Researchers listen for and inquire about the body, time, place, and settings of the phenomena, but the informant is entirely in charge of directing the narratives and story telling. In one example, OT researchers aimed to characterize the experiential features of engagement in creative activity as therapy for elderly people with terminal illness (McMullen & Luborsky, 2006). Using extended discussions about the projects undertaken by older adults in Sweden, the researchers found how creative activity served as a medium that enabled creation of connections to wider culture and daily life, which countered some of the more serious social consequences of terminal illness, such as isolation. The creation of connections to life experience in this study embodied three features: a generous perceptive environment as the foundation for meaningful activity, the creations as an unfolding and evolving liberating process, and a reaching beyond the present for possible meaning horizons. The findings showed that creative activity fosters connections to meanings as an active person, even in the face of uncertain life-threatening illness.

Contributions of Phenomenological Research

As the previous example illustrated, powerful insights relevant to occupational therapy are provided by this perspective. For example, Hasselkus (1998) used a phenomenological approach to illuminate the daily experiences of day-staff who cared for patients with Alzheimer's disease on a

dementia unit. Studies like this that deeply probe the experiences of care providers, be they professionals, family members, or others, are essential for the profession so that we can see how our interventions best fit to support the efforts of others.

A phenomenology method formulated by Karlsson (1993) has been used among some OT researchers. For example, a compelling use of this phenomenological method is reported by Tham, Borell, and Gustavsson (2000). In this study of the experience of unilateral neglect following stroke, research findings strongly supported the value of occupational therapy and clearly illustrated the links between research and effective practice. The following passage from the study illustrates the kind of insights that phenomenological research seeks to achieve (Tham & Kielhofner, 2003):

> The study demonstrated that the participants needed to experience and ultimately come to a practical recognition of their own impairments and the consequences of those impairments during occupational performance, before they learned to handle them in everyday life. However, because neglect represents a particular life-world experience, people with neglect had to learn to stand outside their own experience. Specifically, because unilateral neglect is not directly experienced by the person who has it (e.g., the left half of the world is not "felt" to be absent from perception), persons with neglect must embark on a discovery process. This discovery process involves coming to understand that there exists a half of the world that is not part of their life-world. Once they can comprehend the existence of a part of the world that is outside their experience, they could begin to manage the consequences of their own unilateral neglect during occupational performance. (p. 404)

Summary

In qualitative research there is no single approach. As Patton (2001) suggests, investigators need to use the methods that are most appropriate for the research questions they confront. Quantitative researchers select from a toolkit of methods and frameworks, and they have a wide range of methods from which to select those best suited to their questions, the data required to answer the questions, and the forms of analyses suited to that data.

Although qualitative research is often used as the first or exploratory investigation in a new area, it is also used to address problems that other methods have not been able to unravel in a well-researched area. For the purposes of this chapter, it is sufficient to have begun to appreciate the multiple kinds of stances and goals available to qualitative researchers. Chapters 16 to 18 provide more details of the nuts and bolts of undertaking qualitative research and illustrate in practical ways how to implement the different frameworks outlined in this chapter.

Review Questions

1. How does qualitative research deepen and extend the findings of quantitative research?
2. How does qualitative research provide a foundation for quantitative research?
3. What are the unique aims of qualitative research?
4. What is epistemology, and what role does it play in qualitative research?
5. What are the five major epistemological traditions (or designs) in qualitative research, and how would a researcher choose one for a study?
6. What are some of the unique contributions of qualitative research in occupational therapy?

REFERENCES

American Journal of Public Health. (2003, August). [This issue focuses on public health advocacy and includes an article on challenges and strategies to obtain funding for community-based participatory research.]

American Journal of Public Health. (2003, September). [This issue focuses on the built environment and health. The article "Jemez Pueblo: Built and Social-Cultural Environments and Health Within a Rural American Indian Community in the Southwest" describes a study that used participatory research to uncover sociocultural and environmental factors that indicate capacity for improving health.]

Becker, G., & Kaufman, S. (1995). Managing an uncertain illness trajectory after stroke: Patients' and physicians' views of stroke. *Medical Anthropology Quarterly, 9,* 165–187.

Bertaux, D. (Ed.). (1981). *Biography and society: The life history approach in the social sciences.* Beverly Hills, CA: Sage.

Boas, F. (1966). *Kwakiutl ethnography.* Chicago, IL: University of Chicago Press.

Brush, S. (1977). Myth of the idle peasant: Employment in a subsistence economy. In R. Halperin & J. Dow (Eds.), *Peasant livelihood* (pp. 60–78). New York, NY: St. Martin's Press.

Clements, D., Copeland, L., & Loftus, M. (1990). Critical times for families with a chronically ill child. *Pediatric Nursing, 16*(2), 157–161.

Corbin, J., & Strauss, A. (2014). *Basics of qualitative research: Techniques and procedures for developing grounded theory* (4th ed.). Newbury Park, CA: Sage.

Crist, P., & Kielhofner, G. (2005). *The scholarship of practice: Academic-practice collaborations for promoting occupational therapy.* Binghamton, NY: Hayworth Press.

Csordas, T. (1994). *Embodiment and experience: The existential ground of culture and self.* Cambridge, England: Cambridge University Press.

Dannefer, D., & Sell, R. (1988). Age structure, the life course and "aged heterogeneity": Prospects for research and theory. *Comprehensive Gerontology Series B, 2*(1), 1–10.

Das, V. (2001). *Stigma, contagion, defect: Issues in the anthropology of public health.* Presented at Stigma and Global Health: Developing a Research Agenda, an international conference. Bethesda, MD. Retrieved from http://documents.mx/documents/das-stigma-contagion-defect.html

De Koning, K., & Martin, M. (1996). *Participatory research in health: Issues and experiences.* London, England: Zen Books.

Dijkers, M. (1997). Quality of life after spinal cord injury: A meta-analysis of the effects of disablement components. *Spinal Cord, 35,* 829–840.

Dijkers, M. (1998). Community integration: Conceptual issues and measurement approaches in rehabilitation research. *Topics in Spinal Cord Injury Rehabilitation, 4,* 1–15.

Edgerton, R. B. (1967, 1993). *The cloak of competence: Stigma in the lives of the mentally retarded.* Berkeley, CA: University of California Press.

Embree, L. (Ed.). (1997). *Encyclopedia of phenomenology.* Boston, MA: Kluwer Academic.

Finlayson, M. (2004). Concerns about the future among older adults with multiple sclerosis. *American Journal of Occupational Therapy, 58,* 54–63.

Forsyth, K., Summerfield-Mann, L., & Kielhofner, G. (2005). A scholarship of practice: Making occupation-focused, theory-driven, evidence-based practice a reality. *British Journal of Occupational Therapy, 68,* 261–268.

Geertz, C. (1973). *The interpretation of cultures.* New York, NY: Basic Books.

Gitlin, L., Luborsky, M., & Schemm, R. (1998). Emerging concerns of older stroke patients about assistive device use. *The Gerontologist, 38*(2), 169–180.

Gitlin, L., Lyons, K. J., & Kolodner, E. (1994). A model to build collaborative research or educational teams of health professionals in gerontology. *Educational Gerontology, 20*(1), 15–34.

Glaser, B., & Strauss, A. (1967). *The discovery of grounded theory: Strategies for qualitative research.* Chicago, IL: Aldine.

Gross, D. (1984). Time allocation: A tool for the study of cultural behavior. *Annual Review of Anthropology, 13,* 519–558.

Habermas, J. (1988). *The logic of the social sciences.* Cambridge, MA: MIT Press.

Hammersley, M. (1992). *What's wrong with ethnography? Methodological explorations.* London, England: Routledge.

Hart, E., & Bond, M. (1996). Making sense of action research through the use of a typology. *Journal of Advanced Nursing, 23*(1), 152–159.

Hasselkus, B. R. (1998). Occupation and well-being in dementia: The experience of day-care staff. *American Journal of Occupational Therapy, 52,* 423–434.

Honneth, A. (1991). *The critique of power: Reflective stages in a critical social theory.* Cambridge, MA: MIT Press.

House, J., Kessler, R., & Herzog, A. (1990). Age, socioeconomic status, and health. *Milbank Quarterly, 68*(3), 383–411.

Husserl, E. (2001). *Logical investigations* (vols. 1 and 2), Trans. J. N. Findlay. Edited with translation corrections and with a new Introduction by Dermot Moran. With a new Preface by Michael Dummett. London, England: Routledge. [A new and revised edition of the original English translation by J. N. Findlay. London: Routledge & Kegan Paul, 1970. From the Second Edition of the German. First edition, 1900–01; second edition, 1913, 1920.]

Idler, E., & Benyamini, Y. (1997). Self-rated health and mortality: A review of twenty-seven community studies. *Journal of Health and Social Behavior, 38*(1), 21–37.

Jason, L. A., Keys, C. B., Suarez-Balcazar, Y., Taylor, R. R., Durlak, J., Davis M., & Isenberg, D. (Eds.). (2004). *Participatory community research: Theories and methods in action.* Washington, DC: American Psychological Association.

Karlsson, G. (1993). *Psychological qualitative research from a phenomenological perspective.* Stockholm, Sweden: Almqvist & Wiksell International.

Kaufman, S., & Becker, G. (1986). Stroke: Health care on the periphery. *Social Science and Medicine, 22,* 983–989.

Kayser-Jones, J., Schell, E., Lyons, W., Kris, A., Chan, J., & Beard, R. (2003). Factors that influence end-of-life care in nursing homes: The physical environment, inadequate staffing, and lack of supervision. *Gerontologist, 43*(2), 76–84.

Kielhofner, G. (1995). A meditation on the use of hands. *Scandinavian Journal of Occupational Therapy, 2,* 153–166.

Kielhofner, G. (2008). *A Model of Human Occupation: Theory and application* (4th ed.). Philadelphia, PA: Lippincott, Williams & Wilkins.

Kronenberg, F., Pollard, N., & Sakellariou, D. (2010). *Occupational therapy without borders.* London, England: Churchill Livingstone.

Langness, L., & Levine, G. (Eds.). (1986). *Culture and retardation.* Dordrecht, Netherlands: Reidel.

Law, M. (1998). *Client-centered occupational therapy.* Thorofare, NJ: Slack.

Link, B., & Phelan, J. (2001). Conceptualizing stigma. *Annual Review of Sociology, 27,* 363–385.

Luborsky, M. (1994a). The cultural adversity of physical disability: Erosion of full adult personhood. *Journal of Aging Studies, 8*(3), 239–253.

Luborsky, M. (1994b). The identification and analysis of themes and patterns. In J. Gubrium & A. Sankar (Eds.), *Qualitative methods in aging research* (pp. 189–210). Thousand Oaks, CA: Sage.

Luborsky, M. (1995). The process of self-report of impairment in clinical research. *Social Science & Medicine, 40*(11), 1447–1459.

Luborsky, M. (1997). Attuning assessment to the client: Recent advances in theory and methodology. *Generations, 21*(1), 10–16.

Luborsky, M., & Rubinstein, R. (1995). Sampling in qualitative research: Rationales, issues, and methods. *Research on Aging, 17*(1), 89–113.

Luborsky, M., & Sankar, A. (1993). Extending the critical gerontology perspective: Cultural dimensions. *Gerontologist, 33*(4), 440–444.

Lysack, C., & Kaufert, J. (1994). Comparing the origins and ideologies of the independent living movement and community based rehabilitation. *International Journal of Rehabilitation Research, 17,* 231–240.

Lysack, C., Zafonte, C., Neufeld, S., & Dijkers, M. (2001). Self-care independence after spinal cord injury: Patient and therapist expectations and real life performance. *Journal of Spinal Cord Medicine, 24*(4), 257–265.

Mattingly, C. (1998). *Healing dramas and clinical plots: The narrative structure of experience.* Cambridge, England: Cambridge University Press.

Mays, N., & Pope, C. (1995a). Observational methods in health care settings. *British Medical Journal, 311,* 182–184.

Mays, N., & Pope, C. (1995b). Reaching the parts other methods cannot reach: An introduction to qualitative methods in health and health services research. *British Medical Journal, 311,* 42–45.

Mays, N., & Pope, C. (1995c). Rigour and qualitative research. *British Medical Journal, 311,* 109–112.

Mays, N., & Pope, C. (2000). Qualitative research in health care: Assessing quality in qualitative research. *British Medical Journal, 320,* 50–52.

McDermott, J. (Ed.). (1967). *The writings of William James.* New York, NY: Random House.

McMullen, C., & Luborsky, M. (2006). Self-rated health appraisal as cultural and identity process: African-American elders' health evaluative rationales. *Gerontologist, 46*(4), 431–438.

Minkler, M., Blackwell, A., Thompson, M., & Tamir, H. (2003). Community-based participatory research: Implications for public health funding. *American Journal of Public Health, 93*(8), 1210–1213.

Mishler, E. (1986). *Research interviewing.* Cambridge, MA: Harvard University Press.

Mossey, J., & Shapiro, E. (1982). Self rated health: A predictor of mortality among the elderly. *American Journal of Public Health, 72,* 800–808.

Moustakas, C. (1994). *Phenomenological research methods.* Thousand Oaks, CA: Sage.

Murphy, R. (1987). *The body silent.* New York, NY: Henry Holt.

National Institutes of Health. (2001). *Qualitative methods in health research: Opportunities and considerations in application and review* [NIH Publication No. 02-5046]. Bethesda, MD: Office of Behavioral and Social Sciences Research, National Institutes of Health. Retrieved from http://obssr.od.nih.gov/Publications/Qualitative.PDF

Patton, M. (2001). *Qualitative evaluation and research methods* (3rd ed.), Thousand Oaks, CA: Sage.

Ragin, C., Nagel, J., & White, P. (Eds.). (2004). *Workshop on the scientific foundations of qualitative research* [Document Number: nsf04219]. Arlington, VA: National Science Foundation. Retrieved from http://www.nsf.gov/pubs/2004/nsf04219/start.htm

Reilly, M. (1962). Eleanor Clark Slagle Lecture: Occupational therapy can be one of the great ideas of 20th century medicine. *American Journal of Occupational Therapy, 16,* 1–9.

Rossman, G. B., & Rallis, S. F. (1998). *Learning in the field: An introduction to qualitative research.* Thousand Oaks, CA: Sage.

Schnelle, J. F., Traughber, B., Sowell, V. A., Newman, D. R., Petrilli, C. O., & Ory, M. (1989). Treatment of urinary incontinence in nursing home patients. A behavior management approach for nursing home staff. *Journal of the American Geriatrics Society, 37,* 1051–1057.

Schwandt, T. (1997). *The Sage dictionary of qualitative inquiry.* Thousand Oaks, CA: Sage.

Spradley, J. (1979). *The ethnographic interview.* New York, NY: Holt, Rinehart and Winston.

Spradley, J. (1980). *Participant observation.* New York, NY: Holt, Rinehart and Winston.

Stafford, P. (Ed.). (2003). *Gray areas: Ethnographic encounters with nursing home culture.* Sante Fe, NM: School of American Research Press.

Stringer, E. T. (2014). *Action research* (4th ed.). Thousand Oaks, CA: Sage.

Taylor, R. R., Braveman, B., & Hammel, J. (2004). Developing and evaluating community services through participatory action research: Two case examples. *American Journal of Occupational Therapy, 58,* 73–82.

Tham, K., Borell, L., & Gustavsson, A. (2000). The discovery of disability: A phenomenological study of unilateral neglect. *American Journal of Occupational Therapy, 54,* 398–406.

Tham, K., & Kielhofner, G. (2003). Impact of the social environment on occupational experience and performance among persons with unilateral neglect. *American Journal of Occupational Therapy, 57,* 403–412.

Townsend, E., Langille, L., & Ripley, D. (2003). Professional tensions in client-centered practice: Using institutional ethnography to generate understanding and transformation. *American Journal of Occupational Therapy, 57*(1), 17–28.

Townsend, E. A., & Wilcock, A. A. (2003). Occupational justice. In C. Christiansen & E. Townsend (Eds.), *Introduction to occupation* (pp. 243–273). Upper Saddle River, NJ: Prentice-Hall.

Viswanathan, M., Ammerman, A., Eng, E., Gartlehner, G., Lohr, K., Griffith, D., . . . Whitener, L. (2004). *Community-based participatory research: Assessing the evidence. Summary, Evidence Report/Technology Assessment No. 99* [Prepared by RTI–University of North Carolina Evidence-Based Practice Center under Contract No. 290-02-0016, AHRQ Publication 04-E022-1]. Rockville, MD: Agency for Healthcare Research and Quality. Retrieved from http://www.ahrq.gov/clinic/evrptpdfs .htm#cbpr.

Wark, L. (1992). Qualitative research journals. *The Qualitative Report, 1*(4). Retrieved from http://www.nova.edu/ ssss/QR/QR1-4/wark.html

Whiteford, G., & Wright St. Clair, V. (Eds.). (2004). *Occupation & practice in context.* Sydney, Australia: Elsevier Churchill Livingstone.

Zemke, R., & Clark, F. (Eds.). (1996). *Occupational science: The evolving discipline.* Philadelphia, PA: F.A. Davis.

CHAPTER 17

Collecting Qualitative Data

Cathy Lysack • Mark R. Luborsky • Heather Dillaway

Learning Outcomes

- Define the four primary methods for collecting data within the qualitative tradition.
- Understand the roles of participation and observation in accomplishing the key objectives of data collection in qualitative research studies.
- Compare and contrast approaches to interviewing in qualitative research.
- Describe approaches used to increase the accuracy of data collection in qualitative research.
- List approaches for gaining entry into a qualitative research site and approaches for exiting the site.

Introduction

Qualitative research has become an increasingly important mode of inquiry for occupational therapists. Long dominated by techniques borrowed from the experimental sciences, occupational therapy has embraced many of the methods of the social sciences, particularly from anthropology and sociology, as an alternate means of studying and understanding social phenomena of relevance to the profession. Although valuable in its own right, quantitative research differs substantially from qualitative research. Qualitative methods use the local varieties of languages and words of the participants in the social settings studied. These methods work to discover and describe participant-defined topics of concern and socioculturally constructed worlds within which individuals pursue meaningful actions. In short, qualitative methods seek to discover and describe socioculturally constructed worldviews, values, and sociocultural norms and how these are instilled, enacted, reinforced, or resisted and changed in everyday life. Qualitative researchers go to the field to study the topic in the natural settings where people socially interact.

In its broadest sense, **qualitative research** must be understood as the systematic study of social phenomena. Irrespective of its particular disciplinary roots, qualitative studies ask questions that are rarely specifiable as conventional hypotheses, as is the case in quantitative research. The ultimate goal of qualitative research is to go beyond the *what* of research to explain the *why* and *how*. This empirical pursuit requires concepts and tools that yield such information and approaches.

Major Strategies for Collecting Data

As shown in the studies described in the Case Example, qualitative "methods" use the local varieties of languages and words of the participants in the social settings studied.

There are four main methods for gathering qualitative data:

1. Participation in the setting
2. Direct observation
3. In-depth interviewing
4. Analyzing written documents and material objects

All of these methods fundamentally reflect the core qualities of qualitative research as identified by Rossman and Rallis (1998). This chapter provides a review and discussion of these four methods, highlighting their relative strengths and weaknesses. Given the key role of the qualitative researcher as a data collection instrument, the role and stance of the qualitative researcher are also critically examined.

Participation

Participation is both an overall approach to inquiry and a data gathering method. To some degree, all

CASE EXAMPLE

Faizan is a professor teaching research methods to first-year occupational therapy (OT) students. He wants his students to have a broad understanding of data collection approaches in qualitative research. He assigns his class to conduct a literature review to provide one example of a study that used participant observation as a data collection method and one example of a study that used focus-group interviewing. To make the assignment interesting, he decides to offer a gift certificate to the university bookstore to the student who comes up with the most detailed example of participant observation and one to the student who comes up with the most detailed example of a focus-group interview.

One of Faizan's students, Jordan, comes up with the following example of a study by Siporin and Lysack (2004) in which participant observation was used. Siporin and Lysack (2004) were interested to know how the self-perceived quality of life (QOL) of women with developmental disabilities working in supported employment differed from those working in sheltered workshops. In this study, the principal investigator (Siporin) devoted weeks of inconspicuous observational data collection in the places of employment of her research participants. In the daytime, she accompanied her research participants as they worked in small enclaves as housekeepers in local hotels and as food preparation assistants in fast-food restaurants. In the evenings, she observed their leisure activities with their family and friends.

This design choice provided invaluable data about the structures and routines that characterized her subjects' work and home lives. For example, the pace of work, chain of authority at work, and the complexity of numerous pieces of equipment in the workplace were far more evident to the investigator after observation than before. So were the stresses these women experienced because of unreliable transportation. Frequent but unpredictable disruptions in bus transportation wreaked havoc with the official work schedule to which they were supposed to adhere. This caused tensions and occasionally heated arguments and certainly reduced the more positive attitudes these women might have held toward the supported employment experience. A lack of available safe transportation also curtailed participants' leisure activities (e.g., shopping, going to movies, bowling).

Other observations in the home setting provided essential data with which to understand these women's QOL. These data painted a picture about the love, respect, and acceptance these women enjoyed and what specific roles and responsibilities they assumed within their families. These data also provided a valuable contrast or counterpoint against which to compare the workplace observations. Finally, participant-observation data in this study revealed how agency policies and governmental regulations affected participants' QOL. For example, it was learned that if a supported employment worker actually improved her skills to the extent that she was promoted and received a pay raise, she would likely become Medicaid ineligible, thus putting in jeopardy insurance coverage for significant medical expenses, including, for example, hospital care, durable medical equipment, prescription medications, and eyeglasses. This was not something these women (or their families) were prepared to do. Thus, despite their wishes and efforts to become more self-sufficient, the women with developmental disabilities stopped short of any "success" that would put their Medicaid eligibility at risk. Without the method of participant observation, these policies and regulations would not have been identified, nor would their consequences on the participants' perceived QOL be fully understood.

Another student, Sophia, came up with the following example of focus-group research. Dillaway and a research team from the Barbara Ann Karmanos Cancer Institute in Detroit conducted a study about African American men and prostate cancer (Dillaway et al., 2005). The purposes of this study were:

1. To explore African American men's awareness of prostate cancer,
2. To determine the barriers to their participation in prostate cancer research trials, and
3. To begin to develop new ideas for recruitment strategies to encourage more African American men to participate in research trials.

(case study continues on page 198)

In the pilot stage of the research, focus-group interviews were used because the research team members wanted to make sure that they were exploring a large range of potential barriers to recruitment and were unsure what recruitment strategies would increase African American men's participation in research.

Not wishing to assume they already knew the answers to these questions, focus groups were selected so the investigators could see how African American men themselves conversed about these topics. During the summer of 2003, eight focus groups comprising 61 African American men were conducted. Focus-group participants highlighted a range of barriers to their participation in research trials, many of which were expected. For instance, in every focus group, participants highlighted their mistrust of doctors and researchers as a reason for their reluctance to participate, sometimes referring to the infamous Tuskegee experiment as a reason for this mistrust. In that experiment, African American men with syphilis were not informed that they were taking part in a research study on the long-term consequences of untreated syphilis.

Because the investigators were well aware of the historical injustices perpetrated on this minority population in the name of health research, they expected participants to highlight such barriers. Yet, in the course of conversation, African American men also highlighted reasons why they would participate in research trials. For instance, in all eight focus groups, participants discussed how important it was for African American men to "step up" and be models for future generations. They also discussed how important it was to keep themselves healthy so that they could ensure their ability to finish raising their children. Finally, they highlighted the fact that, in order to remedy the lack of knowledge about African American men's health, they knew they had to overcome their mistrust of research studies and participate in research, if only to make certain that their children would be healthier than they were.

As a result of the focus groups, the research team learned that individual participants had a higher awareness of prostate cancer and a greater desire for more research than any of the team members expected. In addition, although the researchers expected participants to highlight barriers to participation in research, they did not expect participants to highlight so many reasons why they would be willing to participate. Because most existing research only highlights the barriers to African Americans' participation in research, the researchers did not even ask any questions about why individuals might want to participate in research trials. Thus, if the researchers had not conducted focus groups, a method of data collection in which new meanings can be highlighted within group conversation, they may not have realized that individual African American men have many reasons to participate in prostate cancer research and, more specifically, may not have realized that African American men's connections to their families and to racialized communities could directly facilitate individuals' participation in research trials. In this situation, these data would not have been identified without the focus-group method.

qualitative research has a participatory element. Participation demands firsthand involvement in the social world chosen for study. Qualitative researchers work to gain access to modes of understanding and to approximate as closely as possible the lived realities of those studied, knowing that they will rarely (some would say never) truly experience the situation exactly as their participants do. The purpose of engaging in participation is not to become one of the group studied, but rather to use what is seen and heard to help identify what is important to learn about and to discover issues and events that might not be obvious to an outsider using only preconceived ideas.

Ideally, as with the traditions of cultural anthropology and qualitative sociology, researchers will spend considerable time in the field. Depending on the study purpose and the size of the research project, this could mean anywhere from several weeks to a year or more participating in the routine activities of the group and setting. This immersion experience offers the qualitative researcher the opportunity to learn directly from his or her own experience. The implicit premise is that a truer understanding of the phenomenon studied will be obtained. This approach requires the researcher to be very self-aware and reflective, not only observing the actions and behaviors of others, but also appreciating and recording his or her own personal thoughts, experiences, and reactions.

The personal reflections gained from participation in the research setting, as well as the observations made, are systematically recorded and included as an essential part of the study data. Thus, simultaneously, the researcher using participation as a method is challenged to recognize and record how his or her presence in the field may or may not be influencing study participants' behaviors in the field. Major efforts to track the impact of the presence of the investigator in the field are a feature of this methodology. Journals and field notes, recorded both during and after episodes of data collection, are a core source of study data.

Observation

Observation requires careful watching, listening, and recording of events, behaviors, and objects in the social setting chosen for study. The observation record, frequently referred to as field notes, is composed of detailed nonjudgmental, concrete descriptions of what has been observed. For studies relying exclusively on observation, the researcher makes no special effort to have a particular role in the setting other than simply being an unobtrusive observer.

Unlike participation methods, observational methods do not ask the researcher to become actively involved. Rather, the researcher takes a relatively outsider role. Observational studies of in-patient rehabilitation units are one example of this type of study. Of course, without other sources of data, the meaning of observations can only be inferred. That is why, in many qualitative studies in which not only the setting is important but also the interpersonal interactions in persons in those settings and the personal views held by those in the setting, the study may include elements of both observation *and* participation.

Participant observation is a more active data gathering strategy and combines elements of both approaches. In this method, the investigator establishes and sustains a many-sided relationship with a social phenomenon in its natural setting for the purpose of developing a scientific understanding of that phenomenon. Participant observation thus allows qualitative researchers to see how things really are (observation) and also check in (participation) with knowledgeable insiders who can confirm, or disconfirm, the researchers' emergent insights, understandings, and explanations as they experience the social phenomenon firsthand.

There can be several degrees of participant observation, sometimes in sequence. In its earliest stages, the qualitative researcher using a participant-observation approach enters the field with a broad topic of interest but no predetermined categories or strict observational checklists. At this stage, the investigator is intent on identifying and describing the actions of the participants in pursuit of meaningful goals, values, and ideals. Noting these patterns and reviewing them systematically over time leads to the development and use of more highly specified observational checklists and perhaps even some direct questions to key participants in the setting.

The ultimate goal of the qualitative researcher using participant observation is to understand and explain the sociocultural values, norms, and expectations that underlie the personal beliefs and individual actions observed. As time in the field proceeds, it is possible to understand more fully both what one is observing and what it all means. As stated at the beginning of this chapter, qualitative research is responsive to the changing conditions of the research setting and the topic studied. Thus, as new data are obtained and synthesized, the iterative process of uncovering and then confirming emergent understandings (that is, analysis) begins.

Many qualitative studies use observational methods, at least to some degree. For example, when conducting an in-depth interview, a qualitative researcher is engaged in a shared social scene with customs and expectations about how to interact, be respectful, and reciprocate. The nature of the social interaction is part of the data collection and the data to record. Also, investigators are attentive to the participants' body language and affect— not only their words. In whatever ways observation is used, it is demanding on the part of the researcher. Observational researchers confront psychological discomfort and fatigue and unexpected ethical dilemmas, and they may even expose themselves to unanticipated danger. In addition, they are required to responsibly and as completely as possible record the social happenings around them at the same time as they are trying to find the big picture analytically. This is a real challenge because studying human beings in their natural environments (e.g., in home settings, rehabilitation centers, schools, etc.) by definition implies complexity and a fast-paced and ever-changing social scene.

The following are key objectives of qualitative researchers using participation and observation:

- "Gaining entry" to the setting.
- Negotiating and establishing a social identity in the setting.
- Sustained engagement in the research setting over time and learning how to maintain good relationships in that community or group.
- Active and genuine involvement with group members.

- Development of useful observational measures.
- Accurate documentation of observations in distracting conditions.
- Managing requests to align oneself with one person or group versus another.
- Simultaneously participating with and recording observations of study participants at the same time as experiencing the phenomenon oneself and recording it in a complex and ever-changing environment.
- Documenting additional field notes, questions, quandaries, and complexities after each data collection episode.

It must be recognized that qualitative studies utilizing observation and participation have both strengths and weaknesses. Their greatest strength is that they provide very rich and detailed data in settings and situations in which subjects are observed. Whereas other methods such as in-depth interviews would contribute information from one individual's point of view, observation and participation allow the investigator to study interactions between multiple persons and between persons in specific physical and/or social environments. Furthermore, observation and participation methods are necessary when individual interviews are not possible because of the limited capacity of the participants. For example, some research participants may not be able to provide full and complete information about their experiences because of the nature of their disability or health condition itself. When this is the case, alternate or at least supplemental data gathering strategies are necessary.

Clearly, participation and observation studies are very time- and labor-intensive endeavors. These types of studies also require a great deal of advance preparation, including, at times, special permission to allow access to the setting and group members of interest. In addition, the presence of the researcher in both participation and observation studies can lead study participants to alter their behavior in order to "look good" in the eyes of the researcher or provide what they perceive to be as "the right answer" (i.e., **social desirability bias** or **Hawthorne effect,** both of which occur when subjects change their behavior because they know they are being observed). This can pose a serious threat to the validity of study findings.

Qualitative researchers must be aware of the potential for study participants to influence the events that transpire during data collection as well as the potential for those influences to impact the study findings. Fortunately, although individuals being studied may be conscious of the presence of the researcher and consciously edit or restrict their more extreme or controversial opinions and actions, over time study participants will become less concerned about the presence of the investigator and reveal their "true" thoughts and behaviors. As with all data collection methods, however, the investigator faces tradeoffs with every methodological choice. Table 17.1 summarizes the strengths and weaknesses of participant observation. The most successful qualitative researchers will consider all aspects of their topic, its purpose, and the research setting they are in, and then choose their research methods accordingly.

In-Depth Interviews

In-depth interviews are most often conducted in face-to-face situations with one individual, although they can be conducted by telephone and in a group situation (see the following discussion of focus-group interviews). The goal of the in-depth interview is to delve deeply into a particular event, issue, or context. Interviews differ from participation and observation primarily in the nature of the interaction. In the in-depth interview, the purpose is to probe the ideas of the interviewees and obtain the most detailed information possible about the topic at hand. Interviews vary with respect to their a priori structure and in the latitude the interviewee has in responding to questions.

Generally speaking, though, in-depth interviews can be developed along a continuum (Fig. 17.1). At one end of the continuum is the most open-ended and unstructured conversational approach, in which the interview proceeds more like a casual visit. Another, slightly more directed approach includes having some prepared but still unstructured topics about which to inquire. A semi-structured interview provides even more structure by using a combination of fixed-response and open-ended questions. At the far other end of the continuum is the structured interview, in which the questions and response categories are virtually all predetermined.

Irrespective of their specific form, data gathered using in-depth interviewing methods are typically recorded using audiotapes and written notes, and sometimes even video recording when the study purpose demands. Audio and video recording are used to increase the amount of data available for later analyses and to provide verification of data accuracy. For example, audiotapes can be used to collect data ranging from a running paraphrase or summary of a conversation all the way to microscopically detailed data on the voice contours as people speak each word and the length of pauses and speed of talking. With recording, the

Table 17.1 Participant-Observation: Relative Strengths and Limitations

Participant-Observation	Strengths	Weaknesses
	"Rich description," that is, detailed information about the social phenomenon studied is gathered. Very natural (i.e., valid) data are obtained in these normal (versus laboratory) settings. It is the only method that permits study of people's actual behaviors (versus merely their attitudes and beliefs) in a particular physical and social environment. It may be the only form of data collection possible when study participants themselves cannot be interviewed because of their disability.	There are few opportunities to probe the specific meanings of participants' actions and behaviors if data are not supplemented by other methods such as interviews. Responses may be influenced by social desirability bias. It can be complex to analyze these data without other data to confirm the observed and/or investigator-experienced data. Advance planning, special permissions, and more detailed institutional review board/ethics proposals are often required before approval for the study is granted.

Unstructured interview	Semistructured interview	Structured interview
• Open-ended, conversational approach • Guided conversation • Proceeds like a casual visit	• More structure • Fixed-response and open-ended questions	• Even more structure • Questions and response categories are predetermined

Figure 17.1 There are three types of in-depth interviews that are used by researchers in occupational therapy.

researcher obtains a written transcription of the interview, which can be analyzed at a later point in the study, again at varying levels of detail.

Unstructured Interviews

Unstructured interviews resemble guided conversations. Such interviews typically include a relatively short list of "grand tour" general questions (sometimes referred to as an "interview guide"), and interviewers generally respect how the interviewee frames and structures responses. For example, an unstructured interview about the adequacy of home care received by a recently discharged patient who had a stroke may begin with a general question such as, "How is your home care going since you got out of the hospital?" The answer provided may be brief or lengthy, but no matter what the interviewee says, the interviewer accepts the words used and explanations as offered. Still, when appropriate, some gently probing follow-up questions may be used to delve more deeply into interviewees' initial responses, seeking examples, explanations, and rationales for expressed beliefs and behaviors. For example, an

appropriate probe after a question such as, "Have you encountered any unexpected surprises with your home care?" might be something like "Could you describe one or two of these surprises?" Optimally, probes like this are value neutral and function simply to elicit more information. They are not meant to direct the respondent toward any particular topic or value judgment, but rather to encourage the respondent to reveal more specific information about his or her personal experiences and circumstances. Other appropriate probes might be, "Can you tell me more about your reasons for this answer?" and "Could you give an example?" Most importantly, however, the unstructured or conversational interview conveys the attitude that the participant's views are valuable and useful, and the task of the researcher is to capture these views as completely and accurately as possible.

Semistructured and Structured Interviews

Semistructured and structured interviews permit modest to maximum investigator control over the design and sequence of research questions.

Table 17.2   Fixed-Response Versus Open-Ended Interview Questions: Relative Strengths and Limitations

Strengths	Limitations
Fixed-Response Questions	
They are quick to ask and answer. A large cohort of data can be obtained in a short time. By forcing "one best answer," more honest data may be obtained. Responses can be more easily compared across groups. Statistical analysis can be conducted on numerical data.	It is unclear whether the respondent understood the question as the researcher intended. Relevant information may not be collected. Responses may be influenced by social desirability bias.
Open-Ended Questions	
Respondents' interpretation of the question is more obvious. Issues of importance to the participant are more likely to be identified and described. There are sufficient time and interviewer awareness to record nonverbal behaviors and emotional responses (e.g. tears, anger, confusion, etc.). With a skilled interviewer, sensitive topics can be more easily probed and explored.	It can be very time consuming to both gather and analyze data. Respondents may not wish to reveal personal, sensitive, or provocative information. Data from open-ended questions are not easily comparable across groups. Without well-trained interviewers, too much of the data gathered may be "off-topic" and not adequately address the study aims.

Semistructured interviews provide some structure by using a combination of fixed-response and open-ended questions. In **structured interviews,** interviewers are trained to ask each question precisely as written. This does not mean, however, that the interview consists only of fixed-response questions. All interviews, whether unstructured or structured, can include both fixed-response and open-ended questions. For example, a qualitative interview focused on the meaning of disability might include a fixed-response question such as, "Do you think of yourself as the same person you were before your injury?" for which the response set could be limited to "yes" or "no." The response categories could also be categorical and ordered, for example, "Yes, just the same," "Yes, somewhat the same," "No, not really the same," and "No, absolutely not the same at all." Finally, the question could be entirely open-ended.

As their name suggests, semistructured interviews typically include a combination of fixed-response and open-ended questions with a variety of response categories, some of which border on the kinds of response categories typical of surveys. Structured interviews provide the least interviewer flexibility because all of the questions are predetermined and the interviewer is encouraged not to deviate at all from the prescribed interview protocol. Table 17.2 summarizes the strengths and weaknesses of fixed-response versus open-ended interview questions.

Interviewing has strengths and limitations. Interviews involve personal interaction and cooperation, so trust and rapport between interviewer and interviewee are essential. Interviewees may not be comfortable sharing all that the interviewer hopes to explore, or they may be unaware of specific facts and experiences that are relevant to the study purpose but are not revealed in the interview.

Lack of skill and training on the part of the qualitative researcher may also lead to poorly developed questions, and inadequate interviewer training may lead to inadequate probing and follow-up questions during the interview itself. To be successful, qualitative interviewers must work to develop superb listening skills and be skillful at personal interaction, question framing, and gentle probing for elaboration. One of the great benefits of interviews is the volume of detailed data that can be obtained. However, even optimal interview data are time consuming to analyze, and depending on the expertise of the interviewer, some of these data will not be central to the study aims and thus may not illuminate the study topic at hand. Transcribing and analyzing less relevant data is costly and time consuming. Finally, there is the issue of the quality of interview data. When interviewing is the sole method of qualitative data collection, the qualitative researcher obtains the interviewees' perspectives on events and issues. This is usually absolutely appropriate. However, if the study aims require more objective confirmation of events and issues, the qualitative investigator may need to triangulate his or her interview data with data gathered through other methods. The process of triangulation (discussed further later in the chapter) provides an additional methodological check on the validity and reliability of study data.

In certain circumstances, qualitative researchers will have to consider a wider array of factors when planning and carrying out interviews. This is true when interviewing special or vulnerable populations, for example, children or persons with specific types of disabilities. For example, interviews with children require greater care during the construction of interview questions to ensure they are not too complex for a child to understand. Depending on the topic, questions may also pose unique risks to the child. For example, particular interview questions about severe burns they sustained in a traumatic house fire or injuries sustained in a serious car accident may create emotional upset, fear, or even psychological distress, depending on circumstances associated with those events. Similarly, interviews with persons with specific types of physical and cognitive disabilities demand special consideration. Qualitative interviewing in these contexts requires not only more careful interview item construction in advance of the interview, but also training to prepare the interviewer for a range of expected and unexpected challenges during data collection itself. For example, persons with a stroke may have comprehension and speaking difficulties, and it may be necessary to move from more open-ended to more fixed-response-style questions.

In addition, the choice of interviewer is a consideration. Sensitive topics about sexual function or victimization, for example, clearly require attention to who can best make the interaction comfortable, such as a same-sex or same-age person. Alternatively, choosing someone with the same ethnic background may not always provide better data. In studies of minorities there may be unstated assumptions about shared understandings or experiences (true or not) that make it harder to get an informant/participant to fully verbalize and explain experiences or beliefs that are "obvious" or taken for granted. Qualitative investigators conducting interviews with these special populations will need to address a wide array of considerations such as these in the institutional review board (IRB)/ethics approval process that is virtually always required in advance of approvals to conduct research studies sponsored by universities, whether these studies take place in a rehabilitation facility or a person's home, school, or workplace, and so forth.

The following are key activities of qualitative researchers before and during in-depth interviews:

- Identifying an appropriate study sample.
- Logging communication during recruitment efforts.
- Establishing comfort, rapport, and trust with interviewees.
- Developing the interview guide (conversational style) or explicit interview protocol (structured interviews).
- Skillful listening and question asking.
- Judging appropriately when, how, and whether to probe and pursue interesting turns in the interview (e.g., disclosure of unexpected information, controversial or provocative opinions and statements, etc.).
- Presentation of the self as a competent and skillful interviewer.
- Note-taking comprehensively while astutely questioning and listening.
- Writing up summaries and notes about what the interviewee said as well as reflective personal observations.

Table 17.3 summarizes the strengths and weaknesses of qualitative interviewing. In addition, there are two other kinds of interviewing that deserve additional mention because of their frequency of use and potential to contribute unique data to a qualitative research project. These are focus-group interviews and key-informant interviews. Table 17.4 summarizes their strengths and weaknesses.

Focus-Group Interviews

The focus-group interview emerged from consumer research in the 1950s. Consumer research showed that people tended to make decisions with other people; therefore, to understand consumer behavior, consumer preferences needed to be studied in a group setting. The same principle holds in OT research. Occupational therapists recognize that many aspects of decision-making, especially decisions related to health and disability, are made with family members and other valued persons. Thus, the optimal context to gather data can sometimes be a context in which numerous and varied perspectives can be heard at the same time. This is what makes the focus group a popular method of gathering qualitative data.

Focus-group interviews are conducted with a small group of people on a specific topic (Fig. 17.2). Typically, 4 to 6 people participate

Table 17.3 Qualitative Interviewing: Relative Strengths and Limitations

Interviewing	Strengths	Weaknesses
	The researcher can gather detailed information on the topic of interest. This method also permits exploration of additional topics generated by individuals' responses. Optimal confidentiality is provided. Assuming expert interviewers who establish a respectful and trusting relationship, more personal information is revealed in interviews than may be the case in focus-group situations.	Lack of efficiency—it takes much more time to gather data from individuals than from groups. All data are "self-reported." There is no opportunity to confirm or disconfirm the personal values, attitudes, and beliefs or the related background and events described by participants, unless triangulation is used. Vast amounts of data are generated by interviews, and they are very costly to transcribe. Data analysis is costly and time consuming, even with excellent data.

Table 17.4 Focus-Group and Key-Informant Interviews: Relative Strengths and Limitations

	Strengths	Limitations
Focus-Groups Interviews		
	Efficiency—the researcher can gather data from multiple persons instead of only one. Because of the dynamic interactions across group members, there is the potential for contradictory opinions and not only consensual views to be shared. More valid data—group interactions tend to hone in on the most salient issues, therefore making it relatively easy to identify a consistent shared view among interviewees.	The number of questions asked must be minimized because it takes so much more time to gather multiple responses. With six people in a 1-hour focus group, an interviewer would have difficulty asking any more than 10 questions. Responses may be overly "sanitized," that is, negatively influenced by social desirability bias. Difficult to control—unexpected diversions, interpersonal conflicts, and so forth can distract group members from the purpose. Skilled facilitators are essential to quality data. It is difficult to take notes with so much going on. There is limited ability to protect confidentiality.
Key-Informant Interviews		
	Insight—key leaders are well informed and can shed considerable light on the history and policies of groups and organizations.	The interview often requires a referral from a prestigious and respected "other" before access is achieved. It sometimes requires great skill and effort to "manage" the egos and personalities of these important leaders and spokespersons.

in the interview, which lasts about 1 to 2 hours, although focus groups can include 8 to 12 participants, or even more. Participants in focus-group interviews are usually a homogeneous group who are selected because of their knowledge about the study topic. Participants in focus groups get to hear one anothers' responses and contribute their own responses in light of what others have said. Often the questions in a focus group are deceptively simple. The aim is to promote the focus-group participants' expressions of their views through the creation of a supportive environment.

As with other methods, the focus group has countervailing strengths and weaknesses. To a great extent, the advantages of the focus-group interview are the disadvantages of the individual interview, and vice versa. The primary advantage of focus-group interviews is their efficiency. A great deal of information can be gathered quickly. In addition, focus groups provide the opportunity for data to emerge as a result of the dynamic interactions between group members. However, it is a common misperception that focus groups are only, or best, for learning about shared opinions or main themes. Nonetheless, focus-group interviews have high face validity (i.e., the questions are transparently reflective of the topic of focus for the assessment). This is because they are conducted

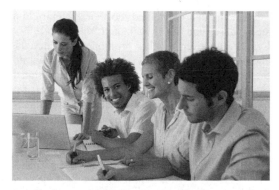

Figure 17.2   Conducting a focus group is an efficient means of collecting data. *(ThinkStock/ Wavebreak Media/Wavebreakmedia LTD.)*

in a natural social setting and under more relaxed circumstances than individual interviews.

The downside, of course, is their management. Particularly strong personalities can dominant the focus group, and some individuals may not have an opportunity to express their views, especially if they are in disagreement with a dominant member of the group. Obtaining optimal data from focus groups requires a skilled facilitator so that there are opportunities for all members to participate and contribute. Because the facilitator/interviewer has less control over what is discussed in the focus group, the interview can result in lost time as irrelevant and dead-end issues are discussed. It may also be difficult to manage the group conversation while simultaneously recording people's opinions on the topic at hand. Finally, data gathered using this method can be very difficult to analyze because context is essential to understanding individual comments, and it is simply not possible to delve into the background context for every opinion offered without the entire focus group grinding to a halt.

Key-Informant Interviews

Key-informant interviews use key informants in at least two ways. In one form, "elite" interviews are conducted with individuals considered to be influential, prominent, and/or well-informed people in an organization or community. For example, if a researcher wanted to collect data on the number of advocacy activities initiated by a prominent center for independent living (i.e., a peer-led infrastructure for advocacy efforts and resources for disabled individuals) in Chicago, she would likely want to approach the chief executive officer or other general manager to obtain this overview. Key informants (elites) are specifically selected for interview on the basis of their expertise in areas

relevant to the research. In the other approach, key informants are selected from the larger sample for more extended and in-depth discussion.

Key-informant interviewing has many advantages. Valuable information can be gained because of the positions these persons hold in social, political, or administrative realms. Key informants can also provide an overall view of the organization and its activities, policies, past history, and future plans from a particular perspective. The disadvantage of key-informant interviewing is that it is often difficult to gain access to this group. They are often very busy people and difficult to contact, especially initially. The interviewer may have to rely on an introduction or recommendation of another elite to gain access/entry to the study setting. Another disadvantage of interviewing key informants or elites is that the interviewer may have to radically adapt the interview to suit the wishes and predilections of the person interviewed. Although this is a possibility with all individual interviewing, elites may be especially bright, thoughtful, and articulate and will resent poorly conceived or ill-phrased questions.

Well practiced at public meetings and persuasive arguments, key informants may desire an active interplay with the interviewer and be unhappy and uncooperative if the interviewer is not superbly prepared or not capable of a pleasing intellectual exchange (see Table 17.4). Thus, conducting key-informant interviews can put a considerable strain on the interviewer, who must demonstrate competence in inquiring about the subject matter at hand and, at some level, be prepared to entertain his or her interviewee with shrewd questioning and even sharp debate. This hard work can pay off, however, because elites are typically intelligent and quick-thinking people and are completely at home in the realm of ideas, policies, and generalizations.

Written Documents and Material Objects

Researchers may choose to gather their data using sources of already existing information, or secondary data. Analysis of available documents (as opposed to primary data newly collected by the researcher, such as interview transcripts) can include diaries and personal journals, historical documents, minutes of meetings, websites, advertisements, annual reports, newspapers, magazines, or political speeches. Analysis can also utilize materials or cultural objects and artifacts.

Researchers who use a review of documents or studies of inanimate objects as their primary or sole method can be described as using an unobtrusive methodology. Observation, described earlier, is also an unobtrusive methodology. It is considered as such because there is minimal investigator disruption to the study participants and setting.

The use of documents often entails a specialized analytic approach called **content analysis.** The raw material of content analysis may be any form of communication or text, although written forms are most common. Historically, content analysis emphasized systematic, objective, and quantitative counts and descriptions of content derived from researcher-developed categories. Today, content analysis can be exclusively numeric or exclusively interpretive—largely dependent on the theoretical traditions dominant within the researcher's discipline. For example, quantitative political scientists might rely exclusively on numerical counts of words in a political speech and use the evidence of the amount of particular forms of speech to argue that a particular politician holds a particular view. In contrast, an anthropologist or a historian will be far more interested in the meaning of the words conveyed by the text than by the number of times a phrase is spoken.

One can easily imagine an OT researcher designing a study using methods of document review and content analysis. For example, if a researcher was interested in understanding the meanings of mobility aids such as walkers, crutches, and wheelchairs to adults with mobility disabilities, the researcher could design a study in which the family photographs of persons who have lived with mobility impairments all of their lives were reviewed and analyzed. The photographs would likely reveal a number of insights, including how the devices were commonly used and what activities these devices were helpful in facilitating.

The qualitative researcher in this type of study would also note who was in the photographs, in what locales the activities occurred, and whether there was any evidence of attempting to hide the mobility devices, perhaps related to embarrassment, shame, or stigma. Of course, a study that supplemented this analysis with individual interviews would result in potentially more useful data than relying on the photographs alone. When multiple methods of data collection are used in the same study, the approach is called triangulation. This is one way of increasing the rigor of a qualitative study; this technique is discussed in more detail later in the chapter.

Reviews of material and cultural objects are not restricted to those provided by individuals in one-on-one situations. Brochures, descriptions of program services, and historical documents developed by organizations, health programs, or social movements can be studied too. For example, in a study described in Lysack and Kaufert (1999), Lysack reviewed books, promotional materials, and educational materials used by activists within the independent living movement and professional proponents of international community-based rehabilitation. The goal of this research was to understand how consumer organizations and professional and policy bodies used the language and imagery of "community" to guide their disability-related educational and rehabilitation activities. Lysack used discourse analysis in this study, a specific method by which special attention is paid to the process of spoken and unspoken communication. This method revealed dramatic tensions between the service-delivery models of the two groups, tensions that were directly linked to the fundamental views held about the meaning of community.

In another example, a study of community integration after spinal cord injury, Lysack and Luborsky's (2004) research team analyzed drawings made by the research participants depicting the meaning of this injury. Although in many cases these drawings were only crude sketches, the visual representations offered a medium by which to express and represent experiences and ideas not readily put into words. Drawing allowed participants a nonverbal way to "tap into" and express deeper feelings. Interviewers on this project were trained to ask questions after the drawing was completed to elicit responses about how and why the drawings were generated as they were. The drawings themselves, coupled with the participants' responses, shed considerable light on topics, including the level of responsibility for the injury felt by participants; the degree of resentment and hostility aimed at those who have provided, or currently provide, medical treatment and care; and in a somewhat more abstract way, the existential place these persons occupy when they assume the label "disabled person" in an able-bodied world.

As stated earlier, methods that use written documents, visual materials, and cultural objects have their advantages. For example, they are usually more quickly moved through the ethical review process because they may be regarded as posing less risk of harm to the participant. On the downside, without supplementation with other data gathering methods, it may be difficult for the qualitative researcher to clarify the meanings of these materials and objects to those who possess them or are influenced by them. As mentioned previously, triangulation of data sources and triangulation of data methods are two ways of increasing the methodological rigor of a qualitative study, issues that are discussed in the next section.

The following are key activities of qualitative researchers engaged in document reviews and analysis of material and cultural objects:

- Selecting appropriate documents or objects
- Gaining permissions to observe and study them
- Selecting and using analytic methods best suited to the kind of data
- Identifying additional means by which to confirm their meanings

Ways of Strengthening the Quality of Qualitative Data

In all research, the question must continuously be asked: "How trustworthy are these data?" The trustworthiness of qualitative data, or how sure we can be that the data are accurate and reflect empirical reality, is essential because the qualitative researcher wants to be confident that the collected data correctly capture the experiences, meanings, and events in the field.

Several important methodological actions can be undertaken to enhance data trustworthiness, including:

- Management of bias
- Interviewer training
- Prolonged engagement in the field
- Reflexivity
- Triangulation
- Member checks
- Audit trails
- Project-based methods

These methods can be employed whether the data are collected via observation, participation, interviews, or review of existing documents, materials, and objects.

Managing Bias in Qualitative Research

Bias is a type of prejudiced consideration or judgment. Several types of bias can negatively impact qualitative studies: (a) overreliance on accessible research participants or favoring of more dramatic events and statements involving research participants and the context of study; (b) biasing effects produced by the presence of the investigator in the research site, that is, the Hawthorne effect; and (c) biases stemming from the influence of the participants and the research site on the investigator. In all of these situations, the investigator may be biased if he or she is unaware of the social influences that various players in the research enterprise exert and are subject to. In qualitative research, biases must be recognized and accounted for. Qualitative investigators have an onus to report on the reasons for having chosen their particular topic for study, their design choices, and their decisions about sample and methods. All need to be transparent so that the reader of the study can judge for themselves the quality of the results.

Interviewer Training

The importance of interviewer training should not be underestimated. The time and financial costs of interviews are great. Thus, significant time spent training interviewers is a critical investment to ensure that data are obtained most efficiently, without compromising their quality.

Interviewer training includes technical skills on how to ask the interview questions and the use of follow-up probes to elicit more detailed explanations. It also includes training on appropriate behaviors needed to gain entry into the research context. The latter includes the interpersonal behaviors with research participants that occur during subject recruitment and data collection. Interviewers must also be carefully trained to ensure a consistent style of data collection across research participants. This requires an element of standardization in question asking and probing. At the same time, however, the interviewer needs to be flexible and responsive when the need arises.

These are skills that can be learned. For example, mock interviews under supervision are an excellent way to learn to ask questions skillfully, to listen carefully, and to pose appropriate follow-up questions (Fig. 17.3). Interviewers especially must learn how to facilitate a somewhat conversational style during the interview at the same time that they communicate respect for the research participant. They must also learn to practice a quiet awareness of the trade-off between patience and efficiency.

Prolonged Engagement in the Field

Prolonged engagement is the phrase used to describe the period of time spent in the field observing the phenomenon of interest. The amount of time in the field varies, depending on the nature of the inquiry and its scope, the design of the study, the time available to the investigator, and the time available to the research participants themselves.

As a rule of thumb, however, data collection continues in the field until saturation is reached.

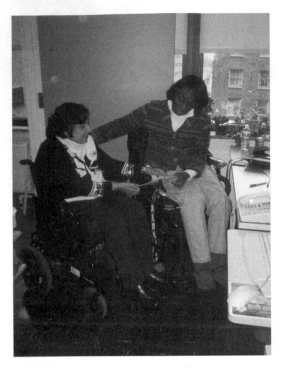

Figure 17.3 Research team members practice conducting a semistructured interview using an interview guide. *(From* Research in Occupational Therapy: Methods of Inquiry for Enhancing Practice, *by Gary Kielhofner, 2006, Philadelphia, PA: F.A. Davis Company, p. 346.)*

Saturation is the point in the data collection period when the researcher is gaining little or no new information. Because the criteria are data based and not time based, there is no knowable ideal duration of time in the field. Investigators need to evaluate their data for signs of diminishing gains or saturation. When investigators are no longer adding new insights or are no longer puzzled by what they observe and are able to predict what is going to happen next, saturation is likely being reached. This means that it is nearing the time to leave the field and begin writing up the results of the observations in the field.

Reflexivity

Reflexivity refers to a deliberate and systematic process of self-examination. It involves a continuous cycle of seeking insights from inward reflection on the experiences of working in the outside world and looking back at what is being learned outside in light of the inner experience.

This process is necessary in qualitative research because the investigator will encounter a wide array of thoughts, feelings, and reactions to people and

events in the course of data collection. Whereas such feelings and reactions are not a major concern of quantitative researchers, they are of great importance to qualitative researchers.

First, these data are important in and of themselves. Especially in observational and participation studies, these are the only data that will be collected and analyzed. Second, the reactions and views of the qualitative researcher—both gleaned as a direct result of participation in the study and brought to the study in the form of preexisting attitudes and values—have the potential to color the data collection and analysis processes. Qualitative researchers acknowledge that this sort of influence is real and has the potential to affect study findings.

They also know that although the "bias" cannot and, in fact, should not be eliminated, it is important to identify it and examine its influence on emerging interpretations. Personal diaries are frequently used by qualitative investigators to note these attitudes, feelings, and reactions. Later, the diaries themselves become a source of data and are an important check on the development of research conclusions.

Triangulation

Triangulation is another technique used to increase the accuracy (or trustworthiness) of data gathered (Fig. 17.4). Triangulation refers to the use of two or more strategies to collect and/or interpret or analyze information. For example, in a single study triangulation may mean using interviews to learn what people say to investigators about using a wheelchair and observation to see what they actually do and tell to others, instead of relying on either method alone. The purpose of triangulation is to validate a particular finding. Triangulation of data methods increases the chances that the conclusions reached are better able to represent the whole set of relevant features, or are "true," as a result of the complementary strengths of the respective methods.

Although triangulation of methods is the most common form of triangulation in qualitative inquiry, there are other forms of triangulation, including triangulation of data gatherers. Triangulation of data gatherers refers to the use of two or more individuals who have independently observed and recorded their own field notes of a phenomenon. Data quality is enhanced by comparing their observations afterward and resolving differences through discussion. The same process can be undertaken during the data analysis stage of a research project. Triangulation in this sense refers to the use of multiple persons to do the data

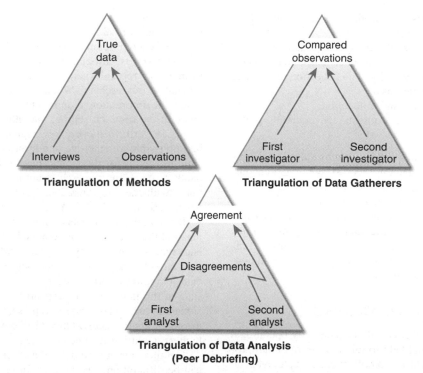

Figure 17.4   Various forms of triangulation are used to increase the accuracy of collected data.

analysis. Sometimes this is called peer debriefing. Irrespective of its title, the process is one of multiple investigators simultaneously but independently engaging in the analytic process.

Peer debriefing is very valuable in qualitative inquiry because it provides a means by which areas of disagreement and controversy are highlighted. Again, as in data collection, the use of multiple analysts provides a mechanism for contrary views to arise and receive careful review. Peer debriefing may be the only way for opposing opinions to be heard and contrary explanations for phenomenon to be aired. The use of peer debriefing sometimes leads to additional data collection as the need to clarify conflicting data and conflicting views becomes apparent. The entire process strengthens the legitimacy of the final version of study findings. It is an important point of departure from more standardized forms of data collection that rely on a standardized fixed set of measures conducted identically with each participant.

Member Checks

Member checks define the process whereby the investigators check out their assumptions and emerging interpretations about the data with the original stakeholders who provided the information. This is vitally important. Not only does it ensure accuracy of the facts and information gathered in the study, but it also helps ensure that the investigator's conclusions make sense from the perspective of the persons who experienced those events.

As with prolonged engagement in the field, there is no magic amount of stakeholder checking that is "right" for every study. In very small studies, it may be possible to return the interview transcript to every person interviewed for checks on accuracy of transcription and to return drafts of emerging research findings to the original participants. In a large study, however, this is usually not possible, and sometimes only a small portion of the data (commonly about 20%) will be returned to the original stakeholders for this sort of check.

Audit Trail

An **audit trail** is a systematically maintained set of documentation, typically including:

- All data generated in the study.
- Explanations of all concepts and models that shaped the study design.

- Explanations of procedures used in data collection and analysis.
- Notes about technical aspects of data collection and analysis as well as decisions taken throughout the study to refine data collection procedures and interpretations.
- Personal notes and reflections.
- Copies of all instruments and interview protocols used to collect study data.

The audit trail can be used by the researcher as a means of managing record-keeping and encouraging reflexivity about a project and its goals. It also permits a third-party examiner to review all aspects of the conduct of a qualitative study and attest to the use of dependable procedures. In this way, the audit trail functions as a means of reliability checking for both the procedures and conclusions of a study.

Project-Based Methods

Project-based methods include daily operational procedures that help to minimize errors in all processes related to data collection, data storage, and data management. Other chapters address these more technical and procedural aspects of actions taken to ensure optimal data quality and data security in detail. However, three final aspects of qualitative data gathering should be reviewed: entry and exit from the research setting and potential pitfalls encountered within the research setting.

Entering the Field Study Site

It is important to address the basic issues of entry and exit from the field, especially the relationships that must be created and then ended with the participants/informants and stakeholders who support access to the research setting. Neglecting these processes can ruin even the best developed scientific design. Thus, entering and exiting relationships with participants at the field site requires careful and full consideration of practical details.

Adequate preparation is necessary to ensure that all members of the research team (subject recruiters, interviewers, etc.) present themselves and treat others professionally. This includes, for example, style of dress and behavior, because appearance and verbal communication send very important messages to the research participants about the importance of the study and the investigator's respect for them as human beings. A reasonable rule of thumb is to dress conservatively but professionally. It is important to be attentive to the values and style of the individuals and organizations where the data are gathered. This can require

"dressing up" in studies conducted in more formal settings and "dressing down" in studies with teenagers or where circumstances dictate.

The hazards associated with being both too formal and too informal can be overlooked by qualitative researchers. When project staff misjudge the impression required to be taken seriously in the research setting, the entire study can be put in peril. In those cases, organizations will be impossible to penetrate and informants impossible to recruit for the simple reason that participants perceive the research is not sufficiently "in tune" with them to reward the project with their participation.

If research participants do not accept the legitimacy of the researchers or do not take the research endeavor seriously, they may not participate, or, alternatively, they may provide only very limited data. Ongoing effort is needed to remind project staff of the importance of appearance and professionalism and to take care to represent the project to others appropriately. Only in this way can the highest quality of data be collected.

Gaining entry to the field of a qualitative study can be difficult and challenging for other reasons. For example, an organization or group may have had a negative experience with a previous project. For example, in the study by Lysack and Luborsky (2004) of community integration after spinal cord injury described earlier, research staff realized that potential study recruits had several misperceptions about what participation in the study really meant. They learned, for example, that for some recruits, spinal cord research meant being "stuck with needles" or "strapped to a machine." Interest and willingness to participate increased significantly once it was understood that the study involved being interviewed and that no invasive procedures would be used.

Another reason that gaining entry into the field can be difficult is because the gatekeepers to the research setting are important and busy people. They may view research participation as less important than many of their other activities. In such a situation, gaining access will require considerable persistence, tact, and possibly assistance from someone who is respected in the setting. At this preliminary level, gaining access requires the investigator to negotiate with those who control access to the research setting or access to the documents or objects that the researcher wishes to study. The investigator must also balance the needs of the study against the concerns of the host group.

Where the investigator expects cooperation, gaining entry may be largely a matter of establishing trust and rapport. A mainstay of the qualitative investigator is saying something like: "I'm here because I would like to understand X better and because we believe your opinions and experiences will help us to learn more about Y and help to improve Z." When access is expected to be more difficult, often the best tack is through the known sponsor approach. In this approach, the qualitative researcher is vouched for by an already familiar and respected person. If the known individual is truly trusted and respected, the qualitative researcher can rely on his or her introduction to facilitate entry and to step in if or when unanticipated bumps arise in the data-collection process over time.

A useful technique in participant-observation studies in particular is to begin observations/fieldwork at the same time that new members begin the activity of study interest or join the group. By using timing to one's advantage, investigators can minimize the disparity between their level of knowledge and that of the study participants. For example, a good time to begin to participate as a participant-observer in a study of the effects of a nonreligious 12-step self-help intervention on rates of alcoholism is when the self-help group is first forming, before members know what the 12 steps are, and when everyone is just beginning the recovery process.

Pitfalls of Field Study

A closely related challenge is obtaining high-quality data once in the field (Dillaway, 2002). Although achieving excellent data quality is not directly linked to gaining access to the research site, it is a topic of high importance. If measures are not taken to ensure smooth operations, data quality will suffer. As mentioned earlier, challenges to data occur when participation in the research is difficult for participants, for whatever reason. This may be due to research questions that participants consider too private, provocative, or controversial. In situations like this, participants may be too embarrassed to reveal their true attitudes and describe their experiences in full detail, even to a well-trained and empathetic interviewer. When participants feel the questions they are answering are too personal or intimate or find the topics studied too emotionally difficult, they may drastically restrict the information they share. Superficial data will result.

On the other hand, the interviewer may cause poor-quality data. An interviewer who is perceived to be overly comfortable or overly intrusive and who creates an unwelcome sense of familiarity with participants can have negative consequences. These interviewer problems can best be avoided by thorough staff training, clearly written recruitment materials, and prepared interview scripts and responses to frequently asked questions to use verbatim when answering the most common queries of prospective research recruits. With complete descriptions of the study purpose, information about the kinds of questions that will be asked, and honest evaluations about the time and effort required of participants provided before data collection, most problems of data collection can be avoided.

Collecting qualitative data can be challenging for reasons beyond the practical issues just reviewed. A qualitative interviewer or qualitative participant-observer is always at some risk of being pulled into the lives of study participants (Dillaway, 2002). This pull can come in the form of requests for assistance, advice, and emotional support, for example. For occupational therapists who are also researchers, the dual role of clinician and researcher can be especially challenging. For example, in the Lysack and Luborsky (2004) study of community integration after spinal cord injury mentioned earlier, office staff and interviewers were frequently asked for advice on the following: where to obtain better home care services, where to socialize to meet someone of the opposite sex, how to find a better medical specialist, where to buy an adapted motor vehicle, how to obtain funding to return to school, how to find research projects that paid more, and how to find a better job. Of course, these requests for advice were predicated on the reasonable assumption that the staff possessed a higher degree of expertise in some of these areas than participants did themselves, although this is not always true. When researchers are also clinicians, they may find themselves in conflict about which role they are playing and what ethical and practical obligations they have to both the project and the research participants. Thus, qualitative researchers should be aware that although they must develop sufficient rapport with and closeness to research participants to elicit useful research data, there will be times when the relationship becomes too close, with the potential for negative consequences to participant and researcher alike.

To be clear, it is commonplace and expected that qualitative researchers will give back to their study participants in at least a modest way. The provision of helpful answers, advice, and assistance is an immediate way of doing this and creates the reciprocity that researchers feel they owe their research participants given their generous contributions of data. Reciprocating research participation (e.g., simple assistance, thank-you cards, educational handouts) can become substantial and frequent, placing more serious demands on the qualitative researcher. When this occurs, the psychological resources of the interviewer/researcher can be stretched and even ethically compromised. In some instances, it can drain the financial, social, and tangible resources of the entire project.

In such situations, team meetings and discussions with the principal investigator of the study are imperative so that clear guidelines are established for what does and does not constitute appropriate action. These guidelines will involve issues of practicality but will also bear directly on a variety of ethical issues and responsibilities, not only to research participants, but also to project staff, the university, and even the agency that funded the research. Regular debriefing sessions with project peers, particularly after difficult data collection episodes, are essential to provide emotional support to data gatherers who can and do face surprising and stressful events during qualitative interviews.

When the interviews take place in the homes and communities of the research participants, the range of unexpected events can be rather remarkable. These surprises can include such diverse things as insect infestations, angry family members, unhealthy pets, and instances of negligent care or abuse. Thus, thorough staff supervision and leadership by the principal investigator of the study is essential to provide guidance in dealing with such situations. This guidance is necessary to ensure that the actions of the staff are as scientifically sound as possible, ethically appropriate, adequate to protect the research staff and the participants in the encounter, and in compliance with legal requirements (e.g., reporting abuse and neglect).

Because qualitative research can involve deep investigations of social experiences and meanings on personal and emotionally difficult topics, there will be occasions when qualitative researchers encounter a study participant who becomes upset or tearful or, more rarely, expresses severe depressive symptoms or suicidal thoughts. Although these instances are infrequent, the qualitative researcher must be knowledgeable and prepared to exercise skill and resourcefulness. On such occasions, qualitative researchers must be appropriately empathetic and also be prepared to offer referrals to professionals for counseling and to relevant agencies for more tangible resources. Confronting these types of challenging interpersonal circumstances repeatedly and over a sustained time frame can lead to fatigue, stress, and potential burnout. Thus, the principal investigator must address such circumstances at the earliest evidence because they not only adversely affect the health and well-being of research staff, but also compromise optimal data quality.

Leaving (Exiting) the Field Study Site

Lofland and Lofland (1995) report that leaving the field is one of the most difficult aspects of research for the qualitative researcher. Leaving the field reminds the qualitative researcher of the unequal power relationships that exist between the researcher and the researched. Not uncommonly, leaving creates feelings of guilt because the researcher walks away with highly prized data and the participants receive little or nothing at all. Of course, this is not completely true. The give-backs mentioned earlier, including small measures of assistance and advice, can have a real and lasting impact on some study participants. Even sending out simple thank-you cards might be appreciated. Although qualitative researchers frequently have at the ready and distribute handouts that list local resources and services relevant to their study participants, these small measures are often perceived as inadequate in the face of the valuable data that study participants share with researchers. Furthermore, every study eventually reaches a final conclusion when there are no longer staff or resources to keep in touch and help out when needed. When this time comes, there are no means of giving back to study participants other than a collective and anonymous acknowledgment of their help in public presentations and in published manuscripts. Although some investigators distribute summaries of study findings to interested study participants, this too can be costly, and not all studies have the financial resources to produce such materials.

In the end, the researchers must say thank you and good-bye. One important reward to research participants is a methodologically rigorous study that yields important new findings that are disseminated to audiences so that changes and improvements can be made. In this way, although the benefits of the research do not accrue to the individuals who originally contributed the data, and they are hardly immediate, there are meaningful benefits to others who share the same health condition, social circumstances, or experience. For all these reasons, qualitative research increasingly involves utilization of participatory approaches (see Chapter 16) that seek in the course of the study to empower participants to effect desired changes in their own circumstances.

Summary

As noted at the outset, qualitative research is a naturalistic, emergent and evolving, and interpretive endeavor (Rossman & Rallis, 1998). Qualitative data collection reflects these characteristics. Moreover, qualitative researchers view social phenomena holistically and are sensitive to their own influence on the study and its findings (Rossman & Rallis, 1998). These two elements always guide how the data collection strategies discussed in this chapter are undertaken in a given study. In this chapter, the following major strategies for collecting data were covered: participation, observation, the various types of in-depth interviews (unstructured, semistructured, structured, focus group, and key informant), and reviewing written documents and material objects. Additionally, the following approaches to strengthening data collection were reviewed: managing bias, interviewer training, prolonged engagement in the field, reflexivity, triangulation, member checks, audit trails, and project-based methods. The chapter also describes establishing entry, addressing pitfalls, and exiting appropriately.

Review Questions

1. Of the four primary approaches to collecting data in qualitative research, which would be the most appropriate in a setting in which direct interaction with study participants was not encouraged?
2. Assuming you have unrestricted entry into a community-based setting, what data collection approach would be most likely to yield detailed, accurate data about the lived experiences of participants?
3. Assuming you have an unlimited amount of time to spend with participants who are highly talkative and have the capacity for self-reflection, which approach to interviewing would be the most desirable as a data collection approach? Which would be the most desirable in a study with limited time or less-talkative participants?
4. In planning various qualitative data collection approaches, what general provisions would you need to make to increase the accuracy of data collection?
5. Provide an example of a sensitive population in a community-based setting in which it might be difficult to gain entry. Describe at least two approaches for gaining entry into that setting.

REFERENCES

Dillaway, H. E. (2002). Menopause in social context: Women's experiences of reproductive aging in the United States. Unpublished doctoral dissertation, Michigan State University, East Lansing, MI.

Dillaway, H., Stengle, W., Miree, C., St. Onge, K., Berry-Bobovski, L., White, J., . . . Brown, D. (2005). Community as paradox: Understanding both barriers and incentives to African American men's participation in prostate cancer prevention trials. Unpublished manuscript. Department of Sociology, Wayne State University.

Lofland, J., & Lofland, L. (1995). *Analyzing social settings: A guide to qualitative analysis and observation.* Belmont, CA: Wadsworth.

Lysack, C., & Kaufert, J. (1999). Disabled consumers' perspectives on provision of community rehabilitation services. *Canadian Journal of Rehabilitation, 12*(3), 157–166.

Lysack, C., & Luborsky, M. (2004). Community living after spinal cord injury: Models and outcomes (R01 #1HD43378, funded by NIH/NICHD/NCMRR).

Rossman, G. B., & Rallis, S. F. (1998). *Learning in the field: An introduction to qualitative research.* Thousand Oaks, CA: Sage.

Siporin, S., & Lysack, C. (2004). Quality of life and supported employment: A case study of three women with developmental disabilities. *American Journal of Occupational Therapy, 58*(4), 455–465.

RESOURCES

Websites Relevant to Gathering Qualitative Research:

http://www.socialresearchmethods.net/kb/

Recommended Readings for Gathering Qualitative Research:

Creswell, J. C. (1998). *Qualitative inquiry and research design: Choosing among five traditions.* Thousand Oaks, CA: Sage.

Denzin, N. K., & Lincoln, Y. S. (2000). *Handbook of qualitative research* (2nd ed.). Thousand Oaks, CA: Sage.

Gubrium, J. F., & Holstein, J. A. (Eds.). (2002). *Handbook of interview research: Context and method.* Thousand Oaks, CA: Sage.

Lincoln, Y. S., & Guba, E. G. (1985). *Naturalistic inquiry.* Beverly Hills, CA: Sage.

Lofland, J., & Lofland, L. (1995). *Analyzing social settings: A guide to qualitative analysis and observation.* Belmont, CA: Wadsworth.

Marshall, C., & Rossman, G. B. (Eds.). (1999). *Designing qualitative research.* Thousand Oaks, CA: Sage.

Office of Behavioral and Social Sciences Research & National Institutes of Health. (n.d.). *Qualitative methods in health research: Opportunities and considerations in application and review.* Retrieved from https://obssr-archive.od.nih.gov/pdf/Qualitative.PDF

Shaffir, W. B., & Stebbins, R. A. (Eds.). (1991). *Experiencing fieldwork: An inside view of qualitative research.* Newbury Park, CA: Sage.

Spradley, J. (1979). *The ethnographic interview.* New York, NY: Holt, Rinehart and Winston.

CHAPTER 18

Contemporary Tools for Managing and Analyzing Qualitative Data

Nadine Peacock • Amy Paul-Ward

Learning Outcomes

■ Identify the major steps involved in qualitative data analysis.
■ Describe quality assurance measures that are specific to qualitative data analysis.
■ List the advantages of computer-assisted approaches to qualitative data analysis.
■ Identify other technologies that can expedite and improve qualitative data analysis.

Introduction

In any research endeavor, raw data must be transformed into coherent, believable, and meaningful findings. In qualitative studies, this transformation requires that the investigator make a number of strategic decisions about data management and analysis, including whether to use specialized technology. These decisions ordinarily require consideration of the following factors:

• The amount of time and funds allocated to the analysis process.
• The volume and structure of the data.
• One's comfort level with using what may be unfamiliar software.
• Epistemological stances guiding one's research.

Qualitative studies can range from those that are exploratory to those designed to test or confirm hypotheses or findings from prior research. They can be performed by an individual investigator using participant observation in extended ethnographic fieldwork or by a team doing rapid assessment with structured checklists and interview guides. The data can take many forms, including:

• Loosely structured, lengthy narratives derived from in-depth interviews
• Short-answer responses to open-ended survey questions
• Field notes taken by participant observers

• Audio or video recordings of events
• Secondary data (e.g., documents, brochures, minutes of meetings) created by persons other than the investigators

The data from a given study may range from a handful of documents to hundreds of them. **Qualitative data analysis** encompasses a range of approaches to the management and analysis of qualitative data. This can be accomplished by an individual researcher or by a team, and it can take a low-technology approach (e.g., reading through data and making note of passages that illustrate useful themes) or a high-technology approach (e.g., one that makes use of sophisticated and specialized software). Finally, analysis and interpretation of qualitative data can reflect a broad spectrum of epistemological stances.

The aim of this chapter is to identify key elements shared by a range of approaches to qualitative data analyses and to describe some of the varied software programs and other types of technological support (such as transcription and editing systems) that are useful for managing and analyzing qualitative data. The resource list at the end of the chapter provides a list of books, websites, and listservs that present and review the various software programs available for analyzing qualitative data.

Common Features of Qualitative Research

Although qualitative research approaches are many and varied, they share certain commonalities. First, qualitative studies tend to have a less formal, less structured purpose. A qualitative study is often built around what Mason (2002) calls an intellectual puzzle—that is, a general question about a social phenomenon that the investigator hopes to understand better. This puzzle can then be expanded into a number of more specific research

CASE EXAMPLE

Master's degree students in a public health qualitative data analysis course at the University of Illinois at Chicago were asked to design a small study to generate data with which they could practice their analysis skills. They decided to conduct interviews with friends, family members, and colleagues on the topic of safe driving. Their prediction was that many people would admit to engaging in practices that they themselves define as unsafe, while still considering themselves "safe drivers." The students engaged in convenience sampling, with an effort to cover a mix of ages, genders, races/ethnicities, and national origins. Interviews were audio-recorded and transcribed. The first part of their analysis assignment was a "low-tech" approach, using the margin area of printed transcripts to label text segments with analytic memos and codes.

Students next used ATLAS.ti®, one of the qualitative data analysis (QDA) software programs described in this chapter, to replicate this "hand-coding" process. Figure 18.1 shows how ATLAS.ti permits the linking of index codes and memos to text segments in a manner that parallels the "low-tech" method but requires much less effort. The electronic coding made it much easier for the students to search for related content across multiple interviews to ascertain whether their predictions were supported, and for whom.

The student investigators also used ATLAS.ti's theory-building functions to develop conceptual models that are grounded in the qualitative data. Figure 18.2 shows an example of a Network View showing code–code relationships.

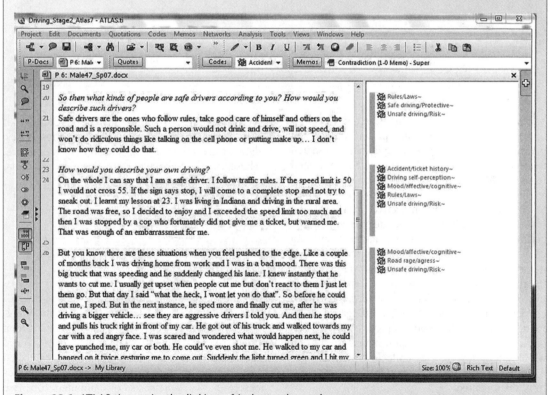

Figure 18.1 ATLAS.ti permits the linking of index codes and memos to text segments.

(case example continues on page 216)

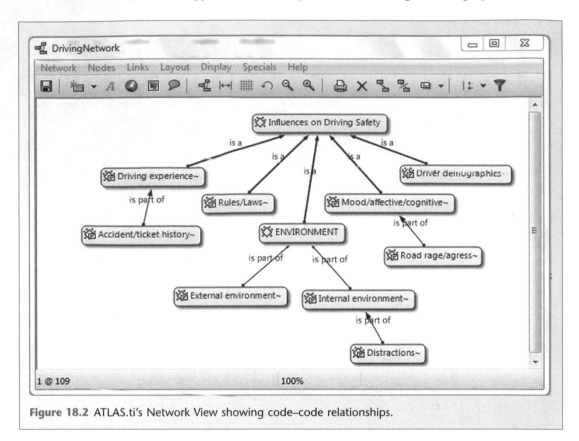

Figure 18.2 ATLAS.ti's Network View showing code–code relationships.

questions, which are usually best addressed by observing, listening, and interpreting rather than measuring and testing. Thus, qualitative research tends to be more inductive than deductive, and leans more toward theory building than theory testing.

A corollary to the inductive nature of the research is the blurring of boundaries among the tasks of data collection, data management, and data analysis. In other words, qualitative research is an iterative process, wherein some data are collected, interim analyses are performed, and research instruments are modified before further data are collected and analyzed (Fig. 18.3). Because of the fluid, nonlinear nature of this process, it becomes particularly important to establish an audit trail, in which study design, data collection and management procedures, and analytic decisions are carefully documented.

Another key feature of qualitative data analysis is the creation of **metadata,** or data about data (Guest & MacQueen, 2008). These are new text and/or graphic products created by the researcher to represent key themes, constructs, and relationships that emerge from and are applied to a body of qualitative data. As such, they are tools for, as

well as products of, data analysis. Examples of metadata in qualitative research are memos, codes, data matrixes, concept maps, and case summaries. These types of metadata are described in more detail in this chapter.

General Principles of Data Management and Analysis

Coding and other metadata are common products of computer-assisted qualitative data analysis. However, it is important to understand that qualitative analysis software simply adds a layer of technology to a process that was a well-established component of qualitative inquiry for decades before the widespread use of computers for these purposes.

Key procedures involved in the qualitative data analysis process include active reading, writing analytic memos, index coding/conceptual labeling, and producing code directories. These steps and their functions, which are outlined in Table 18.1, primarily refer to the more "procedural" aspects of data analysis. How a researcher actually goes about the more "conceptual" aspects of data analysis depends on the particular form of qualitative research performed. These conceptual aspects of data analysis are described in detail in Chapter 19.

To illustrate this point, let us consider a study undertaken in the 1970s, prior to the widespread use of computer-assisted qualitative data analysis systems (CAQDASs). A team of UCLA investigators including anthropologists, sociologists, and occupational therapists studied the experiences of adults with developmental disabilities who were deinstitutionalized from state hospitals into community residential facilities. The investigators were interested in how successfully these adults were integrated into community life, what types of occupational routines they established, and how the organization structures and practices of the residential settings affected their lives (Bercovici, 1983; Goode, 1983; Kielhofner, 1979, 1981; Kielhofner & Takata, 1980).

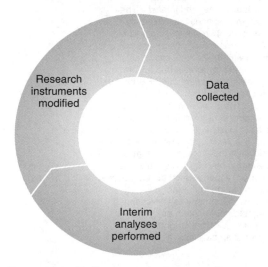

Figure 18.3 Qualitative research is a nonlinear, iterative process.

In the UCLA study, participant observation was selected as the key method of data collection. The investigators accompanied and observed study participants both within the residential facilities and the community, making special note of daily routines and activities, conversations and other social interactions, and participant insights on their daily lives gleaned from informal conversations.

Researchers also conducted interviews with the adults with developmental disabilities as well as with staff in the facilities. Data from the participant observations were recorded as hand-written field notes, which were later typed and supplemented with additional descriptive detail (Fig. 18.4). Interviews were audio-recorded and sometimes video-recorded, and the recordings were later transcribed into typewritten documents.

The researchers routinely included in their expanded field notes and transcripts descriptive comments and explanations that helped complete the "picture" of what was going on during the observed events, reflexive notes on the investigators' actions and reactions in the field, and notes on their role in generating and interpreting the data.

The activities described so far (typing and expanding field notes and transcribing interviews) are data management tasks as well as early steps in analysis, whereby the investigators began to extract meaning from and make sense of their qualitative data.

Other important data management tasks involved identifying the body of products that constituted the investigators' data. In this instance, the data included not only typewritten information from participant observation, interviews, and videotaping, but also documents produced in the residential facility (e.g., mission statements, policies, notices, advertising brochures, and reports), medical records of some of the developmentally disabled adults, and photographic and video records of events. Decisions needed to be made

Table 18.1   Qualitative Data Analysis Procedures and Their Functions

Analysis Procedure	Function
Active reading	The process by which investigators immerse themselves in their qualitative data, reading and rereading while making marginal notes about important themes and constructs
Index codes/conceptual labels	Words or short phrases that serve as a kind of tag for segments of text, categorically describing information the segments contain
Analytic memos	Reflective notes through which the investigators begin to organize their thoughts about the data
Code directory	A list of all codes with clear operational definitions to assure that the coding process is rigorous and reliable

Note, there is a legitimizing affect that those who "appear normal" have in being associated with those who have obvious physical characteristics that lead to stigma.

Physical features that make stigma obvious

Daniel and Michelle had brought their guitars, so naturally Doris was asked to play. Doris began to play and sing with Michelle accompanying her both playing guitar and singing. I was sitting on top of a picnic table a few feet away and Tim sat beside me. From where I sat I could see not only Doris and Doreen, Bill, Shereen, Jess and the UCLA folks, but also the many kids in the background who had noticed us and were curiously looking on. Finally one brave soul (a young man who appeared 10 years old) approached the corner of the area and unobu unobtrusively watched.

Ho appeared almost mesmerized by the whole scene which included: a toothless lady with funny red skin and very obese, wearing a red wig playing a guitar and singing her soul out; Buddy, a 50 year old with Down Syndrome whose appearance approximates a buddha figure, Doreen whose appeances approximate Doris's but who appears older in a black wig. Everyone else could possibly pass for "normal" on appearances alone. Probably the presence of these folks and the 5 UCLA people make the whole scene a little lss less threatening.

Note; an interesting feature of the age differences is that children appear to become increasingly aware with ago that it is okay (perhaps normative) to make fun of people who are different and their sense of shame in responding to stigma seems to correspondingly, disappear

attracting "spectators"

After the first young man had ventured into "our territory" more and more children began to approach. Those who were younger held expressions of curiosity, fear and intensity. They appeared nervous and cautious but inexorably drawn toward the scene. Two little girls looked at Buddy (A downs-syndrome phenotype) whispered to each other, giggled with their hands over their mouths, stopped, stared for a while and so forth over and over. Bobby seemed unaware of their attention; he did not appear to look at them. Most of the others focused on Doris and Doreen (who were doing the singing and guiart guitar playing). Responses were obviously age graded. The younger ones in the group seemed not to know what to make of it. The few who were older recognized that it was a spectactle and laughed obviously, with only mild attempts to hide their response such as turning away sometimes when the laughed harder.

Something about their laughter was interesting- it was nervous laughter, not the open enjoyable laughter of a harmless joke, but laughter which betrayed some sort of ambivalence about the whole sene scene.

Personal reflection: I was uncomfortable initially and then became aware of this. Let me elaborate. The feeling I had was one of "guilt by association" There was this automatic feeling of self protectiveness that arose with the thought that the children would "think ther was something wrong with me too" When I realized this I was ashamed of the feeling

Differential awareness of others' reaction to stigma

Most of the Picadilly people were unaffected by the presence of the children. Doris and Doreen seemed to definitely like them as an audience. Jim is was laughing about their presence and I think he saw them as just an audience to the music. Tim, however, got very nervous from the beginning. More than anyone else from Picadilly, so I think Tim knew what was going on. he turned to me with a mortified look on his face and said he was going to leave the area and join Nancy and Sheryl and Lolita who were playing tennis. I asked him if what was happening was making him nervous and he said yes. I knew that Tim knew and that he clearly wished not to accrue guilt by association. Later when Lisa, and the others joined us from the tennis area, Tim came along. I noted later that he was singing along with the music and appeared much more comfortable and there was definitely less tension on in the air.

Figure 18.4 Field notes from a 1970s UCLA study with index labels and analytic notes.

about where and how these varied types of data were stored, who had access to them, and what role they played in addressing the intellectual puzzle and research questions. All of these tasks are part of the data management process.

Once the investigators had begun to amass typed field notes, interview transcriptions, and other documents, they were ready to delve further into the analytic process. Recall that desktop computers were not available in the 1970s when this study took place. Although mainframe computers were commonly used in the social and behavioral sciences, their use for qualitative data analysis at this time was rare. How, then, did the systematic management and analysis of this data set proceed?

First, the investigators made multiple photocopies of each set of typed field notes and transcripts. An original copy with complete provenance information (e.g., the date and location the observation or interview took place, who gathered the data, who transcribed the tape, etc.) was stored in a reference file that was arranged chronologically and by site. The photocopies of the data were working copies that team members marked up in a process of **active reading** of the data—a key early step in the analysis process by which the reader interacts with the data by making notes in reaction to what is read.

As the investigators first read through the data, they routinely made free-form margin notes, commenting on things that struck them as important and noting consistencies or contradictions in different observations or interviews. This process was facilitated by leaving a wide margin when notes were typed, so that there was ample room for such secondary note-taking. When more room was needed, notes were stapled to the pages to which they pertained. The notes fell into two broad categories (see Fig. 18.4):

• **Conceptual labels,** which were words or short phrases that served as a "tag" for segments of text, categorically describing information the segments contained. These would eventually evolve into a list of index codes used to label and retrieve segments of text that relate to a common theme (see the next heading).

• **Analytic memos,** which were reflective notes through which the investigators began to organize their thoughts about the data. These were the raw materials for later interpretations and findings.

In this study, because several investigators worked together, they routinely met to present and discuss the conceptual labels and analytic memos they had created. These discussions led to the

identification and elaboration of important emerging themes that were captured in additional analytic notes. The discussions also guided the focus of future data gathering sessions, in that special attention could be paid to data that were relevant to emerging concepts and themes. Clearly, the active reading and working discussions described here served as early stages of data analysis.

Conceptual Labels and Index Codes

As these investigators proceeded with multiple readings through the data, descriptive conceptual labels tended to become more systematic and consolidated, eventually culminating in a comprehensive set of what are sometimes referred to as **index codes.** Such codes function much like the index to a book, in that they indicate places in the text where one can retrieve information on a particular topic.

Codes in this study included labels for different types of social behaviors (e.g., approaching, avoiding, staring, demeaning, reproaching, punishing), cognitive/affective states (e.g., embarrassment, frustration, anger, fear), subjective experiences (e.g., helplessness, agency, being "frozen in time"), and issues over which there was often misunderstanding between mainstream culture and those who were the focus of study (e.g., privacy, personal space, scheduling time). The early creation of codes such as "stigmatizing behavior" and "time use" reflect the fact that the study was conceptually grounded in the field of occupational therapy (e.g., Kielhofner, 1977) and that it built on previous research on deinstitutionalization (e.g., Edgerton, 1971).

Index codes can derive from findings of prior studies or from an initial conceptual framework, and additional codes can be added as new concepts emerge from the data. As codes are developed, a **code directory** or codebook is constructed, which includes operational definitions, as well as inclusion and exclusion criteria—that is, instructions about circumstances under which the code should or should not be applied (Bernard & Ryan, 2010; MacQueen, McLellan-Lemal, Bartholow, & Milstein, 2008). Code definitions tend to evolve over time, and with increasing use, the definitions and the inclusion and exclusion criteria become more precise. Codes that represent broad themes may be broken down to component parts, and, conversely, codes that are conceptually very closely related may be merged. Investigators should keep careful records of when codes are created, split, or merged and when their definitions or application criteria are refined. (This is one component of the "audit trail" discussed in Chapter 17.) Investigators may need to go back and recode earlier coded portions of the data set in light of evolving code criteria.

In the UCLA study, the investigators eventually developed a comprehensive indexing system, consisting of a list of concepts grouped together into various themes. For example, one emergent theme was "temporal adaptation" (Kielhofner, 1979). This pertains to how the deinstitutionalized adults experienced time and the ways in which their unique experience of time differed from the mainstream culture. Within this broad conceptual theme of temporality were nested subcategories, such as:

- Time-related behaviors (e.g., waiting, dealing with appointments, filling time).
- Temporal perspectives (e.g., how people talked about the future).
- Temporal misunderstandings (i.e., problematic interactions that emanated from nonnormative views of time held by the participants).

These and other index codes were written in the margins of clean copies of the typed field notes.

Recall that a main purpose of coding is to allow the investigators to retrieve all relevant passages on a given theme so that their content can be further explored. The index code "Time-Related Behaviors" was used in the UCLA study to indicate where in the texts one could find participants' comments about making appointments, waiting, and other factors related to item management. In order to conduct a more in-depth analysis of this content area, the investigators needed to find all passages labeled with this code and look in detail at the selected passages. This could prove difficult, given that any single page of data (field notes, transcribed interview, or other document) can have numerous codes and margin notes, and a single passage might be coded for more than one concept. Looking through hundreds of pages of codes and margin notes would be a cumbersome way of finding all the passages containing information on time-related behaviors.

The investigators chose instead to physically group together all the text segments dealing with the topic of interest. Any passage labeled with the relevant code was physically cut from a photocopy of the original page, tagged with information on its source location, and placed along with all other such text segments in a folder, as shown in Figure 18.5. Typically, multiple copies of a coded page needed to be made because more than one code was often associated with a given text

passage, and therefore the passage would be filed in more than one folder.

By flipping through any folder, the investigators were able to read, grouped together, all the passages in the data in which participants discussed these issues. Passages gathered from different parts of the data set (thus "decontextualized") were used to build an explanation about various ways the participants behaved with reference to time, including how it was related to their life experiences and perspectives and to the organization of the settings where they lived.

Of course it was also important to preserve information concerning where in the document a passage was originally located, because appreciating its full meaning often required viewing it in the context of the surrounding text. Thus, decontextualizing and re-contextualizing of data are important components of the qualitative analysis process.

As data accumulated in the folders representing various concepts, the reading and processing of that material sometimes resulted in the contents of a folder being divided into two or more component concepts. At other times, two folders were collapsed into one. In this way, the coding scheme was continuously refined as the data analysis unfolded.

Memos

Recall that margin notes contain not only index labels, but also longer annotations referred to as **memos** (Mayan, 2009; Strauss & Corbin, 1998). Rather than serving primarily as an indexing function, memos are methodological and analytic notes from which explanations and findings are built. Although these memos may begin as brief notes in the margin, they commonly become longer and more complex as analysis proceeds.

Over time, the investigators in the UCLA study started recording memos in a larger format, using separate sheets of paper that were filed along with text passages in topic folders. Eventually, these memos were integrated into working drafts of the analysis. These working papers were shared in meetings of the research team, which led to discussion, critique, and new insights. Those developing ideas were in turn also recorded as memos. Individual team members or small groups had primary responsibility for generating explanations on a given theme, but the group process allowed for other team members to write memos and share their thoughts on the topic. In this way the analysis was organic, collaborative, and iterative, unfolding in constant interaction with the data.

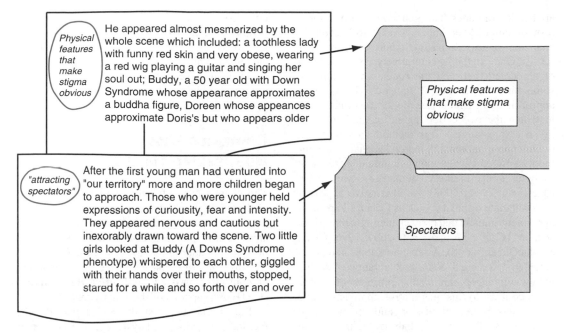

Physical features that make stigma obvious

He appeared almost mesmerized by the whole scene which included: a toothless lady with funny red skin and very obese, wearing a red wig playing a guitar and singing her soul out; Buddy, a 50 year old with Down Syndrome whose appearance approximates a buddha figure, Doreen whose appeances approximate Doris's but who appears older

Physical features that make stigma obvious

"attracting spectators"

After the first young man had ventured into "our territory" more and more children began to approach. Those who were younger held expressions of curiousity, fear and intensity. They appeared nervous and cautious but inexorably drawn toward the scene. Two little girls looked at Buddy (A Downs Syndrome phenotype) whispered to each other, giggled with their hands over their mouths, stopped, stared for a while and so forth over and over

Spectators

Figure 18.5 An example of "decontextualizing" data by grouping text passages related to a common theme.

Interdependence of Codes and Memos

Indexing is fairly simple and mechanical, whereas producing memos is more complex and analytic, yet these methods are interdependent and coordinated. As analysis proceeds, the coding scheme may be elaborated, and perhaps made hierarchical, with some of the index terms reflecting broader conceptual domains. These in turn can serve as cover terms for more detailed analytic categories, which are commonly arrived at inductively after the investigator spends time intellectually processing the data and writing memos.

Quality Assurance in Qualitative Data Analysis

Methods for ensuring the quality and trustworthiness of qualitative data were introduced in Chapter 17. These methods include interviewer training, prolonged engagement in the field, reflexivity, triangulation, stakeholder checks, and audit trails. Because qualitative inquiry is an iterative process involving successive rounds of data collection and interim analyses, these methods are as relevant to data analysis as they are to data collection. There are additional quality assurance measures that are specific to data analysis, particularly to

the process of coding and the concept of interrater reliability. Those two measures are addressed in the following sections.

Coding and Retrieving

The creation of a code directory with clear operational definitions is an important first step in ensuring that the coding process is rigorous and reliable. Particularly when multiple investigators are coding, analyzing, and/or interpreting the data, it is important that these activities take place in a systematic and consistent way (Carey & Gelaud, 2008).

This is not to say that all investigators working on a project should arrive at the same interpretations and explanations of qualitative data. Indeed, the possibility that investigators will bring different perspectives to analysis (in other words, investigator triangulation) is an important reason for conducting collaborative research. However, the mechanics of analytic tasks, such as coding and retrieval of text segments, must be systematic and consistent across researchers and documents. Otherwise, the results are simply a series of independent, individually conducted analyses rather than a coordinated research effort.

Interrater Reliability

There are a number of steps investigators can take to assess and improve interrater reliability in the application of codes. This generally involves some form of redundant coding, in which two researchers code the same text passages and compare their results. One can then quantitatively assess the level of agreement between the coders by calculating some kind of agreement statistic. The simplest approach is to calculate the proportion of instances in which the two coders agree on the coding of given text passages. This method, however, can overestimate agreement for codes that are commonly applied because some degree of agreement by pure chance is likely (Bernard & Ryan, 2010; MacQueen et al., 2008). An alternative approach is to calculate a statistic such as Cohen's kappa, an agreement statistic that takes chance agreement into account (Carey, Morgan, & Oxtoby, 1996; Guest & MacQueen, 2008). A separate kappa statistic is calculated for each code, and a range of kappa values can be reported for the entire set of codes.

In contrast to this quantitative approach, many researchers prefer discussion and reconciliation as a means of ensuring reliability of the coding process. This begins the same way—with the redundant coding of texts by two or more analysts. Differences are identified and discussed. Eventually, the parties reconcile their differences and agree on one set of codes for the document. Many qualitative researchers use only this approach and reject statistical measures, considering them to be unnecessary and even inappropriate because they are borrowed from positivist, quantitative paradigms (Friese, 2012).

Both approaches are useful and important. When code-by-code agreement statistics are collected and scrutinized, the investigators can detect patterns in which types of codes are more or less easily agreed on. For example, they may find that codes that represent affective states are much more difficult to apply consistently than those that capture overt behaviors. Discussions in which coders explain their rationale for applying codes in a particular way can lead not only to reconciliation,

but also to more careful crafting of operational definitions that will make future disagreements less likely. This can be documented by assessing agreement statistics before reconciliation and then again using a new subset of the data after code criteria have been refined.

Computer-Assisted Qualitative Data Analysis

This chapter has so far presented a basic overview of the qualitative data analysis process. Although the low-technology example of qualitative data analysis has not been discussed in its full complexity, it is appropriate to review what the UCLA investigators did and describe high-technology or **computer-assisted qualitative data analysis (CAQDA)** versions of these activities.

Recall that the first thing that was done to facilitate systematic analysis was the conversion of data from one format (hand-written field notes) to another (multiple copies of typed and expanded notes). Likewise, computer-assisted qualitative data analysis almost always requires a preparatory step of data conversion. In this case, the conversion is from data stored in a "hard" or analog form to a digital form. For example, verbatim transcripts of audiotaped interviews are generally prepared by typing them in a word processing program. Other examples of such conversions are listed in Table 18.2 (read further for discussion of technologies that permit the automation or elimination of conversion steps).

If data were being analyzed in 2015 rather than the 1970s in the UCLA study, how might the work proceed in a way that takes advantage of advances in computer technology? First of all, the observers might enter data directly into a laptop or handheld device. If hand-written notes were used (which is still common in many settings), they would likely

Table 18.2   Hard/Analog-to-Digital Data Conversion for Computer-Assisted Analysis

	Hard/Analog	Digital
Text	Hand-written or typed field notes, observation records, pencil-and-paper surveys, brochures/small media	Word processing files, spreadsheet data, text files, PDF files, etc.
Sound	Audiotaped recordings	Word processing files; digital recordings
Images	Photographs, drawings, etc.	Scanned images, PDF files, web pages, etc.
Image and sound	Videotape, film	Digital film, streaming video/sound files, multimedia web pages, etc.

be typed in a word processing program, such as Microsoft Word or Apple Pages, and then imported into a qualitative data analysis (QDA) software program. The first commercially available QDA program, The Ethnograph®, was introduced in the early 1980s. Since then, the selection has greatly expanded, with products such as NVivo®, MaxQDA, ATLAS.ti, HyperRESEARCH, and Dedoose (a web-based program) being among the most popular. AnSWR® and EZ-Text® are programs developed by the Centers for Disease Control and Prevention (CDC), and they have the distinct advantage of being distributed free to the public. Note: When illustrating computer-assisted qualitative data analysis in this chapter, examples from the ATLAS.ti program will be used in most cases. This should not be considered an endorsement of a particular product over others, but simply due to the fact that this is the program most familiar to the authors.

Whereas older versions of QDA programs required conversion of texts from word processing to text-only formats, most products now accept a wide variety of digital text formats. Once files are imported into the QDA program, a variety of data management and analysis tasks can be performed. Some key tasks are described here, including data storage and management, tag and retrieval functions, memo writing, theory building, and quality assurance. Ways in which software programs support team-based analysis and mixed-method approaches are also described.

Low-Technology Data Storage and Management

Recall that in the low-technology type of analysis described previously, a clean copy of all typed documents is stored in a master file organized by some selected criteria. For example, the project data might include transcripts of interviews, filed sequentially by their unique alpha-numeric ID numbers, which carry information about the particular data gathering event. For example, an ID number D022677_3M might indicate that a particular interview was done in a facility labeled "Facility D" on February 26, 1977; that it was the third interview done at that site on that day; and that the respondent was a male. No other interview could have exactly that constellation of attributes, and thus the ID number is unique. Transcripts can be filed by a primary criterion (e.g., the setting); within that grouping, they can then be ordered by a secondary criterion (e.g., the date of the interview).

High-Technology Data Storage and Management

How does computer-assisted data storage and management differ from the process described previously? One major advantage to computers is that one can easily use the software to categorize the data files in multiple ways. For example, the data may be entered and retrieved by any number of criteria, such as gender, age, ethnic group, or disability status. Stored and categorized data such as interview transcripts or field notes can then be imported into an appropriate software program, such as a QDA program.

Text-Based Searches

All of the major QDA programs allow for text-based searches, in which words or strings of text can be located in the original data. Most programs also have the capability to generate word counts, or calculations of the frequency with which specific words appear in the text. Some programs have more specialized features for conducting various types of quantitative content analysis.

Codebook Development

All major QDA programs support the creation of a list of codes to be applied to textual data, as well as a code directory with code definitions or criteria. In ATLAS.ti, the investigator creates codes that are displayed in a drop-down list. Code definitions, instructions for application, examples, and other aspects of the data must either be stored in a generic "comment" window attached to each code or in a separate document such as a spreadsheet or word processing file. Other programs (e.g., the CDC's AnSWR) have more fully developed codebook features, with separate fields for the code name, a brief definition, a full definition, inclusion criteria, exclusion criteria, and examples.

Tagging and Retrieval

Recall that in the low-tech coding example, investigators labeled passages of text with index codes, after which like-labeled passages were extracted and placed together in a folder. QDA software uses the same logic, but accomplishes the tasks with much greater efficiency by using hypertext connections, whereby noncontiguous text or images are electronically linked to one another. In most programs text passages of any size, from a single character to the entire document, can be highlighted and designated as a text segment (called a "quotation" in ATLAS.ti). Text segments can overlap with or be embedded within other segments. Codes stored in a code list can be linked electronically to text segments through keystroke commands, drop-down menus, buttons, or a "drag-and-drop" function. This "tagging" part of the "tag and retrieve" process is one type of hypertext connection. Hypertext links can also be made between one text segment and another, either within a document or between one document and another (Friese, 2012). For example, an interviewee in the student safe driving project described earlier made the following statement: "On the whole I can say that I am a safe driver. I follow traffic rules." But later in the interview he confided: "If I had a bad day at work, or fight with my partner, I tend to become aggressive, race with others on the road, beep if someone cuts me." Even though these statements are separated by several paragraphs in the transcript, they can be connected through a hypertext link, with the link indicating that statement 2 contradicts statement 1. In another example from the UCLA study, a staff member in a residential facility commented that it is acceptable to let oneself into a resident's room unannounced because "they don't really care about privacy." There are other passages in the data set from other interviews and from observations that either support or contradict the statement, along with both the connection and the semantic relationship ("supports" or "contradicts"); this can be established through hypertext links.

QDA programs also include one or more search tools, which constitute the "retrieving" part of tagging and retrieval. These tools allow the investigator to retrieve all text segments labeled with a particular code, so that passages on a given topic or theme can be grouped and viewed together, similar to the topic folders in the low-tech example. However, the QDA programs can go much further, allowing for complex search commands that combine two or more codes or other search criteria. This can be particularly useful with large data sets, when searching on a code that is heavily used may result in a very large volume of retrieved data, not all of which may be relevant to the question at hand. In such cases, the search can be narrowed by retrieving only a subset of the coded segments, either by combining one code with another or by imposing other restrictions on what is retrieved.

Boolean Connectors. A common way to perform these more complex searches is by using **Boolean** connectors (e.g., "and," "or," "not") to combine codes. For example, the investigators might be interested in examining accounts of disability-related stigma in the community, but only when the stigma involves some kind of discriminatory behavior. The search string "stigma AND discrimination" would retrieve the desired material, while ignoring accounts of stigma not associated with discrimination, as well as discrimination linked to race or ethnicity but not disability.

Semantic Connectors. Complex searches can also be conducted using **semantic connectors.** Recall from the earlier discussion that codes reflecting broad conceptual domains can serve as cover terms for more detailed analytic categories. In QDA software programs, semantic relationships can be created that indicate hierarchical or other types of relationships between codes. For example, "waiting," "filling time," and "being stuck in time" can be defined as types of "Temporal Experience." "Temporal Experience" therefore serves as a parent term for the other three, and the three types of experiences are related to one another as sibling terms. This semantic relationship is illustrated in Figure 18.6.

Because these semantic relationships are specified in the software, a researcher can issue a simple search command to, in effect, "retrieve any passage coded with 'Temporal Experience' OR any of its daughter terms." Some programs also allow the grouping of related codes without defining a semantic relationship. In ATLAS.ti, codes can be grouped together in units called "families," which can also be used as search terms. Families of other objects, such as documents and memos, can also be used in searches.

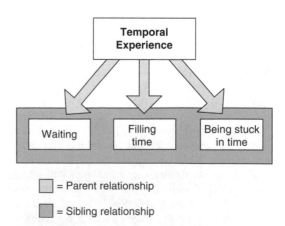

Figure 18.6 An illustration of semantic connectors.

Proximity Connectors. A third kind of complex search uses **proximity connectors,** which analyze spatial relationships between coded segments. Continuing with the earlier example, imagine that the data contain a passage describing a stigmatizing event in the community. This account itself may have had no overt reference to discrimination, but in the text segment immediately following it, an instance of discrimination may be reported. This co-occurrence would not be identified using semantic connectors because the "stigma" and "discrimination" codes aren't attached to a single text segment. Using proximity connectors, however, one could search for all "stigma" segments that are adjacent to (or overlapping or embedded within) a segment coded with "discrimination."

Memoing

All major QDA programs have a mechanism for **memoing,** or writing notes and memos, through which the investigators can record impressions about the data, methodological insights, developing interpretations and theory, and so forth. ATLAS.ti has two mechanisms for such annotations. Memos are one of the four major objects in the program (along with documents, codes, and quotations). These objects have a special status, and they can be ordered, sorted, and displayed in special ways. "Comments" is a more general category of annotation, and it serves as a kind of "sticky note" that can be attached to any object, including the entire project, a document, a code, or a "family."

Theory Building

The most popular QDA programs go beyond simple tagging and retrieval and memoing functions to support theory building. Theory-building functions allow the construction of explanations that are grounded in the qualitative data and include mechanisms for defining relationships among data elements, including original text, codes, memos, and documents. ATLAS.ti has a tool called Network Editor, which is a graphic space in which data and metadata elements can be imported and linked to one another through semantic relationships, as described previously. These "network" views can evolve into formal analytic products such as conceptual models.

Teamwork

All of the major QDA software programs provide some level of support for team-based analysis. Login names can be assigned to multiple users working on the same project so that their contributions can be tracked. Users can be assigned different levels of access, so that, for example, only individuals in supervisory positions can alter or delete data. There are "bundling" procedures to facilitate moving files between users, computers, and networks. Partial analyses performed by different researchers can be combined through merge procedures. The CDC programs (AnSWR and EZ-Text) include a tool for calculating Cohen's kappa, the interrater reliability statistic discussed earlier.

Multimedia Capabilities

Several QDA programs allow for importing and coding not only word processing files, but also PDF documents, graphic files, HTML web pages, and digital audio and video files. There are also specialized programs specifically designed for audio and video editing, some of which include tagging and retrieval functions (e.g., Transana®).

Support for Mixed-Method Analyses

For researchers who are interested in incorporating quantitative methods into their qualitative studies, tools are available in some QDA software programs to support a variety of approaches, including calculating and graphing code frequencies, creating code-by-document tables and other data matrixes, exporting data to statistical analysis or spreadsheet programs, and conducting quantitative content analysis. Beyond basic functions, however, specialized programs may be needed. For example, TextSTAT® is a specialized content analysis program used for tasks such as concordance and cluster analyses of word distributions within texts. Anthropac® is used for exploring cultural domains using data gathered through systematic elicitation techniques such as freelists (where a respondent is asked to list items in a domain, such as types of discrimination), pile sorts (where respondents sort a set of printed cards or items into piles from which taxonomies are built), and paired comparisons (where items in a domain are ranked along some dimension by having respondents compare pairs of items in the domain).

Complex quantitative procedures that typically build on qualitative research are also supported by specialized software. Examples are decision analysis, cultural consensus modeling, and Q Methodology, all of which are systematic decision science tools that attempt to discover the underlying structure of human subjective viewpoints and decisions.

Other Tools and Software Programs That Facilitate QDA

With new technological advances, some of the analog-to-digital conversion steps described previously can be automated or even eliminated. Optical scanning can quickly convert written or typed material to machine-readable text or image files. Audio and video data can be directly recorded in digital format with digital recorders and cameras. Voice-recognition software can directly convert spoken words or voice recordings to digital text. Interview responses may be typed directly into a computer by the respondent in response to recorded questions, as is done with audio-enhanced computer-assisted self-interviewing (audio CASI) technology. E-mail, text messaging, online discussions and forums, voice over Internet protocol (VoIP) technologies, and various types of social networking platforms have all been used in the service of qualitative research (Redlich-Amirav & Higginbottom, 2014). High-speed Internet connections combined with high-capacity cloud storage have made possible a new generation of Internet-based qualitative data analysis.

Summary

Although increasingly common, the use of QDA software has not been universally embraced by qualitative researchers. Some simply have well-established work habits using manual techniques or word processing programs and see no need to change them. There may be concern among some that the programs will be too difficult to learn or not worth the effort for the type of analysis planned. Some, particularly those working within participatory research, may fear that the computers distance the researchers too much from the voices and lived experiences of research participants and make it more difficult for the latter to participate in the data analysis. Still others have a basic philosophical opposition to using technological tools and methodological approaches associated with positivist paradigms that they see as antithetical to the spirit of qualitative research.

Some of these concerns are not without merit. For very small projects it may arguably not be worth a researcher's time to learn a complex QDA program, when the same results could be achieved with low-technology approaches. Some researchers are tempted to use software inappropriately, for example, performing individual-level statistical analyses on focus-group data. Some investigators become so wrapped up in their coding schemes and diagrams that they fail to stay close to the texts that are the true heart of their research findings. Such examples notwithstanding, computer-assisted analysis is appropriate and useful for many types of qualitative research.

As Weitzman (2000) notes, there are software tools to support a wide variety of research and analysis methods. Moreover, there is no single best program to meet all needs, and no program will conduct the data analysis for an investigator. To make the best use of QDA software programs, qualitative researchers must first and foremost understand the fundamentals of qualitative inquiry. They must take time to think about and articulate their intellectual puzzles, research questions, and the type of inquiry needed to answer those questions. Finally, the researcher should take advantage of the considerable volume of resources available to help select an appropriate program. Some of those resources are listed in the Resources section of this chapter.

Review Questions

1. What are the major steps involved in qualitative data analysis?
2. What are some of the quality assurance measures that are specific to qualitative data analysis?
3. From a practical and quality-assurance perspective, what are the advantages of computer-assisted approaches to qualitative data analysis?
4. What other kinds of technologies might expedite and improve qualitative data analysis?

REFERENCES

Bercovici, S. (1983). *Barriers to normalization*. Baltimore, MD: University Park Press.

Bernard, H. R., & Ryan, G. W. (2010). *Analyzing qualitative data*. Los Angeles, CA: Sage.

Carey, J., & Gelaud, D. (2008). Systematic methods for collecting and analyzing multidisciplinary team-based qualitative data. In G. Guest & K. M. MacQueen (Eds.), *Handbook for team-based qualitative research* (pp. 227–274). New York, NY: Altamira Press.

Carey, J. W., Morgan, M., & Oxtoby, M. J. (1996). Intercoder agreement in analysis of responses to open-ended interview questions: Examples from tuberculosis research. *Cultural Anthropology Methods, 8*(3), 1–5.

Edgerton, R. (1971). *The cloak of competence: Stigma in the lives of the mentally retarded*. Berkeley, CA: University of California Press.

Friese, S. (2012). *Qualitative data analysis with ATLAS.ti*. Los Angeles, CA: Sage.

Goode, D. (1983). Who is Bobby? In G. Kielhofner (Ed.), *Health through occupation: Theory and practice in occupational therapy* (pp. 83–101). Philadelphia, PA: F.A. Davis.

Guest, G., & MacQueen, K. M. (2008). Reevaluating guidelines in qualitative research. In G. Guest & K. M. MacQueen (Eds.), *Handbook for team-based qualitative research* (pp. 205–226). New York, NY: Altamira Press.

Kielhofner, G. (1977). Temporal adaptation: A conceptual framework for occupational therapy. *American Journal of Occupational Therapy, 31,* 235–242.

Kielhofner, G. (1979). The temporal dimension in the lives of retarded adults: A problem of interaction and intervention. *American Journal of Occupational Therapy, 33,* 161–168.

Kielhofner, G. (1981). An ethnographic study of deinstitutionalized adults: Their community settings and daily life experiences. *Occupational Therapy Journal of Research, 1,* 125–142.

Kielhofner, G., & Takata, N. (1980). A study of mentally retarded persons: Applied research in occupational therapy. *American Journal of Occupational Therapy, 34,* 252–258.

MacQueen, K. M., McLellan-Lemal, E., Bartholow, K., & Milstein, B. (2008). Codebook development for team-based qualitative analysis. *Cultural Anthropology Methods, 10*(2), 31–36.

Mason, J. (2002). *Qualitative researching* (2nd ed.). Thousand Oaks, CA: Sage.

Mayan, M. J. (2009). *Essentials of qualitative inquiry.* Walnut Creek, CA: Left Coast Press.

Redlich-Amirav, D., & Higginbottom, G. (2014). New emerging technologies in qualitative research. *The Qualitative Report, 19*(12), 1–14.

Strauss, A., & Corbin, J. (1998). *Grounded theory in practice: Procedures and techniques* (2nd ed.). Thousand Oaks, CA: Sage.

Weitzman, E. A. (2000). Software and qualitative research. In N. K. Denzin & Y. S. Lincoln (Eds.), *Handbook of qualitative research* (2nd ed., pp. 803–820). Thousand Oaks, CA: Sage.

RESOURCES

The past decade has seen a dramatic proliferation of books, journals, websites, and listservs dealing with various aspects of qualitative research. The following is a small selection of resources the reader might find useful for learning about computer-assisted qualitative data analysis. Although several of the books contain helpful advice on selecting software programs, developments in these products occur so quickly that it is best to consult Internet resources that are more frequently updated for help with selecting a program. The websites listed here contain links to many software sites in addition to those listed in this section. The software sites in turn contain links to product-specific listservs.

Books

Creswell, J. W. (2013). *Qualitative inquiry and research design: Choosing among five approaches* (3rd ed.). Thousand Oaks, CA: Sage.

Denzin, N. K., & Lincoln, Y. S. (2011). *The Sage handbook of qualitative research* (4th ed.). Thousand Oaks, CA: Sage.

Grbich, C. (2013*). Qualitative data analysis: An introduction.* Thousand Oaks, CA: Sage.

Miles, M. B., Huberman, A. M., & Saldana, J. (2014). *Qualitative data analysis* (2nd ed.). Thousand Oaks, CA: Sage.

Patton, M. Q. (2015). *Qualitative research and evaluation methods.* Thousand Oaks, CA: Sage.

Websites—General

CAQDAS Networking Project—a project housed at the University of Surrey in the United Kingdom that is funded to support the use of software in qualitative data analysis: http://www.surrey.ac.uk www.qualitative-research.net/

Websites—Product Specific

AnSWR, EZ-Text—CDC: http://www.cdc.gov/hiv/library/software/answr/
ANTHROPAC—Analytic Technologies: http://www.analytictech.com/
ATLAS.ti—Scientific Software Development: http://www.atlasti.com/
Dedoose: http://www.dedoose.com
Ethnograph—Qualis Research Assoc.: http://www.qualisresearch.com/
Hyper-Research—ResearchWare: http://www.researchware.com/
MaxQDA: http://www.maxqda.com
NVivo—QSR International: http://www.qsrinternational.com/

CHAPTER 19

Qualitative Approaches to Interpreting and Reporting Data

Heather Dillaway • Cathy Lysack • Mark R. Luborsky

Learning Outcomes

- Define the qualitative approach to interpreting and analyzing data.
- Recognize inductive approaches to qualitative analysis.
- Identify key differences between qualitative approaches to data analysis and quantitative approaches.
- Outline the major steps in the data analysis process.
- Explain how to approach the dissemination of qualitative findings.

Introduction

There are many ways in which qualitative approaches to data analysis are unique. This chapter outlines some of the basic purposes and stages of qualitative analysis, and it covers the broad themes and major characteristics of qualitative analysis and reporting, rather than the specific nuances between them. It enhances an understanding of the general philosophies behind and steps within any type of qualitative data analysis or reporting strategy. Interested readers may wish to explore grounded theory, narrative analysis, phenomenological analysis, discourse analysis, semiotic analysis, and other specific data analysis strategies themselves after reading this chapter.

This first section of this chapter defines the qualitative approach to interpreting or analyzing data and describes the major differences between qualitative and quantitative data analysis, identifying what makes qualitative data analysis unique. The sections that follow explain the process of completing qualitative analysis and reporting qualitative data once analysis is complete. The chapter concludes with reminders about qualitative approaches to analysis and reporting.

The Qualitative Approach to Data Analysis

In broad terms, the qualitative approach to interpreting and analyzing data involves interpreting words, not numbers. These words take the form of observations (e.g., from ethnographic field notes), interviews, or documents (Miles, Huberman, & Saldana, 2014). Note that some qualitative researchers also analyze images (moving or still) as their data, but that form of qualitative analysis is not addressed in this chapter. Instead, it focuses on qualitative analysis of interviewing and observations.

When reading through observational field notes, interview transcripts, or examining documents, the researcher looks for:

- Patterns or common expressions of people's perceptions or understandings of their world.
- The meanings they attach to aspects of the settings in which they live or the behaviors in which they engage.
- The reasons why people think particular things.
- The ways in which people account for or come to particular actions.
- How they organize their day-to-day situations.

At its foundation, then, **qualitative analysis** is about understanding meanings, processes, people, and their thoughts and actions through the interpretation of people's words.

Although qualitative researchers easily could reduce participants' words to numbers, it is important that they do not, in most cases. The reasons for this can be found in the purposes of qualitative research. That is, qualitative researchers aim to describe and explore a particular topic, group, or culture. Qualitative research is often undertaken when a particular topic or group has not been explored before, but it can also be used when much is already known about a topic, and a deeper understanding and explanation is needed to

CASE EXAMPLE

Kate, an occupational therapy (OT) doctoral student, is taking a course in qualitative research methods as an elective in her program. For her first assignment, she is asked to write a brief literature review illustrating how qualitative research extends and sheds a different light upon what is typically found as a result of quantitative research. Kate provides the following summary.

Qualitative research is particularly valuable in providing an understanding of the unique circumstance of different groups of people. For instance, we would never know as much about how poor communities share resources (e.g., cars, child care, money, etc.) if it were not for ethnographies such as *All Our Kin* by Carol Stack (1974). Although this research is not generalizable in the quantitative sense, it is nonetheless very valuable if our goal is to understand the role of kin and community resource networks among poor, racially disadvantaged groups. There are many other seminal contributions of qualitative research of relevance to the health sciences and to occupational therapy.

Many of these qualitative studies are ethnographic in nature and represent relatively prolonged periods of research time in the field. When this is the case, the reporting of the study often takes the form of a book. For example, Sue Estroff documented the lives of the mentally ill in *Making It Crazy* (1981, 1985) and revealed how our society and even medical professionals stigmatize and discriminate against this group. *Boys in White* by Howard Becker and colleagues (1961, 1991) is another classic ethnography in book form. In this study, Becker and his team conducted interviews with a cohort of medical students as they moved through their medical school training. This research focused on the cultural rites of passage and rituals of professional indoctrination that make doctors into the medical practitioners they are. Another excellent ethnography that focuses on cultural practices is *Everyone Here Spoke Sign Language* (Groce, 1985). This book is the result of a study on the islanders of Martha's Vineyard and how they worked to include those with congenital deafness. All of these examples enter the life worlds of social and cultural groups and explore their practices and rituals that help explain how and why things come to be the way they are.

fully comprehend the phenomenon. In both situations, people's presentations or constructions of their own worlds are very important because the researcher's central concern is to describe the phenomenon and gain new insights.

Quantitative analysis is often more about understanding cause and effect, that is, how one independent variable or multiple independent variables may affect a dependent variable. The goal, then, of quantitative research is often more concerned with explanation than description. In this latter case, numerical analyses become fruitful because they can help the researcher explain or predict relationships between two variables. But because qualitative researchers aim to describe and explore and understand, they need to preserve people's voices and the context that surrounds their voices. Ultimately this means that qualitative researchers preserve the original format of their data (or stay as close to the original as possible) so that readers of their analyses can see or experience for themselves as much of the participants' world as possible.

An Inductive Process

Qualitative analysis is often inductive, which is characteristic of several steps and stages in the overall qualitative research enterprise that was emphasized in Chapter 16. The idea behind an **inductive approach** is to allow research findings to emerge from the raw data that has been collected, without the restraints imposed by stricter methodologies or preestablished theories. Miles et al. (2014, p. 10) suggest that the researcher "attempts to capture data on the perceptions of local actors from the inside, through a process of deep attentiveness, of empathetic understanding ..., and of suspending or 'bracketing' preconceptions about the topic under discussion." Emerson, Fretz, and Shaw (2011, p. 36) talk about this same process as being one of "ethnographic participation." For these authors, qualitative research requires the investigator to achieve a "deeper immersion in others' worlds" in order to grasp what they experience as meaningful and important. Mishler (1979) has

ess as being more fundamental
any meaning that is extracted
ctions between the researcher
d is fundamentally social, and
ithout the context from which
it was generated. Mishler argues the researcher
and the researched are inextricably intertwined:
the phenomenon studied cannot even have objective characteristics independent of the observer's
perspectives and methods. Therefore, a researcher
using an inductive naturalistic approach is not only
centrally concerned with the identification of key
themes and findings, but also with epistemology,
or what counts as knowledge.

The following example illustrates some of these
fundamental differences between quantitative and
qualitative research. In the area of adherence to
medications, mostly quantitative approaches have
been used to measure a small set of patient characteristics (e.g., sociodemographic, psychosocial)
and health behaviors (e.g., drug use, risk profile)
to determine the statistical relationship of these
factors to patient medication adherence, where
adherence is generally specified as a percentage
(e.g., 90% adherent). In the literature, adherence
has been variably operationalized as the number of
pills or doses taken over a specified period of time,
numbers of days with no missed doses, or patient
self-report of percent adherence (e.g., "how adherent have you been in the last month?"). Although
many patient characteristics and health behaviors
have been shown to be statistically correlated with
adherence, their explanatory value is low (only
small amounts of the variance in patient adherence is explained), and therefore it has not been
possible to determine, for example, a profile of the
"noncompliant patient."

A qualitative approach to studying medication
adherence, in contrast, may investigate the understandings, meanings, and experiences of living with
a particular disease and adhering to medications.
An example is a study of adherence to HIV anti-
retroviral medications at Wayne State University
(HAART Adherence Among HIV+ African Americans). One finding of the study is that patients
quite frequently do not understand adherence in
the same way as their doctors. Patient understanding of the notion of being completely adherent
often means managing all aspects of the illness the
best one can given the circumstances, which may
mean taking none of the prescribed medications
whatsoever (Sankar, Nevedal, Neufeld, Berry, &
Luborsky, 2011).

Thus, the power of qualitative research in this
case is to explicate the variety of meanings of
adherence held by patients and uncover reasons for
patients' behaviors in relation to compliance with

therapeutic medication regimens. As evident from
this example, qualitative studies focus on uncovering how specific behaviors such as taking medications are understood in the context of people's
daily lives, and very often, this style of research
is the only way to interrogate assumptions that are
taken for granted about what constructs, such as
adherence, really mean in real people's lives.

The Goals of Description and Explanation

Another significant way in which qualitative
research differs from quantitative research is in its
ultimate goal, which is often simply to describe a
particular sample and/or small group that is being
studied. The goal of qualitative analysis is not to
come up with conclusions that could be generalized to populations. Describing a particular sample
or small group can give an in-depth understanding of the topics or people under study, and it
often spurs on larger, future research projects that
could be more population-based studies. In other
instances, as in the example on HIV medication
adherence in the preceding section, the goal is to
gain deeper insight into human behavior across a
larger sample in an effort to achieve full understanding across a wide range of study subjects.

As shown in a related example from the same
study, it has long been observed that many individuals with HIV are diagnosed only when they
are very ill and hospitalized, and this has been
attributed to a failure of public health education
to properly teach people about HIV risk groups
and behaviors. Qualitative research asks the "why"
questions, such as, "Why do some people wait
so long to get tested for HIV?" Answers such as,
"because I didn't think I was at risk," generate
follow-up questions, such as, "Why didn't you
think you were at risk?" Results show that individuals have largely absorbed and internalized
public health messages (i.e., they understand what
risky behavior is and precautions needed to avoid
HIV infection), but they have simply excluded
themselves from the risk categories (Sankar et al.,
2011). Without this very systematic work to interview individuals with HIV and follow their logic,
these insights and understandings would not have
been uncovered. This type of research is clearly
essential in the areas of health-related behaviors
and services.

Depth of understanding and proximity to people's worlds cannot be found in more structured,
deductive, quantitative, population-based research.
In keeping with its purpose, qualitative researchers
depend on recruiting the most informative people
possible to illuminate the topic of interest. Again,

the value of qualitative research lies in the "thick description" (Geertz, 2001), or deep understanding gained.

Data Collection and Analysis Intertwined

Another extremely important characteristic of qualitative analysis is that it begins during data collection and then continues after data collection is completed. Thus, there is a "zigzag" or back-and-forth process of data gathering and data analysis, especially in the early stages. At times, especially in grounded theory studies, data analysis might also be interrelated with sampling and with the choice of setting for the research, as researchers try to find people or settings that will garner them more information about particular themes arising in early field notes, journals, and interview transcripts.

In qualitative research, several steps in the research process (i.e., sampling, recruitment, entry into the field, data collection, analysis, etc.) may be intertwined. For example, in qualitative studies, interviewers might realize early in data collection that a particular theme is arising, and they may vary the main questions and probes that they use in later interviews so that they can explore this theme more fully. In her study of menopausal women, Dillaway (2005) discovered in early in-depth interviews that women did not feel "old" upon entering this life stage; because she began analysis of these early interviews before data collection was over, she was able to explore the reasons why women felt this way overall, finding that many women distinguished between reproductive aging and other types of aging. That is, according to her later interviewees, menopause was positive because it allowed women to let go of a function that they were ready to give up, whereas other aging conditions (e.g., losing eyesight, having Alzheimer disease, etc.) meant the loss of a function they desired to keep (Dillaway, 2005). This theme was fully flushed out only during data analysis because data collection strategies were altered to explore menopausal women's perceptions more deeply through probing and follow-up questions.

In another example, studies have found that older adults may not adopt a mobility aid such as a scooter or a walker just because their occupational therapist tells them it will make them safer and more independent. Issues such as their sense of being seen and treated as a disabled person and "less" than a full adult person actually weigh more heavily on their decision to acquire and utilize a mobility aid than many people, including therapists, realize (Gitlin, Luborsky, & Schemm, 1998; Luborsky, 1997). The fact that individuals'

perceptions of mobility aids differ from occupational therapists' perceptions is something that might be discovered only through a back-and-forth relationship between data collection and data analysis. In early data collection, an OT researcher might not be inclined to ask older individuals about their own perceptions and, instead, may begin by asking about their contact with a therapist and with the therapist's recommendations. Yet, if analysis starts during data collection, researchers could quickly pick up on the fact that they might not be exploring this issue in full and realize that individuals' perceptions of mobility aids may be more important than the recommendations they are given by the occupational therapist.

Finally, it is useful to return once more to the HIV adherence study because it very ably demonstrates how the results obtained from one set of qualitative research questions drive an entirely new set of questions. It should be noted that most, if not all, of these second-round questions are impossible to identify and plan for in advance. For example, in responding to questions about their medication adherence, many patients reported their number of missed doses (during some specified period of time), but later in the interview or in "side talk," they revealed that the meaning of a missed dose may not be straightforward (e.g., "I missed that dose because I did not take it until later"). As a result, a new set of questions about the meaning of a missed dose was developed and given to patients and their clinicians. Results revealed large variability and substantial difference between patients and clinicians in the understanding of what a "missed dose" is and what to do about missed doses (Sankar et al., 2011). The results have implications for the measurement of self-reported adherence, for patient–doctor communication, and for medication adherence itself.

Rigor, Flexibility, Challenge, and Reward

Qualitative analysis—and qualitative research in general—should be thought of as both a flexible and rigorous process. What qualitative researchers select to analyze in their data is not set in stone, and how qualitative researchers interpret these data can depend on many things (e.g., existing literature, the research questions or research problem he or she begins the project with, the kinds of themes that arise in early interviews or early analytic notes, or a combination of all of these). Yet, at the same time, there are particular systematic steps that a qualitative researcher goes through in order to arrive at a final interpretation of the data that can be reported.

Although qualitative research is often touted for its flexibility and subjectivity, it is as important to think about how qualitative research is simultaneously precise, detailed, and valid or trustworthy because of the process that researchers undertake in data collection and analysis. Qualitative researchers follow particular steps and verify their findings. At the same time, they adapt to the data that are arising in front of them.

Qualitative data analysis is a complex process that can be both time consuming and exhausting; thus, it can be challenging. In qualitative research, and largely because data collection does not occur in controlled situations, data collection and especially data analysis will take considerable energy and time. Simply put, qualitative analysis is not for the faint of heart. Perseverance is key. Often, the hardest thing for researchers is pushing through data analysis to see the final results they may come up with. The important thing to remember is that although qualitative analysis can be challenging and time consuming, it is a rewarding process as researchers see participants' voices and lives come into focus and as they share these voices with a larger audience. Those who engage in qualitative research will acknowledge the difficulties that others have in qualitative analysis, but these difficulties do remain somewhat hidden from those who do not engage in this research.

Carrying Out Qualitative Data Analysis

Although this section focuses on analysis and not on data collection, the reader should keep in mind that the two processes are intertwined, not separate. A key to good qualitative analysis is knowing that it is not a time-bound process and that data collection and data analysis are not partitioned from each other. There is a reflexivity that develops between data collection and data analysis in qualitative research that specifically creates the ability to achieve new and deeper understandings of particular perceptions, behaviors, and ways of human living.

The Importance of Data Processing

Data processing must occur for data analysis to begin; in some ways it is the first step researchers take in interpreting and reporting data. Chapter 17 covered many of the mechanics of data processing, so they are only briefly noted

here. Data processing includes making permanent records of interviews, field notes, or other documents that count as data (Rubin & Rubin, 2011). For example, data processing might be turning handwritten field notes into typed computer notes or transcribing audio-recorded (and/or video-recorded) data from in-depth interviews. Transcribing is the process by which the researcher listens to digitalized recordings of interviews and either stores automatically transcribed data or types verbatim what is said during the recorded interview so that the original data are preserved in a computer file. Many researchers also take handwritten notes during in-depth interviews or as part of textual analysis in addition to audio recordings, so those notes would need to be typed as well. Data processing might also include making multiple digital and paper copies of all original data files stored in a computer so that original data are not lost during data collection, data analysis, or afterward.

When analysis starts, the analytic work should take place with or on a duplicate copy of the original data so there is no chance to ruin the original data; this also allows the researcher to backtrack and start an analysis over if need be. At base, numerous attempts should be made to preserve data in their original format in multiple copies (and stored in multiple safe locations) so that the researcher can always find and access the data. This is particularly true of computer files—backing up data means not only peace of mind but also assurance against corrupted files, computers that crash and ruin files, stolen or damaged computers, and the like.

Just as importantly, data processing should at least begin alongside data collection, so that important themes in early interviews are not lost and the benefits of the reflexive, back-and-forth process between data collection and data analysis can be captured. The earlier the researcher completes the processing of data, the earlier the analysis process can be started. Moreover, the earlier the researcher starts the analysis process, the more likely it is that the researcher is able to grasp and gain a deep understanding of the themes that might be arising out of samples gathered in early data collection. With early data processing, researchers make the best use of the strengths of the qualitative approach to interpreting and analyzing data.

Regardless of the fact that data has been processed, when starting analysis, the researcher should be looking at and interpreting collected data in their original form. Thus, transcriptions and typed notes should be as precise as possible. Certain types of qualitative analysis in particular (e.g., phenomenology, narrative analysis, or semiotic analysis) require that processed data mirror exactly what was said in an interview or what was typed in an original field note, but all qualitative analysis should be initiated with data in as close to their original format as possible. When and how an interviewee laughs during a conversation, for example, may be important in telling the researcher about the interviewee's feelings of nervousness when discussing a particular topic or about the level of trust the researcher has gained during the interview. How quickly an interviewee answers a particular interview question may tell the researcher how strongly that person feels about the topic. For those using semiotics, or a linguistic approach to data analyses, even more detailed attention to the level of words and even syllables is undertaken. Thus, interview transcriptions should record laughs, hesitations, interruptions, emphases on particular words and phrases, and other speech patterns as much as possible, alongside the actual words of the conversation.

Riessman (1993) also notes that when an interviewee or informant appears to be going off on a side topic or tangent in conversation, the researcher must make every effort to follow and keep records of that side conversation because later on a researcher might realize that the conversation was an entry into a story that is relevant and answers a research question. Particular care should be taken during data processing so that all of these data are completely and systematically captured so that original data are maintained.

As noted in previous chapters, researchers can and do expand upon their primary data (e.g., handwritten field notes, audiotaped interview data) by keeping informal notes, memos, or a field journal during data collection. Notes could be about important ideas that interviewees or participants are suggesting about the topic or their culture, their experiences, or their behavior, as well as general ideas that the researcher begins to have about what the researcher is observing and hearing and would like to analyze as complex themes later in analysis (after the researcher is out of the field). The researcher might also record key quotes from interviews or overheard conversations that might be important in the data analyses later on. Notes could detail the researcher's personal assessments or opinions about how interviews or field observations are going and the ways in which data collection needs to be altered in order to secure a deep understanding of the topic/group at hand. In addition, notes include researchers' reactions to being in the field if they are doing participant observation, or feelings about the course of any type of data collection experience.

The purpose of this extra data can be threefold; they can:

1. Highlight key events during observations or interviews and thereby serve as a check on one's primary data source.
2. Serve as an emotional outlet for researchers during data collection and analysis when things get particularly frustrating (and details recorded here may become helpful later in writing up one's methods or research experiences).
3. Serve as the first step to data analysis by getting one's main ideas out on paper to propel more advanced analytic thinking about the study topic.

For these reasons, all qualitative researchers should keep some sort of informal notes or a journal as they engage in qualitative data collection. These notes or journal entries will help in the interpretation and documentation of one's research experiences and one's data (Emerson et al., 2011; Rubin & Rubin, 2011). They can be typed or handwritten, but, optimally, they should be made immediately after leaving the research setting for the day. Researchers may also have thoughts about how data collection is proceeding or about the types of patterns arising in interviews, and these thoughts may occur at random times (e.g., in the shower, lying in bed at night, driving). Thus, keeping a journal or a set of informal electronic notes that can be accessed easily at all times is a way of documenting such thoughts, no matter when they occur. These informal notes or journals become important sources for ideas of how to analyze and report about the significant amount of data that investigators accumulate over time. This informal data source can make the analysis stage less cumbersome, especially at the beginning.

Next Steps After Accumulating Processed Data

Rubin and Rubin (2011) suggest that it is helpful to think about data sources being broken down into data units, or blocks of information that will eventually be examined together. Investigators must begin their analysis by figuring out what blocks of information are appropriate to analyze. These blocks of information could be:

- Stories that interviewees tell that span several typed pages
- A paragraph of typed text from an interview or field note in which an individual describes

a particular encounter with a therapist or discussion of a particular health condition and its meaning

- A phrase or term used over and over by interviewees or informants or members of a particular organization, clinical team, or profession

The characteristic of these blocks of information is that they signify a key concept or theme. Thus, initial analyses consist of multiple readings of the data sources to look for the blocks of information that might be worth analyzing. Once the researcher finds a block of information that seems to emerge as important, then she or he might look to see if a similar block of information exists in a second data source, whether that data source is an individual or a large group of individuals. Then, the researcher begins a process of comparing and contrasting across data sources to see whether this data unit is important across a particular sample, as well as how and why it is important to the people interviewed or observed.

Four Steps in the Data Analytic Process

The analytic or interpretive process is discussed as four separate steps in this section. What follows is only one, albeit a common, approach to data analysis. Although data analysis frequently does begin with a singular data source as discussed here, it can also begin with responses to an entire set of interview questions across a group of study participants. Furthermore, when the latter is the case, "codes and coding" refer to an analytic category and not merely the words of one single study participant. These distinctions are drawn in the following discussion.

Step 1: Perform a Formal Analysis or Interpretation of One Data Source

Formal analysis or interpretation of qualitative data often begins with one data source. This may be one interview or one field note, for example. The researcher reads through this data source multiple times, gaining comfort with what it includes. Rubin and Rubin (2011) explain how, in this step, the researcher gains recognition of the concepts, events, feelings, and behaviors recorded, as well as the patterns within that particular data source. For instance, an investigator may ask whether an interviewee continually referred back to family history, situating the disability experience within the context of the extended family, or whether the

informant characterized the disability experience as owing very little to the extended family.

Once researchers are familiar with the initial data source, they should begin coding it. That is, investigators should come up with brief terms that can be written in the margins or recorded within a computer program that summarize blocks of information in that data source. Schwandt (2015) defines coding as a procedure that disaggregates the data, breaks the data down into manageable segments, and identifies or names those segments. It is impossible to undertake coding without at least some conceptual structure in mind. Nonetheless, coding can be undertaken in a more descriptive mode or in a more analytic mode, depending on the level of interpretation involved (refer back to Chapter 17 for more information on coding).

The most troublesome tendency in the act of coding, according to Strauss (1987), is to code too much at the descriptive level instead of coding for the purposes of explaining or developing an understanding of what is going on. This understanding is the heart of data analysis for thoughtful, reflective, and critical qualitative researchers. It is very easy to be mechanical in the coding process, but it is much more difficult to address the theoretical concepts that are involved in understanding social phenomena. Returning to the example alluded to previously, descriptive coding could thus take place every time a person refers to his or her family history during an interview; for instance, "family history" (even "fam. hist." or "FH") could be recorded or "coded" next to that data unit. At this descriptive level, the goal is to find a way to track similar blocks of information through a coding system, finding brief terms that categorize multiple areas of text. Miles et al. (2014) refer to this process as within-case analysis, in that one is doing all one can to master an understanding of a particular interview transcription or a set of observational field notes.

If, on the other hand, the research is less exploratory and more conceptual (i.e., theory and literature driven), qualitative investigators may utilize more semistructured interviews, and as a result, they may be in a position to focus on a clearly defined set of data provided in response to a clearly delineated subset of interview questions. In this case the single data source is somewhat more broadly construed. When this is the case, the researchers undertake a systematic process of comparisons across study participants simultaneously. They are also engaging in a deeper level of explanatory coding. In essence, the researchers are looking beyond the words and descriptions of their interview subjects to understand more fundamental conceptualizations of how people experience what they do.

Geertz (2001) has referred to this process as **inscribing social discourse;** it is a deliberate act to ensure that interactional details are fully captured. This level of detail in both the collection of data in field notes and in the interpretive process of data analysis is demanding, but it holds the potential to explain categories of meaning in a way that more superficial attention to words alone cannot.

Irrespective of the stance taken, it is generally accepted that investigators should code everything in the data source that is relevant to the research questions or research problem. However, this does not mean that researchers will code everything within a data source (Rubin & Rubin, 2011). Researchers must make a great many decisions about what data units are related to their initial goals in the research project and whether/how particular data units address the research questions. Certainly, some research questions take on greater priority, as is the case when a particular manuscript on a specific topic is planned. Thus, at times, coding must be strategically undertaken in response to practicalities such as available time and energy.

Once data are coded, important and related blocks of information are easy to find and access for further analysis and for reporting. Codes essentially flag patterns or themes that rest within the data. By defining and labeling codes, and through the act of assigning codes to their data, qualitative researchers begin to identify salient analytical connections among data units (even within the same data source). Thus, regardless of whether coding is undertaken on an informant-by-informant basis or is done across subjects simultaneously at a more conceptual level, coding must be done with great care because it forms the bedrock of subsequent interpretations.

For example, an investigator may wish to know how interviewees understand and describe a particular health problem such as hip fracture in old age. The investigator may further be interested to determine whether particular symptoms of hip fracture are more salient than others or whether certain meanings of having a hip fracture manifest over and over again in the same data source. To address these concerns, a specific code should be created for each issue to intimate what is important about each data unit. A researcher may go back and recode this data source at a later point, but these initial analytic steps are essential to establishing a systematic and theoretically informed analytic

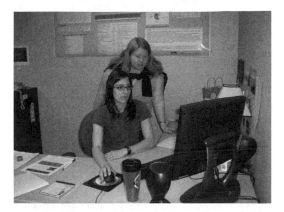

Figure 19.1   Members of a qualitative research team discuss their coding and analysis of an interview transcript.

strategy and for selecting particular data units to explore further (Fig. 19.1).

Step 2: Select a Particular Code for Further Analysis

After the researcher completes the coding of one particular data source, the next step is to select a particular code (and thus a particular set of data units or pattern among data units) for further analysis. How researchers select a particular code/pattern in the data for this second step of analysis is variable. Researchers could select a particular code to analyze based on their reading of literature on their topic of study or based on the research questions with which they began their project. However, qualitative researchers are often urged not to rely too much on past research or even research questions to dictate the specific data units they'll analyze. Relying too much on past literature and preconceived research questions can constrict the ways in which one is reading the data source as a whole and/or how one interprets particular blocks of information (Emerson et al., 2011; Miles et al., 2014; Riessman, 1993).

Thus, investigators should pay attention to codes/patterns that simply emerge out of the data source themselves, upon the investigators' critical reflection. For example, Siporin and Lysack (2004) studied the work and home settings of adults with developmental disabilities. They relied on prolonged engagement in the field and in-depth interviews to illuminate how different the experience of working in a sheltered workshop was from working in more community-based supported employment programs. This study relied on prolonged periods of observation in the workplace of clients to show how factors in the physical and social environment operated to enhance or limit the quality of life perceived by the clients.

Specifically, the investigators learned that the type of work characteristic of sheltered workshops as opposed to supported employment settings accounted for only a small amount of the clients' subjective quality of life. This finding contradicted the investigators' expectations that type of work would matter much more. Other factors, such as the personalities of agency staff and life coaches and the types of social opportunities linked to each distinctive type of worksite, turned out to be more powerful influences on clients' expressed quality of life. If these investigators had not paid attention to the codes they attached to these other aspects of the work environment (besides the ones they expected would be important based on existing literature), they would not likely have discovered the importance of personally meaningful interactions with agency staff and fun opportunities outside of work as key factors in clients' perceptions of a good life.

Other things may also influence what analytic strategy an investigator chooses to pursue. For instance, the way in which current media is framing an issue/topic/cultural group may be important in shaping a researcher's analytic strategy. A qualitative researcher engaged in a study on aging may note that aging is being characterized negatively by the mainstream media; in response, the researcher will develop and assign one or more codes that speak to this issue. On the other hand, ideas from a researcher's informal notes or field journal may generate some new codes. There are numerous ways in which researchers select the codes and data units they analyze. Qualitative investigators must be aware of and open to a range of different strategies when developing their approach to data analysis and coding.

An important strategy for simplifying the oftentimes complex task of data analysis is picking only one code to analyze at a time. This strategy can be particularly useful advice for novice qualitative researchers. Because qualitative data include so many different patterns and themes (and because these patterns and themes probably are not mutually exclusive), the easiest way to navigate qualitative analysis is to keep one's attention on one pattern in the data at a time. There is always time to go back and analyze other sets of data units at other times. As will be discussed later, the process of qualitative analysis is never completely over. Thus, researchers might as well dedicate themselves to just one specific analytic task and carry it through to completion before undertaking another.

Step 3: Compare and Contrast Data Sources Utilizing a Particular Code

After reading and coding one particular data source and selecting one code or pattern to highlight in further analysis, the next step is to compare and contrast data sources utilizing a particular code. Miles et al. (2014) call this step cross-case analysis. In this step the researcher asks whether it is possible to move to the next data source and find similar ideas or topics and code that second data source in similar ways (i.e., using the same code selected in step 2).

In step 3, the researcher is essentially clarifying what is meant by a particular data unit or coded block of text (Rubin & Rubin, 2011). As investigators compare blocks of information in the first and second data sources, they begin to understand the similar and different ways interviewees or field notes discuss a particular topic. Thus, the information stored within each code is analyzed for nuances, and the meaning of the original code becomes clearer than it was in previous steps.

Going back to the example of how people might talk about the role of their family history in explicating their disability experience, the researcher might find that one interviewee felt that family history led directly to his or her own health condition. Therefore, such an interviewee might characterize the impact of family history as negative. However, a second interviewee might also talk about family history, but consider his or her own health problems to be an anomaly. In this second data source, then, the interviewee may have characterized family history more positively. In this example, the comparison of similarly coded text across two data sources leads to a greater understanding of how individuals attach importance or meaning to their family histories. It may become clearer when comparing and contrasting similarly coded text that although importance is placed on family history across interviewees, the particular meanings they attach to family history vary. In such an instance, the codes may be adjusted to fit the new understanding of these data units as they are compared and contrasted. This is a repeated process, comparing and contrasting each data source to others until all cases in a sample have been analyzed (Miles et al.,1994).

The decisions researchers make during initial coding and coding revisions shape what they will be able to conclude at the end of the analysis. Thus, the process of coding and then comparing, contrasting, and revising understanding of codes is key to the analytic or interpretive process. The emphasis should be on either finding ways of relating coded blocks of data together (similarities) or finding differences in the way data units uphold a particular code, so that the nuances underneath a code can be brought to the surface.

Step 4: Draw Some General Conclusions About What a Coding Strategy or Arising Data Pattern Means

In a final step of analysis, investigators stop specific cross-case comparisons and zoom out, so to speak, on what has been found thus far. In this step, the investigator will draw some general conclusions about what a coding strategy or arising data pattern means. This allows both the consistencies and differences among a particular set of data units to be described and understood. Therefore, this step is about arriving at a kind of final synthesis (Rubin & Rubin, 2011) or a thematic narrative (Emerson et al., 2011) that illuminates the theme or pattern that has been recognized or identified in the cross-case analyses completed in step 3.

The goal of this step is to develop a way to refer to the theme or pattern and the subthemes and subpatterns beneath it (if one has created subcodes underneath a main code, which is often the case). This is very much a reflective analytic step, one in which the researcher must step back and find a way to evaluate all data units underneath a specifically coded theme. The key questions that need to be answered in this step are:

- What am I going to call this theme as I move into a reporting stage?
- How am I going to define the nuances I found within it as I looked at different data units and in different data sources?
- What are the examples of variations under the umbrella of this coded theme, and how can I explain them? Why do these variations matter?
- What are examples of the commonalities across all data units I have labeled with a given theme, and how do I explain them? Why do they matter?
- What is the significance of this theme overall for my research topic, and how might my analysis of this particular topic/theme add to previous literature on this subject?

If one's coding strategy and previous levels of analysis can hold as one answers these questions, then it is probably the case that one has arrived at what resembles a complete analysis. Perhaps the most important question in the list is the last one. A researcher must think about the broader significance of the analysis just completed and whether or not there are general implications of what has

been learned. Thus, one should ask how far the thematic analysis (and thus codes/coding strategies one has developed) might extend.

For example, Lysack and Seipke (2002) found that oldest-old women often defined aging well differently than policymakers and health-care providers. They defined their own well-being in terms of whether they could still complete gendered household tasks rather than in terms of established health or independence scales that a therapist or policymaker might use to determine their need for services. Although individuals' definitions of aging well were interesting as findings in and of themselves, Lysack and Seipke (2002) concluded that their findings had policy and health-care implications. Moreover, they suggested that traditional notions of successful aging and independence among the elderly needed to be rethought at the national and local levels. Thus, although qualitative research is not generalizable in that it cannot speak to a heterogeneous population's attitudes or behaviors, qualitative analyses can still hint at ideas that must be explored further and broader implications that might have meaning outside of any particular research sample.

Although this is a final step in analysis, it should be acknowledged that an investigator may return again and again (often in response to reviewers', editors', and particular audiences' comments) to clarify what is meant by particular data units explained by particular themes. Investigators may also add further nuances to the understanding of how data units fit (or do not fit) together at a later date.

It is also important to note that researchers typically move back and forth among these major steps as they attempt to make sense of the data units relevant to their research question or research problem. In the grounded theory tradition, this iterative process is called the constant comparative method (Glaser & Strauss, 1967).

Just as data collection and analysis can be a back-and-forth process, so too is the analysis process. Investigators will move back and forth between looking at individual data sources, looking at multiple data sources, and then making tentative interpretations of the data. Only at the point when researchers are no longer finding new interpretations or new similarities and differences should they move to conclude that saturation has been reached and begin to write the findings. When researchers can draw a small set of conclusions about the interpretations that help to answer the initial research questions (and that would be acceptable to the people studied), the analysis is complete.

Enhancing Rigor Through the Steps of Qualitative Data Analysis

Emerson et al. (2011) urge qualitative researchers to utilize a variety of organizational strategies to enhance the rigor of their analyses. These authors and others (Strauss, 1987) devote entire chapters to strategies undertaken in the field to capture scene depictions, to communicate dialogue and interpersonal exchanges, to elucidate indigenous meanings with and without verbal data, to develop and analyze integrative memos, and many other tasks in the qualitative data collection and analysis process. All such measures contribute to achieving greater quality in the end product of qualitative research.

There are various ways to check analysis during the analytic process or verify the patterns or themes found in the original data. First, some researchers have multiple coders and/or analysts on their research projects to ensure that they are reading data units in similar and valid ways. This is a check on the reliability of the emerging interpretations (read more about interrater reliability in Chapter 17). Second, qualitative researchers sometimes also give copies of their initial analyses back to their interviewees or informants in the field to assess how closely they have captured what participants' voices and worlds are. This is called member checking or stakeholder checking in some qualitative traditions (refer to Chapter 16 for more information on stakeholder checking). Third, it is often easy to look to previous literature to evaluate whether initial results make sense (although this does not mean that findings need to mirror the results of past studies!). Fourth, the researcher might reflect on whether, intuitively, initial findings make sense. Finally, within the analysis process itself, if the coding holds up across multiple data sources and back-and-forth processes of within-case and cross-case analysis, then the researchers probably have reasonable grounds to conclude that the coding strategy and larger analytic strategy are valuable and the results generated from the qualitative data analysis are worth reporting.

How and Where to Report Findings

Researchers should make the transition from analysis to reporting by thinking about why they initiated their projects and what their goals were. For instance, qualitative research may be undertaken with a purely academic goal of adding to existing literature on the topic or group, or a more applied goal of coming up with ways to make the lives of members of a particular group better in some way. Investigators also need to consider what form the results need to be in to reach the initial goals of the research. This may include, for example, a peer-reviewed journal article, book or other lengthy manuscript, policy brief, oral presentation, or poster.

Determining the Audience

Based on the initial goals of the research, investigators should determine the audience for their findings—that is, the group of people who will be reading and reacting to the findings. Different audiences will find different presentations of the analysis more or less important and will require different kinds of information. For instance, if the researchers seek to influence policy for the developmentally disabled, they need to think critically about the policy implications in the final steps of analysis and make them understandable and believable to policymakers, who are typically not well versed in academic literature or research methodology. On the other hand, if researchers have an academic audience, it will be more important to spend time reporting all the similarities and differences found across data sources when coding for a particular topic or theme. For this latter audience, researchers would also need to spend more time detailing past literature on the subject. Thus, the audience of the report will determine how the analysis is communicated.

Retaining Voice

Another important issue to think about at the beginning of the reporting process is how best to retain participants' voices and/or the original data when communicating themes in the data to an audience. As noted earlier, one of the key goals of qualitative research is to report what group members' thoughts, behaviors, and lives look like from the inside (Miles et al., 2014). To stay close to this goal, researchers must maintain a commitment to reporting original data. This means, for instance, reporting participants' actual words from interview conversations or verbatim field notes so that the audience can immerse themselves in the original research setting alongside the researcher.

Because the qualitative researcher is the research instrument, great care must be taken to include both what is observed or heard and what is thought and interpreted by the researcher.

This means that within a report or presentation, examples of original data must be provided along with interpretations of these data. Thus, although a researcher may provide an interpretation of how to read or make sense of the data, the actual data are also in the report for readers to interpret on their own.

How to Report the Analysis

Typically, qualitative researchers select a broad pattern or theme to introduce in the report or presentation. This theme is directly related to the codes that are analyzed first in one data source, then across data sources. How researchers present this theme is usually related to the answers to the questions presented under step 4 of the analysis. That is, the researcher must first name and define what the finding or theme is. This is often about defining the coding strategy. After a theme is presented and summarized, the researcher should present an example of original data.

For instance, in reporting the quality of nursing care in their report, Williams and Irurita (1998) discuss how nurses initiate rapport with their patients; "initiating rapport" was a code they defined during the analysis stage of their research. In their report, they first define this concept: "Rapport was established by informal, social communication that enabled the nurse and the patient to get to know each other as persons" (p. 38). Then they present an example by stating, "One of the nurses interviewed described this interaction" (p. 38). The nurse's description is then provided:

> "Just by introducing yourself, by chatting along as you're doing things...with the patient. Asking them...questions about themselves...like 'how are you feeling about being in hospital? How are you feeling about the operation tomorrow?' And then they'll sort of give you a clue...and actually then tell you how they're feeling about things...just general chit chat..." (Nurse). (Williams & Irurita, 1998, p. 38)

The sequence used by Williams and Irurita (1998) to describe and elaborate on the data patterns they analyzed is an effective format for reporting qualitative analyses. This format consists of:

- A name or label for the category,
- The authors' description of the meaning attached to the category, and
- A quotation from the raw text or original data to elaborate on the meaning of the category and to show the type of text coded into the category.

After presenting this sequence of information, the researcher goes on to present the nuances underneath each thematic category. This includes, perhaps, presenting the ways in which particular data sources are grouped together under that category or theme during analysis. If the researchers found, for example, that the way in which interviewees talked about family history varied depended on whether or not they felt family factors determined a current health condition, they could present first those who felt positively about their family history (defining this group and then presenting examples of original data) and subsequently present those who felt negatively about the same. Then the researchers might speculate about the reasons why there were differences in the meanings attached to family histories.

The presentation of nuances underneath a theme or code illustrates the rigorous process by which the researchers arrived at conclusions about the important aspects of their data, and it also helps shape a deeper understanding of the topic at hand. By presenting nuances underneath a theme, researchers show how thorough the analysis has been and bring the audience into the description as much as possible. The presentation of a theme or coding strategy begins broadly and then becomes more specific. This pattern of reporting qualitative data is widely accepted and well understood as an adequate way to present complex analyses and, at the same time, remain as close as possible to participants' voices.

Researchers should try to keep their reports of qualitative analysis as simple as possible. This means presenting very few themes or findings in each report. The definition and discussion of qualitative analyses is a lengthy process because it requires:

- The definition and discussion of the finding,
- The presentation of original data,
- The presentation of nuances within that finding, and
- The presentation of more original data (to provide evidence of these nuances).

Thus, there is often not enough room within any one written document or oral presentation to communicate more than one or a few themes or findings. Thus, qualitative researchers should keep reports simple so that they can report specific findings in full, following the format of starting with a broad theme and then defining its specific nuances.

Regardless of the type of reporting qualitative researchers produce (e.g., poster, oral presentation, published paper, or written report), they must stand ready to explain the qualitative approach and its

	Title of Poster Author & Affiliation	
Introduction (perhaps 1–2 paragraphs)	Definition of Broad Theme/Code	Definition of Specific Nuances
Methods (perhaps 1–2 paragraphs and charts/graphs)	Examples of Original Data	Examples of Original Data
		Some Basic Conclusions

Figure 19.2 General layout for a poster illustrating a qualitative study.

benefits because this approach is still misunderstood and less valued than quantitative approaches in most arenas (anthropology being an important exception). Thus, when making a report of qualitative analyses and/or responding to audience members' or readers' questions, researchers should be ready to discuss the following issues:

• Why they chose to do qualitative over quantitative research,
• The unique benefits of qualitative data, or why researchers might engage in qualitative research,
• The rigor of the qualitative data collection and analysis strategies and the specific steps completed to arrive at results, and
• The implications and/or significance of the results—that is, how the results can be used to promote future research, advocacy efforts, or policy efforts, even if the analyses are based on a limited sample. In other words, why do the results matter even if they are not generalizable and/or based on a random sample and numerical data?

If researchers prepare statements or answers in response to these issues before finalizing the report, they can guarantee a better reception of the qualitative analyses and conclusions. Laypersons often value quantitative research more highly than qualitative research. Thus, qualitative researchers need to be prepared to deal with these societal views in public forums.

Common Ways to Report Qualitative Analyses

There are many ways to report data. This section focuses on the three most common ways: poster presentations, oral presentations, and written reports.

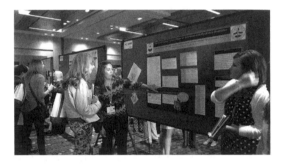

Figure 19.3 A poster presentation at a conference. *(Courtesy of Catana Brown.)*

Poster Presentations

Poster presentations can be made easily in software programs such as PowerPoint or Microsoft Word. Although various styles and formats for organizing a poster are possible, typically, the poster layout should permit readers to move from left to right as they view the poster, as if they were reading a book. Thus, on the left, the researcher should start with a small introduction of the topic/study and some brief information about the research methods undertaken. As readers move to the middle area of the poster, they should see information about basic results or findings, that is, a presentation of the broad themes found within the analysis, which should include the name and definition of the theme/code and then original data examples to back up the definitions. As readers move to the right-hand side of the poster, they should then see the specific nuances within the findings, or ways in which particular groups of one sample or groups of data sources allowed for a deeper understanding of that theme/code. Figure 19.2 is an illustration of how a poster might be organized, and Figure 19.3 shows a completed poster presented at a conference.

One variation of this basic example is to place the key research question and the main study findings and conclusions in the top center of the poster. This can be eye-catching and effective. Another variation might be undertaken to address particular needs of the audience. That is, if this is a poster presented in an academic setting, the researcher might want to present more details on prior research literature on the topic on the left-hand side of the poster, after the introductory section and before the presentation of methods. If the poster is for an advocacy organization's event or for a group of health-care providers or policymakers, it might be less important to provide the results of prior research and instead highlight more salient take-home messages for policy decision-makers.

Oral Presentations

In presenting results orally, researchers typically describe and provide visual depictions (e.g., slides) of the same data as in a poster format. Variations would be based on the audience, and this is very similar to poster presentation as well, with the academic audiences being accustomed to hearing more about past literature than policy audiences or consumer/lay audiences. Thus, the researcher should know both the disciplinary backgrounds of the audience and the level of interest they might have in the components of the presentation. Novice researchers should query prior conference participants on facts like these to ensure that their presentation "hits the mark" with respect to the audience's needs.

Typically, 10 to 20 minutes will be allotted for an oral presentation at a scholarly or professional conference or other public forum, followed by 5 to 10 minutes of audience questions. Researchers should determine the allocated length of time and ensure their presentation is of appropriate length. Oral presentations of qualitative data analyses are often quite difficult to complete in a short amount of time. Introducing the topic and briefly discussing the research methods may require one-third to one-half of the time allotted for an oral presentation. Moreover, because the presenter often needs to read examples of original data out loud (or at least summarize what pieces of original data suggest) for the audience, time is quickly spent. Thus, to skillfully complete an oral presentation of qualitative analyses, the researcher must prepare for the specific time allotted and present few findings. Keeping things simple and presenting as few themes/findings as possible is extremely important. Researchers should expect that in a 10-minute presentation, for example, they might be able to present only two or three examples of original data to illustrate a broad theme and then may only be able to present one or two nuances under that theme.

Formal Written Reports for Academic Audiences

When completing a thesis dissertation, preparing a funded report, or publishing in an academic forum, researchers can present a fuller picture of the topic under study and the past literature on the topic, a broad description of the research methods that were used, and more detail on actual findings. In a formal written report, there is also considerably more emphasis on formalizing conclusions and the implications of completed analyses. Thus, this type of report is the most complete version of a qualitative analysis. The standard format for a formal written report, especially for an academic audience, is as follows:

- An introduction to the topic or group under study, including a discussion of the research purpose and the relevance of the research;
- A literature review or "background" section, illustrating past research on the topic, including a discussion of any gaps in this past literature that might be filled by the current analyses;
- A methods section that details the sample, data collection and processing procedures, analytic strategies, and potential biases/limitations of the research;
- A findings section (referred to as a results section in quantitative studies) detailing one or a few broad findings and all the specific nuances found within these findings; for both broad and specific sets of findings, numerous examples of original data should be presented and explained in full;
- A discussion and/or conclusion section, summarizing what was found in the results and the implications of the findings; attention may be paid to avenues for future research, especially based on particular limitations of the current study;
- Any tables, charts, graphs, or other appendices that make the discussion of methods or findings clearer to the reader; and
- References to past research on the topic.

These sections may vary in length, depending on the audience for the written report. By following this standard format, there is a greater chance that the qualitative research and analytic procedures will be considered credible or believable. This is particularly important when presenting qualitative analyses to audiences who value numerical results more than original data or people's voices or those who value explanation over description and exploration.

Summary

This chapter illustrates how both qualitative analysis and reporting of qualitative research findings are multilayered enterprises. Investigators start with a particular data unit in a particular data source and then connect it to other data units in other data sources during a complex and flexible, yet rigorous, analytic process. Once connections are found (i.e., patterns or themes across multiple interviews or observations), investigators think about what those patterns mean and create a way to not only understand, but also to talk about those connections (i.e., a reporting strategy). Qualitative reporting then involves sharing information about the research process and about both broad and specific information found in the research.

Qualitative analysis and reporting are ongoing as well. Although the researcher may come to the end of a cycle of analysis or the end of a particular report, there are always more data to analyze and more analyses to report. The researcher should be ready to continue analyzing the same data sources over and over again for more and deeper insights and explanations. Qualitative researchers should also be ready to go back and analyze the very same coded themes and patterns, for there is always more they can discover about previously coded data units. Each time the researcher starts a particular analysis or reporting cycle, she or he makes choices about what to concentrate on, which, ultimately, means some analysis and reporting is left for later.

This means, then, that the conclusions qualitative researchers discuss are partial, and they always warrant further exploration. Thus, researchers should always be thinking about how they can extend the data they have with just a bit more data analysis. Researchers should think about ways in which to push the boundaries of interpretation and understanding to facilitate insights that are needed to answer the range of study questions. This may include a search for ways of broadening the analytic strategy, but it can also mean finding ways to be more specific and insightful. Finally, because data collection and analysis should always be reflexive and iterative, researchers should never stop thinking about the next steps that could be taken in data collection. Such reflection can lay the groundwork for yet another new phase of the research project.

Although this chapter discusses the major steps or processes that all qualitative researchers complete to interpret and report qualitative data, there are necessarily and inevitably variations in how each researcher moves through the analysis and reporting processes. By no means does everyone analyze or report their data in the same way, nor should they. As highlighted many times, a benefit to qualitative research is the flexibility that characterizes it. Thus, although this chapter details particular ways in which qualitative analyses and reports can be completed, they should be seen only as a guide. They should not be taken as a prescription for how to complete qualitative analysis and reporting.

Finally, because qualitative research—and, in particular, analysis—is time consuming and conceptually demanding, completing a qualitative analysis and getting to the reporting stage is a feat in and of itself. Still, researchers must be able to take constructive criticism and seek to make future analyses and reports better. The goals of qualitative research—to describe, to explore, to present people's voices—can be realized only if individuals are dedicated to the complexities involved in data collection, analysis, and reporting. Researchers should be mindful of this during the arduous process of qualitative analysis and reporting.

Relatively little is known about the wide range of factors that contribute to individuals' health and disability, about individuals' use of particular therapeutic treatments, and about the processes by which occupational therapists facilitate health and wellness through their interventions. Consequently, *the initiation of more qualitative research in OT settings is critical.* Although there have been important qualitative studies in recent years in occupational therapy, there is a need for much more description and exploration of both clients' conditions and of clients' and therapists' attitudes and behaviors.

Review Questions

1. What are the key features of qualitative analysis?
2. How can you demonstrate an inductive approach to qualitative analysis?
3. What are the key differences between qualitative approaches to data analysis and quantitative approaches?
4. What are the major steps in the data analysis process?
5. What are the key considerations in disseminating qualitative findings?

REFERENCES

Becker, H. S., Geer, B., Hughes, E. C., & Strauss, A. L. (1961, 1991). *Boys in white: Student culture in medical school.* Somerset, NJ: Transaction.

Dillaway, H. E. (2005). Menopause is the "good old": Women's thoughts about reproductive aging. *Gender & Society, 19*(3), 398–417.

Emerson, R. M., Fretz, R. I., & Shaw, L. (2011). *Writing ethnographic fieldnotes* (2nd ed.). Chicago, IL: University of Chicago Press.

Estroff, S. (1981, 1985). *Making it crazy: An ethnography of psychiatric clients in an American community.* Berkeley, CA: University of California Press.

Geertz, C. (2001). Thick description: Toward an interpretive theory of culture. In R. M. Emerson (Ed.), *Contemporary field research* (2nd ed., pp. 55–75). Long Grove, IL: Waveland Press.

Gitlin, L., Luborsky, M., & Schemm, R. (1998). Emerging concerns of older stroke patients about assistive device use. *The Gerontologist, 38*(2), 169–180.

Glaser, B., & Strauss, A. (1967). *The discovery of grounded theory: Strategies for qualitative research.* Chicago, IL: Aldine Press.

Groce, N. (1985). *Everyone here spoke sign language: Hereditary deafness on Martha's Vineyard.* Cambridge, MA: Harvard University Press.

Luborsky, M. (1997). Attuning assessment to the client: Recent advances in theory and methodology. *Generations, 21*(1), 10–16.

Lysack, C., & Seipke, H. (2002). Communicating the occupational self: A qualitative study of oldest-old American women. *Scandinavian Journal of Occupational Therapy, 9,* 130–139.

Miles, M. B., Huberman, A. M., & Saldana, J. (2014). *Qualitative data analysis: A methods sourcebook* (3rd ed.). Thousand Oaks, CA: Sage.

Mishler, E. G. (1979). Meaning in context: Is there any other kind? *Harvard Educational Review, 49,* 1–19.

Riessman, C. K. (1993). *Narrative analysis.* Thousand Oaks, CA: Sage.

Rubin, H., & Rubin, I. (2011). *Qualitative interviewing: The art of hearing data* (3rd ed.). Thousand Oaks, CA: Sage.

Sankar, A., Nevedal, A., Neufeld, S., Berry, R., & Luborsky, M. (2011). Cultural rationales guiding medication adherence among African Americans with HIV/AIDS. *AIDS Patient Care and STDs, 25*(9), 547–555.

Schwandt, T. A. (2015). *The Sage dictionary of qualitative inquiry* (4th ed.). Thousand Oaks, CA: Sage.

Siporin, S., & Lysack, C. (2004). Quality of life and supported employment: A case study of three women with developmental disabilities. *American Journal of Occupational Therapy, 58*(4), 455–465.

Stack, C. (1974). *All our kin: Strategies for survival in a black community.* New York, NY: Harper & Row.

Strauss, A. (1987). *Qualitative analysis for social scientists.* Cambridge, England: Cambridge University Press.

Williams, A. M., & Irurita, I. F. (1998). Therapeutically conducive relationships between nurses and patients: An important component of quality nursing care. *Australian Journal of Advanced Nursing, 16*(2), 36–44.

CHAPTER 20

Quantitative Research Designs: Defining Variables and Their Relationships With One Another

David L. Nelson • Gary Kielhofner • Renée R. Taylor

Learning Outcomes

■ Outline the two major types of quantitative research designs used in occupational therapy research and their applications.
■ Compare and contrast univariate and correlational descriptive research designs.
■ Outline the steps of a basic experiment.
■ Compare and contrast type I errors and type II errors.
■ Describe the characteristics and major types of group comparison designs.

Introduction

As discussed earlier in this text, quantitative research designs are those that translate information from assessments and observations into numerical data that are analyzed statistically according to a preestablished plan. In this chapter we provide more detailed coverage of a range of designs that fall into two broad categories of quantitative research: descriptive research designs and comparative group designs. **Descriptive research** is common in occupational therapy and serves a number of purposes. Descriptive research depicts naturally occurring events or characteristics of research participants (e.g., behaviors, attitudes, and other attributes; DePoy & Gitlin, 2010; Polit & Hungler, 1999; Portney & Watkins, 2009). **Group comparison designs** compare groups of subjects and are among the most common in quantitative research. Group comparison designs may be classified in terms of two major categories: experimental designs comparing subjects deliberately assigned to groups (random assignment)

and nonexperimental designs comparing naturally occurring groups.

Descriptive Research

In many situations, too little is known to undertake studies in which independent variables are manipulated and their effects on dependent variables are observed. For this reason, descriptive research takes advantage of naturally occurring events or available information to generate new insights through inductive processes. Consequently, descriptive investigations often serve an exploratory purpose. Such studies typically lead to greater understanding of phenomena, and the resulting conceptualizations are then later tested through more rigorous research designs. Sometimes basic descriptive information is needed to indicate norms, trends, needs, and circumstances that inform and guide practice. Finally, descriptive research is a component of all research studies because it is used to characterize subjects and other relevant circumstances that surround the research.

There are two types of descriptive research designs:

• **Univariate research designs,** in which data are collected on a single variable or a series of single variables and then characterized with descriptive statistics; and
• **Correlational research designs,** in which relationships between two or more variables are examined.

These two types of descriptive studies and their uses in occupational therapy (OT) research are presented in the following sections.

CASE EXAMPLE

Jabil, a new assistant professor of occupational therapy at a Carnegie-ranked research-intensive university, studied motor control in post-stroke elders as a quantitative researcher in his doctoral program and during his postdoctoral fellowship. Now that he has been hired in a junior faculty role, he decides to conduct research on a topic that is completely different than what he studied during his doctoral and postdoctoral work. Against his mentor's advice (which is to remain focused on motor control in post-stroke elders), Jabil now wants to study a completely different topic: the behavioral risk factors associated with cardiovascular disease in urban-dwelling Native American adults. Knowing that this topic is Jabil's new passion, his mentor recommends that he map out a 5-year research plan and timeline describing how he will build his trajectory of scholarship as he works toward obtaining grant funding and tenure at his university. Struck by the enormity of this assignment, Jabil begins by thinking about the major classifications of quantitative research and how certain types of research designs might be used to build upon one another. He knows that he must first conduct descriptive studies that will eventually lead to group comparison studies.

Having conducted no prior studies on this topic, with little information about cardiovascular disease in urban-dwelling Native American elders in the existing literature, and with few funds to support his budding research program, Jabil knows he must begin at the very beginning. He writes into his plan a series of small pilot studies that follow descriptive research designs. First, Jabil decides to conduct a prevalence study in a local primary-care sample extracted from a large urban health-care network affiliated with his university. A prevalence study would yield data on the number of elders affected by cardiovascular disease and the social-demographic characteristics of those elders. A prevalence study could also provide information about the nature and course of the disease in the sample. Next, he decides to conduct a study according to a univariate research design that would reveal the demographic characteristics of elders who have developed cardiovascular disease as well as their behaviors and occupational participation. He anticipates that this descriptive study would have identified a series of variables associated with cardiovascular disease. Knowing the literature on behavioral correlates for cardiovascular disease in non–Native American elders, he predicts that the study will reveal characteristics such as obesity, inactivity, dietary factors, stress, tobacco use, and comorbid health conditions, such as diabetes and other metabolic conditions.

Based on this prediction, Jabil plans a third descriptive study that employs a correlational research design. This study will allow him to evaluate the strength of the relationships between the various behavioral characteristics that he identified through his univariate studies and the strength of the relationships between each of those characteristics and the type and extent of cardiovascular disease in the elders. A correlational study would also yield the extent to which each of these characteristics is associated with cardiovascular disease. Once a correlational study is complete, Jabil can then plan interventions to address the behavioral correlates that emerge as most strongly associated with cardiovascular disease. A pilot group comparison study with nonrandom assignment would then allow him to test the outcomes of those interventions in a convenience sample of Native American elders. A visual depiction of Jabil's research trajectory is presented in Figure 20.1.

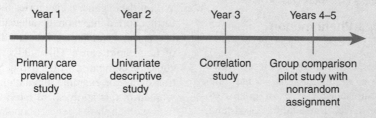

Figure 20.1 Jabil's 5-year research plan.

Univariate Descriptive Studies

Univariate investigations are typically used to:

- Characterize the sample or circumstances that make up any study,
- Characterize a problem or phenomenon,
- Document incidence and prevalence of health-related conditions,
- Establish norms,
- Document developmental phenomena, and
- Document case studies.

These univariate descriptions are ordinarily in the form of frequencies, central tendencies (e.g., mean), and dispersion (e.g., range or standard deviation). In the following sections, the nature and purposes of these types of descriptive research designs are discussed.

Defining a Study Sample and Characteristics

No matter how complex the design of a study, all investigations include components of basic descriptive design through which the participants and other relevant circumstances in the study are characterized. Basic descriptive data are always collected, analyzed, and reported in any research. This is true for qualitative research as well, where basic quantitative information is typically used along with qualitative information to characterize the study participants.

Essential to any study report is information about the subjects of a study on key demographic variables (e.g., age, sex, race or ethnicity, diagnosis, type of impairment). In addition to characterizing research participants, it is also important to characterize other conditions that make up a study. For example, in a study of intervention outcomes, the investigator would describe the types of services provided, the length of time over which the service was provided, the frequency of service provision, and how much service in total was provided.

Characterizing a Phenomenon or Problem

Descriptive studies in occupational therapy often serve the purpose of illuminating some phenomenon or circumstance that is of interest to the field. For instance, Bar-Shalita, Goldstand, Hahn-Markowitz, and Parush (2005) studied the response patterns of typical 3- and 4-year-old Israeli children to tactile and vestibular stimulation. This study was undertaken to generate basic knowledge about the response patterns of typically developing children to sensory stimuli. The investigators sought to describe sensory response patterns and to determine whether they changed from age 3 to age 4.

The study results indicated that these children were neither hypo- nor hyperresponsive to tactile and vestibular stimuli. By providing evidence that typically developing children do not swing between hyper- and hyporesponsivity, this study provided a framework for identifying children whose sensory responsiveness is atypical. The investigators also found no evidence of change in responsiveness from the 3- to 4-year-olds. This finding suggested that children's patterns of response to tactile and vestibular stimulation have stabilized by age 3. As this investigation illustrates, descriptive research that characterizes typical phenomena, such as sensory responsiveness, can be very useful in occupational therapy.

In addition, descriptive studies are often used in occupational therapy to characterize functional aspects of a disability. Such investigations are helpful in understanding what types of occupational challenges are faced by certain populations. When such studies describe ways that individuals with disabilities adapt, they are helpful as guidelines for practitioners.

For example, Liedberg, Hesselstrand, and Henriksson (2004) used a diary method to collect data on the time use and activity patterns of women with long-term pain (diagnosed with fibromyalgia). The women were asked to fill in a diary for 7 consecutive days and again 3 months later over 4 consecutive days. In the diary, they noted what they were doing during each time period, where they were, with whom they were doing the activity, whether they had physical problems, and their mood. The investigators then coded the diary entries in a number of ways. For example, they coded activities as belonging to one of seven spheres of activity (care of self, care of others, household care, recreation, travel, food procurement or preparation, and gainful employment). Within these general categories the activities were further sorted into more detailed activity categories (e.g., sweep, vacuum, scrub, and dust as categories of household care). This study yielded data that could be compared with existing Swedish population data. For example, the authors found that the women in this study spent more time in self-care than women in the general population.

Incidence and Prevalence Studies

Another important purpose of descriptive studies is to document the incidence and prevalence of health-related conditions. Studies that address this purpose are referred to as epidemiological studies. Although incidence and prevalence studies are usually conducted by public health and medical researchers, their results are widely used in occupational therapy. Additionally, OT researchers are increasingly contributing to and conducting incidence and prevalence studies that focus on functional aspects of impairment.

Prevalence is defined as a proportion of a total population of people who have a particular health-related condition (Polit & Hungler, 1999; Portney & Watkins, 2009). Prevalence (P) is calculated as:

$$P = \frac{\text{Number of observed cases of a condition at a given time point or during a given interval}}{\text{Total population at risk}}$$

When prevalence is examined at a specific time point, it is referred to as point prevalence. When it is calculated based on observed cases during a time period (e.g., over a year), it is referred to as period prevalence (Portney & Watkins, 2009). Prevalence is calculated without reference to the onset of the condition; thus, it aims to characterize what proportion of a population has a condition at a point or period of time without consideration of when the condition began.

Incidence is concerned with how many persons have onset of a condition during a given span of time. Incidence refers to the number of new cases of a disease or disability in a population during the specified time period. It can be calculated as either cumulative incidence or incidence rate (MacMahon & Trichopoulos, 1996).

Cumulative incidence (CI) is calculated as:

$$CI = \frac{\text{Number of observed new cases during a specified period}}{\text{Total population at risk}}$$

Incidence rate (IR) is calculated as:

$$IR = \frac{\text{Number of observed new cases during a specified period}}{\text{Total person-time}}$$

In the formula for IR, the denominator is calculated as person-periods. For example, if a condition was studied over a 10-year period and 100 persons were enrolled, the total possible person-years is 1,000 (100 persons observed over 10 years). However, if two persons died and were no longer in the sample after 5 years, they would contribute only 10 person-years (5 years × 2 persons) to the formula, reducing the denominator by 10 person-years. Unlike cumulative incidence, which assumes all subjects are at risk during the entire period studied, incidence rate characterizes the number of new cases as a proportion of persons who were actually at risk during each of the identified segments of the total period studied (e.g., for each year of a 10-year period).

Prevalence and incidence rates are important to providing both an understanding of the magnitude of a health-related condition (i.e., how common or prevalent it is) and risk (i.e., what are the chances of someone incurring a given health-related condition). For example, the Centers for Disease Control and Prevention (CDC) reported that at the end of 2012 there were an estimated 1.2 million people living with HIV in the United States (CDC, 2015b). Calculated as a proportion of the population, these existing cases would represent the prevalence of HIV in the United States. At that time, the CDC also estimated that approximately 50,000 new HIV infections occur annually in the United States (CDC, 2015a). When calculated as a proportion of the total U.S. population, these cases would represent the cumulative incidence of HIV infection. The prevalence of HIV infection provides researchers and health-care providers with an understanding of the magnitude of the problem of HIV infection in the United States because it provides information about both the absolute number of cases and the proportion of the total population affected by the condition. The incidence estimate provides an understanding of risk.

Incidence and prevalence are ordinarily calculated for subpopulations as well (e.g., different ages, males versus females) because the occurrence of new and existing cases of conditions is not evenly distributed across the population. For example, early studies of HIV in the United States indicated that men who have sex with men were at highest risk. Although individuals in this group are still at highest risk, over the past 30 years, the incidence of the disease has changed: HIV increasingly affects women, individuals from minority populations, individuals with histories of substance abuse, and young people ages 13 to 24 (AIDS. gov, 2014; Karon, Fleming, Steketee, & DeCock, 2001; Kates, Sorian, Crowley, & Summers, 2002; Orenstein, 2002). Findings on the incidence of new cases thus help identify which populations are at greatest risk.

Normative Research

Investigators undertake **normative research** to establish usual or average values for specific variables. This type of research is helpful for identifying and characterizing performance problems (i.e., knowing how extreme a person's deviation from a norm is) and doing treatment planning. As Portney and Watkins (2009) note, norms are often used as a basis for prescribing corrective intervention or predicting future performance. For example, research that led to the description of what is normal strength for different populations is used routinely in OT practice. These types of norms serve as a basis for evaluating the performance of a given individual by comparing that individual with what is typical for someone with the same characteristics (e.g., age and sex). Research that aims to establish norms must be particularly careful to avoid sampling bias. For this reason, normative studies use random samples and ordinarily rely on large sample sizes.

Developmental Research

Developmental research seeks to describe patterns of growth or change over time within selected segments of a population (Portney & Watkins, 2009). Such studies may describe patterns of change that characterize typical growth and development. Developmental research has been important in documenting the course of acquiring functional abilities in childhood (e.g., crawling, walking, talking, grasping) as well as the functional changes associated with aging.

Other developmental investigations seek to characterize the course of disease or disability over time (e.g., the course of functional recovery from a traumatic event or the course of functional decline in degenerative conditions).

Developmental research usually involves a **cohort design** in which a sample of participants is followed over time and repeated measures are taken at certain intervals to describe how the variable or variables under study have changed (Stein & Cutler, 2012). Sometimes developmental research is accomplished through a **cross-sectional design** in which the investigator collects data at one time point from a sample that is stratified into different groups, such as age groups (e.g., children who are 6, 12, 18, and 24 months of age or older adults who are 60 to 64, 65 to 69, 70 to 74, 75 to 79, etc.). Observed differences between the samples in each age strata are then attributed to the process of development or aging. Cohort studies have the advantage of eliminating effects of sample bias on observed changes, but they are subject to the influence of historical events that are unrelated to the course of development. Cross-sectional designs avoid the latter problem but are prone to cohort

effects (i.e., effects that are unrelated to age and are due to some circumstance unique to a particular age cohort). In both cases, random sampling is critical to generalize from the sample to the population the study is intended to characterize.

Descriptive Case Studies

Descriptive case studies are in-depth descriptions of the experiences or behaviors of a particular individual or a series of individuals. Case studies are most typically undertaken to describe some new phenomenon or to document a client's response to a new intervention. Although many case studies in occupational therapy are qualitative in nature, quantitative case studies can also be useful in characterizing how an individual has responded following a traumatic event and/or intervention. Typically, a series of numeric statistics is presented, describing different dimensions of a topic at issue. In some cases, the same sets of statistics are presented over time at evenly increasing time points to illustrate either stability or change over time, depending on the topic.

Descriptive case studies differ from single-subject designs in that there is no experimental manipulation of an independent variable. Rather, the investigator documents variables as they naturally occur or documents an intervention and what happens following it (but without the comparison to the absence of the intervention or to another intervention). Case studies are most valuable when the information reported is comprehensive. Thus, investigators undertaking a case study will either attempt to provide numeric data on several variables of interest or provide repeated measures of some variable over time.

Although such case studies are readily related to practice, they are one of the least rigorous forms of research because they lack control and generalizability (Portney & Watkins, 2009). For this reason, a series of, or several, case studies with numeric data will often be used as the basis from which to generalize concepts, which then lead to more controlled studies.

Case studies can be particularly useful for investigating new interventions or interventions that require substantial individualization or trial and error. For example, Gillen (2002) reported a case in which OT services based on concepts of motor control were used to improve mobility and community access in an adult with ataxia. The study reported baseline information from the Functional Index Measure (FIM™) and then reported OT techniques of "adapted positioning, orthotic prescription, adapted movement patterns, and assistive technology" that were used to address client-centered functional goals (Gillen, 2002, p. 465). The study reported positive changes in the client's FIM score following the intervention.

Correlational Research Designs

Correlational research aims to demonstrate relationships between variables under study (Portney & Watkins, 2009). Correlation refers to an interrelationship or association between two variables (i.e., the tendency for variation in one variable to be either directly or inversely related to variation in another variable). This type of research is sometimes referred to as exploratory, because it is frequently undertaken to identify whether specified variables are related or to determine which variables are related in a multivariable study. For example, the Model of Human Occupation (Kielhofner, 2008) argues that volition leads to choices about occupational participation. Based on this theoretical argument, it can be hypothesized that volitional traits should be associated with observed patterns of occupational participation. Correlational studies have been implemented to test this proposed relationship.

Neville-Jan (1994) examined the correlation between volition and patterns of occupation among 100 individuals with varying degrees of depression. Her study found, as hypothesized, a relationship between the adaptiveness of the subjects' routines and a measure of their personal causation, independent of the level of depression. Another example is a study by Peterson et al. (1999) that examined the relationship between personal causation (feelings of efficacy related to falling) and the pattern of occupational engagement in 270 older adults. They found, as expected, that lower personal causation (i.e., lower falls-self-efficacy) was related to reduced participation in leisure and social occupations. These two studies thus provided evidence in support of the proposition that volitional traits (in this case, personal causation) influence the choices persons make about engaging in occupations. However, these correlations are consistent with, but cannot be taken as proof of, causation.

Correlational studies such as these may provide evidence that is consistent or inconsistent with causal assertions. They can provide important evidence for developing theoretical propositions that assert causal relationships between variables. An important limitation of correlational studies with reference to making causal assertions is that, without experimental control, there is no way to rule out the possibility that two variables might be related by virtue of their association with a third, unobserved variable. Correlational studies can serve as helpful first steps in sorting out causal relationships (that is, if two variables are not correlated, then there is no reason to anticipate or test for a causal relationship between them). Many correlational studies serve as precursors to experimental studies that exert experimental control over independent and dependent variables to draw inferences about causation.

Although many correlational studies are concerned with relationships between pairs of variables, investigators are often interested to know the relationship among several variables that are hypothesized or presumed to have a causal relationship with a dependent variable. For example, many studies have examined factors that influence return to work following an injury. In this case, whether or not a person returns to work is the dependent variable of interest, and a study may examine the influence of a number of supposed causal or predictive variables (e.g., age, education, extent of impairment, personality, worker identity, and previous work history) on return to work. This type of study ordinarily uses regression analysis. The aim of such studies is to identify the amount of variance in the dependent variable that is explained by a set of predictor variables.

In correlational research, there may or may not be a temporal sequence between the hypothesized predictor variables and the dependent variable of interest. Sometimes correlational studies are retrospective, and the information on all variables is collected simultaneously. However, in prospective studies data on the predictor variables are collected first, and the dependent variable is observed at a later time or at several later time points. Obviously, when there is a temporal sequence, inferences about causal relationships have greater weight.

Group Comparison Studies

In this section, we begin with a discussion of experimental designs and proceed through other types of group comparison designs. A basic premise is that no design is best for all research questions; each has its advantages and disadvantages. **Experimental designs** test if–then statements and provide evidence about probable causality. Probable causality tests the probability that an intervention has an effect on an outcome or the probability that one intervention has a different effect on an outcome than another intervention. Pioneers such as psychologists Thorndike and Woodworth (1901); statistician R. A. Fisher (1935); and physicians Amberson, McMahon, and Pinner (1931) integrated concepts such as randomization and controls with probabilistic statistics, and the result is a rational and logical basis for if–then statements. When if–then statements are drawn from theory or from clinical observations and transformed into testable hypotheses, science advances. Embedded in this chapter are procedures to enhance validity as well as practical discussions about the assumptions that must be made in quantitative research.

Nonexperimental group comparison designs (sometimes called quasi-experimental designs or nonrandom designs) lack the degree of control achieved by experimental designs. In some cases, these kinds of designs can lay the groundwork for subsequent experimental investigations. In other cases, where the researcher needs to know about the differences between different kinds of people, true experimentation is impossible. The researcher must build other kinds of controls into these designs.

Basic Experiments

The **basic experimental design** is the most rigorous type of group comparison study. The elements of a basic experiment include the following:

1. There is one sample that is drawn representatively from one population.
2. There is one categorical independent variable.
3. Study participants are randomly assigned to as many groups as there are conditions to the independent variable.
4. The independent variable is administered as planned.
5. Potentially confounding variables are minimized, and otherwise uncontrollable events are equally likely across the groups.
6. There is one dependent variable on which all subjects are measured or categorized.
7. The experimental hypothesis tested is the probability of a causal effect of the independent variable on the dependent variable within the population.

In the following sections, each element of the basic experiment is examined in detail.

1. Using a Representative Sample

As discussed in earlier chapters, a population is any set of people (or in some cases, animals) who share common features. "Americans 70 years of age or older residing in extended care facilities (ECFs)" is a population. Similarly, "persons with Parkinson disease (stage II through IV)" and "6-year-old children with autism (but not mental retardation) attending special education classes" also make up populations.

A sample consists of the persons (participants or subjects) who are in the study. The sample is a subset of some population. A study sample could consist of 120 persons 70 years of age or older, who reside in ECFs in the United States. This subset of 120 persons is drawn from the entire population (hundreds of thousands of people) who are older than 70 years of age and reside in American ECFs. It is critical that the persons who make up the sample in an experiment are representative of the population from which they are drawn.

2. Using One Categorical Independent Variable

There are two kinds of variables: categorical and continuous. The conditions of a categorical variable are qualitatively different from each other, whereas the conditions of a continuous variable are quantitatively different from each other. Type of intervention is an example of a categorical variable. Neurodevelopmental therapy is one type of intervention, and biomechanically based therapy is a different kind of intervention. Each of these interventions could be a condition of a categorical variable; in this case, the categorical variable would have two qualitatively different conditions. Another example of a categorical variable could have three conditions: authoritarian group structure, laissez-faire group structure, and democratic group structure.

In contrast, continuous variables involve quantitative, ordered relationships. Measured height is a continuous variable. The score on a sensory integration test is also a continuous variable.

A categorical variable is an independent variable when the researcher examines its probable effects on an outcome (called a dependent variable). The independent variable is the possible cause, and the dependent variable is the possible effect. In an OT study designed to test whether an occupationally embedded exercise protocol produces a different outcome from a rote exercise protocol, one condition of the categorical independent variable might be stirring cookie batter, and another condition might be the same kind of stirring but with no batter. The dependent variable could be the number of times that the circular motion is completed.

3. Assigning Randomly to as Many Groups as There Are Conditions to the Independent Variable

Study participants are assigned by the researcher into groups, each of which receives one condition of the independent variable. For example, if there are 120 study participants and if there are two conditions of the independent variable, 60 persons could be assigned to one condition and 60 to the other condition. For an experiment with four conditions to the independent variable and with N (overall sample size) = 120, 30 persons could be assigned to each group.

As in the previous examples, a 1-to-1 ratio is usually used in assigning participants to groups, but not always. For example, a researcher might have a good reason for assigning more participants to one group than to another. Regardless of ratio, randomization is absolutely essential. In a 1-to-1 ratio, randomization means that every participant in the sample will have an equal chance of being in each of the groups. Randomization ensures that there is no bias that favors one group over the other. If randomization is done properly, then the rules of chance make it probable that the groups are equivalent to each other at the beginning of the experiment.

Each of the conditions of the independent variable might consist of alternative, previously untested interventions or stimuli (e.g., comparing a parallel group task to a project group task). A second option is to compare an intervention to a control condition (i.e., the absence of any research-induced intervention or stimulus). For example, the control group in a study of an occupation-based wellness program for middle-aged, overweight male professors could be given no special intervention as a way of finding out if the wellness program is effective.

A third option is to compare an intervention or stimulus to an attention-placebo condition. A placebo condition in drug studies involves administration of a nonactive substance (e.g., a pill) that looks, smells, and tastes the same as the active drug in the study. An attention-placebo condition involves administration of human contact that mimics the intervention under study, without involving the essence of what is under study. For example, in a study of neurodevelopmental therapy (NDT), the children in the attention-placebo condition receive the same amount of touching and time with an adult as the children receiving NDT. A technique to ensure equality of attention is yoking, whereby each person in the attention-placebo group receives the same amount of attention as a specific person in the intervention group. With reference to the previous NDT study example, this technique would mean that each child in the attention-placebo condition would receive the same amount of touching and time as a specific child in the NDT group. Fourth, a common type of comparison condition involves usual care or standard care, which is compared to some new type of intervention. For ethical reasons, subjects in any of these different types of comparison conditions often receive the intervention condition (if found effective) after the experiment is completed.

4. Administering the Independent Variable as Planned

A study is said to have **fidelity** if there is documentation that the independent variable is administered just as planned (Moncher & Prinz, 1991). Using the earlier example of a study of occupationally embedded exercise, a problem of fidelity occurs if the research assistant by mistake tells a participant in the rote exercise condition to "make cookies." Also, a subject in the image-based condition might become distracted, fail to think about stirring cookies, and just do the stirring as a rote exercise. Both of these situations exemplify *bleeding,* in which a participant assigned to one condition actually experiences some or all of the comparison condition.

In addition to bleeding, there are other problems of fidelity. Consider an experiment whereby each participant is supposed to attend four specially designed family education sessions (versus a usual-care condition), and some subjects arrive late and miss part of the sessions. Here the problem is that some of the subjects simply are not experiencing what they are supposed to be experiencing. A problem of delivery occurs, for instance, when the interventionist fails to spend the required time with the participant or forgets to administer all of the protocol (e.g., leaving out a component of one of the family education sessions). A problem of receipt is a failure of the participant to pay attention to the therapist's instructions (e.g., a subject is present at the educational session but is distracted because of a problem at work). A problem of enactment is a failure of participants to do something they are supposed to do (e.g., following the advice given in the educational session). Documentation of fidelity is especially important in studies that involve complex interventions administered over long periods of time and in studies involving the participant's generalization of learning from one context to application in another.

5. Minimizing Confounding Variables and Equalizing Uncontrollable Events

In an ideal experimental world, the independent variable is the only thing affecting the participants while they are in the experiment. But in the real world, there are many potentially **confounding variables** (things that could affect the participants in addition to the conditions of the independent variable). Potentially confounding variables are also sometimes called *confounds, extraneous variables, nuisance variables,* and *sources of error.* For example, in a study comparing occupationally embedded exercise to rote exercise in older nursing home residents, a nursing aide could interrupt the participant while stirring the cookie dough, or the older person could lose attentiveness because of poor sleep the night before. Therefore, good experimental design incorporates practical strategies for minimizing the chances of potentially confounding variables. For example, the researcher can explain the need for privacy to the staff; select a quiet, out-of-the-way room for the study; and put up a do-not-disturb sign.

Despite any researcher's best efforts, there are always events that cannot be controlled. This is especially true of intervention studies taking place over many months. For example, a study of the effects of a multisite, school-year-long, occupation-based fitness program for overweight children (versus an attention-placebo control condition) involves potentially confounding variables such as differing school-based practices, differing levels of family participation, family and community events (positive as well as negative), differing exposures to mass media, differing opportunities for sports participation, changes resulting from growing older, and illnesses that may occur. Experimental design cannot eliminate all these potentially confounding variables, and there are practical limitations even on monitoring them. The researcher's goal is that these potentially confounding variables are equally likely to occur in each of the comparison groups. In other words, the researcher tries to ensure that bias does not occur (where one of the conditions is systematically favored). Other terms used to refer to a biasing confounding variable are *artifact* and *sources of systematic error.*

To eliminate certain artifacts, researchers frequently use *masking* (also called *blinding*). In a *double-blind* study, neither the participants (one blind) nor the researcher (the other blind) is aware of which groups receive which condition of the independent variable. This is usually done through use of a placebo. However, total double-blinds are impossible in most OT studies because the participant is usually aware of what is happening, and the administrators of the independent variable (often occupational therapists) are professionally responsible for being aware of the service they are providing. In OT research, other types of blinding may sometimes be used:

- The person conducting the randomization can be masked from the subsequent randomization sequence;
- The person measuring the dependent variable (see following section) can be masked from knowing who has received which condition; and
- The statistician can be masked from knowing who has received which condition.

6. Measuring All Subjects on the Dependent Variable

The dependent variable is the criterion used to compare the conditions of the independent variable to each other. All participants are measured or categorized on the dependent variable. For example, for an independent variable involving a comparison between occupationally embedded exercise and rote exercise, the dependent variable might be the number of exercise repetitions (a continuous variable that can be measured). Alternatively, the dependent variable in a special skin protection program for individuals who use a wheelchair (compared to a usual-care condition) might be the presence or absence of skin breakdown (a categorical variable).

The method used to collect data on the dependent variable must be valid and reliable. Experimenters often try to improve reliability and validity through a variety of strategies:

- Measuring each participant several times so that the dependent variable is the mean;
- Providing training that exceeds the minimum specified in the measurement protocol;
- Using multiple, simultaneous raters or judges in measuring or judging the dependent variable; and
- Masking the measurers/judges.

In selecting a dependent variable for a study, the researcher has to be especially concerned about its responsiveness. **Responsiveness** (also called *sensitivity* in the nonmedical literature) is the degree to which a dependent variable shows appropriately small but meaningful increments of change over time. For example, a responsive measure might solicit a number on a continuous scale that can detect small achievements in bathing. In contrast, a nonresponsive measure might be a 3-point scale for measuring self-care: independent, partly dependent, and dependent. A research participant can make meaningful progress in taking care of herself, but her progress might not show up in the measure; if she starts out with the ability to do very little self-care and ends with the ability to take care of herself except for one or two things, her rating would not change because she is still partly dependent.

Another kind of nonresponsive measure is one that has ceiling or floor effects. A **ceiling effect** occurs where the sample's scores are already so high on the scale that little improvement is possible. A **floor effect** occurs when the opposite is the case. For example, adolescents with conduct disorders are unlikely to demonstrate a reduction in aggressive episodes in a 1-day study if the typical participant engages in only a few aggressive incidents per week.

Ideally, the experimenter–researcher uses a method of capturing the dependent variable that is recognized as the **criterion standard** (sometimes called the *gold standard*) in the field. Thus, in selecting a data collection procedure for the dependent variable, the investigator asks whether there is a consensus in the field concerning the best way to measure or categorize that variable. For example, 5-year survival rate is a criterion standard for interventions addressing certain types of cancers. However, OT researchers frequently address research questions that have not been studied adequately in the past. An excellent way to address this problem is for the designer of an experiment to ask experts in the field to confirm the validity of a dependent variable. At the same time, the investigator can ask the experts to identify how much of a difference between comparison groups at the end of the study is required to be meaningful. For example, the investigator might ask whether a 10% reduction in rehospitalization rates is a meaningful difference in a study of interventions for participants with chronic schizophrenia.

Knowing how much change investigators can expect to see in the dependent variable can be factored into a decision about the number of subjects needed in the study. There is a calculation called *power analysis* that allows researchers to make this determination.

7. Developing the Experimental Hypothesis

A **hypothesis** is a prediction about the relationship between variables within a population. The end result of an experiment can have only two possibilities: support for this hypothesis or a lack of support. The first thing about this definition to notice is the word *prediction*. It is a hallmark of quantitative research that all the variables under study and their possible relationships, one way or the other, are determined in advance.

Consider the following experimental hypothesis: Occupationally embedded exercise elicits more exercise repetitions than rote exercise in nursing home residents aged 65 years or more. Even though the present tense (*elicits,* not *will elicit*) is used, a prediction is implied because the hypothesis is stated before the research starts. The independent variable has two conditions: occupationally embedded exercise versus a control condition. The dependent variable consists of exercise repetitions. And the sample is drawn from the population of nursing home residents 65 years of age or older. The type of relationship between the variables under study is the hypothesized effect of the independent variable on the dependent variable. Probable causality is involved: The independent variable is the hypothesized cause, and the dependent variable is the hypothesized effect. Quantitative research deals with probability, not with certainty or truth.

The logic of the basic experiment is as follows: If groups assigned to conditions of the independent variable are probably equal at the start of the experiment (the chance processes of randomization ensure probable equivalence), if groups are treated the same except for the independent variable, and if there are differences between groups at the end of the experiment, then the differences were probably caused by the independent variable acting on the dependent variable. This is the basis for experimental design's claim to study probable causality.

The following is another experimental hypothesis: In nursing home residents 65 years of age or older, there are differences among occupationally embedded exercise, imagery-based exercise, and rote exercise in terms of exercise repetitions. Here, the independent variable has three conditions that are compared with each other. This is also an example of a nondirectional hypothesis. A nondirectional hypothesis does not predict which condition will end up with the superior outcome; it simply predicts that one of the conditions will be superior. Still implied is probable causality. In contrast, a directional hypothesis is clear as to which group is predicted to have higher scores (or higher proportions in the case of categorical variables). Figures 20.2 to 20.4 illustrate three basic experimental designs.

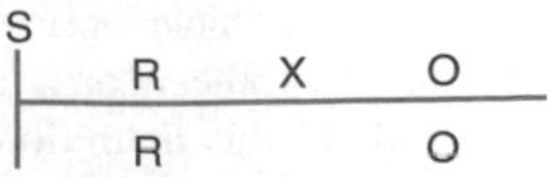

S = Start
R = Randomization
X = Condition of independent variable
O = Observation (measurement or categorization used
    for dependent variable)

Figure 20.2 Basic experimental design, with true control group, one intervention, and no pretest. After the sample is randomized (R) into two groups, one group receives an intervention (X), whereas the control group does not. Both groups are measured or categorized (O) in the same way. *The symbolic format for these figures is adapted from Campbell and Stanley (1963).

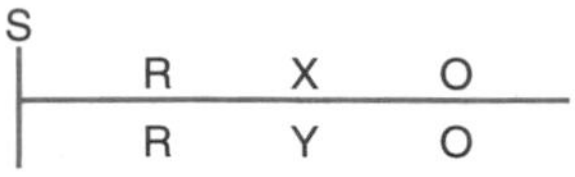

S = Start
R = Randomization
X = Condition of independent variable
Y = A different intervention, usual care, or attention-
    placebo
O = Observation (measurement or categorization used
    for dependent variable)

Figure 20.3 Basic experimental design comparing two conditions of the independent variable, with no pretest. After the sample is randomized (R) into two groups, one group receives an intervention (X), whereas the other group receives (a) a different intervention, (b) usual care, or (c) an attention-placebo (Y). Both groups are measured or categorized (O) in the same way.

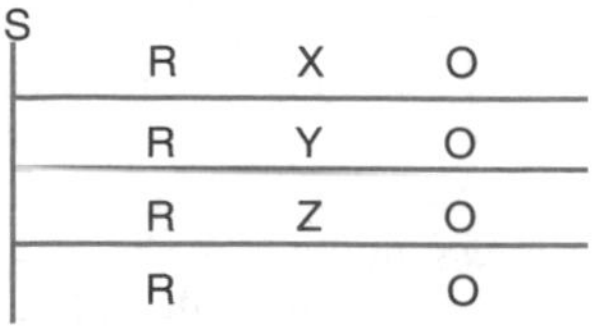

Threats to Methodological Rigor in a Study

The rigor of group comparison designs may be measured through an assessment of internal validity and external validity and through an assessment of the risk for type I and type II errors.

Internal Validity

One of the most important points to keep in mind when designing a quantitative research study is that just because one is able to quantify an association (or nonzero correlation) between two variables (i.e., that X *is associated with* Y), it does not mean that one can confidently conclude that an independent variable caused the dependent variable to change (i.e., that X *caused* Y). The extent

S = Start
R = Randomization
X = An intervention
Y = A different intervention or usual care
Z = A different intervention, usual care, or attention-
    placebo
O = Observation (measurement or categorization used
    for dependent variable)

Figure 20.4 Basic experimental design (posttest only), comparing three conditions of the independent variable to each other and to a control group. After the sample is randomized (R) into four groups, three groups receive X, Y, and Z, respectively, whereas the fourth receives nothing. All groups are measured or categorized (O) in the same way.

of causality is estimated by a statistic that reflects the probability of cause, rather than cause itself. **Internal validity** refers to the extent to which one variable is directly implicated in an outcome, or change, in a second variable and is free from the influence of extraneous (confounding) variables. For example, if one wants to study the effects of a persuasive smartphone app on increasing hydration and decreasing overexertion in high-risk adolescents with the sickle-cell trait, then one must do one's best to either control for or measure the coexistence of all of the other potential variables that might influence hydration and exertion in the adolescent sample. For example, hydration might be influenced by the teen's access to fluids, preference and availability of fluids that have taste appeal, and time to actually drink the fluids. Similarly, exertion levels might be influenced by the teen's access to transportation, general fitness level, the actual altitude of the location where the teen is engaging in activity, and other factors. The extent to which one can control for or reduce these other explanations for a teen's hydration and activity levels through rigor in the research design determines the extent of internal validity of the study.

Type I Error. **Type I error** involves reporting a relationship when there really is no relationship. A reader of a research report can never be absolutely certain that a type I error has been made. However, the reader may reason that weaknesses in the research design make the chances of a type I error unacceptably large.

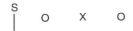

S = Start
X = An intervention
O = Observation (measurement or categorization used for dependent variable)

Figure 20.5 Pretest–posttest design with no control or comparison group. After a pretest, an intervention is given, to be followed by a posttest. It is important to note that this design is not recommended except for pilot testing in advance of future research.

To understand this point, consider the following nonexperimental research design that is highly prone to type I error: the pretest–posttest no-control group design (Fig. 20.5). In this design, a single group of participants receives a test, an intervention, and another test after the intervention. Consider the statement: Manipulation of the spine decreases pain in adult males with acute lumbar pain secondary to lifting-related injuries. The researcher following this design simply:

- Selects persons with acute lumbar pain secondary to lifting-related injuries,
- Measures the level of pain (a pretest),
- Administers a series of manipulation interventions,
- Measures the level of pain once again (a posttest), and
- Compares the pretest to the posttest.

If pain decreases significantly from the pretest to the posttest, the researcher concludes that the spinal manipulation is effective. The problem with the researcher's logic is that the design does not protect against type I error: It is quite likely (no one knows exactly how likely) that the manipulation has nothing to do with the improvement in pain levels. The following potentially confounding variables unrelated to manipulation may have caused the improvement:

- Acutely ill persons might recover without any intervention through natural healing.
- The research participants might have received other interventions between the pretest and the posttest.
- There might have been something about being tested twice on the pain scale that resulted in lower scores the second time around.

There are many possible explanations for the observed change, and so the bottom line is that we do not know anything more than we knew before

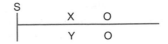

S = Start
X = An intervention
Y = A different intervention, usual care, or attention-placebo
O = Observation (measurement or categorization used for dependent variable)

Figure 20.6 Nonrandomized comparison group design (no pretest). The subjects in one naturally occurring group receive one intervention (X), and the subjects in a different naturally occurring group receive a different intervention. A measurement or categorization is then done (O). It is important to note that this design is not recommended except for pilot testing in advance of future research.

the research study. Possible sources of type I error are not controlled in this study design.

Another nonexperimental research design often highly at risk for a type I error is the nonrandomized control group design (Fig. 20.6). Consider the following hypothesis: Splinting technique A is superior to splinting technique B in improving wrist range of motion for persons with carpal tunnel syndrome. Instead of randomly assigning participants to groups, the researcher assigns one naturally occurring group (e.g., patients at one hand clinic) to receive technique A and assigns another naturally occurring group (e.g., patients in a different hand clinic) to receive technique B. At the end of 2 weeks of being splinted, the patients in the first clinic who received technique A actually have greater wrist range of motion than the patients in the other clinic who received technique B. Consequently, the researcher reports the superiority of splinting technique A.

However, the chances of a type I error are unacceptably high. The problem is that the patients at the first clinic might have been different from, or nonequivalent to, the patients in the second clinic (even before splinting, they might have been less severely disabled). Also, they might have had special opportunities for progress based on the quality of the clinic's staff or on demographic factors, or they might have had less risk for reinjury. Even if the researcher uses a pretest–posttest nonrandomized control group design and finds that the two groups do not differ on the baseline, there is still a high chance of a type I error. Patients at the first clinic might have a greater potential for change than the patients at the second clinic. For example, it is possible that the range-of-motion scores are equal at pretest even though the patients at the first clinic have relatively recent, acute injuries, whereas the patients at the second clinic have chronic injuries unlikely to change in a short period of time.

The basic experiment was invented to reduce the chances of a type I error to some small, controllable amount. Randomization ensures that the comparison groups are probably equivalent at the outset of the study. A comparison condition balances potentially confounding variables (thereby preventing systematic bias). For example, both groups in a basic experiment are equally likely to be exposed to the same processes of healing, maturation, extraneous interventions, repeated testing, and other factors. The basic experiment was developed within the tradition of scientific skepticism: the biggest danger to scientific development is to report a relationship when one does not exist.

Type II Error. **Type II error** is the failure to find and report a relationship when the relationship actually exists. As with type I errors, the reader of a research report can never be certain that a type II error has occurred. But certain research designs and situations are prone to increasing the risks of type II error to unacceptable levels. Recommendations by Ottenbacher (1995) and Ottenbacher and Maas (1998) for identifying risks of type II error and for how to avoid type II error are particularly recommended for those who wish to understand more about this issue.

Sources of type II error include:

- A small sample size.
- A subtle (yet real) independent variable.
- Much dispersion on the dependent variable within groups.
  - Dispersion due to individual differences among subjects.
  - Dispersion due to measurement error.
- A stringent or nonrobust statistical test of the hypothesis.

Although the basic experiment provides the best protection against type I error, it sometimes provides poor protection against type II error. Consider a study with the following hypothesis: An OT program will increase the organizational skills of clients with traumatic brain injury (versus an attention-control condition). The OT program takes place once a week for 4 weeks, and the measurement of organizational ability involves a nonstandardized rating system whereby a therapist makes judgments concerning the client's organizational ability while shopping from a list in the supermarket. The researcher has ensured a lack of bias by selecting 20 clients for the study, randomizing

them to groups, making sure of high fidelity within groups and no bleeding between groups, ensuring that the measurer remains masked (i.e., unaware of the intervention condition of the participants), and following the plan for statistical analysis.

Following the logic discussed earlier, this design allows little chance of a type I error because neither group is favored by biasing variables. However, the chances of a type II error are so great that it is very unlikely that a difference will be found between groups even if the type of intervention under study is actually effective. This is because:

- The number of subjects in each group is small.
- The intervention is not intensive enough to produce a large effect.
- The quality of the measure of the dependent variable is unknown and may not be reliable or sensitive.

To decrease the chances of a type II error, the researcher can:

- Increase the sample size by extending the study over time or by finding additional sites for the research.
- Increase the effect of the independent variable by providing therapy more often per week and over a longer period of time.
- Decrease dispersion due to measurement error by using a test of organizational ability that has been demonstrated to be accurate (reliable) yet sensitive to change (responsive) in past studies.

In fact, all three strategies are warranted in this case to avoid type II error.

There are several strategies to decrease dispersion on the dependent variable that is due to individual differences. The most straightforward way to decrease dispersion is to select participants who are homogeneous (similar to each other, as opposed to heterogeneous). In our example of persons with brain injury, the researcher could decide in advance that research participants are included only if at a similar stage of recovery.

Another way to decrease dispersion is to use a pretest–posttest experimental design, as opposed to a posttest-only experimental design. Figures 20.7 and 20.8 illustrate two such designs. To use the same example again, a pretest of organization ability administered before the independent variable would permit statistical procedures that control for individual differences in the final analysis. The dependent variable is adjusted, correcting for the individual differences. This is done in an unbiased way, so that neither group being compared to each other receives a special advantage.

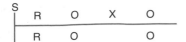

S = Start
R = Randomization
X = Condition of independent variable
O = Observation (measurement or categorization used for dependent variable)

Figure 20.7 Basic experimental design (pretest–posttest), with true control group and one intervention. After the sample is randomized (R) into two groups, both groups are pretested (O to left) in the same way. Next, one group receives an intervention (X), whereas the control group does not. Finally, both groups are posttested (O to right).

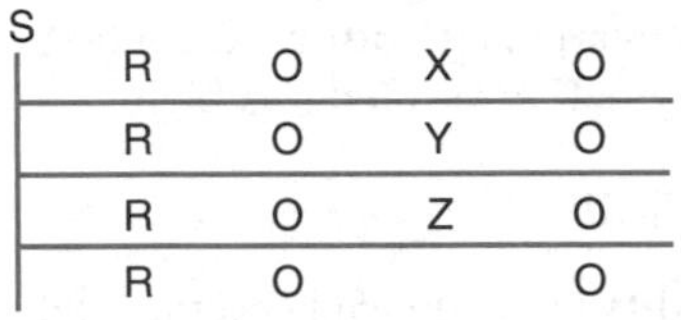

S
	R	O	X	O
	R	O	Y	O
	R	O	Z	O
	R	O		O

S = Start
R = Randomization
X = An intervention
Y = A different intervention, usual care, or attention-placebo
Z = A different intervention, usual care, or attention-placebo
O = Observation (measurement or categorization used for dependent variable)

Figure 20.8 Basic experimental design (pretest–posttest) comparing three conditions of the independent variable to each other and to a control group. After the sample is randomized (R) into four groups, groups are pretested (O to left) in the same way. Next, three groups receive X, Y, and Z, respectively, whereas the fourth receives nothing. Finally, all groups are measured or categorized (O to right) in the same way.

Several different statistical procedures are capable of making this adjustment.

Sometimes it is impossible to do a pretest. For example, in a study of occupationally embedded exercise, it is impossible to do a pretest of repetitions because the repetitions can be counted only in the simultaneous context of the independent variable (e.g., while actually stirring). In this case, some other variable can be measured in advance that is probably associated with the dependent variable. This kind of variable is called a *covariate*. For example, in a study in which the dependent variable involves stirring repetitions, a likely covariate is grip strength. Individual differences

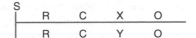

S = Start
R = Randomization
C = Covariate(s) reflecting variable(s) associated with the dependent variable
X = Condition of independent variable
Y = A different intervention, usual care, or attention-placebo
O = Observation (measurement or categorization used for dependent variable)

Figure 20.9 Experimental design comparing two conditions of the independent variable, with planned covariate(s). After the sample is randomized (R) into two groups, the covariate (C) is measured. Next, each group receives intervention X or Y. Both groups are measured or categorized (O) in the same way.

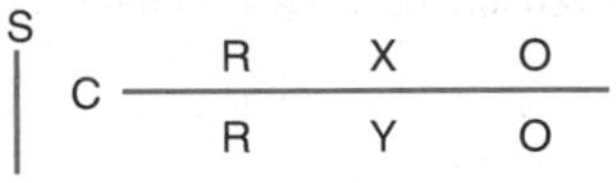

S
	C	R	X	O
		R	Y	O

S = Start
R = Randomization
C = Covariate reflecting variable associated with the dependent variable
X = An intervention
Y = A different intervention, usual care, or attention-placebo
O = Observation (measurement or categorization used for dependent variable)

Figure 20.10 Experimental design comparing two conditions of the independent variable, with a planned covariate available prior to randomization. After the sample is randomized (R), each group receives X or Y. Both groups are measured or categorized (O) in the same way.

reflecting grip strength can be controlled through analysis of covariance. The point here is that a covariate, properly chosen in advance of the study, can reduce individual differences and thereby reduce dispersion on the dependent variable. The result is less of a chance of a type II error, making it possible to demonstrate that the independent variable probably makes a real difference. Figures 20.9 and 20.10 illustrate two such designs.

Yet another strategy to decrease individual differences is to use a randomized matched-subjects design (Fig. 20.11); it is called a randomized matched pairs design when there are two conditions of the independent variable. This design is also referred to as a type of randomized block design. In this instance, participants are matched to each other in advance on some relevant variable, and then they are randomly assigned to groups (each of which receives a different condition of the independent variable). Consider the following hypothesis: Community-dwelling persons with dementia who receive added home-based occupational therapy are less likely to enter extended care facilities than community-dwelling persons with dementia receiving usual care. Participants can be paired to each other in terms of level of dementia and then randomly assigned to either the OT

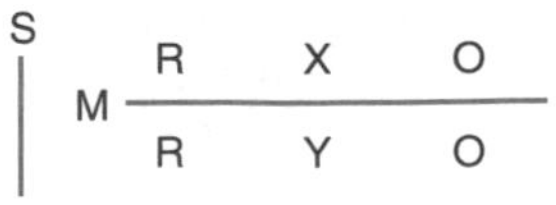

$$
\begin{array}{c}
S \\
| \quad\quad R \quad X \quad O \\
M \,\rule{2cm}{0.4pt} \\
| \quad\quad R \quad Y \quad O
\end{array}
$$

S = Start
M = Matching
R = Randomization
X = Condition of independent variable
Y = A different intervention, usual care, or attention-placebo
O = Observation (measurement or categorization used for dependent variable)

Figure 20.11 Matched-subjects (matched-pairs) experimental design comparing two conditions of the independent variable. First, subjects are paired based on some relevant similarity. Randomization (R) is done in blocks of two (randomized block design). Next, one group receives X or Y. Both groups are measured or categorized (O) in the same way.

condition or to usual care. The statistical analysis for this design involves comparisons of persons who are similar to each other, thereby reducing unsystematic error due to individual differences.

In summary of our discussion of type I and type II errors, the basic experiment is a great means of preventing type I error. But special adjustments must often be made to prevent type II error. Table 20.1 describes a way of depicting how likely a type II error is in OT research in comparison to research in some other fields. But we are not alone. Researchers in psychotherapy, special education, and many branches of medicine must overcome the same disadvantages. Statistical texts discuss the importance of reporting the effect size of a comparison, not just the P value. What is important to note here is that an experiment reporting a substantial but statistically nonsignificant difference must be interpreted with great caution: The chances of a type II error might be high.

External Validity

External validity has to do with generalizability—whether the results of a research project can be applied to the nonresearch environment (the real world). Unfortunately, it is possible that an experiment can avoid making type I and type II errors (i.e., it could have internal validity) and yet have no external validity. For example, a laboratory study of how people interact under experimental conditions might have excellent internal validity

Table 20.1 Inherent Dangers of Type II Error in Occupational Therapy Research

Common Causes of Type II Error	Laboratory Animal Studies	Occupational Therapy Studies
Small sample size	Animals are readily available at reasonable cost.	Persons with disabilities are small minorities of the population, often with major health and financial problems.
Dispersion due to individual differences	Healthy animals are highly homogeneous (often genetically matched).	Persons with disabilities vary from each other more than the general population; all persons respond somewhat differently to occupational forms.
Dispersion due to measurement error	Measurement systems in most animal research are highly precise.	Most measurement systems in occupational therapy generate high levels of error.
Dispersion due to random events	Highly controlled environments are typical.	People's lives are full of chance events that cannot be eliminated in multisession studies.
Robustness of the independent variable	Biological interventions are often powerful; subtle effects can be investigated after robust effects are demonstrated.	A single short-term occupation usually has few long-term effects; ethical considerations preclude risky interventions.
Powerful statistical procedures	Biostatisticians are familiar with techniques to reduce unsystematic error.	Much occupational therapy research in the past has not employed sophisticated procedures to reduce unsystematic error.

but might not reflect how people interact when not under close examination.

External validity can be threatened by two main factors: artificiality in the experimental environment (things are so different that subjects behave differently from how they do in everyday life) and unrepresentative samples (a mismatch exists between the intended population and the actual sample that is studied).

Artificialty. Artificiality can apply to the independent variable or the dependent variable. Laboratory coats, unusual settings, excessively complex informed consent procedures, and unusual equipment can threaten external validity. For example, in studies of perception, participants asked to discriminate among carefully projected images might make discriminations that they cannot make in the blooming and buzzing confusion of everyday life, where they focus on individually meaningful things. An example of artificiality in measuring the dependent variable can be seen in an electro-goniometer strapped onto the participant's arm to measure elbow flexion. The participant might reach differently when wearing this bulky contraption (e.g., he or she might lean forward more than usual, thereby decreasing elbow flexion artificially).

To decrease artificiality, the researcher can strive to design the independent variable so that it takes place (as much as possible) under everyday conditions. Instead of studying perception in a controlled laboratory, it can be studied in the participant's home. The problem in this instance is that naturalistic settings involve potentially confounding variables (the ring of the telephone or the voices of others in the home) that threaten to cause type II errors. For this reason, careful investigators may gather preliminary evidence under controlled laboratory conditions, then later in subsequent experiments show that the effect also can be demonstrated in the everyday world. As for artificiality of the dependent variable, unobtrusive measurements can sometimes be used. For example, there are motion-detection systems that do not involve strapping objects to participants' arms.

Unrepresentative Samples. Unrepresentativeness of the sample can be addressed in two ways: subject selection procedures and dealing with study dropouts. The basic idea of this strategy is to ensure that the participants in the study do not represent some special subpopulation that responds differently to the independent variable from the population that is supposedly under study. Examples of unrepresentative samples are studies of U.S. nursing home residents where the sample is 80% male and studies of children with autism

where the sample is 80% female. A proper experimental write-up details the relevant demographic characteristics of the sample so that the reader can decide to whom the study can be generalized. There is nothing wrong with a study of male nursing home residents as long as the researcher does not say that the results can be generalized to all nursing home residents.

Dropouts are particularly likely in long-term experiments; participants might lose interest over time, become ill in ways that are not relevant to the experiment, or move away. The danger to external validity is that the participants who drop out might be different from the participants who remain in the study (e.g., dropping out might be a way of avoiding unpleasant side effects of the intervention under study, or dropping out might reflect special frailty). Strategies to prevent dropouts include careful explanation of the study in advance, frequent positive communications over the course of the study, and due consideration for the inconveniences participants experience (e.g., lost time, transportation, etc.). The experimental plan should include procedures for recording and reporting any dropouts; ideally, dropouts can be compared to nondropouts to see if differences exist.

Variations on Randomized Designs

We have already discussed three variations on basic posttest-only experimental design:

- Pretest–posttest experimental design,
- Use of a covariate to adjust for individual differences, and
- Randomized matched subjects design.

There are other variations that can be helpful, given particular research problems, which are discussed in the following sections.

Interim Repeated Measures, Post-Posttests, and Long-Term Follow-Up Tests

Sometimes it is desirable to measure the outcome repeatedly over the course of an experiment. This is referred to as a **repeated-measures design.** For example, in a study in which sensory integrative therapy is administered to children with learning disabilities over a full year (compared to a true control group), the researcher might measure school achievement each quarter. In this way, the researcher can gain insight as to quarter-by-quarter rates of change. It is possible that there might be little difference between groups at the end of the

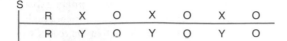

S

	R	X	O	X	O	X	O
	R	Y	O	Y	O	Y	O

S = Start
R = Randomization
X = An intervention
Y = A different intervention, usual care, or attention-
placebo
O = Observation (measurement or categorization used
for dependent variable)

Figure 20.12 Experimental design (no pretest) comparing two conditions of the independent variable with repeated observations (repeated measures). After the sample is randomized (R) into two groups, each group receives X or Y. Both groups are observed (O) in the same way. Observations (O) occurring before the designated primary endpoint are called interim measures. Observations (O) occurring after the primary endpoint are called post-posttests.

first quarter, but there is a large difference at the end of the second quarter. This provides important information concerning the duration required for this intervention to have an effect. The researcher using repeated measures should be clear in advance as to the primary (most important) endpoint, the measurement that will be used to test the main hypothesis of the study. For example, in the study of sensory integration, the primary endpoint might be the final quarter's measurement of school performance at the end of the school year. In this case, the earlier quarter-by-quarter measures are interim measures. However, if the researcher designates the second-quarter measurement of school performance as the primary endpoint, then the third- and fourth-quarter measurements are called post-posttests. Figure 20.12 illustrates a repeated-measures design.

Sometimes the organizations responsible for the protection of human subjects require interim measurements. For example, in a study of a daily-walking intervention to reduce falls in community-dwelling older persons (versus an attention-control condition), the institutional review board wants to rule out the possibility that the daily walking might actually increase the rate of falling. There are unique statistical procedures for analyzing the dependent variable when there are repeated measures. The more statistical tests that are done, the more likely it is that some of those tests appear to be statistically significant by chance alone.

The difference between post-posttests and long-term follow-up tests is that a long-term follow-up test occurs after a period of no intervention. To

S

	R	O	X	O	O	O
	R	O	Y	O	O	O
	R	O	Z	O	O	O

S = Start
R = Randomization
X = Condition of independent variable
Y = A different intervention, usual care, or attention-
placebo
Z = A different intervention, usual care, or attention-
placebo
O = Observation (measurement or categorization used
for dependent variable)

Figure 20.13 Experimental design (pretest–posttest) comparing three conditions of the independent variable with repeated observations (repeated measures) and two long-term follow-ups. After the sample is randomized (R) into three groups, each group is pretested. Next, each group receives X, Y, or Z. Groups are observed (O) in the same way immediately after the intervention and at two additional points in time.

take the example of the year-long program of sensory integration, a long-term follow-up test can take place a year after the conclusion of intervention and the posttest. The long-term follow-up test sheds light as to whether the effects of the intervention are still detectable a year after the withdrawal of the intervention. Figure 20.13 illustrates an experimental design with long-term follow-ups.

Multiple Dependent Variables Tested in Reference to the Same Independent Variable

Researchers frequently want to know whether an intervention affects several dependent variables. For example, in a study of the effects of added levels of occupational therapy in comparison to usual care in subacute rehabilitation patients, the researcher might want to know if the added sessions affect three separate outcomes: objectively measured self-care, discharge outcome, and patients' self-reports of goal achievement. There is a statistically testable hypothesis for each of the dependent variables, and there is also a way to do a single test of the effectiveness of the intervention across all three dependent variables (multivariate analysis of variance). Figure 20.14 illustrates an experimental design with three dependent variables.

The advantage of having multiple dependent variables is obvious. It is great to know about all three outcomes without having to do three studies.

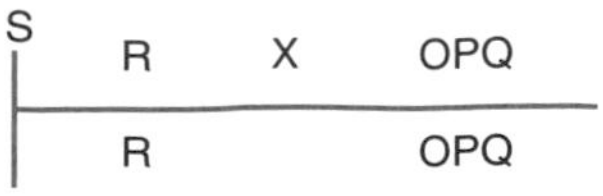

S = Start
R = Randomization
X = An intervention
O = Observation (a dependent variable)
P = Observation (another dependent variable)
Q = Observation (yet another dependent variable)

Figure 20.14 Experimental design (posttest only), with three dependent variables (O, P, Q) and a true control group. After the sample is randomized (R) into two groups, one group receives an intervention (X), whereas the control group does not. Both groups are measured or categorized (O, P, Q) in the same way.

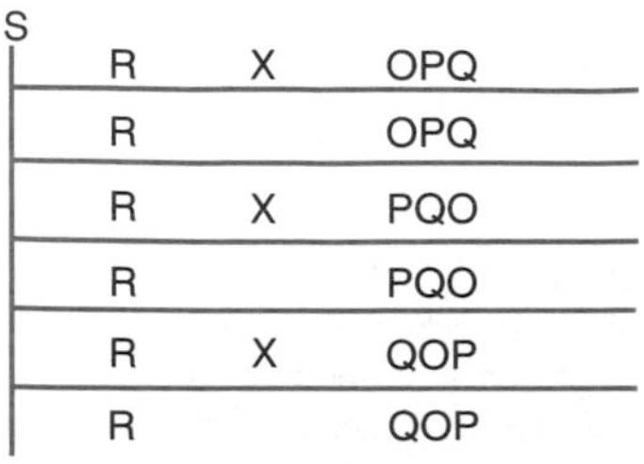

S = Start
R = Randomization
X = An intervention
O = Observation (a dependent variable)
P = Observation (another dependent variable)
Q = Observation (yet another dependent variable)

Figure 20.15 Experimental design (posttest only), with true control group and three dependent variables (O, P, Q) that are counterbalanced according to a Latin square. After the sample is randomized (R) into six groups, three groups receive an intervention (X), whereas three groups serve as controls. All groups are measured or categorized on O, P, and Q, but in different sequences, so that two groups receive O first, two receive P first, and two receive Q first. The alternative is to assign subjects to all possible sequences of the three measurements (which would result in 12 groups).

A possible problem, however, is that measurement of the first dependent variable has an effect on the second dependent variable. A person could have fatigue after the first measurement, or the first measurement might sensitize the person to the second measurement (a measurement of vestibular ability might artificially inflate a subsequent measure of alertness). A design strategy to deal with this problem is **counterbalancing of the dependent variables** (Fig. 20.15), where the different variables are experienced in different sequences, so each dependent variable sometimes occurs early in the testing protocol and sometimes late. Note that this counterbalancing of the dependent variables should not be confused with counterbalancing of the independent variables, to be discussed later in the section on crossover designs.

Another problem encountered by having several outcomes is **multiplicity:** the increase in type I error due to multiple statistical tests on the same participants. The more tests that are done, by chance alone it is likely that some of those tests will appear to be statistically significant. Unless special care is taken, the chances of a type I error increase for multiple statistical tests, especially if these tests are done on the same participants. For instance, a study might have 20 dependent variables if the researcher wishes to look at each aspect of self-care (tooth-brushing, hair-combing, buttoning, etc.) individually. If each of these 20 variables is tested independently, the chances are that at least 1 of the 20 tests will be found significant even if the independent variable had no effect at all (a type I error). Therefore, investigators use special corrective procedures. It is also good practice that a researcher interested in multiple outcomes must clearly identify and justify a primary dependent

variable and discriminate in statistical procedures between analysis of the primary dependent variable and secondary dependent variables.

Mechanisms of Change. **Mechanisms of change** is a special type of argument in favor of multiple dependent variables. This occurs when the researcher theorizes that the intervention under study works in a chain-reaction style, in which first one aspect of the person is affected, which in turn influences some other aspect (Gitlin et al., 2000). For example, consider a comparison between a client-centered approach to occupational therapy and an impairment-reduction approach, in which the primary dependent variable is functional outcome. The researcher may theorize that the reason the former approach is superior is that it increases the patient's sense of volition. Therefore, the researcher not only measures functional outcome but also measures volition. Depending on the researcher's theory, volition might be measured at the midpoint of the study, at the end of the study when functional outcome is measured, or at multiple points. The measurement of hypothesized mechanisms of change strengthens the interpretation of the results and contributes to theory confirmation. Figure 20.16 illustrates such a design.

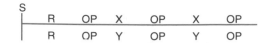

S = Start
R = Randomization
X = Condition of independent variable
O = Observation (primary dependent variable)
P = Observation (measurement indicating theory-
    based mechanism of change)

Figure 20.16 Experimental design comparing two
interventions, with pretest and interim repeated
measure on primary dependent variable (O) as
well as on a measure indicating a theory-based
mechanism of change (P).

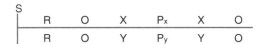

S = Start
R = Randomization
X = An intervention
Y = A different intervention
O = Observation (primary dependent variable)
P_x = Measure of fidelity of intervention X
P_y = Measure of fidelity of intervention Y

Figure 20.17 Experimental design (pretest–
posttest) comparing two interventions, with an
interim measure of the degree to which the
conditions of the independent variable were
administered as called for by the research
protocol (P_x and P_y).

Tests of Fidelity. A desirable feature of the research design is to conduct quantitative tests for
intervention **fidelity.** Fidelity defines the degree to
which an intervention is loyal to itself in terms of
the intended content and process of the intervention. Figure 20.17 illustrates this type of design. In
the comparison between the client-centered and
impairment-reduction approaches to therapy discussed previously, the researcher could document
that the therapists administering the two types of
intervention actually follow the intended protocol,
with no bleeding from condition to condition and
with adherence to "doses" (i.e., amount of intervention) called for in the protocol. Another example is to compare statistically the amount of
time spent with subjects in an attention-control
group to the amount of time spent with intervention subjects. The researcher in this instance generates a methodological hypothesis (a test of the
validity of the research procedures).

Completely Randomized Factorial Designs

Completely randomized factorial designs have
more than one independent variable; otherwise,
they resemble basic experiments. For example,
a researcher may want to test the effects of a
home safety program on falls prevention in older
community-dwelling persons, while also testing
the effects of a lower extremity strengthening
program on falls prevention in the same population. In a completely randomized factorial design,
the researcher randomly assigns participants to one
of four groups:

- A group that receives the lower extremity
  strengthening program only.
- A group that receives the home safety program
  only.
- A group that receives both interventions.
- A group that receives attention-control only.

In a factorial design, both interventions can be
tested, and a special bonus is that the interaction
of the two interventions can be studied. An interaction occurs when the effects of one intervention
depend on (i.e., augment or decrease) the effects
of the other intervention. For example, one kind
of interaction is that the home safety program
is effective only when combined with the lower
extremity strengthening program, such that the two
interventions together are more effective than the
lower extremity strengthening program alone.

When two independent variables each have two
conditions (as in our falls prevention example), we
call it a 2×2 factorial design. If one of the independent variables has three conditions (e.g., lower
extremity weight training versus tai chi training
versus attention-placebo) and the other has two
conditions, then we call it a 2×3 factorial design
(Fig. 20.18). In this case, subjects are randomly
assigned to six groups. If there are three independent variables (let us say that we are adding
a vision-training program to the 2×3 design),
then we call it a $2 \times 2 \times 3$ factorial design. Here
participants are randomly assigned to 12 groups.
Some interesting interactions can be studied in
such an instance. Still another factorial design
($2 \times 2 \times 2$) is shown in Figure 20.19. Another
advantage of factorial designs is that statistical analysis (through analysis of variance) often
reduces error, thus tending to prevent type II error.
The main problems with factorial design are that
many more subjects are needed to fill up all those
groups, and there are many more things that can
go wrong in a complex factorial design than in a
relatively straightforward basic experiment.

S				
	R	O	XY$_1$	O
	R	O	XY$_2$	O
	R	O	X	O
	R	O	Y$_1$	O
	R	O	Y$_2$	O
	R	O		O

S = Start
R = Randomization
X = An intervention (one of two conditions of an independent variable—the other condition is control)
Y$_1$ = An intervention of type Y (one of three conditions of an independent variable—the other conditions are Y$_2$ and control)
Y$_2$ = An intervention of type Y (one of three conditions of an independent variable—the other conditions are Y$_1$ and control)
O = Observation (a dependent variable)

Figure 20.18 Completely randomized 2×3 factorial design (pretest–posttest), with true control condition. After randomization (R) and the pretest (O), one group receives a combination of two interventions (X and Y$_1$), the next group receives a combination of X and Y$_2$, three groups receive a single intervention (respectively, X, Y$_1$, or Y$_2$), and one group serves as a true control. The posttest follows.

Randomized Treatments by Levels Design

Randomized treatments by levels design is a different kind of factorial design that involves a randomized independent variable along with another independent variable that reflects two or more types of persons (Fig. 20.20). This kind of independent variable is sometimes called an **organismic variable,** a fixed variable, a nonmanipulated variable, or a variable consisting of preexisting conditions. Basically, this kind of variable cannot be randomly assigned (e.g., you cannot randomly assign some people to the older group and others to the younger group). Gender is a commonly studied organismic variable. Consider a study of men and women wherein the randomized independent variable is a parallel group (in which each person completes a task in the presence of others) versus a project group (in which each person works together on a shared, common project). The dependent variable in this study is a measure of nonverbal socialization (e.g., the frequency with which participants make eye contact). The researcher recruits an equal number of men and women. A positive design

S				
	R	C	X$_1$Y$_1$Z$_1$	O
	R	C	X$_2$Y$_1$Z$_1$	O
	R	C	X$_1$Y$_2$Z$_1$	O
	R	C	X$_2$Y$_2$Z$_1$	O
	R	C	X$_1$Y$_1$Z$_2$	O
	R	C	X$_2$Y$_1$Z$_2$	O
	R	C	X$_1$Y$_2$Z$_2$	O
	R	C	X$_2$Y$_2$Z$_2$	O

S = Start
R = Randomization
C = Covariate (a variable associated with the dependent variable)
X$_1$ = An intervention of type X (one of two conditions of an independent variable—the other condition is X$_2$)
X$_2$ = An intervention of type X (one of two conditions of an independent variable—the other condition is X$_1$)
Y$_1$ = An intervention of type Y (one of two conditions of an independent variable—the other condition is Y$_2$)
Y$_2$ = An intervention of type Y (one of two conditions of an independent variable—the other condition is Y$_1$)
Z$_1$ = An intervention of type Z (one of two conditions of an independent variable—the other condition is Z$_2$)
Z$_2$ = An intervention of type Z (one of two conditions of an independent variable—the other condition is Z$_1$)
O = Observation (a dependent variable)

Figure 20.19 Completely randomized $2 \times 2 \times 2$ factorial design (posttest only with covariate). After randomization (R) and measurement of the covariate (C), the eight groups receive all possible combinations of the three types of interventions, each of which has two conditions. The posttest follows.

feature is to ensure that the men and women match up well to each other on potentially confounding variables, such as age and socioeconomic status. Next, the research assigns half the men to the parallel condition and half to the project condition, then proceeds to assign half the women to the parallel condition and half to the project condition. This design permits the study of the interaction of gender and parallel/project group status. For example, it could be found that women interact nonverbally more when working in a parallel situation, whereas men interact nonverbally more in a project situation.

The following are other examples of randomized treatments by levels design:

S

		R	O	X	O
T_1	M	R	O	Y	O
T_2	M	R	O	X	O
		R	O	Y	O

T_1 = One type of person (e.g., persons with a specific health problem, or persons of one gender)
T_2 = A different type of person (e.g., persons with a different health problem/persons with no health problem, or persons of the other gender)
S = Start
M = Matching of the two types of persons on potentially confounding variables
R = Randomization
X = An intervention
Y = A different intervention
O = Observation (a dependent variable)

Figure 20.20 Randomized treatments by levels design (2 × 2) (pretest–posttest with matching on potentially confounding variables). There are two types of people before the start of the research (T_1 and T_2). The two types of people are matched (M) in relevant ways. The first type of people are then randomly assigned to one of two interventions, and the second type of people are also assigned to one of the two interventions.

- Studying the effects of an intervention (versus usual care) in persons with left hemiparesis in comparison to persons with right hemiparesis.
- Comparing the effectiveness of an educational strategy (versus typical classroom strategy) in first-year versus second-year OT students.
- Studying the effects of an intervention (versus a usual-care condition) at multiple sites, whereby subjects are randomly assigned within each site.

Randomized Controlled Trials

A **randomized controlled trial (RCT)** (sometimes called a *clinical trial*) is an experiment wherein an important health outcome is the dependent variable, a clinical intervention is part of the independent variable, and research participants are recruited and randomly assigned over time as they become available. Many of the examples used already in this chapter reflect hypotheses that could be studied by RCTs (e.g., falls prevention studies, the effects of various OT interventions on functional outcomes). However, not all the examples discussed in this chapter dealt with outcomes; several dealt with short-term effects of theoretical interest to occupational therapy (e.g., the effects of occupationally embedded exercise on exercise repetitions, or the comparison of parallel versus project groups in terms of nonverbal socialization).

These theory-based studies of short-term effects are experiments but not RCTs. These non-RCT experiments add to the theoretical base of occupational therapy and OT models of practice, but they do not directly test whether occupational therapy produces health outcomes or not.

RCTs reflect a tradition of experimentation that developed in medicine and pharmacology. A major problem faced in drug outcome studies that is not so much of a problem in short-term, non-RCT experimentation is the fact that dropouts can threaten the validity of results. Another problem in studying long-term outcomes is that bias can easily be introduced if there are not special procedures for masking randomization codes. For example, if a research assistant is screening a particularly weak patient who nevertheless meets the criteria for inclusion, and if the research assistant knows that the randomization code indicates that the next person accepted into the study is assigned to the research assistant's preferred intervention, the temptation (conscious or unconscious) is for the research assistant to reject the patient from the study. Another feature of RCTs is that outcomes are often categorical (e.g., life or death) rather than measurable; therefore, biostatisticians have paid particular attention to branches of statistics dealing with categorical outcomes (e.g., survival rates).

Authors within the RCT tradition often use different terms from other experimenters (e.g., in psychology, agriculture, or sociology). Instead of saying independent variable, they often say interventions. Instead of saying that participants are randomly assigned to conditions of the independent variable, they often say that subjects are randomly assigned to arms. Instead of saying dependent variable, they often say outcome. In the RCT literature, a distinction has been made between studies of efficacy and studies of effectiveness. Efficacy deals with the study of an intervention under nearly ideal conditions (where random error is highly controlled, where interventionists have special training, and where costs are not considered). On the other hand, studies of effectiveness test whether the intervention works in typical clinical conditions.

A special issue related to dropouts involves a choice between intention-to-treat analysis and per-protocol analysis. In **intention-to-treat analysis,** dropouts are sought out for outcomes testing even if they discontinued the intervention to which they were assigned, and even if they ended up experiencing the opposing intervention (the other condition of the independent variable). Part of the rationale for intention-to-treat analysis is that participants who drop out or choose the opposite intervention might do so because of adverse side effects brought about by the intervention to which they were originally assigned. Advocates of intention-to-treat analysis argue that the clinician and the patient need to know the likelihood that a particular intervention will be effective in advance of a prescription. In contrast, **per-protocol analysis** excludes dropouts, with the rationale that inclusion of dropouts only causes random error and increases the chances of a type II error. Currently, intention-to-treat analysis tends to be the favored methodology, with the possibility of a secondary test on a per-protocol basis after the primary test.

Much effort has been devoted to the improvement of RCT design and RCT reporting. A result of this effort is the **CONSORT** (Consolidated Standards of Reporting Trials) Statement. The current version of CONSORT (Moher, Schulz, & Altman, 2001) provides a checklist of essential items that should be included in an RCT (Table 20.2) and a diagram for documenting the flow of participants through a trial (Fig. 20.21).

Cluster Randomized Controlled Trials

A **cluster randomized controlled trial** (Fig. 20.22) is a special kind of RCT in which clinical sites are randomly assigned to arms (conditions of the independent variable), as opposed to randomly assigning individual participants. For example, in a study of the effects of intensive, repeated home evaluations on patients in acute rehabilitation after hip fracture (versus usual care), 20 rehabilitation hospitals can be involved. Ten are randomly assigned to the special home evaluation condition, with the other 10 assigned to usual care. Perhaps each hospital can supply 15 patients, and all patients at a given site are treated the same because they are in the same experimental condition. Sometimes this is called a *nested design* (participants are "nested" together within each site). One advantage of this design is the prevention of bleeding from one condition to the other (e.g., when patients see their roommates getting special treatment). Another advantage is that differing skill levels and possible biases of those administering the interventions can be assumed to be more balanced across conditions than is the case when interventionists observe each other in close quarters. The main disadvantage is complexity, given expanded training, fidelity issues, and ethical compliance within the rules and cultures of many different organizations. Another disadvantage is a loss of power in the statistical analysis caused by within-site similarity. It is important to distinguish

this design from the multisite design discussed earlier in the section on randomized treatments by levels design, in which participants at each site are randomized (as opposed to being nested, as in this design).

Crossover Design

A **crossover design,** also known as a **counterbalanced design,** starts off like a basic experiment, in which participants are randomly assigned to as many groups as there are conditions of the independent variable. But each group then goes on to experience both conditions of the independent variable. In the case of two conditions of the independent variable, one randomly assigned group receives condition X first, is measured on the dependent variable, then receives condition Y, and then is measured again. The other randomly assigned group receives condition Y first, then X. If Y consistently leads to different effects of the dependent variable, regardless of order, it is concluded that the independent variable is probably responsible for the difference.

Consider the following hypothesis: A specially designed wheelchair seat will increase work productivity in adults with cerebral palsy and mental retardation (in comparison to an off-the-shelf, standard sling-seat wheelchair). Half the participants are randomly assigned to experiencing the special seating system first, then experiencing the standard seating system. The other half of the participants are randomly assigned to the standard system first, then to the special system. If productivity is greater for both groups when seated in the special system, the directional hypothesis is supported.

This design controls against type I error through counterbalancing the conditions of the independent variable. A faulty design not controlling for type I error is the administration of one condition of the independent variable to all participants first, followed by the administration of the other condition second. The difference on the dependent variable might be due to many factors other than the independent variable. For example, participants might have scored high on the second condition because they were warmed up on the first, or because they learned what they have to do to score well on the dependent variable. On the other hand, participants might have scored low on the second condition because of fatigue or boredom. These are potentially biasing confounding variables. In contrast to this faulty design, the counterbalancing of order in a crossover design addresses all of these causes of type I error. If participants score higher when experiencing one intervention than another,

Table 20.2 CONSORT Criteria for Randomized Control Trials

PAPER SECTION/Topic	Item	Description
TITLE AND ABSTRACT	1	How participants were allocated to interventions (e.g., "random allocation," "randomized," or "randomly assigned")
INTRODUCTION	2	Scientific background and explanation of rationale
METHOD		
Participants	3	Eligibility criteria for participants and the settings and locations where the data were collected
Interventions	4	Precise details of the interventions intended for each group and how and when they were actually administered
Objectives	5	Specific objectives and hypotheses
Outcomes	6	Clearly defined primary and secondary outcome measures and, when applicable, any methods used to enhance the quality of measurements (e.g., multiple observations, training of assessors)
Sample size	7	How sample size was determined and, when applicable, explanation of any interim analyses and stopping rules
Randomization: Sequence generation	8	Method used to generate the random allocation sequence, including details of any restriction (e.g., blocking, stratification)
Randomization: allocation concealment	9	Method used to implement the random allocation sequence (e.g., numbered containers or central telephone), clarifying whether the sequence was concealed until interventions were assigned
Randomization: implementation	10	Who generated the allocation sequence, who enrolled participants, and who assigned participants to their groups
Blinding (masking)	11	Whether or not participants, those administering the interventions, and those assessing the outcomes were blinded to group assignment; when relevant, how the success of blinding was evaluated
Statistical methods	12	Statistical methods used to compare groups for primary outcome(s); methods for additional analyses, such as subgroup analyses and adjusted analyses
RESULTS		
Participant flow	13	Flow of participants through each stage (a diagram is strongly recommended). Specifically, for each group report the numbers of participants randomly assigned, receiving intended treatment, completing the study protocol, and analyzed for the primary outcome. Describe protocol deviations from the study as planned, together with reasons.
Recruitment	14	Dates defining the periods of recruitment and follow-up
Baseline data	15	Baseline demographic and clinical characteristics of each group
Numbers analyzed	16	Number of participants (denominator) in each group included in each analysis and whether the analysis was by "intention to treat." State the results in absolute numbers when feasible (e.g., 10/20, not 50%).
Outcomes and estimation	17	For each primary and secondary outcome, report a summary of results for each group, and the estimated effect size and its precision
Ancillary analyses	18	Address multiplicity by reporting any other analyses performed, including subgroup analyses and adjusted analyses, indicating those prespecified and those exploratory.
Adverse events	19	All important adverse events or side effects in each intervention group
DISCUSSION		
Interpretation	20	Interpretation of the results, taking into account study hypotheses, sources of potential bias or imprecision, and the dangers associated with multiplicity of analyses and outcomes
Generalizability	21	Generalizability (external validity) of the trial findings
Overall evidence	22	General interpretation of the results in the context of current evidence

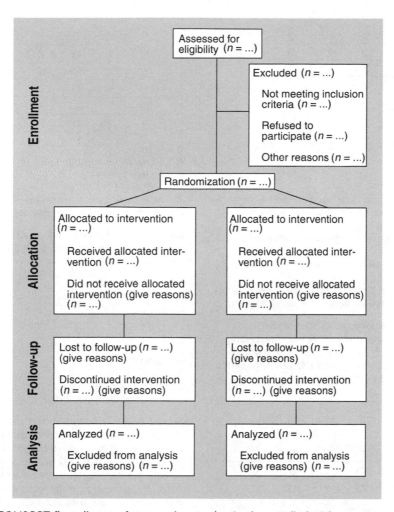

Figure 20.21 CONSORT flow diagram for reporting randomized controlled trials.

regardless of order of presentation, factors such as warming up, learning, fatigue, and boredom probably cannot account for the results.

The advantage of crossover design is the reduction of the chances of a type II error. Dispersion due to individual differences is controlled because each participant is compared to him- or herself. In addition, two measurements per person increase statistical power in comparison to designs in which each person is measured once. The disadvantage of this design is that a sequence effect or a carryover effect can prevent a clear interpretation that one intervention is superior, regardless of order. For example, the researcher must be hesitant to conclude that the special seating system is superior if productivity was approximately equal between conditions for the group that experienced the special seating system second. Crossover design is therefore not recommended for studies of interventions

that are hypothesized to lead to enduring changes within the person. Crossover designs are also not recommended for studies in which the dependent variable involves certain kinds of learning (in which participants tend to do better the second time through a problem). On the other hand, this design is particularly appropriate for studies of assistive technology and compensatory methods and for the study of stimuli that have short-term effects (e.g., effects on mood or arousal).

If there are three or more conditions to the independent variable, a counterbalanced design offers two options: the Latin square (Fig. 20.23) or random assignment to all possible sequences (Fig. 20.24). Consider the hypothesis of comparing occupationally embedded exercise (coded O), imagery-based exercise (coded I), and rote exercise (coded R). One-third of the sample is randomly assigned to an O–I–R sequence, another

S

Rs	O	X	O
Rs	O	X	O
Rs	O	X	O
Rs	O	X	O
Rs	O	Y	O
Rs	O	Y	O
Rs	O	Y	O
Rs	O	Y	O

(Eight Sites)

S = Start
Rs = Randomization by site (each site and all persons at that site have an equal chance of being assigned to X or Y)
X = An intervention administered to each subject at the site
Y = A different intervention administered to each subject at the site
O = Observation of each person (measurement or categorization used for dependent variable)

Figure 20.22 Randomized cluster design comparing two interventions at eight research sites. Four research sites are randomly assigned (R$_s$) to one condition (X), and the other four sites are assigned to the other condition (Y).

S

R	X	O	Y	O	Z	O
R	Y	O	Z	O	X	O
R	Z	O	X	O	Y	O

S = Start
R = Randomization
X = An intervention
Y = A different intervention
Z = Another different intervention
O = Observation (primary dependent variable)

Figure 20.23 Randomized counterbalanced design (Latin square), with an independent variable consisting of three conditions (X, Y, Z).

S

R	X	O	Y	O	Z	O
R	Y	O	Z	O	X	O
R	Z	O	X	O	Y	O
R	X	O	Z	O	Y	O
R	Y	O	X	O	Z	O
R	Z	O	Y	O	X	O

S = Start
R = Randomization
X = An intervention
Y = A different intervention
Z = Another different intervention
O = Observation (primary dependent variable)

Figure 20.24 Randomized counterbalanced design (fully randomized), with an independent variable consisting of three conditions (X, Y, Z).

S

O	X	O
O		O

S = Start
X = Intervention
O = Observation (measurement or categorization used for dependent variable)

Figure 20.25 Nonrandomized comparison group design (pretest–posttest, with true control group). After a pretest and before the posttest (O), the subjects in one naturally occurring group receive an intervention (X), and the subjects in a different naturally occurring group receive nothing. It is important to note that this design is not recommended except for pilot testing in advance of future research.

Group Designs Not Involving Randomization

Nonrandomized Comparison Group Design

The **nonrandomized comparison group design** (Fig. 20.25) is also called a nonrandomized trial when the dependent variable is a valued health outcome. When type I error was discussed earlier, nonrandomized comparison group designs were described as similar to experiments but as using convenient preexisting groupings as the method of assigning participants to conditions of the independent variable, as opposed to randomization. For example, classrooms of children make up convenient preexisting groups, so that all the children in two classrooms can be assigned to one condition, and all the children in two different classrooms can

one-third is assigned to I–R–O, and the rest of the sample is assigned to R–O–I. This is a Latin square. Note that each of the interventions occurs first once, second once, and third once. The Latin square uses three of the six possible sequences; other possible sequences are I–O–R, O–R–I, and R–I–O. The alternative counterbalancing strategy is to randomly assign the sample into six groups, each of which experiences one of the six possible sequences.

be assigned to the other condition. The problem is that the children in two sets of classrooms might be systematically different from each other (e.g., due to class placement procedures, such as grouping the academically talented children in one classroom). Confounding variables might account for any difference found for the dependent variable. Hence, this design is often called the nonequivalent group design.

A variation on this kind of design is the **wait-list control-group design,** sometimes called a *delayed-treatment control,* in which those at the top of a waiting list for an intervention are assigned to an intervention, and those at the bottom of the list serve as the control group. After the completion of the study, those at the bottom of the list receive the intervention, so this design is favored for humanitarian reasons. Another advantage of this design is that it permits the study of expensive interventions (e.g., home modifications) without the researcher having to fund the intervention because all the persons on the waiting list will ultimately receive the intervention. However, as with other nonrandomized designs, it is possible that the people at the bottom of the list are systematically different from those at the top (e.g., those at the top might be more knowledgeable on how to work the system, more resourceful, and/or more assertive).

An important design strategy when conducting nonrandomized designs is to match the groups at the outset on potentially confounding variables, as illustrated in Fig. 20.26. Consider the hypothesis

S
| M   X   O
| M   Y   O

S = Start
M = Matching on the dependent variable or some
    variable associated with the dependent variable
X = Intervention
Y = A different intervention
O = Observation (measurement or categorization used
    for dependent variable)

Figure 20.26 Nonrandomized comparison group design, with matching. The subjects in one naturally occurring group are matched to the subjects in another group, either on the dependent variable (O) or on a variable associated with the dependent variable. Each group then receives X or Y. Although the matching procedure improves the design somewhat over other nonrandomized designs, it is always possible that some relevant variable has not been matched. It is important to note that this design is not recommended except for pilot testing in advance of future research.

that an OT handwriting program increases legibility in first-grade children identified as educationally at risk because of poverty. The school principal and teachers welcome the research and offer four classrooms of children, but only if classes are not disrupted by randomization. The researcher gathers data on exact age and standardized educational scores. Then the researcher makes sure that the children in the two classrooms to receive the intervention are matched to the children in the other two classrooms. Means and dispersions of age and standardized educational scores as well as proportions of gender are approximately equal between children receiving the intervention and those not receiving it. This process of matching necessarily involves the exclusion of some children at the extremes of the ranges who are preventing an overall match. Ideally, the matching and exclusion are done by someone masked to the hypothesis and to knowledge of which group will receive which condition of the independent variable (dealing only with numbers). Despite all this, it is still possible that the two groups are systematically different from each other in some way that the researcher did not or could not measure. For example, one of the classroom teachers might emphasize penmanship in ways that the other classroom teachers do not.

An alternative strategy to matching is the use of special statistical procedures designed to correct for initial differences between groups. Here, potentially confounding variables must be identified, measured, and entered into statistical calculations. These procedures are controversial (Huitema, 1980, p. 100). On the one hand, it can be argued that appropriate statistical control permits a researcher to make an end-of-study claim that an independent variable probably affected the dependent variable. However, others place little confidence in the results of nonrandomized comparison designs and claim that the write-ups of these designs should not infer probable causality. Perhaps the best use of this design is in the collection of pilot data to justify a much more expensive randomized controlled trial.

Cross-Sectional Design

The purpose of a **cross-sectional design** (also called *immediate ex post facto comparison*) is to compare different types of persons in terms of some immediately measurable dependent variable (Fig. 20.27). For example, the researcher might want to compare children with cerebral palsy to children without a known disorder in terms of spatial perception. The researcher wants to know if children

	S	
T₁		MO
T₂		MO
T₃		MO

T_1 = One type of person (e.g., persons with a specific health problem)
T_2 = A different type of person (e.g., persons with a different health problem)
T_3 = Another different type of person (e.g., persons with a different health problem or persons with no health problem)
S = Start
O = Observation (a dependent variable)

Figure 20.27 Cross-sectional design (three conditions), with matching. The nonmanipulated independent variable (three types of persons to be compared) preexists the research. The three types of persons are matched (M) on potentially confounding variables, then immediately observed (O) for possible differences.

		S		
E or no E	T₁		M	O_E
E or no E	T₂		M	O_E

E = An event hypothesized to be a risk factor
T_1 = A type of person with a specific health problem
T_2 = A type of person without the health problem
S = Start
M = Matching of the two types of persons on potentially confounding variables
O_E = Observation (dependent variable) of the hypothesized risk factor through retrospective documentation

Figure 20.28 Case-control design investigating a single risk factor in a single health condition (in comparison to a matched group of persons without the health condition). A group with a health problem (T_1) is identified and matched (M) to a group without the health problem (T_2). The researcher documents (O_E) whether or not each group experienced a specific risk factor event (E) prior to the development of the health problem in T_1.

with cerebral palsy have a special problem with spatial perception. Another example is the cross-sectional developmental study, where children of different age groups (let us say 36-month-olds, 42-month-olds, and 48-month-olds) are compared in terms of attention to task. A third example is to compare persons with left hemiplegia to persons with right hemiplegia in terms of standing balance.

In this design, the researcher does not manipulate the assignment of subjects to groups, as in experiments. This kind of independent variable is sometimes called an organismic variable or a variable consisting of preexisting conditions. Because the independent variable took place in the past, before the researcher came along, the Latin phrase ex post facto is also used to describe this design.

Cross-sectional designs are needed to answer questions concerning the special characteristics of disability groups. The problem, of course, is that a difference on the dependent variable might well be due to some confounding variable (a type I error). For example, a difference in spatial perception between children with cerebral palsy and nondisabled children might be due to factors that have nothing to do with cerebral palsy (e.g., parental skill, access to older siblings, etc.). As with other nonrandomized designs, cross-sectional designs require careful matching on potentially confounding variables (i.e., matching means, dispersions, and proportions). Usually a sample from the relatively rare population (e.g., the disability group) is selected in some representative way, and then members of the comparison group (e.g., matched nondisabled controls) are assembled. Once again,

masking the matcher is a positive strategy. The other strategy employed with this and all other nonrandomized designs is to use statistical methods to make adjustments on the dependent variable when comparison groups differ in relevant ways. It is important to remind ourselves that this strategy has vigorous adherents as well as vigorous critics.

In the field of human development, aspects of cross-sectional designs are frequently combined with **longitudinal approaches** (in which the same sample is repeatedly measured at planned intervals over time). The general idea is that the researcher can have a relatively high degree of confidence if the cross-sectional and longitudinal approaches confirm each other. The longitudinal approach eliminates the possible bias likely in comparing different populations, and the cross-sectional approach eliminates the possible bias of repeated testing. The same logic could be applied to studies of the progression of specific disabilities.

Case-Control Design

The **case-control design,** also called **cross-referent design** or **case comparison design,** was developed in the field of epidemiology (Fig. 20.28). The purpose of the design is to find out if some specific variable from the past discriminates between people who today have a disease (or disability) and people who do not. The classic example is to investigate past levels of smoking habits of persons with lung cancer and matched controls that do not have lung cancer. An example that is more relevant to occupational therapy is to compare newly admitted patients with hip fracture to matched controls in terms of past injurious falls requiring medical care. Because the data collected refer to past events, case-control designs are termed *retrospective* studies.

The advantage of this design is the relative ease with which possible causal or risk factors can be explored, without waiting for years to see how events unfold. As with many other kinds of nonrandomized designs, research questions can be studied in humans that are unethical or impossible to study through random assignment. However, in addition to the possibility that the comparison groups might be different from each other in other ways than the dependent variable, retrospective studies frequently depend on unreliable data. For example, one common way to collect data concerning past events is to interview the participant. As a general rule, self-reports become less accurate as distance in time increases. In addition, the interviewer may be biased, consciously or unconsciously, in the way that questions are asked to the participant. Another type of measurement error occurs when using archival information (e.g., medical records). In prospective studies (involving measurement of future events), a plan can be formulated to collect data that includes special training for raters and tests of interrater independent agreement. This is impossible in retrospective studies. Another common problem with case-control studies involves multiplicity, in which the researcher investigates a host of past events, some of which might discriminate between currently assembled groups by pure chance. Special statistical procedures are needed to deal with specificity and the possibility of complex interactions.

Multigroup Cohort Design

In a **multigroup cohort design** (also called cohort analytic study), the researcher matches a sample that has a hypothesized risk factor to a sample that does not (Fig. 20.29). Then the researcher picks a future point in time (or a series of points if using repeated measures) to see if the hypothesized risk factor truly predicts the disease or disability. A classic example in epidemiology is to see if high levels of cholesterol in middle age predict heart disease in old age. An example more relevant to occupational therapy is to investigate if mild left hemiplegia predicts automobile accidents in comparison to matched cohorts of (a) persons with mild right hemiplegia and (b) healthy controls.

This design is similar to nonrandomized comparison group design. Indeed, some authors use the

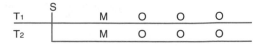

T_1 = Persons with a specific risk factor
T_2 = Persons without the risk factor
S = Start
M = Matching of the two types of persons on potentially confounding variables
O = Observation (a dependent variable)

Figure 20.29 Multigroup cohort design (two conditions), with matching and longitudinal follow-ups. Persons with (T_1) and without (T_2) a possible risk factor are matched on potentially confounding variables. Repeated observations (O) over time indicate whether or not the hypothesized risk factor leads to the health problem.

term *cohort design* for what we earlier defined as nonrandomized comparison group design. A difference between the designs is that a multigroup cohort design deals with the study of risk factors not under the researcher's control and resulting in poor outcomes, whereas a nonrandomized comparison group design deals with interventions under the control of the researcher and hypothesized to have positive outcomes. Given this logic, a study of whether brain injury predicts psychiatric disorders (at higher rates than controls) is a multigroup cohort design, whereas a study of a special intervention designed to prevent psychiatric disorders in persons with brain injury is a nonrandomized comparison group design if participants are assigned to conditions in some way other than randomization.

Prospective multigroup cohort studies generally have stronger claims to validity than retrospective studies because measurements can be planned, and possible confounding variables can be monitored. Multigroup cohort studies are stronger than single-cohort studies because the presence of a matched control group makes it possible to estimate not only the rate of the outcome but also the differential rate in comparison to a control group. This controls for the possibility that the outcome will develop whether or not the risk factor is present. Another weak alternative to the multigroup cohort study is the use of previously collected demographic data on the healthy population as a control condition, as opposed to using matched controls. Problems with previously collected demographic data are as follows: (a) the data were collected under different circumstances by different data collectors, and (b) the life experiences of a prospective cohort are different from archival information collected at a different point in time.

Summary

In this chapter, we outline the two major types of quantitative research designs: descriptive research designs and group comparison designs. Descriptive research is common in occupational therapy. As noted in this chapter, it serves a number of important purposes, not the least of which is leading to more sophisticated research designs. This chapter focuses on descriptive research in which investigators obtain observational data directly from subjects. Other types of studies, including retrospective studies that examine existing data sets and survey research, also sometimes employ designs with a descriptive purpose. When that is the case, the underlying logic of these studies is the same that as described in this chapter.

Selection of a group comparison research design depends on five factors: prevention of type I error, prevention of type II error, external validity, the resources available to the researcher, and the theoretical or clinical importance of the research question. If the researcher wishes to study the effects of a powerful independent variable (i.e., one that produces a large effect in the dependent variable) and if generous resources are available, the basic posttest-only experimental design (perhaps configured as a randomized controlled trial) provides the strongest evidence. However, the researcher is often unaware of how powerful the independent variable is until years of study have passed. Therefore, the desire for protection against type II error (which is almost always more likely in the best of designs than type I error) enhances the attractiveness of alternative randomized research designs. Each of these has its advantages and disadvantages, depending on the research question and resources available. Although questionable in terms of type I error, nonrandomized designs are important as cost-efficient pilot studies. Nonrandomized designs can also address research questions of special importance to the field of occupational therapy and to the understanding of persons with disability. No single design is best for all circumstances. Hopefully, this chapter provides an introduction to the advantages and disadvantages of the main group comparison designs.

Review Questions

1. What are the advantages and limitations of using descriptive research designs in occupational therapy?

2. What criteria are used when choosing among group comparison research designs?
3. What is the difference between a crossover design and counterbalancing the dependent variable?
4. How are type I errors different from type II errors?
5. Why might an occupational therapy researcher choose to use an experimental design (RCT)?

REFERENCES

AIDS.gov. (2014). *U.S. statistics.* Retrieved from https://www.aids.gov/hiv-aids-basics/hiv-aids-101/statistics/

Amberson, J. B., McMahon, B. T., & Pinner, M. (1931). A clinical trial of sanocrysin in pulmonary tuberculosis. *American Review of Tuberculosis, 24,* 401–435.

Bar-Shalita, T., Goldstand, S., Hahn-Markowitz, J., & Parush, S. (2005). Typical children's responsivity patterns of the tactile and vestibular systems. *American Journal of Occupational Therapy, 59,* 148–156.

Campbell, D. T., & Stanley, J. C. (1963). *Experimental and quasi-experimental designs for research.* Chicago, IL: Rand McNally.

Centers for Disease Control and Prevention (CDC). (2015a). *HIV in the United States: At a glance.* Retrieved from http://www.cdc.gov/hiv/statistics/overview/ataglance.html

Centers for Disease Control and Prevention (CDC). (2015b). Prevalence of diagnosed and undiagnosed HIV infections—United States, 2008-1012. *Morbidity and Mortality Weekly Report (MMWR), 64*(24), 657–662. Retrieved from http://www.cdc.gov/mmwr/preview/mmwrhtml/mm6424a2.htm?s_cid=mm6424a2_e

DePoy, E., & Gitlin, L. N. (2010). *Introduction to research: Understanding and applying multiple strategies* (4th ed.). St. Louis, MO: C.V. Mosby.

Fisher, R. A. (1935). *The design of experiments.* London, England: Oliver and Boyd.

Gillen, G. (2002). Improving mobility and community access in an adult with ataxia. *American Journal of Occupational Therapy, 56,* 462–465.

Gitlin, L. N., Corcoran, M., Martindale-Adams, J., Malone, C., Stevens, A., & Winter, L. (2000). Identifying mechanisms of action: Why and how does intervention work? In R. Schulz (Ed.), *Handbook on dementia caregiving: Evidence-based interventions for family caregivers* (pp. 225–248). New York, NY: Springer.

Huitema, B. E. (1980). *The analysis of covariance and alternatives.* New York, NY: John Wiley & Sons.

Karon, J. M., Fleming, P. L., Steketee, R. W., & DeCock, K. M. (2001). HIV in the United States at the turn of the century: An epidemic in transition. *American Journal of Public Health, 91*(7), 1060–1068.

Kates, J., Sorian, R., Crowley, J. S., & Summers, T. A. (2002). Critical policy challenges in the third decade of the HIV/AIDS epidemic. *American Journal of Public Health, 92*(7), 1060–1063.

Kielhofner, G. (2008). *A Model of Human Occupation: Theory and application* (4th ed.). Baltimore, MD: Lippincott Williams & Wilkins.

Liedberg, G., Hesselstrand, M., & Henriksson, C. M. (2004). Time use and activity patterns in women with long-term pain. *Scandinavian Journal of Occupational Therapy, 11,* 26–35.

MacMahon, B., & Trichopoulos, D. (1996). *Epidemiology: Principles and methods* (2nd ed.). Boston, MA: Little, Brown, and Company.

Moher, D., Schulz, K. F., & Altman, D. G. (2001). The CONSORT statement: Revised recommendations for improving the quality of reports of parallel-group randomized trials. *Annals of Internal Medicine, 134,* 657–662.

Moncher, F. J., & Prinz, R. J. (1991). Treatment fidelity in outcome studies. *Clinical Psychology Review, 11,* 247–266.

Neville-Jan, A. (1994). The relationship of volition to adaptive occupational behavior among individuals with varying degrees of depression. *Occupational Therapy in Mental Health, 12*(4), 1–18.

Orenstein, R. (2002). Presenting syndromes of human immunodeficiency virus. *Mayo Clinic Proceedings, 77*(10), 1097–1102.

Ottenbacher, K. J. (1995). Why rehabilitation research does not work (as well as we think it should). *Archives of Physical Medicine and Rehabilitation, 76,* 123–129.

Ottenbacher, K. J., & Maas, F. (1998). How to detect effects: Statistical power and evidence-based practice in occupational therapy research. *American Journal of Occupational Therapy, 53*(2), 181–188.

Peterson, E., Howland, J., Kielhofner, G., Lachman, M. E., Assmann, S., Cote, J., & Jette, A. (1999). Falls self-efficacy and occupational adaptation among elders. *Physical & Occupational Therapy in Geriatrics, 16*(1/2), 1–16.

Polit, D. F., & Hungler, B. P. (1999). *Nursing research: Principles and methods* (6th ed.). Philadelphia, PA: Lippincott.

Portney, L. G., & Watkins, M. P. (2009). *Foundations of clinical research: Applications to practice* (3rd ed.). Upper Saddle River, NJ: Prentice-Hall.

Stein, F., & Cutler, S. (2012). *Clinical research in occupational therapy.* San Diego, CA: Singular Press.

Thorndike, E. L., & Woodworth, R. S. (1901). The influence of improvement in one mental function upon the efficiency of other functions. *Psychological Review, 8,* 247–261, 384–395, 553–564.

RESOURCES

Websites

http://consort-statement.org/OTseeker.com

Publications

Altman, D. G., Schulz, K. F., Moher, D., Egger, M., Davidoff, F., Elbourne, D., . . . Lang, T. (2001). *The revised CONSORT statement for reporting randomized trials: Explanation and elaboration.* Retrieved from https://www.ncbi.nlm.nih.gov/pubmed/11304107

Begg, C., Cho, M., Eastwood, S., Horton, R., Moher, D., Olkin, I., . . . Stroup, D.F. (1996). Improving the quality of reporting of randomized controlled trials: The CONSORT statement. *Journal of the American Medical Association, 276,* 637–639.

Berk, P. D., & Sacks, H. S. (1999). Assessing the quality of randomized control trials: Quality of design is not the only relevant variable. *Hepatology, 30,* 1332–1334.

Huwiler-Muntener, K., Juni, P., Junker, C., & Egger, M. (2002). Quality of reporting of randomized trials as a measure of methodological quality. *Journal of the American Medical Association, 287,* 2801–2804.

Kazdin, A. E. (2003). *Research design in clinical psychology* (3rd ed.). Boston, MA: Allyn & Bacon.

Moher, D., Jones, A. J., & Lepage, L. (2001). Use of CONSORT statement and quality of reports of randomized trials: A comparative before-and after evaluation. *Journal of the American Medical Association, 285,* 1992–1995.

Montori, V. M., & Guyatt, G. (2001). Intention-to-treat principle. *Canadian Medical Association Journal, 165,* 1339–1341.

Portney, L. G., & Watkins, M. P. (2009). *Foundations of clinical research: Applications to practice* (3rd ed.). Upper Saddle River, NJ: Prentice-Hall.

Rennie, D. (2001). CONSORT revised: Improving the reporting of randomized trials. *Journal of the American Medical Association, 285,* 2006–2007.

Developing and Evaluating Quantitative Data Collection Instruments

Gary Kielhofner • Wendy J. Coster

Learning Outcomes

▪ Describe different types of quantitative measures that are commonly utilized in occupational therapy research.
▪ Describe the scales of measurement.
▪ Explain the two types of measurement error.
▪ Identify three ways to reduce measurement error when developing an assessment.
▪ Define four ways to ensure the reliability of an assessment.
▪ Outline the four types of validity evidence to consider when evaluating or developing an assessment.
▪ Explain the relationship between reliability and validity.
▪ Discuss issues of voice and sociocultural perspective that are pertinent to the selection or development of assessments.

Introduction

Both everyday practice and research in occupational therapy require the use of sound quantitative data collection assessments. Examples of assessments include:

• Self-report forms
• Interviews with rating scales
• Observational checklists or rating scales
• Calibrated measurement devices
• Tests

The purpose of this chapter is to examine the concepts and methods that underlie the development of assessments and the criteria that may be applied to examine the quality of those assessments.

In this chapter, we discuss an approach to quantitative assessment development and analysis that is based in the perspective of classical test theory (Hambleton & Jones, 1993; Nunally, 1978). **Classical test theory (CTT)** refers to a set of psychometric approaches that aim to define and improve the reliability of assessments and predict other outcomes, such as item difficulty or the score of a test-taker on a given variable. We also present a set of considerations for choosing or developing an assessment that are not always introduced in traditional discussions of this topic, including issues of congruity of voice and sociocultural perspective.

Quantifying Information

Many of the things that occupational therapists seek to measure can be directly observed and judged in a commonsense way. For example, one can readily recognize strength and coordination (i.e., some persons are obviously stronger or more coordinated than others). However, everyday powers of observation are not very precise or reliable. For example, when two persons have similar strength, it may be difficult to say who is stronger. Moreover, if two different people are asked to judge who of a small group of individuals is the most coordinated, they are likely to arrive at different judgments. This kind of imprecision and inaccuracy of judgment is unacceptable in research and clinical practice. Both situations require that occupational therapists make much more precise judgments than are possible through everyday powers of observation.

Quantitative measures seek to achieve accuracy and consistency by translating information about some aspect of a person into numbers (Cronbach, 1990; Guilford, 1979). This process of measurement is classically defined as a rule-bound procedure by which one assigns numbers to variables to quantify some characteristic.

All measurement requires a specific procedure and instrumentation that allow for quantification of the characteristic of interest. For example, occupational therapists measure muscle strength using assessments that quantify strength as an amount of pressure generated or an amount of weight lifted. Similarly, coordination can be quantified by

CASE EXAMPLE

Koning and Magill-Evans (2001) sought to study the construct validity of the Child and Adolescent Social Perception Measure (CASP) (Magill-Evans, Koning, Cameron-Sadava, & Manyk, 1995), an assessment that measures the ability to use nonverbal cues to identify the emotions of others. **Construct validity** defines whether an assessment measures the phenomenon that it is believed to measure, and it is the ultimate objective of all forms of empirically assessing validity. The CASP involves 10 videotaped scenes that depict situations that children and adolescents frequently encounter (with verbal content removed). After viewing each scene, the persons being tested are asked to identify the emotions portrayed by each of the characters and to note which cues they used to identify the emotions. The assessment generates two scores: an emotion score (ES), which reflects the ability to correctly identify emotions, and a nonverbal cues score (ESC), which reflects the ability to correctly identify the cues that were present in the scene for inferring emotions.

In this study, the authors used a known-groups approach. Participants were 32 adolescent males who had social skills deficits consistent with the diagnosis of Asperger syndrome and 29 controls who were matched on gender, age, and intelligence quotient (IQ). The means score for both the ES and ESC scores on the CASP was higher for the control group than the group with social skills deficits ($p < .001$). The investigators also used discriminant analysis to determine how well the two CASP scores together could discriminate the subjects into the two groups. They found that 96.9% of the children with social skills deficits and 86.2% of the controls were correctly classified in their respective groups.

The investigators further examined the correlation between the CASP and the Social Skills Rating System (SSRS), a standardized assessment of general social skills (which does not measure social perception). This assessment can be used by a parent, administered by a teacher, or completed via self-report. Because it measures a construct (general social skills) that is related to (but not identical to) the construct of social perception measured by the CASP, moderate correlations were predicted. Correlations between the ES and ESC and the parent, child, and teacher ratings on the SSRS ranged from .34 to .63, as expected. The pattern of correlations (stronger association for parent and teacher than for students) was as expected because children with social skills problems tend to have difficulty admitting their problems with peers. Similarly, moderate correlations were predicted with IQ (i.e., .59 for both the ES and ESC).

Correlations with three scores from the Clinical Evaluation of Language Fundamentals-Revised (CELF-R), a standardized evaluation of expressive and receptive language skills (a construct not expected to be highly related to social perception), ranged from .29 to .40. Correlations of the CASP with scores obtained from the Child Behavior Checklist (CBCL), a standardized questionnaire in which the teacher or parent reports the frequency of problem behaviors, ranged from .38 to .57. Because some problem behaviors are related to difficulties in reading social cues, these somewhat higher correlations were also consistent with expectations.

This study illustrates a systematic approach to evaluating the CASP in terms of construct validity. The investigators used a known-groups method, along with convergent and divergent methods. They demonstrated patterns of difference/discrimination and association that fit based on theoretical arguments about the construct under study (i.e., the ability to use nonverbal cues).

transforming the observed speed and accuracy of standardized task performance into a score.

Returning to the earlier example, the problems that occur in everyday judgments about who is stronger or more coordinated are linked to the fact that strength or coordination might mean different things to different persons, and each person may have a different procedure or criteria for arriving at judgments about strength or coordination.

For example, one person may think of strength as an observable muscle mass. Another person may think of strength in terms of some performance (e.g., winning an arm-wrestling contest). In each instance, the person who seeks to make a judgment about strength is working with an idea of what strength is (e.g., muscularity or ability to demonstrate strength in performance) and has some way to observe that idea (e.g., looking at who appears more muscular or watching to see who lifts more or wins an arm-wrestling contest).

These two elements tend to be implicit in everyday judgments, leading to the kinds of inaccuracy or disagreement noted earlier. Consequently, they are made explicit in measurement. That is, underlying all measurement are two essential steps:

1. Definition of the construct to be measured, and
2. Operationalization of the construct through formal instrumentation.

Defining Constructs

All variables that are measured must first be conceptualized as constructs. A **construct** is an abstract idea that exists in the absence of quantification. For example, consider the phenomenon "movement." If one wishes to measure some aspect of movement, one must first conceptualize or define the specific characteristic of movement that one wishes to measure. For example, the measurement of movement could involve such things as freedom of movement, speed of movement, and efficiency of movement.

Once one has chosen an element of movement for measurement (e.g., freedom of movement), then one must clearly define or conceptualize what will be measured. The most common measure of the freedom of movement is joint range of motion, which is defined as the movement about the axis of a joint. Joint range is further specified as active and passive. Active range of motion refers to the range of movement about the axis of a joint that a person can produce using his or her own strength.

Operationalizing Constructs

Once a very specific definition of a construct is developed, then a procedure and/or assessment for operationalizing that construct can be developed. **Operationalizing a construct** refers to assigning a concrete means of defining an abstract idea, such as a measurement. In the case of active range of motion, the procedure involves asking a client or research participant to move the part of the body of interest and then applying an assessment that operationalizes the movement and represents it in terms of numbers. In this case, a goniometer would be the assessment (in this case, instrument) used to operationalize the movement about the axis of a joint, and the unit of measurement would be degrees of a circle (i.e., 0 to 360 degrees).

If one wished to measure another aspect of movement, such as efficiency of movement, then a specific construct would need to be defined and an appropriate method of operationalizing that construct developed. Consequently, all measurement begins with identifying the construct that one intends to measure and proceeds to a specific method of operationalizing that construct.

The very process of using an assessment from which one derives a score rests on an important assumption, which is that functional skills, capability, emotional experience, or whatever construct is the focus of the assessment can be quantified. When we observe behavior in the natural environment, it typically appears fluid and seamless, but when we use a scale such as the Functional Independence Measure (FIM; UDSMR, 2015) we accept for the moment that meaningful differences between people in their dressing, bathing, or walking can be described using one of seven distinct categories of assistance.

Similarly, when we ask a parent to complete the Functional Skills section of the Pediatric Evaluation of Disability Inventory (PEDI; Haley, Coster, Ludlow, Haltiwanger, & Andrellos, 1992), we accept for the moment that there is a clear (observable) difference between children who are and are not capable of "using a fork well," and that this difference can be represented by a score of 1 or 0. This assumption is necessary to conduct any kind of quantitative measurement of behavior. However, like all assumptions, the plausibility of its application in a particular measurement situation should be carefully evaluated.

A second assumption is that a sample of a person's behavior, thoughts, or opinions taken at one point in time can serve as a legitimate representation of his or her "true" situation or experience. This assumption rests on the interesting proposition, strongly reflected in Western culture, that there is such a thing as the person's "true" situation or experience. In other words, an investigator who had the correct methods would be able to pinpoint the person's "true" level of function, understanding, judgment, and so forth. For example, if an investigator samples a subject's level of physical fitness at one point in time, one would assume that the finding that results from the assessment reflects the subject's true fitness level. Some form of this assumption is also necessary to engage in measurement. However, assessment developers and users may vary in how they interpret the meaning of information derived from a particular sample of behavior.

Until the past decade or so, users of measures of skill performance or ability (both clinicians and researchers) accepted that administration under standard, controlled conditions yielded the best approximation of the person's "true" capability.

This assumption confounds two important but distinct issues. By having persons perform under standard conditions, we do help ensure that the scores for each person were obtained under reasonably similar conditions, which is necessary for a fair comparison. However, it does not follow that this standard performance context necessarily reveals more about the person's abilities than his or her performance in a different context, for example, in one that is more familiar.

Scales of Measurement

Measurement is rule bound in that there are specific rules or laws that govern how numbers can be used to stand for some quality of the construct that is being measured. Physical measurements of human traits (e.g., height, weight, strength, and range of motion) build on physical measures that have been developed for characterizing a whole range of objects. Other human traits (e.g., abilities, attitudes, aspects of the personality, and so on) rely on the development of unique new forms of measurement. For the most part, it is these latter forms of measurement that are discussed in this chapter.

The rules of measurement reflect the basic scales of measurement. That is, numbers may be used to:

- Differentiate one characteristic from another,
- Indicate order from less to more of a characteristic,
- Indicate an amount of a characteristic on a continuum from less to more, and
- Indicate an absolute amount of a characteristic.

These purposes correspond to the nominal, ordinal, interval, and ratio level scales. Each of these scales of measurement has a specific purpose, meaning of the number, and rules that govern how numbers are assigned and how they can be mathematically manipulated, as summarized in Table 21.1.

Nominal Scales

Nominal scales are used to classify characteristics such as gender. In this case numbers are used to identify a specific category (e.g., 1 = female; 2 = male). In nominal scales numbers have no meaning other than identifying the category or characteristic to which a person belongs. The basic rule underlying nominal scales is that each category must be exclusive of the other categories. The

Table 21.1   Scales of Measurement

Type of Scale	Purpose of Scale	Meaning of Numbers	Requirement	Possible Mathematical Manipulation	Examples
Nominal	Classification	Identify a category	Mutual exclusivity	Counting (i.e., compilation of frequencies)	Sex, ethnicity/race, religion, diagnosis
Ordinal	Ranking (i.e., position within a distribution of categories)	Indicate rank order	Mutual exclusivity/ ordinality	Strictly speaking, same as nominal; in practice, often used as if they are interval	Degree of independence, grade of muscle strength (i.e., good, fair, poor)
Interval	Represents continuum of a characteristic using equal-interval units	Indicate position on a continuum partitioned into equal-unit intervals	Mutual exclusivity, ordinality, and equivalency of units	Can be added and subtracted	Pounds of pressure generated as a measure of strength
Ratio	Indicates amount	Indicate absolute amount (with zero equal to total absence of the characteristic measured)	Mutual exclusivity, ordinality, equivalency of units, and absolute zero point	All mathematical and statistical operations	Height, weight

only mathematical operation that is allowed with nominal scales is that they can be counted. Thus, research variables based on nominal characteristics are usually represented as frequency counts and proportions derived from those counts (e.g., 20 males and 80 females = 1/5 male).

Ordinal Scales

Ordinal scales are used to classify ranked categories. A typical example of ranking in occupational therapy is degree of dependence and independence (e.g., 1 = totally independent, 2 = needs minimal assistance, 3 = needs moderate assistance, 4 = needs maximal assistance, 5 = totally dependent). In ordinal scales, the number refers to a rank order. Using the previous example, 2 is the second most independent rating.

Importantly, in ordinal scales the intervals between ranks are not necessarily the same. That is, the difference between "totally independent" and "needs minimal assistance" may not be the same as the distance between "needs moderate assistance" and "needs maximal assistance." This means that the numbers used in ordinal scales do not represent an amount. Rather, they are categorical labels that indicate ranking within a distribution of categories.

Strictly speaking, then, ordinal scales are descriptive scales like categorical scales, and the numbers used are not true quantities. Thus, the mathematical operations to which they can be subjected in the strictest sense are the same as nominal variables. Although it is common to calculate such numbers as an average rank or a change score that involves mathematical operations (i.e., addition, subtraction, multiplication, and division), the resulting numbers are not meaningful as true quantities (Portney & Watkins, 2009). Thus, when ordinal scores are subjected to these mathematical operations, they are treated "as if" they had the properties of interval scales. This common practice is considered controversial by some researchers. To an extent, the widespread treatment of ordinal data as if it were interval data reflects the fact that in occupational therapy, like other disciplines that seek to measure a range of human traits, ordinal scales are the most commonly used scales.

Interval Scales

Interval scales demonstrate equal distances (i.e., intervals) between the units of measurement. Interval scales represent the continuum of a characteristic (from less to more) using equal interval units. They allow the investigator or practitioners

to determine relative difference. For example, on an interval scale, the difference between 2 and 3 is the same as the difference between 3 and 4, 4 and 5, and so on. An example from occupational therapy would be an observational assessment of the number of times a child engages in self-stimulatory behavior in the classroom. In this case, the assumed difference between a single count and two counts of the behavior is the same as the assumed difference between two counts and three counts of the behavior.

Interval scales do not indicate the absolute amount or magnitude of a characteristic because they do not have a true zero point indicating the absence of any of the characteristics. It should be noted that although some interval scales do have a zero point (along with plus and minus values), these are arbitrarily zero points without meaning. A true zero point must represent the absence of the characteristic being measured.

Importantly, interval scales are additive because the intervals between numbers are the same. Thus, total scores (addition) and change scores (subtraction) can be calculated. Because interval scales can be subjected to a number of mathematical operations without violating the underlying rules, they are preferable to ordinal scales.

Ratio Scales

Ratio scales demonstrate equal distances between units of measurement, and they also have an absolute zero point. Therefore, they indicate absolute amounts of the characteristics measured. Unlike interval scales, numbers from ratio level scales can be interpreted as ratios; for example, someone who is 6 feet tall can be said to be twice as tall as someone who is 3 feet tall. Moreover, all forms of mathematical and statistical operations are permissible with ratio scales. An example of ratio scales used in occupational therapy is strength measures (e.g., a dynamometer), where the zero point represents a total lack of strength (i.e., inability to generate any pressure).

Measurement Error

Returning again to the example of estimating strength and coordination, the underlying problem was inaccuracy of judgment. The aim of measurement is to achieve the most accurate judgment possible. Theoretically, there is always some error present in measurement, but measurement seeks to minimize the amount of measurement error. **Measurement error** represents the general degree of error present in measurement. There are three areas where measurement error can occur, as described in the following subsections.

Classical Test Theory

To think about and minimize error, classical test theory (CTT) uses two concepts:

- True score, which refers to the actual quality or amount of the underlying characteristic measured that a person has, and
- Observed score, which refers to the number that the observer assigns to the individual using an assessment.

In CTT, the observed score is considered to be a function of two factors: the true score and the error of measurement (Hambleton & Jones, 1993).

Errors When Using Assessments

There are two types of errors that can occur when using assessments: systematic error and random error.

Systematic errors are consistent or predictable errors; they occur when an assessment misestimates the true score by a consistent amount and in the same direction (too low or too high). For example, a systematic error may occur when a client self-report assessment consistently overestimates the extent to which a therapist effectively communicates with her clients because there are not enough questions to capture the smaller details that differentiate highly effective versus moderately effective communicators. Classical test theory ordinarily conceptualizes systematic error as a problem of validity (Portney & Watkins, 2009).

Random error occurs by chance and is thus unpredictable. For example, in a study of therapeutic communication, random error might manifest when construction at the medical center creates additional stress on the occupational therapists due to a temporary lack of treatment areas and the relocation of key equipment. The awkwardness of not having the familiar treatment areas and equipment available may show in terms of subtle missteps in therapeutic communication, thus affecting the accurate measurement of a person's capacity for therapeutic communication during that construction period.

Errors Involving Assessment Use

Typical sources of error when administering an assessment include:

- The assessment itself,
- The individual who is administering the assessment (i.e., rater or tester error), and
- Fluctuations in the characteristic measured.

A variety of assessment-related variables contribute to measurement error. These include such things as:

- Problems in the conceptualization of the construct being measured and how it is translated into an assessment,
- Lack of precision that requires the person administering or taking the assessment to estimate or guess,
- Complexity or lack of clarity in how the assessment is to be used, and
- Ambiguity that leads to differential interpretation of items or tests that are part of the assessment.

In summary, the choice and use of assessments is highly important when planning and executing a research study. The following section outlines a number of strategies and points of consideration to reduce the multiple types and sources of error that can occur when administering an assessment.

Strategies for Reducing Measurement Error

There are a number of ways that developers and users of assessments seek to reduce measurement error. The most common are:

- Standardization of the assessment,
- Methods of informing, training, and ensuring accuracy of raters, and
- Taking repeated measures.

Standardization

One of the most important and effective ways to reduce the measurement error of an assessment is to standardize it. **Standardization** refers to specifying a process or protocol for administering the assessment. Assessments may involve varying degrees of standardization, depending on the nature of the assessment. The following are examples. Tests such as the Minnesota Rate of Manipulation Test (Lafayette Instruments, 1969) or the Sensory Integration and Praxis Tests (Ayres, 1989) require a specific administration protocol along with a standard test kit. Observational assessments such as the Assessment of Motor and Process Skills (Fisher, 1993) may require standardized situations while allowing a certain amount of discretion on the part of the administrator. Semistructured clinical interviews such as the Occupational Circumstances Interview and Rating Scales (Forsyth et al., 2005) may allow substantial flexibility in how the interview is conducted but require the therapist to complete a standardized rating scale. Self-administered assessments rely on the structure of the paper-and-pencil form and clear instructions and guidance on the part of the therapist administering the assessment.

In each of these instances, the developer of the assessment considered and often completed many trials to determine what procedures would optimize gathering comprehensive and stable information. In the case of testing sensorimotor abilities, a set of specific, highly structured motor tasks was considered optimal. In the case of doing an interview, flexibility to respond to clients and make them feel comfortable was considered optimal for gathering the personal information for which the interview asks.

Reducing Rater or Tester Error

Rater or tester error is ordinarily caused by such factors as mistakes, guessing, or variability in test administration or circumstances. This source of error is minimized by ensuring that the person using the assessment:

- Understands the construct the assessment is designed to measure,
- Knows the administration protocol, and
- Understands the content of the assessment.

Standardization of assessments helps to reduce variability in how raters administer a test. Other approaches to minimizing rater or tester error are:

- Providing detailed assessment instructions or an administration manual,
- Training, and
- Credentialing those who will administer an assessment (credentialing ordinarily involves both formal training and some kind of practical test or other demonstration that the person is competent to administer the assessment).

Repeated Measurement

In instances in which the characteristic that the assessment seeks to measure tends to fluctuate, testers typically take multiple measurements to note the range and central tendency of the variability. In this way the practitioner or investigator can avoid using only an extreme or unusual score and

thus misestimating the true or more usual value of the characteristic being measured. **Regression toward the mean** (the tendency for extreme scores to be followed with scores that are more average) makes taking repeated measures a good strategy for reducing error. Use of this strategy depends, of course, on how feasible it is to take multiple measures and on how much the fluctuation affects the precision of the measure.

Evaluation of Assessment Reliability

Reliability refers to the property of consistency in a measure. Implied in the definition of reliability is that any difference in the score obtained (e.g., from time to time or from different individuals) should be due to true differences in the underlying characteristic and not due to error. Reliability, then, reflects the extent to which an assessment is free from sources of error.

The Reliability Coefficient

Reliability is expressed as a ratio of the variance of the true score to the total variance observed on an assessment. The value of this ratio is referred to as the **reliability coefficient.** It ranges from 0.0 to 1.0, with 1.0 indicating there is no error. The larger the error, the more the reliability coefficient will deviate from a perfect coefficient of 1.0.

The reliability coefficient is interpreted as the proportion of observed variance that is attributed to true score variance (Bensen & Schell, 1997). Thus, for example, a reliability coefficient of .90 is considered to be an estimate that 90% of the variance observed can be attributed to variance in the characteristic measured (true score) as opposed to error variance. When the reliability of assessments is being investigated, reliability coefficients are calculated as correlation coefficients.

Empirical Evaluation

When assessments are being developed or evaluated for particular use, their reliability is empirically investigated. In the context of classic test theory, the reliability of an assessment is empirically assessed using the following methods:

- Test–retest reliability,
- Split-half reliability,
- Alternate forms or equivalency reliability, and
- Internal consistency.

Test–Retest Reliability

One of the most common ways of determining whether an assessment provides consistent results is to administer the same assessment on two different occasions. When readministering an assessment to assess reliability, there is no empirical way to separate differences that are due to changes in the underlying trait and changes that are due to error.

Therefore, consideration has to be given to how likely it is that the underlying trait will change or has changed in the period between administrations. This defines **test-retest reliability.** This is a consideration in both choosing the period of time between administrations and in interpreting the statistical results.

Choosing the period for readministration also requires consideration of possible effects of the first administration on subsequent administration. For example, memory can inflate agreement if the subject recalls and repeats the responses given on an assessment when taking the assessment a second time. In tests of ability, the practice effect of taking the test the first time may inflate the score the individual receives on the second administration. For this reason, investigators generally want to include a period that is long enough to erase the effects of memory or practice, yet not so long as to result in a genuine change in the underlying characteristic that will be confounded with error.

Moreover, when reporting findings on test–retest reliability, investigators should indicate both the time interval between administrations and any rationale for whether the underlying trait is expected to change during that period.

Test–retest reliability correlations are calculated based on the two administrations of the assessment; the time 1 score is the first variable, and the time 2 score is the second variable. The Pearson product moment correlation is typically used for test–retest reliability. Generally, correlations (r-values) above .60 for longer time intervals, and higher values for shorter intervals, are considered evidence of reliability. In the end, interpretation of the statistic should be based on theoretical expectations. If there is no reason to suspect that the underlying characteristic changed, then a higher correlation will be expected.

The following is an example of test–retest reliability. Doble, Fisk, Lewis, and Rockwood (1999) examined the test–retest reliability of the Assessment of Motor and Process Skills (AMPS; Fisher, 1993). They administered the AMPS to a sample of 55 elderly adults and then reassessed them within 1 to 10 days, calculating Pearson product moment

correlations. The two administrations of the AMPS were highly correlated (i.e., Motor $r = .88$ and Process $r = .86$), providing evidence of good test–retest reliability.

Split-Half Reliability

Split-half reliability is a technique most often used when testing the reliability of questionnaires. It is preferred because the alternative way to test reliability is to readminister the entire questionnaire. If it is readministered too soon, reliability may be overestimated because of memory (i.e., the respondents fill it out based on how they recall having filled it out before). If it is readministered too far apart, then the underlying characteristic may have changed, leading to an underestimation of reliability because true score change is confounded with error.

To avoid these problems, investigators divide the items into two smaller questionnaires (usually by dividing it into odd and even items, or first half and last half) and then correlate the scores obtained from the two halves of the assessment. In this case, the Spearman–Brown prophecy statistic is typically used. The correlation (r) should be .80 or higher.

Parallel Forms of Reliability

For some assessments, it is important to be able to administer different versions of the assessment. For example, national certification tests or aptitude tests use different combinations of items to avoid cheating and also to ensure that the item pool reflects contemporary material (Benson & Schell, 1997). In other cases, investigators are concerned with different administration formats of an assessment (e.g., an assessment that can be administered as a paper-and-pencil checklist or a card-sort procedure). In these instances, it is important that different versions, or forms, of an assessment provide consistent results.

Parallel forms reliability involves administration of the alternative forms to subjects at the same time. To avoid the effects of sequence (e.g., fatigue), the order in which the forms are administered may be counterbalanced (i.e., half the subjects take one assessment first and the other half take the other assessment first), or the items that make up the two forms may be integrated randomly or in alternating sequence in a single test. Parallel forms reliability is assessed using the Pearson product moment correlation. It is generally accepted that the correlation (r) should be .80 or higher.

Internal Consistency

Internal consistency defines the extent to which the items that make up an assessment covary or correlate with each other. This property is often referred to as homogeneity. This is tested by asking whether the items covary. For example, if the items on a scale of cognition all reliably measure cognition, then a person with low cognition would tend to score lower on all the items, and a person with high cognition would tend to score higher on the items. If this is the case across a sample, then the items will demonstrate consistent variance.

It should be noted that internal consistency and construct validity, which is discussed later, are closely related. However, internal consistency is considered an issue of reliability because if many items measure the underlying construct and some do not, the latter will be adding error to the assessment. Consequently, internal consistency is generally taken as evidence of both reliability and validity.

Internal consistency is typically assessed using Cronbach's coefficient alpha (α) (Cronbach, 1951). Alpha is the average of all split-half reliabilities for the items that make up the assessment. It can be used with both nominal, two-choice rating scales (i.e., dichotomous) and ordinal scales (i.e., three or more choice ratings). Like other correlations, alpha ranges from 0.0 to 1.0, and the larger the alpha coefficient, the stronger the intercorrelation among items and, therefore, the homogeneity of the scale as a whole. Generally, alpha values that approach .90 are indications of high homogeneity. Because alpha is affected by the number of items, longer scales will tend to generate higher coefficients. Although alpha gives an indication of overall consistency, it does not provide information about which items may be inconsistent and, therefore, contributing error to the assessment.

Another approach to examining internal consistency or homogeneity is item-to-total correlations. In this method, each item is correlated to the total test score. Pearson product moment correlations are used unless items are dichotomous, in which case a point-biserial correlation coefficient is used. Generally, authors suggest that item-total correlations should yield correlations between .70 and .90 (Streiner & Norman, 2008). The advantage of item-total correlations over alpha is that they allow an assessment developer to identify individual items that may be inconsistent with the total score and contributing error to the assessment.

The choice of which of the four approaches to use for evaluating reliability depends on what sources of measurement error are relevant to the assessment. For example, if an assessment targets a characteristic that is somewhat variable from time to time (e.g., mood state or fatigue), test–retest is not a very good estimate of reliability because there is no way to empirically sort out what variability is due to error versus fluctuation in the underlying trait. In this case, split-half reliability is a more relevant approach. On the other hand, if an assessment measures a characteristic that is relatively stable, then test–retest is a relevant form of reliability to examine.

In cases in which different items or administration formats are used in versions of an assessment (e.g., the national certification examination taken by occupational therapists), the approach of choice is parallel forms. Thus, in developing or assessing evidence about the reliability of an assessment, consideration needs to be given to what the assessment measures and how the assessment is intended to be used.

It is important to recognize that reliability assessment based on classical test theory is sample dependent. This means that the obtained reliability coefficient will differ from sample to sample, largely because of differences in the variability of different samples drawn from the same population. For this reason, Benson and Schell (1997) recommend that whenever an assessment is used within a study, reliability evidence should be reported for that sample. In practice, it is often the case that if an assessment is used with a group for which there has previously been reported reliability data, investigators will make reference to this previous research, but not reevaluate reliability in the context of the study. However, it is common practice and highly desirable to report reliability findings when an investigation uses an assessment with a population that differs from previous research or when some aspect of the administration varies from previously reported studies. For example, an assessment of fatigue severity that originally demonstrated reliability using a population of individuals with lupus erythematosus who have not been treated with chemotherapy may or may not demonstrate reliability in a sample of individuals with post-chemotherapy fatigue. For this reason, it would be important to reestablish reliability in the post-chemotherapy population.

Rater/Observer Effects on Reliability

In occupational therapy many types of assessment require the administrator to complete a checklist, form, or rating scale based on information gathered about a client based on observation, testing, or interview. As noted earlier, the rater or observer can be a source of error, and certain strategies can be used to reduce rater error. Rater or observer error is also assessed empirically. For this purpose, there are two sources of observer/rater error that are typically examined: the biasing effects of observer presence or observer characteristics and rater bias.

- **Observer presence or characteristics** may have an impact on the behavior of or information provided by the client. For instance, clients who are aware of being observed may alter their behavior to influence the observer's conclusion. In addition, the characteristics of an observer (e.g., gender, race, age) may influence how a person behaves. For example, in responding to an interview, clients who perceive the interviewer to be more able to understand their situation may give more complete information or note problems that would be withheld from another interviewer who is not perceived to be as capable of understanding. Moreover, a client may seek to create a particular impression on the part of the interviewer based on perceived characteristics of the interviewer.
- **Rater bias** may occur when the rater translates the information obtained into a classification or rating. In this situation, any number of characteristics of the rater may introduce error. Rater characteristics that might result in error include demographic characteristics, experience, training, and theoretical orientation of the rater. Rater demographics might result in error, for example, when the rater shares characteristics with the person rated and overempathizes or judges the person too harshly or with too much leniency because of personal experience. Differences in experience, training, and theoretical orientation may result in raters bringing different perspectives or understandings to the assessment, thereby introducing error.

Assessing Interrater Reliability

The extent of rater bias is assessed through investigations of interrater reliability. **Interrater reliability** is typically studied by having two or more raters observe the same clients, either directly or through videotape or audiotape. The interrater reliability coefficient that is used depends on the nature of rating that is done.

For example, when raters classify clients on characteristics, investigators sometimes calculate percent agreement. Although percent agreement can provide some information about rater agreement, it tends to inflate agreement when fewer

categories are used. For example, when there are only two categories, raters will agree 50% of the time just by chance. Thus, 75% agreement represents only a 25% agreement above chance. For this reason, a more accurate estimate of agreement takes chance agreement into consideration. Thus, investigators use the kappa statistic (Cohen, 1960), which corrects for chance. When there is concern about magnitude of disagreement, a weighted kappa statistic is used because kappa assumes all disagreements are of equal weight or importance. For example, if raters were classifying client mood states as depressed, anxious, happy, or tranquil, there would be more concern about two raters who judged a client to be happy and depressed, respectively, than if they rated the client depressed and anxious, respectively. The latter is a smaller amount of disagreement than the former. In this instance a weighted kappa (Cohen, 1968) can be used to consider the extent of disagreements; it would distinguish between the two types of disagreements given in the example.

The kappa statistic is influenced by sample size, subject variability, and the number of categories used, so it must be interpreted with care. Fleiss (1981) provides the following guidelines for interpretation of kappa values:

- Greater than 0.75 = excellent agreement,
- 0.40 to 0.75 = fair to good agreement, and
- Less than 0.40 = poor agreement.

The following is an example of the use of the kappa statistic. Clemson, Fitzgerald, Heard, and Cumming (1999) examined the interrater reliability of the Westmead Home Safety Assessment (WeHSA), a checklist of categories of potential fall hazards. Because this is a dichotomous assessment (i.e., items are assessed as to whether or not they present a potential fall hazard), kappa is an appropriate statistic for assessing interrater reliability.

A previous study had shown inadequate reliability for a third of the items. Therefore, the assessment was revised to clarify items, and a manual and a training program were developed. In this study, pairs of therapists, who were trained in the use of the assessment, completed normally scheduled home visits during which one therapist administered, the other observed, and both independently scored the WeHSA. Based on evaluations of 21 homes of clients who were referred for home modification assessment, falls risk management, and other functional reasons, kappa statistics were calculated. The investigator reported that:

- 52 of the items received kappa values greater than 0.75,

Table 21.2 A Hypothetical Illustration of Systematic Disagreement Due to Differences in Rater Severity/Leniency		
Observation	Rater 1	Rater 2
1	2	5
2	3	6
3	5	8
4	1	4
5	6	9
6	4	7

- 48 of the items received kappa values between 0.40 and 0.75, and
- None of the items received kappa values lower than 0.40.

The results of this study indicated that the assessment's interrater reliability had improved and met recommended criteria for reliability.

When ordinal scales are used, the most appropriate assessment of agreement is a nonparametric correlation coefficient, the Spearman rho. For interval and ratio scales, the parametric Pearson product moment correlation is typically used.

An important limitation of correlation coefficients in estimating rater agreement is systematic disagreement, which occurs when there are differences in rater severity or leniency. For example, on a 10-point rating scale, two raters may consistently give different ratings that covary, as shown in Table 21.2. Although the two raters are always in disagreement about the appropriate rating, their disagreement is systematic (i.e., rater 2 always gives a higher score that is 3 points higher than rater 1's score). For this reason, investigators increasingly estimate interrater reliability with more powerful statistics than these traditional correlations.

Generalizabilty Theory and Intraclass Correlations

Alternatives to traditional correlational approaches to estimating interrater reliability include item-response theory and the variance components approach of generalizability theory (Benson & Schell, 1997). The latter approach allows for the estimation of multiple sources of error in addition to the random error considered in classical test theory. Moreover, classical approaches to assessing reliability estimate reliability only by examining one source of error at a time, whereas the variance components approach estimates, reliability while

accounting for several different sources of error simultaneously. Thus, this method can be used to calculate the reliability of an observed score in estimating the true score by partitioning error due to several factors (referred to as facets), such as variations in the raters and testing conditions, alternate forms, and administration at different times. This approach uses analysis of variance (ANOVA) to estimate sources of variation and their interactions. A reliability coefficient, called the intraclass correlation coefficient (ICC), can be computed. Unlike other reliability estimates, it is not sample dependent; therefore, the components approach is also referred to as generalizability theory. Another important value of this statistic is that it reflects the extent of agreement between raters, including systematic disagreement, which is not reflected in other estimates of reliability (Ottenbacher & Tomchek, 1993).

Evaluation of Assessment Validity

Validity means that a measure derived from an assessment represents the underlying construct that the assessment is designed to measure. Strictly speaking, an assessment is never validated. Rather, investigators seek to validate an interpretation of the scores the assessment yields (Benson & Schell, 1997; Cronbach, 1971; Nunally, 1978). This distinction underscores the fact that all assessments are used to make inferences about a specific characteristic of a person (or group in the case of community or group assessments). It is the validity of that inference that is ultimately of concern. Thus, when an assessment is said to have validity, it means that the interpretation of the measurement that is made with the assessment is correct in its meaning.

As noted earlier, all assessments are designed to measure some abstract characteristic or construct. A construct is a theoretical creation, and so it is important to demonstrate the usefulness of the construct for explanation and for practice (e.g., making sense of a client's behavior, identifying a client's problems or strengths, predicting future functioning). Inevitably, concerns for validity also interrelate with the intended use and demonstrated utility of the results obtained from an assessment.

Validity is not an all-or-nothing property of an assessment; rather, it is a matter of degree (Benson & Schell, 1997). The validity of an assessment is demonstrated by the accumulation of several types of evidence produced over many studies.

An assessment should be judged by a body of evidence that provides or fails to provide support for its validity. Moreover, ongoing research should continue to provide evidence about the validity of an assessment long after it is published and in use.

How one goes about generating or assessing the evidence of validity depends on both the underlying trait it seeks to measure and the intended use of the assessment. Generally, the following are indices that are used to develop and assess validity of an assessment:

• Face validity,
• Content validity,
• Criterion validity, and
• Construct validity.

Each is discussed and illustrated in the following subsections.

Face Validity

Face validity means that an assessment has the appearance of measuring an underlying construct. For example, if an assessment is designed to measure an attitude about leisure (i.e., how important leisure is), and the items all are made up of statements about leisure, the assessment can be said to have face validity. Face validity is, however, the weakest evidence of validity. For example, consider the following statements about leisure:

• I always try to make time for leisure activities.
• I often feel there is not enough time to do the things I enjoy.
• Doing leisure activities helps one achieve relaxation and refreshment.
• Engaging in leisure always enhances my mood.

On the face of it, the items all ask about leisure and, arguably, reflect how much a person values leisure. However, the second item may reflect more about how much a person works or fulfills other nonleisure obligations than how much leisure is important to that person. Similarly, the last item may reflect whether a person is depressed instead of how much leisure is valued.

Consequently, face validity alone is insufficient to demonstrate the validity of an assessment. However, it is often a good place to start when one is trying to generate or create items to make up an assessment. Moreover, face validity can be helpful in deciding whether or not to use an assessment. If the items that make up an assessment are not, on the face of it, relevant or meaningful to what one aims to measure or to the intended audience, then the assessment is not likely to be valid for

that purpose. Finally, in the absence of any other evidence about the validity of an assessment, face validity is the minimum criterion that one should apply when deciding whether to use an assessment. However, because there is no formal way of evaluating face validity, it is ultimately an informal process. Consequently, two experts may review the same assessment, and one might say it has face validity and the other may not.

Content Validity

Content validity refers to the adequacy with which an assessment captures the domain or universe of the construct it aims to measure. The constructs that assessments are intended to measure inevitably include a range of content. For example, self-care includes such content as brushing teeth, bathing, and dressing. When developing or judging an assessment, one must ask whether the universe of content represented by the underlying construct is adequately reflected in the assessment.

In addition to the concern about whether all the relevant content is included in an assessment, content validity is also concerned that irrelevant content be excluded from the assessment. So, for example, an assessment of self-care should not have items that reflect socializing with friends or performance at work because these occupations are not part of the occupation of self-care.

Content validation requires one to conceptually define the domain that is being measured and specify how this domain is to be operationally defined (i.e., making concrete the elements of the conceptual definition) (Benson & Schell, 1997). Only then can one determine that the items that make up an assessment adequately represent the universe of the construct.

Assessing content validity often begins with developing a set of specifications about what domains make up the construct of interest. This can be done by:

• Reviewing relevant literature,
• Reviewing existing assessments that target the construct to see what content is included, and
• Seeking the opinions of an expert panel (i.e., a group of individuals who have in-depth knowledge or expertise concerning the domain of interest).

Sometimes expert panels are consulted in several rounds as an assessment is being developed. For example, in the first round members of the panel may be asked to brainstorm content that should be included. In the second round they may be asked to examine a list of content for its comprehensiveness and focus. In a third round they may be asked to generate or evaluate specific items that reflect the content.

The following is an example of how one group of assessment developers approached the issue of content validity. In developing the Volitional Questionnaire (de las Heras, Geist, Kielhofner, & Li, 2003), investigators first identified the broad construct of volition that includes a person's thoughts and feelings about personal causation (effectiveness and capacity), interests, and values. Moreover, included in the definition of the construct was that volition was manifest across a continuum of exploratory, competency, and achievement motivation. This assessment was designed to capture volition as it is manifested in behavior. Thus, to operationalize the construct of volition, the authors had to specify ways that a person demonstrated a sense of capacity and efficacy, interest, and value or meaningfulness in action across the continuum from exploration to competency to achievement. Items were generated based on clinical experience and using feedback from a panel of experts who used the concept of volition in practice (Chern, Kielhofner, de las Heras, & Magalhaes, 1996). The resulting items that were designed to capture the universe of volition are shown in Table 21.3.

One important consideration in identifying the universe or domain of a construct is how broadly it is defined because this will affect the degree of inference that someone using the assessment must make. Borg and Gall (2006) note that a low-inference construct is one that is readily or easily

Table 21.3 Items That Make Up the Volitional Questionnaire

Items	Continuum of Motivation
Seeks challenges	ACHIEVEMENT
Seeks additional responsibilities	
Invests additional energy/emotion/attention	
Pursues an activity to completion/accomplishment	
Tries to solve problems	COMPETENCY
Shows pride	
Tries to correct mistakes/failures	
Indicates goals	
Stays engaged	
Shows that an activity is special or significant	EXPLORATION
Tries new things	
Initiates actions/tasks	
Shows curiosity	
Shows preferences	

observed and that requires only limited judgment on the part of the observer. In contrast, a high-inference item may involve a series of events or behaviors and/or one that requires the observer to assemble different aspects of a client's behavior into a judgment. High-inference items tend to produce less reliable observation. Therefore, low-inference items have the virtue of making observational scales more reliable. This is often the case when the trait of interest is relatively concrete.

However, in occupational therapy there are variables of interest that are more difficult to translate into low-inference items. The Volitional Questionnaire, which was described earlier, is an example of this situation. The developers of this assessment wanted to measure volition from observations of the behavior of individuals who could not self-report their volitional thoughts and feelings. Making inferences about motivation based on behavior requires a level of abstraction and judgment. Consequently, the assessment's developers had to create a detailed manual with definitions and examples of each item. Moreover, it is important that the person using the Volitional Questionnaire have a theoretical understanding of volition, the construct that the assessment seeks to measure.

As this example illustrates, it is important in high-inference assessments that the observer/rater have adequate background and understanding of the intended construct and how it is operationalized. Sometimes, this need can be addressed though a detailed user's manual. Moreover, in some instances, training in how to use the assessment is also desirable or necessary (Benson & Schell, 1997). It also seems that in these types of assessments, the user must have both a solid theoretical background and commitment to applying theory in practice.

Assessing content validity is inherently a subjective and conceptual process that involves consideration of the various domains that make up a construct. Sometimes these domains are specified by consensus, as in the case of self-care. Other times, the domains must be identified from a particular theoretical perspective, as in the earlier examples of the Volitional Questionnaire.

Finally, when developing a questionnaire or self-report, it is often important to identify the domain from the perspective of persons who will be responding to the assessment. For example, if the intention of a self-report assessment is to capture environmental barriers to disabled persons' independent living, content validity would require that it include all the things that persons with disabilities encounter as barriers. In this case, using focus groups of persons with disabilities to generate ideas about and to evaluate the content of such an assessment would be advisable.

Criterion Validity

Unlike face and content validity, **criterion validity** involves collecting objective evidence about the validity of an assessment. Criterion validity refers to the ability of an assessment to produce results that concur with or predict a known criterion assessment or known variable. As the definition implies, criterion validity includes two types of evidence: concurrent validity and predictive validity.

When assessing criterion validity, it is important to select a criterion assessment that is recognized and demonstrated to have good reliability and validity. Often such an assessment is referred to as the "gold standard" assessment (i.e., an assessment that is widely recognized and empirically demonstrated to be a reliable and valid measure of the intended construct). Benson and Schell (1997) also recommend and provide a formula for estimating the upper bound (highest possible value) of a validity coefficient. If it is too low, they recommend improving one of the two measures or selecting a different criterion measure. They also provide a related formula for estimating how high a validity coefficient would be if the two measures were perfectly correlated; if the value of this estimate is too low, they recommend choosing a different criterion measure.

Concurrent Validity

Concurrent validity is an approach to establishing criterion validity that refers to evidence that the assessment under development or investigation concurs or covaries with the result of another assessment that is known to measure the intended construct or with another criterion. Concurrent validity is often the method of choice when there is an existing "gold standard" assessment. One may ask, if such an assessment exists, why develop a new assessment? There may be a variety of reasons. For example, the existing assessment(s) may be too lengthy or costly to administer regularly. Moreover, the existing assessments may demand capabilities for participation that the intended clients do not possess. Finally, the existing assessments may simply not be practical for use in the situation for which the new assessment is intended.

Concurrent validity is assessed by administering the new assessment that is under development or investigation at the same time as the criterion assessment or variable and then calculating

a correlation. If the two assessments are found to be highly correlated, then there is evidence of concurrent validity. For example, Sudsawad, Trombly, Henderson, and Tickle-Degnen (2000) studied the relationship between the Evaluation Tool of Children's Handwriting (ETCH) and teachers' perceptions of handwriting legibility (the criterion variable) using a questionnaire that asked about the student's handwriting performance in the classroom. Contrary to expectations, there was no significant relationship between the ETCH and teacher questionnaire scores in legibility or task-specific legibility. The findings of this study brought into question whether the ETCH validly measures handwriting legibility.

Predictive Validity

Predictive validity is an approach to establishing criterion validity that involves generating evidence that an assessment is a predictor of a future criterion. Assessment of predictive validity is achieved by administering the assessment under question first and then collecting data on the criterion variable at a later time. For example, if an assessment is designed to capture a client's ability for independent living or return to work, then the appropriate criteria would be whether the person is living independently or employed at a future date.

Predictive validity is often challenging to demonstrate because it requires a longitudinal study. All other forms of validity and reliability testing can essentially be done through simultaneous data collection. Nonetheless, it can be powerful evidence of validity.

Construct Validity

Construct validity refers to the capacity of an assessment to measure the intended underlying construct. In reality, construct validity is the ultimate objective of all forms of empirically assessing validity, but the process of empirically assessing construct validity involves a series of studies that provide cumulative evidence. Construct validity is ultimately concerned with the underlying construct that the assessment targets. Construct validity is crucial when the "interpretation to be made of the scores implies an explanation of the behavior or trait" (Benson & Schell, 1997, p. 11).

As noted earlier, a construct is a theoretical conceptualization. As such, it is tied to a network of explanatory ideas that make sense of the trait. This network of explanation is foundational to how construct validation is accomplished. It includes not only a clear definition of the construct, but also how it is related to other constructs. A well-articulated theory that explains a construct and its relationship to other constructs allows for a stronger approach to validation. Construct validity testing is sometimes referred to as hypothesis driven because studies that provide evidence of construct validity test hypotheses that are based on theoretical assertions about the construct and its relationship to other variables.

There are several approaches to demonstrating construct validity; the most common include:

- Known-groups method,
- Convergent and divergent methods, and
- Factor analytic method.

Each is discussed in the following subsections.

Known-Groups Method

The **known-groups method** involves identifying subjects who are demonstrated to differ on the characteristic the assessment aims to measure. So, for example, if an assessment is designed to measure capacity of independent living, it might be administered to people who are living in nursing homes and those living independently in the community. In this instance, the assessment should produce different scores for the two groups of persons (i.e., document differences known to exist in the two different groups).

With the known-groups method, it is also common to perform a discriminant analysis to evaluate the ability of the measure(s) derived from the assessment to correctly classify the subjects into their known groups. Discriminant analysis is a form of regression analysis in which independent variables (in this case, test scores) and categorical dependent variables (group membership) are analyzed. Based on an equation generated by the discriminant analysis, individuals are assigned to groups in the analysis. If the assessment accurately discriminates subjects into known groups, there is evidence of validity.

Convergent and Divergent Methods

Assessment of convergent and divergent validity involves theoretically derived comparisons. **Convergence** is the principle that two measures intended to capture the same underlying trait should be highly correlated. Convergence obviously overlaps with the concept of concurrent validity. Implied in the concept of concurrent validity is that the association between two measures of the same construct should be demonstrated across different circumstances of place, sample, and time.

Divergence (or discriminant validity) measures whether different traits show patterns of association that discriminate between the traits. Thus, for example, two measures of unrelated traits such as attitudes toward leisure and motor capacity should be unrelated. Similarly, measures of associated but not identical constructs should be moderately related. Thus, in using convergent and divergent methods, investigators examine how closely the results of an assessment measure the characteristics that are closer and more distant conceptually from the intended construct and ask whether the strength of association is related.

Campbell and Fiske (1959) proposed a combination of convergent and divergent validity for assessing validity; it is referred to as the multitrait–multimethod approach. According to this approach an investigator would examine two or more traits using two or more assessments (methods) for measuring each trait. For example, if one is developing an assessment to measure problem-solving, it should correlate strongly with another test of problem-solving and moderately with a test of attention. Similarly, two tests of attention should correlate more strongly than tests of different traits, such as a test of attention and a test of problem-solving. The logic is that the two tests designed to measure the same thing should be more correlated than two tests designed to measure concepts whose functions overlap, as illustrated in Figure 21.1.

Factor Analytic Method

When investigators believe that a construct is or may be multidimensional, factor analysis is

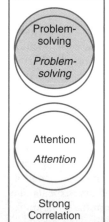
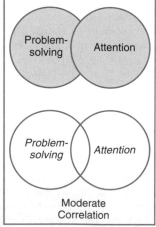

Figure 21.1 An illustration of the multitrait–multimethod matrix: expected pattern of concurrence–divergence based on theoretical associations of problem-solving and attention.

sometimes used to empirically demonstrate the dimensions of the construct. **Factor analysis** is an approach to demonstrating construct validity that examines a set of items that make up an assessment and determines whether there are one or more clusters of items.

Sachs and Josman (2003) used factor analysis to study the Activity Card Sort (ACS), a standardized assessment that aims to measure the amount and level of involvement in various activities. The ACS requires persons to sort cards depicting people engaged in real-life activities into categories. The investigators administered the ACS to 184 participants (53 students and 131 elderly persons). Factor analysis revealed five factors (i.e., demanding leisure, instrumental activities of daily living, maintenance, leisure, and social recreation) for students and four factors (i.e., instrumental activities of daily living, leisure, demanding leisure, and maintenance) for older persons based on 60 pictures. The results of this study indicate an important feature of factor analysis: its sample dependency. Factors from an assessment identified for one group cannot be assumed to be the same for another group. Moreover, factors should be previously hypothesized based on the underlying theory. Exploratory factor analysis that looks for patterns after the fact does not provide evidence of validity. As noted earlier, evidence about construct validity is ordinarily reflected in a number of the types of construct validity just discussed.

Interrelationship of Reliability and Validity

The reliability and validity of assessments are interrelated. If an assessment is unreliable because of random measurement error, it cannot be valid. However, a reliable assessment is not, de facto, valid. That is, an assessment might produce consistent results, but the items may not be targeted to the intended variable; in this instance, the items would consistently measure something other than the intended construct.

In the end, a desirable assessment achieves consistent results that clearly target the underlying construct the assessment is designed to measure. Factors that make for a weak assessment generally affect both reliability and validity. For example, if an assessment includes several items that are ambiguous, the assessment will have high error (unreliability) and will fail to consistently target the underlying characteristic of interest (invalidity). Efforts to enhance any assessment ordinarily target both reliability and validity simultaneously.

As noted earlier, validity is always a matter of degree that is reflected in the extent of accumulated evidence about an assessment. Moreover, the more variability in evidence (e.g., across types of validity, populations, and situations), the more confidence one can have in the validity of a measure.

Deciding how to go about validating an assessment or judging the evidence on behalf of an assessment depends in part on the intended use of the assessment. For example, Law (1987) argues that different approaches are relevant depending on whether the purpose of an assessment is descriptive, predictive, or evaluative. If the purpose is descriptive, then evidence of content and construct validity is most relevant. If the purpose is predictive, then content and criterion-related validity are important to assess. If the purpose is evaluative, content and construct validity are most important.

In the end, each assessment developer must pursue a logic and strategy that provides evidence connected to:

• The nature of the intended construct,
• The purpose to which the assessment will be put,
• The population(s) with whom the assessment is intended to be used, and
• The types of circumstances in which the assessment will be applied.

When all these factors are reflected in the evidence of validity, one can have a degree of confidence in the validity of the assessment.

Other Psychometric Properties and Additional Considerations

Reliability and validity are fundamental to any good assessment. However, because assessments are used in practice and research to measure traits in ways that influence clinical and research decisions, a good assessment must have other properties, including:

• Precision,
• Sensitivity and specificity,
• Criterion or norm referencing, and
• Standardized scores and standard error of measurement.

Each of these psychometric properties is discussed in the following subsections.

Precision

Precision refers to the exactness of an assessment (i.e., the extent of its ability to discriminate differing amounts of a variable). The more precise an assessment is, the finer is its ability to discriminate between different amounts. For example, a ruler that is calibrated only to 1/8 of an inch cannot accurately discriminate smaller amounts. A ruler that is calibrated to 1/16 of an inch is more sensitive in measuring distance and, thus, has more precision. Similarly, a scale that measures only pounds is less precise than a scale that measures pounds and ounces. The precision of physical measures is determined by the fineness of the calibration they use.

All other things being equal, the precision of measures of psychological or behavioral traits (e.g., measures that are based on self-reports or rating scales) is generally related to the number of items on the scale. If each item is conceptualized as an "estimate" of the underlying trait, precision increases with each estimate. Of course, other factors affect precision, including the error associated with each item and how well the items are targeted to the person being measured.

Because more items increase precision, it would seem logical to compose assessments of as many items as possible. However, lengthy assessments are often not feasible in either practice or research. Moreover, when assessments are too lengthy, error can be increased because of such factors as fatigue. Thus, in constructing an assessment, a balance must be struck between enhancing precision through increased items and practical issues of instrumentation (e.g., time, cost demands on the client or subject).

Precision is closely linked to the ability of an assessment to measure change (sometimes referred to as responsiveness to change) as well as to power and effect size. For instance, if a scale is calibrated to the nearest pound, and a child grows by gaining 7 ounces, no change will be detected. In choosing or developing an assessment for research or practice, one will need to consider how much change is relevant or important to detect and select an assessment with the appropriate level of sensitivity. For example, if one were studying the influence of an intervention on the growth rates of premature infants, a scale calibrated to ounces might be very important. On the other hand, a study of weight loss among obese adults would not require the same level of sensitivity.

There is no standard way to assess the precision of an assessment because desired precision is always a function of the purpose to which an assessment is being applied. One common approach is to readminister an assessment following a time interval or circumstance that is expected to produce a change and determine through statistical testing whether a change in the mean score is detected. Another solution is to calculate an effect size in the same circumstances.

Sensitivity and Specificity

When assessments are used to determine the existence of a problem or the need for therapy, sensitivity and specificity are concerns. **Sensitivity** refers to the ability of an assessment to detect the presence of a problem or condition when it is present. **Specificity** is the ability of an assessment to produce negative results when the problem or condition is not present.

Most occupational therapy (OT) assessments do not result in simple dichotomous decisions about the presence or absence of a problem. Rather, they typically produce continuous data that illustrate where the individual falls on a continuum of less to more of the trait measured. Assessments require a cutoff score when they are used to make a clinical decision about whether a problem is present (or sufficiently present to warrant intervention or some other decisions, such as discharge placement).

A cutoff score is the point beyond which a person is determined to have a problem or to be unable to perform an activity or achieve a level of independence. In establishing a cutoff score, one has to take into consideration the sensitivity and specificity of the cutoff. That is, one does not want to detect the presence of a problem when it does not exist, nor does one want to incorrectly decide a problem is not present. For example, an assessment of clinically significant fatigue must detect fatigue severity and functional incapacity levels within a certain range to meet a threshold for what would be considered clinically significant. It must be sensitive enough to capture the scores of those within the clinically significant population but specific enough to exclude individuals who have fatigue that is not clinically significant.

In establishing the cutoff, increasing sensitivity will also likely reduce specificity. In other words, if a higher score means a problem is present and the cutoff is set at a lower level, then sensitivity is increased (persons with the problem will likely be detected), but at the same time, specificity is probably reduced (some persons without the condition will be judged to have it). If the cutoff is set higher, specificity can be increased (fewer or no persons will be incorrectly judged to have the problem), but sensitivity will be increased (some persons with the problem may not be detected). The extent to which this is an issue depends on how precise an assessment is, but because all assessments have limited precision and some error, one has to decide in which direction it is better to err.

Norm Referencing and Criterion Referencing

The aim of any assessment is to allow the user to make judgments. Two typical ways that judgments are formed are through norm referencing and criterion referencing. **Criterion referencing** refers to making judgments or interpretations of a score with reference to what is considered adequate or acceptable performance (Portney & Watkins, 2009). In occupational therapy, a criterion may be typically linked to such factors as performance (i.e., adequacy for completing a task), participation (i.e., ability to partake in an occupation such as work or leisure or live independently in the community), and quality of life or well-being (e.g., adequate feelings of efficacy).

Sometimes a criterion is clearly linked to the content of a scale (e.g., if a scale includes all the abilities that are necessary to drive safely, then passing all the items may be the criterion). In other cases, a criterion is tied to a level of knowledge or ability, such as passing a certain percentage of items on a test. Criterion referencing works best when it is clearly linked to a relevant outcome. In some instances it will be necessary to gather empirical data on the assessment and compare it to the criterion to determine the logic for the criterion.

Norm-referenced measures are those that are standardized according to statistical norms established within certain groups of people. Norms are summarized data from the sample on which an assessment is developed (Benson & Schell, 1997). Norms are created by administering an assessment in a standardized way and then combining and summarizing the scores obtained from all those on whom data were collected. Norms should be created by testing a large sample that meets a profile (e.g., that proportionally represents all those with whom the assessment is intended to be used).

Norms are usually reported in terms of means, standard deviations, percentiles, and standard scores. It is important to recognize that norms are sample dependent, and thus it is important that the sample on which norms are based is thoroughly described (Benson & Schell, 1997). When considering the usefulness of norms, one should consider whether the sample on which norms are based is sufficiently similar to the intended population. For instance, one might ask whether the age, cultural background, and gender of the sample are the same as in the target population.

Considerable misunderstanding and controversy exist over the use of norm- versus criterion-referenced tests. Proponents of norm-referencing argue that norms provide important points of reference from which to judge whether or not a person's performance or characteristic is of concern or warrants intervention. Critics of norm-referencing point out that norms often fail to take into consideration variability in development and performance, and they argue that use of norms unfairly devalues or stigmatizes persons who are different from the average. Proponents of criterion referencing point out that criteria are more "objective" in that they link judgments to something that is rational and not biased by a preference for the typical. Critics of criterion referencing point out that a criterion can sometimes be arbitrarily imposed. In the end, the use of both norm- and criterion-referencing should be done with clear attention to the purposes for which they are being used and the consequences of making judgments.

In clinical practice, these considerations must be individualized for a client. For example, identifying a child's deviation from developmental motor or cognitive norms may be important to determining the need for early intervention services for one child with developmental disability. On the other hand, some developmental norms may be much less useful than criteria for making judgments about intervention with a child who is severely developmentally delayed.

Standardized Scores and Standard Error of Measurement

Standardized scores (i.e., t-scores) are sometimes developed for assessment scores to facilitate comparison of an individual's score to that of others on whom norms have been developed for the assessment. The t-scores are computed by setting the mean at 50 and the standard deviation at 10. They allow a person's raw score to be converted to a percentile for comparison to normative data.

If any assessment was applied to an individual an infinite number of times, it is reasonable to assume that the scores obtained would vary somewhat each time. Theoretically, the distribution of these scores would resemble a normal curve. Moreover, the mean of all these measures would be equal to the person's true score (i.e., the actual amount of the variable or characteristics in the person being measured), and the scores would be evenly distributed on either side of this mean, with fewer and fewer obtained scores the more extreme the deviation from the mean. The more accurate or error-free a measure is, the more closely the obtained scores will be distributed around the mean.

The standard deviation of all the measurement errors is referred to as the standard error of measurement (SEM; Portney & Watkins, 2009). The SEM can be interpreted according to the characteristics of the normal curve. That is, there is a 68% chance that an individual's true score falls within ± 1 SEM of the obtained score and a 95% chance that the true score falls within ± 2 SEM of the obtained score. An important limitation of the SEM is that its interpretation is dependent on the type of reliability coefficient that is used to compute it. So, for example, if it is based on test–retest reliability, the SEM reflects the error expected based on readministration; it will not take into consideration error related to rater bias.

In addition to psychometric considerations, there exist key ethical, practical, and theoretical issues that carry equal weight when a researcher is selecting or developing a quantitative measure. They include the fundamental assumptions that are reflected in the assessment and sociocultural perspectives.

Sociocultural Perspectives

A researcher or practitioner selecting or developing an assessment must also think about what source of information is appropriate for the question being asked. The source should be congruent with the definition or model of the construct, as well as with the purpose of the assessment. For example, in her discussion of *participation* as defined in the *International Classification of Functioning, Disability, and Health* (World Health Organization, 2001), Law (2002) notes that a person's preferences for and satisfaction with engagement in occupations are important dimensions of this construct. To be consistent with this definition, the only appropriate respondent for assessment of these aspects of participation is the person him- or herself.

However, an assessment also reflects the developer's idea of *what's important to measure about another person*. Therefore, decisions are not just conceptually based, but are also value based. Often, the values behind these decisions are implicit and may go unexamined for a long period of time. For example, the child development literature contains many studies that describe themselves as reporting on *parents'* effects on development, or *parents'* perceptions of their children's behavior, or *parents'*

beliefs. A closer examination of the studies reveals that most or all of the *parents* providing this information are mothers and that fathers (even in two-parent families) often are not included. This design decision may have been made for practical reasons (e.g., fathers were less available during working hours than mothers; the project did not have sufficient funds to interview both parents). However, the value implicit in the studies' titles and descriptions is that mothers' voices are more important to listen to and that they can speak for both parents' experience.

Thus, when we are evaluating evidence to incorporate into practice decisions, we want to look at where that evidence comes from (Brown & Gordon, 2004). We need to think about the following concerns: Whose voice are we hearing? Is that the appropriate voice? Are we using the correct vehicle to bring us that voice? These questions have been asked with much more frequency in recent years. As noted in the following discussion, there are some excellent examples in the literature that illustrate the importance of, for example, making more effort to include the consumer's voice in the design of assessments or including the voices of children and others with more limited communication skills rather than substituting proxy respondents.

Meyers and Andresen (2000) have critiqued the design of assessments and data collection methods from a universal design perspective. They note that population survey research (the kind of research, for example, used to identify the health status or service needs for a city, state, or nation's population) often relies on random-digit dialing methods, with specific restrictions on the number of rings allowed before terminating a call and against leaving messages. What impact does this methodology (which is quite rigorous in the traditional sense) have on obtaining the perspective of persons who may take a longer time to reach the phone, persons who cannot afford a phone, or persons who communicate through assistive technology?

Other limitations may be less conspicuous. For example, many health status questionnaires ask the respondents to make statements about their general health over a specific time period, such as "in the past 12 months" or "in the past month." How will a person with a variable condition such as multiple sclerosis or Parkinson's disease, whose ability to engage in various life activities may have varied dramatically over the period in question, respond to such an assessment? Or, how should a middle-aged man who sustained a spinal cord injury as an adolescent respond to a question that asks: "As a result of your health, have you been limited in your ability to complete your tasks at work?" This question probably was written by someone without a disability whose definition of *health conditions* includes all variations from "typical," including the mobility limitations that follow spinal cord injury. That may not be the perspective of the person with the disability, who may reserve the term *health condition* for more acute physiological conditions, such as flu or pressure sores, and may view limitations at work as resulting from inadequate accommodations in that environment. Finally, if the highest item on a scale (that is, the item that would identify those with the greatest health) is the ability to *walk* a mile, how will the scale give voice to the experiences of those who may have skied, white-water-rafted, or traveled extensively without ever *walking* a mile?

Researchers who have begun the measurement development process by asking consumers about their perspectives often hear different issues than what is represented on available assessments. For example, Laliberte-Rudman, Yu, Scott, and Pajou-handeh (2000) conducted a qualitative study using focus groups on the perspectives of persons with psychiatric disabilities of what constitutes *quality of life*. The participants identified key themes of managing time, connecting and belonging, and making choices and having control, each of which had several subthemes. The authors compared the themes identified by the participants to the content of existing quality-of-life assessments and identified a number of gaps. Interestingly, not only were some areas identified as important by the participants with disabilities not represented in the assessments, but even when certain content was included, the assessment often did not emphasize the aspects that were important to the participants. For example, many assessments ask about the number of friends a person has or how frequently the person interacts with others, but the participants indicated that the important element to them was the *quality* of the interactions they had and whether it enhanced their sense of connectedness and belonging. Other authors have also questioned the use of *quantity* as an appropriate indicator of the *quality* of a person's social life (Dijkers, Whiteneck, & El-Jaroudi, 2000).

One group whose voice is not as frequently heard as that of adults is children. It is more convenient to hear the voices of concerned adults—parents, teachers, clinicians—who report on the activities and participation of the children. However, studies have shown that by ages 7 and up, children can respond to many of the typical response formats used in self-report assessments

(e.g., Juniper et al., 1996), that they can reliably report on their own functional performance (e.g., Young, Yoshida, Williams, Bombardier, & Wright, 1995), and that they can identify meaningful dimensions of their quality of life (e.g., Ronen, Rosenbaum, & Law, 1999). As has been reported for adults, children's own perceptions of their function, distress, or difficulties may differ significantly from the perceptions of adult proxies (e.g., Achenbach, McConaughy, & Howell, 1987; Ronen, Streiner, Rosenbaum, & the Canadian Pediatric Epilepsy Network, 2003), and reports of children's function may also differ as a function of the context in which they are observed (Haley, Coster, & Binda-Sundberg, 1994).

Not surprisingly, populations with developmental or intellectual disabilities have also been frequently excluded from having a "voice," often because persons with disabilities were assumed to be unable to report reliably on their own experience. However, this assumption is being challenged increasingly as new, better adapted methods are used for the design of measures (e.g., see Cummins, 1997).

Equally salient and discussed elsewhere in this text, individuals from a range of races, ethnicities, nationalities, economic strata, and cultures have not been adequately represented in norm-referenced measures and in the groups upon which many measures used in occupational therapy have been tested in terms of reliability and validity. This needs to change, for ethical reasons and for practical reasons. Within the United States and the world, populations are becoming increasingly heterogeneous, such that in the developed countries where many of these assessments are used, there are many races, ethnicities, nationalities, economic strata, and cultural groups.

In evaluating or planning an assessment, it is important to consider the social forces and issues of voice that affect its design and use. With respect to social forces, researchers should ask the following questions:

- Who (what group of users) was the assessment intended for?
- What purpose was the assessment designed for?
- How has this purpose affected the content and design of the assessment?
- What values are reflected in this measure?
- Are these values and purposes consistent with *my* purpose and values?

With respect to voice, consider the following:

- Whose perspective guided the selection of content and the scoring metric of the assessment?

• Who is the respondent? If someone other than the client is the respondent, is this an appropriate source of information for the purpose?

Summary

This chapter provides an overview of the main issues of concern in the development and evaluation of assessments. Entire books are devoted to detailed discussions of the concepts and methods of measurement and assessment construction. Therefore, this chapter is best taken as a basic orientation to these issues (from the perspective of classical test theory) and as a guide for examining literature that reports the development and empirical study of assessments. This chapter discusses a series of important considerations regarding assessment use in practice and in clinical research. They all, in some way, concern validity, or the meaning that can justifiably be assigned to numbers generated by our assessments. The chapter began by describing the different types of quantitative assessments that are commonly utilized in OT research, including the scales of measurement that are used within those assessments. Types of measurement error were explained, and strategies for reducing measurement error were discussed. Additionally, approaches to ensuring reliability were covered, as well as the types of validity relevant to assessment development and use. The relationship between reliability and validity was explicated, and issues of voice and sociocultural perspectives in assessment use and development were emphasized.

Review Questions

1. What are the two major types of measurement error, and what is the role of measurement error in evaluating an occupational therapy assessment?
2. How would a researcher go about ensuring the reliability of an assessment?
3. Discuss the interrelationship between reliability and validity when deciding whether to select an assessment for a given study.
4. Explain the difference between criterion-referenced and norm-referenced measures, including their strengths and limitations in occupational therapy research.
5. Why are issues of voice and sociocultural perspective important in the development and evaluation of assessments?

REFERENCES

Achenbach, T. M., McConaughy, S. H., & Howell, C. T. (1987). Child/adolescent behavioral and emotional problems: Implications for cross-informant correlations. *Psychological Bulletin, 101,* 213–232.

Ayres, A. J. (1989). *Sensory integration and Praxis texts (manual).* Los Angeles, CA: Western Psychological Services.

Benson J., & Schell, B. A. (1997). Measurement theory: Application to occupational and physical therapy. In J. Van Deusen & D. Brunt (Eds.), *Assessment in occupational therapy and physical therapy* (pp. 3–24). Philadelphia, PA: W. B. Saunders.

Borg, W., & Gall, M. (2006). *Educational research: An introduction* (8th ed.). Upper Saddle River, NJ: Pearson.

Brown, M., & Gordon, W. A. (2004). Empowerment in measurement: "Muscle," "voice," and subjective quality of life as a gold standard. *Archives of Physical Medicine and Rehabilitation, 85*(Supp. 2), S13–S20.

Campbell, D. T., & Fiske, D. W. (1959). Convergent and discriminant validation for the multitrait-multimethod matrix. *Psychological Bulletin, 56,* 81–105.

Chern, J., Kielhofner, G., de las Heras, C., & Magalhaes, L. (1996). The Volitional Questionnaire: Psychometric development and practical use. *American Journal of Occupational Therapy, 50,* 516–525.

Clemson, L., Fitzgerald, M. H., Heard, R., & Cumming, R. G. (1999). Inter-rater reliability of a home fall hazards assessment tool. *Occupational Therapy Journal of Research, 19,* 83–100.

Cohen, J. (1960). Coefficient of agreement for nominal scales. *Educational and Psychological Measurement, 20,* 37–46.

Cohen, J. (1968). Weighted kappa: Nominal scale agreement with provision for scaled disagreement or partial credit. *Psychological Bulletin, 70,* 213–220.

Cronbach, L. J. (1951). Coefficient alpha and the internal structure of tests. *Psychometrika, 16,* 297–334.

Cronbach, L. J. (1971). Test validation. In R. L. Thorndike (Ed.), *Educational measurement* (2nd ed., pp. 443–507). Washington, DC: American Council on Education.

Cronbach, L. J. (1990). *Essentials of psychological testing* (5th ed.). New York, NY: Harper and Row.

Cummins, R. A. (1997). Self-rated quality of life scales for people with an intellectual disability: A review. *Journal of Applied Research in Intellectual Disabilities, 10,* 199–216.

de las Heras, C. G., Geist, R., Kielhofner, G., & Li, Y. (2003). *The Volitional Questionnaire* (Version 4.0). Chicago, IL: Model of Human Occupation Clearinghouse, Department of Occupational Therapy, College of Applied Health Sciences, University of Illinois at Chicago.

Dijkers, M. P. J. M., Whiteneck, G., & El-Jaroudi, R. (2000). Measures of social outcomes in disability research. *Archives of Physical Medicine & Rehabilitation, 81*(Suppl. 2), S63–S80.

Doble, S., Fisk, J. D., Lewis, N., & Rockwood, K. (1999). Test–retest reliability of the assessment of motor and process skills in elderly adults. *Occupational Therapy Journal of Research, 19,* 203–219.

Fisher, A. G. (1993). The assessment of IADL motor skills: An application of many faceted Rasch analysis. *American Journal of Occupational Therapy, 47,* 319–329.

Fleiss, J. L. (1981). *Statistical methods for rates and proportions.* New York, NY: John Wiley & Sons.

Forsyth, K., Deshpande, S., Kielhofner, G., Henriksson, C., Haglund, L., Olson, L., ... Kulkarni, S. (2005). *The Occupational Circumstances Assessment Interview and Rating Scale* (Version 4.0). Chicago, IL: Model of Human Occupation Clearinghouse, Department of

Occupational Therapy, College of Applied Health Sciences, University of Illinois at Chicago.

Guilford, J. (1979). *Psychometric methods* (2nd ed.). New York, NY: McGraw-Hill.

Haley, S. M., Coster, W. J., & Binda-Sundberg, K. (1994). Measuring physical disablement: The contextual challenge. *Physical Therapy, 74,* 443–451.

Haley, S. M., Coster, W. J., Ludlow, L., Haltiwanger, J., & Andrellos, P. (1992). *Pediatric Evaluation of Disability Inventory (PEDI).* Boston, MA: Boston University Center for Rehabilitation Effectiveness.

Hambleton, R. K., & Jones, R. W. (1993). Comparison of classical test theory and item response theory and their applications to test development. *Educational Measurement: Issues and Practice, 12,* 38–47.

Juniper, E. F., Guyatt, G. H., Feeny, D. H., Ferrie, P.J., Griffith, L.E., ... Townsend, M. (1996). Measuring quality of life in children with asthma. *Quality of Life Research, 5,* 35–46.

Koning, C., & Magill-Evans, J. (2001). Validation of the child and adolescent social perception. *Occupational Therapy Journal of Research, 21,* 41–67.

Lafayette Instruments. (1969). *The Complete Minnesota Dexterity Test. Examiner's manual.* Lafayette, IN: Author.

Laliberte-Rudman, D., Yu, B., Scott, E., & Pajouhandeh, P. (2000). Exploration of the perspectives of persons with schizophrenia regarding quality of life. *American Journal of Occupational Therapy, 54,* 137–147.

Law, M. (1987). Measurement in occupational therapy: Scientific criteria for evaluation. *Canadian Journal of Occupational Therapy, 54*(3), 133–138.

Law, M. (2002). Participation in the occupations of everyday life. *American Journal of Occupational Therapy, 56,* 640–649.

Magill-Evans, J., Koning, C., Cameron-Sadava, A., & Manyk, K. (1995). The child and adolescent social perception measure. *Journal of Nonverbal Behavior, 19,* 151–169.

Meyers, A. R., & Andresen, E. M. (2000). Enabling our instruments: Accommodation, universal design, and access to participation in research. *Archives of Physical Medicine & Rehabilitation, 81*(Suppl. 2), S5–S9.

Nunally, J. C. (1978). *Psychometric theory* (2nd ed.). New York, NY: McGraw-Hill.

Ottenbacher, K. J., & Tomchek, S. D. (1993). Measurement in rehabilitation research: Consistency versus consensus. In C. V. Granger & G. E. Gresham (Eds.), *New developments in functional assessment* (pp. 463–473). Philadelphia, PA: W. B. Saunders.

Portney, L. G., & Watkins, M. P. (2009). *Foundations of clinical research: Applications to practice* (3rd ed.). Upper Saddle River, NJ: Prentice-Hall.

Ronen, G. M., Rosenbaum, P., & Law, M., (1999). Health-related quality of life in childhood epilepsy: The results of children participating in identifying the components. *Developmental Medicine and Child Neurology, 41,* 554–559.

Ronen, G. M., Streiner, D. L., Rosenbaum, P., & the Canadian Pediatric Epilepsy Network. (2003). Health-related quality of life in children with epilepsy: Development and validation of self-report and parent proxy measures. *Epilepsia, 44,* 598–612.

Sachs, D., & Josman, N. (2003). The Activity Card Sort: A factor analysis. *OTJR: Occupation, Participation and Health, 23,* 165–174.

Streiner, D. L., & Norman, G. R. (2008). *Health measurement scales: A practical guide to their development and use* (4th ed.). New York, NY: Oxford University Press.

Sudsawad, P., Trombly, C. A., Henderson, A., & Tickle-Degnen, L. (2000). The relationship between the evaluation tool of children's handwriting and teachers' perceptions of handwriting legibility. *American Journal of Occupational Therapy, 55,* 518–523.

Uniform Data System for Medical Rehabilitation (UDSMR). (2015). About the FIM system. Retrieved from http://www.udsmr.org/WebModules/FIM/Fim_About.aspx.

World Health Organization. (2001). *International Classification of Functioning, Disability, and Health (ICF).* Geneva, Switzerland: WHO Press.

Young, N. L., Yoshida, K. K., Williams, J. I., Bombardier, C., & Wright, J. (1995). The role of children in reporting their physical disability. *Archives of Physical Medicine & Rehabilitation, 76,* 913–918.

Resources

General Resources

Benson, J., & Clark, F. (1982). A guide for instrument development and validation. *American Journal of Occupational Therapy, 36,* 789–800. Retrieved from http://www.cosmin.nl/cosmin_checklist.html

Cronbach, L. J. (1990). *Essentials of psychological testing* (5th ed.). New York, NY: Harper and Row.

Nunally, J., & Bernstein I. H. (1994). *Psychometric theory* (3rd ed.). New York, NY: McGraw-Hill.

Terwee, C. B., Mokkink, L. B., Knol, D. L., Ostelo, R. W. J. G., Bouter, L. M., & de Viet, H. C. W. (2012). Rating the methodological quality in systematic reviews of studies on measurement properties: A scoring system for the COSMIN checklist. *Quality of Life Research, 21,* 651–657.

Thorndike, R. L., & Hagen, E. (1990). *Measurement and evaluation in psychology and education* (5th ed.). New York, NY: John Wiley and Sons.

Van Deusen J., & Brunt D. (Eds.). (1997). *Assessment in occupational therapy and physical therapy.* Philadelphia, PA: W. B. Saunders.

Listings and Samples of Assessments

Asher, I. E. (1996). *Occupational therapy assessment tools: An annotated index* (2nd ed.). Bethesda, MD: American Occupational Therapy Association.

*Dittmar, S. S., & Gresham, G. E. (1997). *Functional assessment and outcome measures for the rehabilitation health professional.* Gaithersburg, MD: Aspen.

*Finch, E., Brooks, D., Stratford, P. W., & Mayo, N. E. (2002). *Physical rehabilitation outcome measures: A guide to enhanced clinical decision making* (2nd ed.) [with CD-ROM]. Hamilton, Ontario, Canda: BC Decker.

Law, M., Baum, C., & Dunn, W. (2001). *Measuring occupational performance: Supporting best practice in occupational therapy.* Thorofare, NJ: Slack.

Law, M., King, G., MacKinnon, E., Russell, D., Murphy, C., & Hurley, P. (1999). *All about outcomes* [CD-ROM]. Thorofare, NJ: Slack.

* These resources include actual assessments.

Law, M. (Ed.) (2002). *Evidence-based rehabilitation: A guide to practice.* Thorofare, NJ: Slack.

Forms are also available on the CanChild website: http://www.fhs.mcmaster.ca/canchild

CHAPTER 22

Collecting Quantitative Data

Renée R. Taylor • Gary Kielhofner

Learning Outcomes

- Identify commonly used approaches to data collection in occupational therapy.
- Understand the pros and cons of utilizing an existing validated measure for data collection versus developing your own measure.
- Discuss the central considerations involving the reliability of data collection procedures.
- Explain how to achieve valid data collection procedures.
- Define the steps involved in planning a data collection process for a given study.
- List professional and ethical considerations to follow when collecting data.

Introduction

All research depends on data. Data are pieces of information that have been gathered according to specified rules and procedures to answer questions under investigation in a study (Crotty, 1998; DePoy & Gitlin, 2010; Neuman, 2009; Portney & Watkins, 2009). Answering the research questions requires that information be gathered on the phenomena or variables under study. In the end, the dependability of the research findings is linked to whether the data collected are reliable and valid.

The purpose of this chapter is to discuss the process of data collection within a quantitative research study. It begins with a brief review of how issues of data reliability are approached in the quantitative tradition. Then, approaches to data collection are discussed. Next, the steps involved in research data collection are identified and discussed. The chapter concludes with a discussion of professional and ethical issues that involve the treatment of research participants during data collection.

Quantitative Data

Data can be either quantitative (i.e., numeric) or qualitative (e.g., narrative) in nature. How investigators think about and ensure the dependability (i.e., reliability and validity) of data will depend on whether the data are being collected within the quantitative and/or qualitative traditions (Neuman, 2009). In this chapter, we focus on issues surrounding the collection of quantitative data.

Quantitative Data Collection

Quantitative approaches to data collection are basically concerned with judgments of category or amount (Portney & Watkins, 2009). In quantitative data collection, variables of interest are assigned a numeric value that reflects the category or amount of that variable. Numeric quantities of one variable can then be examined in isolation or compared to those of other variables.

Levels of Data

As a review from the previous chapter, quantitative data may be scaled in one of four major ways:

1. Nominal or categorical, in which case numeric labels are assigned to designate specific categories of a given variable (e.g., determining whether a research participant belongs to a category pertaining to sex, race, religion, or political affiliation);
2. Ordinal, which determines the rank order of a variable (e.g., the rating, 1 = never, 2 = sometimes, 3 = frequently, 4 = always, is a rank order of frequency);
3. Interval (also described as continuous), which is characterized by the assignment of numbers along a continuum of less to more of a variable divided into equal intervals;
4. Ratio (also described as continuous), which differs from interval data only in that there is a true zero point at which none of what is being measured exists.

CASE EXAMPLE

Belinda is an occupational therapy (OT) student enrolled in a research methods course. One of her course requirements is to develop a data collection plan for a study of the use of graded exercise to decrease symptoms of fatigue in otherwise ambulatory adults with post-cancer-treatment fatigue. The desired outcomes of the client's engagement in graded exercise include (a) decreased symptoms of fatigue and (b) increased community mobility. The budget for the imagined study is very low. There is only enough money to cover basic photocopying expenses and labor costs involving a research assistant, paid at an hourly rate. Belinda must take all of these variables into consideration when planning her data collection approach.

Belinda knows this is a challenging assignment because there are many ways to define fatigue, none of which is as complex and comprehensive as the experience of fatigue because fatigue is a subjectively experienced phenomenon that is often difficult for researchers to quantify. Similarly, community mobility may be defined in multiple ways. How shall Belinda define mobility in this study? Does mobility refer to walking (measured by gait velocity, endurance, a pedometer, or actigraph) or a global functional mobility measure? Does it refer to the use of powered mobility (measured by wheelchair data-logging devices)? Does it refer to both walking and wheelchair use?

Belinda decides to look into the literature on the topics of fatigue and community mobility to explore how other researchers have chosen to define and measure these constructs. The literature on fatigue reveals that fatigue may be measured in two major ways: by self-report of subjects' perceived experience of physical and mental fatigue or by the assessment of fatigue using primarily biometric measures (e.g., electromyography [EMG] accompanied by a physical stress test to measure muscle fatigue or functional magnetic resonance imaging [fMRI] accompanied by a cognitive stress test to measure cognitive fatigue). Based upon her clinical experience during her practicum at a local cancer treatment center, Belinda knows that the experience of fatigue in people who have recently completed cancer treatment is pervasive and often experienced both mentally and physically. She hypothesizes that the definition of fatigue that best matches the study question concerns clients' subjective experiences of both physical and mental fatigue. Moreover, the clients she is studying are outpatients who, as they recover from their treatment, will continue functioning within the occupational roles in which they were functioning prior to their treatment episodes.

For these reasons and because of her limited budget, Belinda elects to measure both outcomes (fatigue and community mobility) using low-cost measures. In terms of fatigue, she elects to use a self-report measure of the functional consequences of fatigue that has demonstrated validity and reliability in measuring post-cancer-treatment fatigue and captures both the physical and cognitive aspects. In terms of community mobility, Belinda decides to define this variable as it relates to walking because she cannot afford to purchase enough wheelchair-tracking devices, pedometers, or actigraphs for all 30 participants in the study. She decides to measure community mobility using an activity diary that has been validated in the same population of people with post-cancer-treatment fatigue. She elects to use an activity diary, rather than a global measure of functional mobility, because she predicts that the activity diary will better capture the construct of an individual's mobility throughout the community. She receives an A on her assignment.

Approach to Data Collection

Ordinarily, in quantitative research the same data will be collected from all subjects, or there will be a specific plan for more in-depth data collection depending on subjects' responses or scores from the first phase of data collection. For example, a study may be structured so that only clients who report or demonstrate the presence of a trait will be asked to engage in more in-depth data collection. In quantitative research, investigators will also undertake data collection so as to minimize the amount of missing data because statistical analyses are most rigorous when there are no or few missing data points.

Within occupational therapy, quantitative data collection that focuses on human behavior, thought, attitude, or emotions primarily uses structured methods of collecting data, such as observational rating scales, self-report questionnaires, structured interviews, and standardized tests. In our field, quantitative research also involves the use of functional performance data collection procedures (e.g., motor coordination, self-care, driver safety, and work capacity). These data collection procedures ordinarily require equipment or standardized tests for collecting data. Finally, quantitative research also can involve biometric data collection, which ranges from procedures such as measuring the kinematics of movement to imaging techniques that capture brain activity.

Methodological Rigor and Dependability of Quantitative Data

In quantitative research, investigators carefully choose and justify their data collection procedures when planning the research. Researchers either choose instruments that have previously been developed and investigated or spend substantial time prior to or in the early stages of the research developing instruments and refining and documenting the reliability and validity of those instruments.

Although it is sometimes necessary to construct instruments for research, a wide array of suitable instruments is increasingly available that have been previously developed and studied. Typically, it is more efficient and desirable to use an existing measure that has already been tested for reliability and validity than it is to develop and subsequently test your own measure. Additionally, utilizing a measure that has already undergone psychometric testing and validation maximizes the chances that findings from your study will be comparable to findings from similar studies that have employed the same assessment. This becomes particularly important in outcomes research because defining and assessing an outcome using the same measure across studies is more informative than defining and assessing an outcome with many different measures.

When it is necessary to create a new instrument for a study, the development of that instrument is, in itself, a substantial research undertaking. In many research-intensive institutions there are centers or laboratories that provide technical assistance to investigators who need to develop new data collection instruments. Investigators often seek the resources of such entities when developing an instrument.

Concerns with the dependability of quantitative data are centered on reliability and validity (Benson & Schell, 1997). Questions about the **reliability of data** seek to ensure that the accuracy of information collected was not unduly affected by any extraneous circumstances surrounding data collection. Reliability is typically concerned with how accuracy may be affected by circumstances of data collection (i.e., who collects it, what kind of instrument is used to collect it, and how and when it was collected).

Questions involving the **validity of data** basically ask whether the data collected actually represent the variable under study. Empirical assessment of validity focuses on such factors as the extent to which items used to quantify a variable coalesce together and whether the instrument's scores converge with measures of variables that are theoretically related to the variable the instrument intends to measure.

When collecting quantitative data for a study, investigators who wish to ensure the reliability and validity of their data ordinarily select data collection methods for which there are published reliability and validity findings relevant to the intended study population and/or test the reliability and validity of the data collection procedure in their own investigation.

There is reason to question the reliability and validity of data collection procedures when:

- There is not sufficient previous research on the reliability and validity of the instrument;
- The sample under study differs from those on which the instrument has been studied;
- An aspect of how the instrument will be used varies from its standard use or how it has been used in previous research; and
- A new data collection procedure has been developed specifically for the study, for which reliability and validity are unknown.

In these cases, investigators will ordinarily test the reliability and/or validity prior to using an instrument to collect data in the study, or collect data within the study that simultaneously provide evidence pertinent to the reliability or validity of the instrument.

For example, consider a data collection procedure (e.g., administering a self-report measure by telephone) that has been shown to be reliable and valid with an adult sample. An investigator who wishes to use it in a study of adolescents must consider two questions:

- Will the self-report measure provide valid measures for an adolescent sample?
- Does administering the measure by telephone still yield reliable data in an adolescent sample, or is there something unique about adolescents that would make telephone administration an unreliable data collection procedure in a given study?

Under these circumstances, an investigator may do a pilot study to investigate whether adolescents give stable responses (e.g., test–retest reliability) or whether obtained measures correlate with another means of collecting the same information (i.e., concurrent validity).

As the example illustrates, rigor in quantitative data collection emphasizes determining the dependability of data collection procedures before or at the beginning of the research process.

Approaches to Data Collection

Data can be collected in a wide variety of ways. The most common forms of data collection are:

* Observation,
* Interviews,
* Self-report measures,
* Standardized tests and performance measures,
* Contextual/environmental assessment,
* Focus groups and town hall meetings,
* Biometric measures, and
* Document/records review.

Although many of these methods are used in both quantitative and qualitative research, some are more or less exclusively used in one approach or the other.

Observation

Observational approaches to data collection are suited to both qualitative and quantitative studies. When the aim of research is to answer questions related to performance or behavior, observation is frequently the data collection method of choice. Observational data also provide a richer understanding of an unfolding or ongoing behavior, process, or other situation in real-time. Observation is most straightforward when there is tangible physical evidence, outcomes, or products that can be seen or heard.

In some circumstances, observational methods are used to corroborate data that have been collected through other assessment methods, such as interviews or self-report measures. In other cases, observational methods are used when subjects lack insight or self-evaluation skills or are not able to participate in an interview or provide an accurate self-report (e.g., infants or individuals with severe cognitive limitations).

Observational data collection methods are also useful in providing direct information about a variable under study that is not filtered through the perceptual lens of the person under observation. For example, in occupational therapy, home visits to assess features of an individual's physical environment are a more reliable and valid means of assessing the risk for falls than gathering this information through self-report (Clemson, Fitzgerald, Heard, & Cumming, 1999).

Types of Information Gathered Through Observation

The information typically sought through observation includes:

* Subjects' characteristics or affective states (e.g., whether a person is sad, anxious, agitated, calm);
* Behavior (e.g., what a person does in a given situation, how a person performs a task, level of endurance to activity, or whether a person shows signs of restlessness, inattention, hyperactivity, fatigue, etc.);
* Communication (e.g., what a person says to others, how a person acts toward others, or what a person expresses to others through gestures and facial expressions); and
* Environmental circumstances (e.g., objects and their arrangement in space, social conditions, safety, task demands).

The observer ordinarily watches and/or listens to participants, recording the information. Methods of recording information include:

* Observational guides (i.e., highly structured printed forms or booklets that provide probes or codes for various topic areas and corresponding space to record observations). These can be used for both qualitative and quantitative research.
* Structured checklists (i.e., paper-and-pencil forms used primarily to indicate the presence versus absence or frequency of certain states, behaviors, or communication). These yield categorical data most often used in quantitative research.
* Quantitative rating scales (i.e., forms that assign ordinal numerical scores to a number of items designed to represent the variable under study). The most common is the Likert or Likert-type scale, which uses an ordinal rating technique in which qualitative statements are used to differentiate positions along a continuum (e.g., frequently = 1, sometimes = 2, never = 3).
* Semistructured or unstructured note taking (field notes). This involves taking notes based on broad topics or thematic areas (semistructured)

or based on spontaneous observations (unstructured). This approach is most common to qualitative research, although it is used in quantitative research to provide supportive anecdotal data.

- Electronic/digital recording of data: Data can be collected using audiotape or videotape recording. Recording can occur in any stage of the research depending on the aims and nature of the study. For example, recording can be used as an investigator's "third eye" to gather observational data that involve interaction between the subject(s) and the investigator.

Another advantage of recording is that playbacks can allow the researcher to view the data at any speed and as many times as he or she desires. Thus, it is best used in circumstances where the question under study must be rated in a very detailed manner and a given behavior must be slowed down or replayed to ensure that the researcher has observed and understood all aspects of the behavior correctly.

Forms of Observation

There are two widely known types of observation, passive observation and participant-observation. The first and most commonly utilized form of observation in quantitative research is passive observation. Passive observation involves the investigator observing subjects and recording data on the variables of interest with little to no interaction with the subjects, in the interest of maintaining objectivity and minimizing any biasing influence on what is being observed.

The second general form of observation is participant observation; it is commonly utilized in qualitative research. When using participant observation, the investigator joins the subjects and participates in the same discussion or activities as the subjects. The aim of the participatory process is for the investigator to gain understanding of the phenomena under study as experienced by the participants.

Role of the Observer

In general, the observer's role is to capture certain details about the subject, discern important from unimportant observational data, interpret the observed data accurately and in light of the environmental context, and validate observations over time. In studies that utilize observation, the role of the observer also depends largely on whether the study is quantitative or qualitative. In quantitative

research, the aim of the data collection is ordinarily for the observer to:

- Remain as objective as possible in gathering/recording the data to prevent any biases in data interpretation or other personal expectations imposed on the data by the observer.
- Prevent artificiality or other changes in subjects' behavior due to the presence of the observer. In circumstances where the question under study does not involve interaction with the investigator, the investigator is to remain as unobtrusive and uninvolved as possible so as to avoid contaminating the observational context or influencing the behavior of the subjects. In some cases, this involves observing through a one-way mirror or from a location that is outside of a subject's vision or awareness.
- Take precautionary measures to ensure the reliability and validity involved in recording the data, particularly if the nature of the observation involves subtle changes in behavior, rapidly changing behavior, or some other highly detailed or nuanced aspect of behavior. Precautionary measures include audiotaping, videotaping, and/or corroborative rating checks by an independent rater.

Observational Context

Observation can take place in a number of contexts, including:

- Natural contexts,
- Semistructured (e.g., clinical) contexts, and
- Standardized or laboratory contexts.

In its purest form, observational research takes place within the natural environment or context in which subjects live and function. Natural contexts may include, but are not limited to, a subject's home, workplace, neighborhood, and/or general community environment (e.g., in a grocery store or on public transportation).

In the field of occupational therapy, observational data are often collected in semistructured settings, such as within an inpatient or outpatient clinical setting. Unlike a subject's natural environment, a semistructured setting introduces the following structures:

- Time (i.e., length of therapy session),
- Space (i.e., size and configuration of the therapy space),
- Objects (i.e., therapeutic equipment, assessment tools, assistive technologies, arts and crafts, and other objects within the clinical setting),
- Sensory variation (i.e., different lighting, sounds, smells), and

- People (i.e., therapists, support staff, administrators, other clients) who are artificial to a subject's natural environment.

Standardized or laboratory contexts offer the highest degree of control over confounding factors. Within OT research, a standardized context is typically created within a staged or highly structured treatment room in a clinical setting or within a standardized laboratory space. Depending on the research question, any variety of characteristics of these settings can be controlled, including room temperature, lighting, sound, contents, and space configuration. In addition, standardized or laboratory contexts allow use of specialized measurement devices or test situations.

Advantages and Disadvantages of Different Observational Contexts

The primary advantage of collecting data within a natural environment is the ability to gather data that are authentic and ecologically valid. Natural environments do not introduce extraneous variables that might otherwise be imposed by an artificial laboratory or clinical environment. Semistructured and structured settings can raise questions of ecological validity. However, unlike a highly structured laboratory setting, a semistructured clinical context may be construed in such a way as to simulate enough of a subject's natural environment to increase ecological validity.

For example, a researcher seeking to answer an observational research question pertaining to environmental impact on attentional problems in persons with schizophrenia might compare the subject's attention within three semistructured clinical contexts that simulate aspects of everyday settings. First, the researcher might take the subject into the dining room of the hospital during lunchtime and test the subject's ability to follow a conversation in a highly stimulating environment. Then, the researcher might take the subject into the waiting room of the outpatient rehabilitation clinic to test the subject's ability to follow a conversation in a moderately stimulating environment. Finally, the research might test the subject's ability to follow a conversation in a private therapy room.

Distinct from variation that would be inherent in observing subjects in their natural settings, semistructured settings can be applied uniformly across subjects. However, in contrast to a laboratory setting in which even more control can be imposed over the level of environmental stimulation, semistructured environments still introduce certain risks for confounding the research question. The obvious advantage of standardization is

that it allows the researcher to control the environment across subjects. The disadvantages include limitations to the generalizability to the subject's natural environment and elicitation of responses to the artificiality of the environment.

In deciding the level of control over observational context, a researcher must consider a number of variables. These include, but are not limited to, the nature of the research question and the vulnerability of the research subjects to the influence of environmental variation on their behavior. Finally, the researcher must consider the feasibility of conducting the observation within different types of environments.

Interviews

Interviews typically allow a researcher to collect information that leads to a broader, more holistic, or more integrative view of a subject's impairment or life situation. In OT research, interviews are most commonly utilized to obtain the following types of information:

- Sociodemographic and sociocultural information about subjects (e.g., age, ethnic identification, educational status, annual income, and extent to which culturally diverse clients identify with and practice health-related beliefs and behaviors that are related to their culture of origin);
- Historical information (e.g., health history, history of events leading up to the impairment);
- Information about a subject's experience of his or her current impairment and its functional consequences (this may include information about a subject's volition, habits, roles, and performance capacity);
- Psychosocial information (e.g., available social support, other resources and coping abilities, available sources of assistance within a subject's social network, sources of stress or conflict within a subject's social network);
- Information about a subject's physical living environment (e.g., safety and accessibility within home, work, and community environments); and
- Employment information (e.g., work history, current work status, work performance issues, need for and access to reasonable accommodation).

Methods of Recording Interview Data

There are three general methods of interviewing:

- Structured interviews,
- Semistructured interviews, and
- Unstructured interviews.

Structured interviews are comprised of a set of preestablished questions that follow strict administration and scoring rules. They are used in quantitative research and mostly gather ordinal and nominal data. In many cases, the scoring of structured interviews follows a very rigid and well-defined set of rules or template. In many instances, these interviews ask subjects to select from among responses provided by the interviewer. Questions that ask interviewees to give an open-ended response are generally focused, and the interviewer either records or codes the response using a standard coding scheme. Structured interviews may contain skip patterns that tell an interviewer that he or she may skip certain questions based on a subject's responses to prior questions. They also may contain allowable probing questions or explanations that interviewers can use when subjects do not respond accurately or fully or when they do not understand a question.

The high level of structure is designed to minimize interviewer bias. The structured interview also helps eliminate inaccuracies in scoring or subjective interpretation of responses on the part of the interviewer. Other advantages of structured interviews include their ease of administration (particularly for beginning therapists or researchers), their time-limited nature, and their ease in scoring.

Semistructured interviews may be used in quantitative research to generate data that are later coded or categorized. They are also used to generate more narrative accounts for qualitative research. These interviews use a preestablished schedule of open-ended questions, but they allow considerable flexibility in how they are administered. Semistructured interviews typically also allow interviewers to tailor questions and probes to obtain more in-depth and trustworthy information. When administering a semistructured interview, an interviewer may pursue questioning in a related area to obtain a different perspective or to shed light on the subject's responses to the interview questions at hand. Semistructured interviews require a higher level of clinical judgment, interpersonal skill, knowledge, and expertise on the part of the interviewer. Because scoring or coding rules are much less rigid, interviewers must decide:

- Whether a respondent's answer to each item is accurate, detailed, and comprehensive enough;
- What additional information is needed;
- What kinds of questions are required to probe for that information; and
- How to limit tangential or overly lengthy responses.

The advantages of semistructured interviews are that they allow for better rapport-building and more detailed and in-depth understanding of the variables of interest. The disadvantages can include length of administration and greater vulnerability to interviewer bias.

Unstructured interviews are used in qualitative research. These interviews may be guided by only a general topic or short list of topics that the interviewer pursues. Alternatively, the content of the interview may depend on an issue that is raised by a participant or a recent observation. Although investigators conducting this type of interview are usually guided by a broad study question, they remain open to new topics that may emerge in the interview itself.

Unstructured interviews have the advantage of being able to discover new information and establish a sense of trust (that the investigator really wants to understand and hear the participant's perspective). They require substantial time, interviewing skill, and contextual knowledge. Because, however, unstructured interviews ordinarily take place as part of an ongoing qualitative study in which the investigator is also a participant observer, they benefit from the background knowledge of the interviewer.

Sources of Interview Data

In every interview, there are three possible sources of data:

- Verbal data provided by the subject/respondent,
- Behavioral data, and
- Proxy verbal data provided by significant others, family, friends, and coworkers.

When interviews are used in occupational therapy, the most common source of interview data is the subject. During an interview, a subject is required to respond to questions based on some degree of reflection about his or her experience and/or needs. All interviews require subjects to have the ability to reflect honestly upon their impairments and experiences with a reasonable level of accuracy. Depending on the variables of interest in a research study, participating in an interview may require varying degrees of self-awareness or insight.

Depending on the nature of the interview and the variables under study, behavioral information may also be generated during an interview. In some cases, it may be factored into the overall outcome or score of the interview. Nonverbal information may include subjects' behavioral and affective responses to interview questions, their facility in processing auditory information, and their communication/interpersonal skills.

In many circumstances, a researcher may wish to obtain information about a subject through reports from significant others, family, friends, or coworkers. Data provided on behalf of a subject by others who are close to the subject may be used to corroborate information provided by a subject or to fill in informational gaps within the subject's self-report. In some cases, it is not possible to obtain self-reported interview information from a subject directly because of impairment-related issues. Under these circumstances, interview data from proxy sources may be helpful.

Role of the Interviewer

Establishing rapport is fundamental to every interview. Depending on the preferences and reactions of the subject, achieving rapport can be a relatively straightforward process, or it can be rather lengthy and complex. Some individuals will respond well to a brief period of introductions and small talk before an explanation of interview procedures is provided. Others will prefer that the researcher assume a more professional stance and explain the procedures upfront without preliminary chatter. The interviewer's first role is to make his or her best estimate of the interpersonal preferences of any given subject and act accordingly.

Because there is a potential for the researcher to be viewed as an authority figure in any interview situation, it is important to know or predict how the subject might respond given the automatic power differential involved in an interview situation. Some subjects will feel uncomfortable providing difficult or intimate information to a relative stranger. In such circumstances the researcher must do everything possible to ensure confidentiality and to create an atmosphere of unconditional acceptance and positive regard.

Although the role of an interviewer is clear with respect to the nature of the task, the need to establish rapport, and the power differential involved, interviewers can differ in significant ways in terms of their more nuanced behavior and roles. For example, an interviewer's role may vary according to whether the research is quantitative or qualitative. During an interview that seeks to obtain quantitative data, an interviewer may assume a more formal role. The interviewer may ask the subject to select an answer among a limited number of options, set more limits on side conversations, and/or discourage the interviewee from providing unnecessary details or extraneous information when answering open-ended questions.

Self-Report Measures

Self-report measures are written instruments on which subjects are asked to record information. They typically ask the subject to self-reflect on his or her experience or needs and select the best option from a finite number of categories or to provide an open-ended explanation as a response. Self-report measures are typically self-administered by subjects, and responses are usually provided in writing. However, under certain circumstances (e.g., subjects that require accommodations) subjects may provide verbal responses that the researcher records.

When asking for factual information, self-reports may ask a subject to:

- Report demographic characteristics (e.g., age, gender, race);
- Rate the severity or frequency of certain symptoms or impairments (e.g., "I am able to walk a flight of stairs with no pain" never, sometimes, frequently, always);
- Respond to open-ended questions (e.g., what one typically does at a specific time of the day or what types of difficulties one has performing a given task); or
- Respond to dichotomous questions (e.g., yes–no questions as to whether one can or does perform a given task).

Self-Rating Scales

Some self-reports involve completing self-rating scales. Self-rating scales are used to capture constructs such as personality characteristics (e.g., degree of assertiveness in relationships), attitudes (e.g., how much value one attaches to leisure or work), emotional states (whether one is depressed or anxious), and behavior patterns (to what extent exercise is part of an individual's daily routine).

They can also ask an individual to evaluate him- or herself more directly in terms of his or her performance capacity (e.g., how competent one is at performing a task). The most common form of a unidimensional rating scale is the Likert scale. It most frequently uses a five-category ordinal rating technique in which qualitative statements are used to differentiate positions on a continuum. One example of a commonly utilized self-report measure in OT research that utilizes Likert scaling is the Medical Outcomes Survey Short-Form 36 (SF-36). The eight subscales of this measure each contain Likert scale items that are designed to assess self-reported health-related quality of life and functional impairment.

Semantic Differential, Q-Sort, and Visual Analogue Scales

In addition to instruments that utilize Likert scales, another type of self-report instrument is the semantic differential. The semantic differential asks the respondent to rate a given concept on a series of bipolar adjectives that are used to characterize one's reaction or feelings (e.g., free versus constrained, dull versus exciting). The Q-sort is a self-report method that encourages respondents to organize data into visual categories (e.g., adjectives written on index cards are sorted into piles). During the Q-sort procedure, respondents are expected to sort the visual data into piles that represent meaningful categories. Visual analogue scales employ a straight line with labels to anchor each end. Subjects are then asked to mark the point on the line that corresponds most closely to their experience. Visual analogue scales typically employ a line that is 100 mm in length so that scoring can be accomplished with use of a standard ruler. Semantic differentials, Q-sorts, and visual analogue scales are typically used in the assessment of subjective experiences or less tangible phenomena that are sometimes difficult to describe verbally, such as pain or fatigue.

Unstandardized Questionnaires

No data exist on the reliability and validity of unstandardized questionnaires. They are typically created by investigators for their own use in preliminary studies to gather wide-ranging information about a novel variable or to gather information about a novel population. Researchers are more likely to use unstandardized questionnaires when existing measures do not address the variables of interest and a new measure must be generated. For example, an OT researcher interested in gathering general information about practitioners' attitudes and knowledge about treating a new type of disability in practice might wish to administer a preliminary survey questionnaire that contains items that assess a broad range of variables.

The benefit of unstandardized questionnaires includes their potential to provide rough preliminary information about a wide range of variables. Because of the need for standardized instruments to contain items that cohere with one another and reflect a general construct or constructs, reliable and valid questionnaires tend to be more limited in their breadth and scope. Despite this, unstandardized questionnaires carry a number of limitations. Generally, their accepted use in research is limited to descriptive studies that are preliminary in nature and aim to report general information about a single sample. They are less frequently used in experimental and clinical outcome studies.

Administration of Self-Reports

The most common method of administration of a self-report measure is to provide individuals with a written form. Forms may be given to a subject to be filled out in the presence of the investigator or to be completed at the respondent's discretion and returned later. In addition, forms may be mailed to individuals for responses. Instructions for completing the form may be given verbally or provided in writing on the form itself. When self-reports are mailed to respondents, the instructions are typically provided in writing.

Increasingly, self-reports are being administered using computer-based technologies. For example, researchers who work with relatively large samples of subjects are increasingly posting and administering self-report measures online via the Web. An advantage to online administration is that it can be organized so that subjects' responses are automatically downloaded and scored using a data entry and scoring program. Depending on sample size, online administration may save costs that would otherwise be incurred through printing and postage. However, one must weigh the overall cost of the computer software and programming required to develop, post, protect, and manage the survey and the data records of each of the respondents. This approach requires that subjects in the study have computer access and computer aptitude. There are also a number of considerations regarding the confidentiality and overall security of the data that must be taken into account.

Portable approaches to computer-based administration can be used to gather repeated self-report measurements. Subjects are typically provided with a handheld personal computer or a small data recording device. They can be programmed to cue (e.g., beep) an individual to provide his or her self-report at various times throughout the day, week, or month. Studies that aim to measure an outcome variable that is subject to change periodically throughout the day typically use this approach. For example, if an investigator wished to measure the effects of overall activity levels on the subjective experience of pain, subjects might be provided with a handheld device that would cue the person periodically (e.g., at fixed or random time points) throughout the day to answer questions about what the subject is currently doing and to rate pain level on a visual analogue scale.

Standardized Tests and Performance Measures

Standardized tests involve contrived cognitive or motor tasks that are administered and scored under strictly standardized conditions and typically generate norm-referenced or criterion-referenced scores. Examples of standardized tests include intelligence and aptitude tests, tests of motor proficiency, and cognitive performance tests. A substantial amount of research goes into developing these tests.

Performance measures commonly involve everyday tasks (although they may be somewhat standardized) that are observed to allow researchers to measure performance in the task. For example, the Assessment of Motor and Process Skills (AMPS; Center for Innovative OT Solutions, 2015) is used to observe clients in selected activities of daily living (ADLs) and instrumental activities of daily living (IADLs). It measures the quality of an individual's performance (i.e., motor and process skills).

Advantages and Disadvantages of Standardized Tests and Performance Measures

One advantage of standardized tests and performance measures is that they are widely used and widely accepted as rigorous measures of outcomes. Because they are widely used, they facilitate comparison of any investigator's findings from a given study with those of another investigator from a different study. Disadvantages of standardized tests and performance measures are that they are sometimes too general or broad to answer the more detailed questions that a researcher may have. In addition, not all are cross-cultural in nature and may not be relevant to all sociodemographic and sociocultural groups.

Administration of Standardized Tests and Performance Measures

Standardized tests are typically administered under standardized conditions that are consistent with those that were set when the test was initially developed. Depending on the nature of the test, these conditions might involve having a subject sit at a desk within a research office to respond to a written questionnaire or having a subject perform certain behaviors or tasks in a laboratory or clinical area using standard equipment.

Contextual and Environmental Assessments

In occupational therapy, **contextual and environmental assessments** typically measure aspects of physical, social, educational, or work-related settings in which subjects perform daily life occupations. An example of a contextual assessment that measures the extent to which an individual's physical environment facilitates or thwarts his or her occupational adaptation is the School Setting Interview (Hoffman, Hemmingsson, & Kielhofner, 2005), a semistructured interview that measures the extent to which all of a child's educational environments support engagement and participation in learning activities. Similarly, the Work Environment Impact Scale (WEIS; Moore-Corner, Kielhofner, & Olson, 1998) is a semistructured interview scale that evaluates features of an individual's work environment as they support or interfere with job functioning.

OT researchers who incorporate qualitative strategies may focus on the social and cultural aspects of a subject's occupational context. For example, a researcher interested in the daily routines of homeless individuals with mental illness might observe and document the effects of a number of contextual and environmental variables.

Focus Groups and Town Hall Meetings

A **focus group** is a group discussion conducted by an investigator who serves as a moderator, guiding the discussion by introducing questions, usually from a written set of questions or topics. Ordinarily, data are recorded in the form of audiotapes, which are then transcribed, as well as notes taken by the moderator or another investigator whose role is to record information.

Focus groups ordinarily include between 5 and 15 participants; the aim of the group size is to achieve a balance between ensuring that all members have an opportunity to share their views while including enough members to represent the diversity of existing viewpoints (Krueger & Casey, 2008). Focus groups are used to explore people's perceptions and attitudes regarding topics in which the participants have some investment or stake (Bernard, 2011; Krueger & Casey, 2008; Morgan & Spanish, 1984; Nabors, Ramos, & Weist, 2001).

The advantages of focus groups are that data can be collected from several people at once and that the interaction between members can stimulate data that the investigator might not otherwise have gained. One of the main reasons for using focus groups is to obtain the kind of data that emerge when participants interact with and modify each other's responses. One disadvantage is that some persons, especially those with minority opinions, might be discouraged from sharing their views. Therefore, the researcher aims to create a milieu that encourages participants to share their perceptions and views without the need for overall group consensus (Krueger & Casey, 2008).

Within a single study, researchers may replicate the focus group with different sets of participants who represent a particular constituency. Replication of focus groups representing a particular constituency can reveal common themes, trends, and patterns (Krueger & Casey, 2008). Investigators will also sometimes conduct different focus groups composed of persons who represent different constituencies in a setting (e.g., a focus group composed of staff and a focus group composed of clients in a health-care setting). In this instance the focus groups are designed to emphasize differences in the perceptions of different constituencies.

Focus groups are increasingly used as a method of data collection in both qualitative and quantitative research. In quantitative research, focus groups often serve as a first stage of research or as a pilot study to ensure that later data collection procedures will focus on relevant questions, reflect the perspectives, and be understandable to subjects.

Focus groups are increasingly used to develop and evaluate health-related interventions and programs (Heary & Hennessy, 2002; Hildebrandt, 1999). The following is an example. Ivanoff (2002) used focus groups to develop an occupation-based health education program for adults with macular degeneration. Focus groups were conducted to gain an insider perspective on how vision problems affected their daily lives. The focus group revealed both these elders' insecurities regarding their daily occupations and the strategies they employed to be able to perform their occupations. Findings generated from the focus groups informed the development of the intervention. Postintervention focus groups were used to evaluate the program and to generate ideas for further program development.

Biometry and Physiological Measures

Biometry and physiological measures are objective means of assessing any range of variables that involve physical, biological, or physiological functioning. Examples of biometric measures of physical functioning that are commonly used by OT researchers include measures of grip strength (e.g., dynamometer), endurance (e.g., how long an individual can sustain a motor movement), and range of motion (e.g., joint range of motion specific to seating). Increasingly, OT researchers are beginning to conduct interdisciplinary and translational studies in which they collaborate with researchers from other disciplines to measure relationships between occupationally based variables and other biological or physiological variables, such as immune function, physical fitness, and/or cardiovascular functioning. For example, a study by Taylor and colleagues (2010) quantified the occupational and quality-of-life consequences of postinfectious fatigue following infectious mononucleosis. Adolescents with fatigue reported significantly lower rates of perceived competency, more difficulties with physical functioning, and poorer general health status than those who recovered.

Document Review

In many cases an important source of research data is **preexisting documents** or records. In health care, an important source of information is the medical record. Medical records can be used to extract a wide range of information that might be important to a researcher, including, but not limited to:

- Sociodemographic information;
- Medical and psychiatric diagnoses;
- Access to health insurance;
- Number, reason, and nature of contacts with medical care providers;
- Prior treatment plans;
- Treatments prescribed, provided, or recommended; and
- Treatment follow-through and outcomes.

Within health care, access to historical information of this nature, particularly without direct consent from the subject, is becoming increasingly difficult because of the necessity to protect the confidentiality and rights of the subjects on whom the documentation or records are based (refer to the section on Health Insurance Portability and Accountability Act [HIPAA] in Chapter 14).

Planning and Implementing Data Collection

The next section of this chapter reviews three steps generally taken by researchers to plan and implement data collection:

1. Selecting instruments and procedures for data collection,
2. Developing a data collection plan, and
3. Selecting and preparing personnel for data collection.

Each of these steps is discussed in detail in the following sections. Box 22.1 contains a checklist that can be used by researchers to facilitate self-evaluation of their selected approach to data collection.

Selecting Instruments and Strategies for Data Collection

One of the most important steps in the data collection process involves choosing the appropriate instrument and/or strategy for data collection. This choice has implications for the ease and efficiency of data collection and the quality of the data that are ultimately collected.

Generally, identification of data collection procedures requires careful and sometimes extensive investigation. Some useful strategies are:

- Examining the research literature and attending conference presentations to identify strategies and instruments being used by other investigators in one's topic area.
- Corresponding with other researchers about the state-of-the-art strategies and instruments being used in a given topic area. This allows one to have a more extensive dialogue about the strengths, limitations, and receptivity of a given procedure or instrument. It also allows an investigator to ask other researchers about details such as logistical considerations in administration, preferred approaches to scoring, and issues involving the instrument's sensitivity to change.
- Consulting Web-based and published compilations of assessments (see Resources at the end of the chapter).

When a tradition of research exists on a topic, there are often one or more quantitative instruments that

---

BOX 22.1   A Checklist for Preparing for Data Collection

1. Has the appropriate data collection procedure been selected? ____
(Check off only if all of the following questions are endorsed.)
- Is the information gathered relevant and sufficient to answer the study question? ___
- Is the data collection approach methodologically rigorous enough to adequately address the study question? ___
- Have all relevant logistical variables related to the overall study design, available resources, and subject characteristics been accounted for?

___
- Are norms or other criteria for interpreting the instrument needed and available? ___
- Is the type of data that the instrument yields appropriate for the study question, and will it need to be normalized or transformed? ___
2. Has a data collection plan or protocol been developed? ___
(Check only if all of the following questions have been answered.)
- What data are to be collected?
- Who will obtain the necessary equipment, examination space, and instruments for data collection, and by when will they be obtained?

- Who will be collecting which types of data? Who will be administering each of the instruments?
- What training and qualifications will data collectors need, and by when will they be expected to have completed this training?
- At what time point in the study will data collection be initiated for each instrument or type of data that will need to be collected?
- What are the deadlines for completion of data collection for each data collection time point, instrument, or procedure?
- How will data be identified and coded for data entry? Who will enter the data, how will it be entered, and by when will it be entered? What program will be used for data entry?
- Who will analyze the data, and how will they be analyzed?
- How will data be disseminated? To what audiences?
3. Are the personnel involved in data collection adequately trained and prepared? ___
4. Have all relevant professional and ethical considerations been met? ___

are considered gold standards for collecting data on certain variables. For example, in rehabilitation-related outcome studies of health-related quality of life, the SF-36 (Ware & Sherbourne, 1992) is frequently the measure of choice, but the Quality of Life Index (Ferrans & Powers, 1992) is an equally valid and reliable instrument that measures somewhat distinct dimensions of health-related quality of life.

In choosing one instrument or strategy over another, the following criteria have been identified as important in guiding the selection of one's means of data collection (Depoy & Gitlin, 2010). Each is covered in detail in the following sections.

- Relevance and sufficiency of the information gathered to answer the study question;
- Extent to which the instrument or strategy conforms to standards of methodological rigor;
- Logistical considerations related to the overall study design, available resources, and subject characteristics;
- Availability of norms or criteria for interpreting the information gathered; and
- Type of data the instrument or strategy yields.

Relevance and Sufficiency of Data

In selecting an overall approach to data collection, the first consideration involves whether the approach is relevant to the research question on which the study is based. For example, an observational approach to data collection should be used when one is studying a question that involves a concretely observable phenomenon or behavior. If the research question involves a variable that is highly complex or difficult to observe, self-report or interview may be the correct approach. In the case of a complex research question or variable, a self-report approach may be combined with an observational approach to triangulate measurement.

A second important consideration when selecting an approach to data collection is whether the instrument or strategy represents an accurate reflection of the research question. Consider, for example, investigators studying the outcomes of an OT program designed to improve fine-motor skills in children or one designed to improve communication/interaction skills in adults. These investigators should select sound instruments that specifically measure the dependent variables (i.e., fine motor skills and communication/interaction skills) identified in the research questions.

In addition to these considerations, the way in which an investigator approaches the questions of relevance and sufficiency of data collection approaches depends on the methodology of the study. In quantitative studies, the primary focus of relevance is whether the method of data collection provides accurate data that reflects the variable(s) under investigation and is suitable to the anticipated sample.

Methodological Rigor

The methodological rigor of data collection depends on whether there is evidence in the literature that a quantitative instrument is valid and reliable or that a qualitative strategy is trustworthy. Researchers should ask themselves four questions in evaluating whether a given instrument or strategy for data collection is indicated:

1. What does this evidence say about the reliability and validity of the instrument or about the trustworthiness of a strategy?
2. Does research evidence of reliability, validity, or trustworthiness of the instrument/strategy have relevance for the proposed study sample? Are there any reasons to expect that this sample may respond differently to the procedure than those with which the procedure has been studied?
3. If there is not sufficient evidence for dependability of the procedure with the proposed study sample, then is there some precedent in the literature for successful use of the instrument or strategy with the proposed study population?
4. Are there any logistical aspects of the study that would preclude recommended administration of an instrument or strategy?

One should examine what strategies or instruments have been successfully used by other researchers studying the same or similar research question or population. Consideration should be given to what strategies or instruments are most likely to give reliable and valid data given the particular phenomena to be studied and who the study participants will be. Sometimes preliminary pilot testing of strategies or instruments can give useful information about what are likely to be the best data collection strategies in a given context.

Logistical Considerations

In selecting appropriate instruments and strategies for data collection, researchers must also consider logistical elements of the study. The first logistical consideration is what the planned strategies and/or instruments require of participants in terms of their mental and physical performance capacity, personal time, and level of effort. One should also consider the impact of any strategies or instruments on their health and well-being. Participants should be asked to do only what is within their capacity and absolutely necessary to obtain necessary data. For ethical reasons, any inconvenience, stress, or risk involved in data collection must be clearly outweighed by the importance of the research question.

A second logistical consideration involves the resources that a given data collection procedure would require. Human resources (i.e., time and effort of the investigator or other study personnel) required by data collection procedures is the first major resource that must be considered. The anticipated number and length of different collection instruments or strategies should be examined in light of sample constraints (e.g., the schedules, locations, and availability of participants).

Economic resources are also important when selecting an appropriate data collection procedure. Considerations include the level of education or specialized training data collectors need because they have salary and cost implications. Moreover, the availability or cost of instruments, test kits and forms, scoring and data management and analysis software packages, necessary space, computers, telephones, and other equipment should be considered. If a study will involve data collection within the field, transportation resources and costs must also be considered.

A final logistical consideration in data collection involves the appropriateness of the data collection procedures for any unique characteristics of the sample and the subject burden posed by the data collection procedures. A particular concern in OT research is whether the intended participants have impairments that affect their ability to participate in any of the data collection methods to be utilized in the study. In some cases, the investigator may resolve this issue by removing barriers (e.g., providing a sign language interpreter or a written instrument in interview format, on audiotape, or in Braille). In other cases, the investigator will select a data collection method that does not require skills affected by the impairment.

Subject burden refers to the effort, inconvenience, pain, risk, and other factors that affect what will be required for or may be a consequence of data collection procedures. Subject burden increases with the time involved in data collection, the number of data collection instruments utilized, and the negative effects of any data collection procedure on a participant's emotional or physical well-being.

If subject burden is unduly high in a study, it will lead to low participation rates and high dropout rates. In turn, this will limit sample size and introduce sampling bias, which limits the degree to which the sample is representative of all individuals in the population under study. Researchers must constantly balance the need to obtain adequate, detailed, and comprehensive information against human and other costs involved in actually obtaining that information.

Availability of Norms or Criteria for Interpretation

A consideration in selecting an appropriate quantitative instrument for data collection involves whether norm-referenced scores are available for a given instrument. For many research questions, the availability of norms for a particular instrument may not be required. For example, if a researcher wishes to examine attitudes among occupational therapists regarding the importance of therapeutic use of self to OT outcomes, he or she does not need to utilize an instrument with norm-referenced scores. Alternatively, if the same researcher wishes to examine the extent of impairment in physical functioning among adults with cardiovascular disease over time, he or she may wish to compare subjects' baseline physical functioning scores against the instrument's available norms for individuals with cardiovascular disease on the physical functioning domain. This would yield added information about the comparability of the baseline physical functioning of the sample against national norms. If physical functioning findings are comparable, findings from the researcher's study are more likely to have greater generalizability to the larger population of individuals with cardiovascular disease.

In other instances, investigators may wish to use instruments that are criterion referenced. There are different approaches to criterion referencing. In some cases, there will be cutoff points assigned to scores that may indicate the presence of a problem or the point beyond which a person will be incapable of some criterion (e.g., independent living). Instruments based on item-response theory have built-in criteria because the items serve to represent a hierarchy of capacities, skills, attributes, and so forth. For example, the Volitional Questionnaire (de las Heras, Geist, Kielhofner, & Li, 2003) measures motivation for occupation, and it can indicate the level of motivation as indexed by items that range from low to high motivation. A person at a basic exploratory level shows interest but does not seek out challenges (a higher level, achievement motivation behavior). A person's score on this instrument indicates, then, which of the items on the instrument are below and which are above the person's level of motivation. This kind of criterion referencing is very helpful in interpreting a score.

Type of Data the Instrument Yields

The final consideration in selecting an approach to data collection involves examining the type of data that an instrument or strategy yields. By definition, quantitative instruments yield numeric data, and researchers need to consider whether the type of numeric output is sufficient for the kinds of analyses that will be needed to answer the research question (e.g., scale of measurement, sensitivity of the instrument so that its scores will detect change). Quantitative researchers also need to consider whether the type of numeric output yielded by a given instrument will require transformation to make it consistent with the numeric output yielded by other instruments used in the study.

Developing a Data Collection Plan or Protocol

After evaluating all of the considerations involved in selecting the appropriate procedures and instruments for data collection, a researcher must develop a data collection plan or protocol. This can often be incorporated into an overall study timeline. This plan should answer the following questions:

- What data are to be collected?
- Who will obtain the necessary equipment, examination space, and instruments for data collection and by when will they be obtained?
- Who will be collecting which types of data? Who will be administering each of the instruments?
- What training and qualifications will data collectors need, and by when will they be expected to have completed this training?
- At what time point in the study will data collection be initiated for each instrument or type of data that will need to be collected?
- What are the deadlines for completion of data collection for each data collection time point, instrument, or procedure?
- How will data be identified and coded for data entry? Who will enter the data, how will it be entered, and by when will it be entered? What program will be used for data entry?
- Who will analyze the data, and how will it be analyzed?
- How will data be disseminated? To what audiences?

To the greatest extent possible, all of these questions should be answered prior to initiating data collection.

Selecting and Preparing Personnel for Data Collection

In selecting and preparing personnel for data collection, a number of considerations need to be taken into account. For example, in some studies the quality of data collection is higher when data collectors share as many characteristics in common with study participants as possible. Depending on the research question and the degree of interpersonal interaction required in a given study, similarities in language, age, racial or ethnic background, and disability status can facilitate rapport and trust during data collection procedures. Other characteristics that will enhance data collection are good clinical judgment, interpersonal skills, observational skills, and the ability to grasp and understand the theoretical foundations for the data collection procedures.

In addition to these more fundamental qualities, data collectors should have adequate training and experience required for the data collection procedure. This may include generic training and more specialized training associated with the particular procedure. In most instances study-specific training and ongoing supervision of data collectors will be necessary. These measures help ensure that the particular approach to data collection is fully understood and implemented correctly. They also are useful to ensure that data collectors can relate well with the study population.

Professional and Ethical Considerations in Data Collection

Professional and ethical considerations ensure the safe and humane treatment of research participants. In addition to the required steps for obtaining ethical approval and complying with ethical procedures as outlined in Chapter 14 (e.g., informed consent and risk management), researchers need to take special precautions to limit subject burden. Although most institutions out of which research is conducted have internal review boards that ensure appropriate treatment of research participants, a number of more subtle issues must be considered during data collection.

Before beginning any data collection procedure, adequate rapport with subjects must be established. It is also the data collector's responsibility to maintain rapport throughout the procedure to the extent that it does not distract the participant or interfere with or confound the quality and efficiency of the data collection procedures. Rapport can be maintained during data collection by responding humanely and empathically to any uncomfortable circumstances or difficult disclosures made by the subject during data collection. Empathic responding involves:

• Naming, witnessing, and/or verbally acknowledging a difficult circumstance;
• Questioning the participant about his or her emotional or physical well-being; and
• Following through with any necessary actions to ensure the participant's safety and/or physical and emotional well-being.

Maintaining professional boundaries during data collection is equally important for the protection of research subjects. This means that researchers should avoid nonprofessional relationships with participants. Researchers should avoid unplanned disclosure of highly personal information to participants, and they should not accept personal gifts or money from participants. Researchers must ensure that participants are clear in their understanding of the limits to the researcher's role and availability in their care.

Summary

This chapter reviews the process of data collection, beginning with an overview of how data collection is viewed and approached within the quantitative methodological tradition. It defines and evaluates a wide range of procedures and approaches used for data collection within this tradition and reviews the three steps involved in the actual implementation of data collection within an investigation. The chapter concludes with a discussion of professional and ethical issues that involve the treatment of research participants during data collection. Although this chapter overviews the major considerations involved in selecting and using data collection procedures, readers who are planning data collection for a study should also refer to other chapters in the text as supplemental.

Review Questions

1. What data collection approaches are used in the field of OT research?
2. What are the pros and cons of utilizing an existing validated measure for data collection versus developing your own measure?
3. What must a researcher consider when ensuring the reliability and validity of data collection procedures for a study?
4. What are the key steps involved in planning a data collection process for a given study?
5. What are some of the professional and ethical considerations to follow when collecting data?

REFERENCES

Benson, J., & Schell, B. A. (1997). Measurement theory: Application to occupational and physical therapy. In J. Van Deusen & D. Brunt (Eds.), *Assessment in occupational therapy and physical therapy* (pp. 3–24). Philadelphia, PA: W. B. Saunders.

Bernard, H. R. (2011). *Research methods in anthropology: Qualitative and quantitative approaches* (5th ed). Thousand Oaks, CA: Sage.

Center for Innovative OT Solutions. (2015). *Assessment of Motor and Process Skills (AMPS)*. Retrieved from http://www.innovativeotsolutions.com/content/amps/

Clemson, L., Fitzgerald, M. H., Heard, R., & Cumming, R. G. (1999). Inter-rater reliability of a home fall hazards assessment tool. *Occupational Therapy Journal of Research, 19,* 83–100.

Crotty, M. (1998). *The foundations of social research: Meaning and perspective in the research process.* Crows Nest, Australia: Allen & Unwin.

de las Heras, C. G., Geist, R., Kielhofner, G., & Li, Y. (2003). *The Volitional Questionnaire.* Chicago, IL: University of Illinois at Chicago.

DePoy, E., & Gitlin, L. N. (2010). *Introduction to research: Understanding and applying multiple strategies* (4th ed.). St. Louis, MO: C. V. Mosby.

Ferrans, C. E., & Powers, M. J. (1992). Psychometric assessment of the Quality of Life Index. *Research in Nursing and Health, 15,* 29–38.

Heary, C. M., & Hennessy, E. (2002). The use of focus group interviews in pediatric health care research. *Journal of Pediatric Psychology, 27*(1), 47–57.

Hildebrandt, E. (1999). Focus groups and vulnerable populations: Insights into client strengths and needs in complex community health care environments. *Nursing and Health Care Perspectives, 20*(5), 256–259.

Hoffman, O. R., Hemmingsson, H., & Kielhofner, G. (2005). *The School Setting Interview* (Version 3.0). Nacka, Sweden: The Swedish Association of Occupational Therapists

Ivanoff, S. D. (2002). Focus group discussions as a tool for developing a health education programme for elderly persons with visual impairment. *Scandinavian Journal of Occupational Therapy, 9*(1), 3–9.

Krueger, R. A., & Casey, M. A. (2008). *Focus groups: A practical guide for applied research* (4th ed.). Thousand Oaks, CA: Sage.

Moore-Corner, R. A., Kielhofner, G., & Olson, L. (1998). *Work Environment Impact Scale.* Chicago, IL: Model of Human Occupation Clearinghouse, Department of Occupational Therapy, College of Applied Health Sciences, University of Illinois at Chicago.

Morgan, D. L., & Spanish, M. T. (1984). Focus groups: A new tool for qualitative research. *Qualitative Sociology, 7,* 253–270.

Nabors, L. A., Ramos, V., & Weist, M. D. (2001). Use of focus groups as a tool for evaluating programs for children and families. *Journal of Educational and Psychological Consultation, 12*(3), 243–256.

Neuman, W. L. (2009). *Social research methods: Qualitative and quantitative approaches* (7th ed.). Needham Heights, MA: Allyn and Bacon.

Portney, L. G., & Watkins, M. P. (2009). *Foundations of clinical research: Applications to practice* (3rd ed.). Upper Saddle River, NJ: Prentice-Hall.

Taylor, R. R., O'Brien, J., Kielhofner, G., Lee, S. W., Katz, B., & Meares, C. (2010). The occupational and quality of life consequences of chronic fatigue syndrome/myalgic encephalomyelitis in young people. *British Journal of Occupational Therapy, 73,* 524–530.

Ware, J. J., & Sherbourne, C. D. (1992). The MOS 36-Item Short-Form Health Survey (SF-36). Conceptual framework and item selection. *Medical Care, 30,* 473–483.

RESOURCES

There are useful publications that identify and review occupational therapy and related instruments for data collection. The following are two examples:

• Law, M., Baum, C., & Dunn, W. (2001). *Measuring occupational performance.* Thoroughfare, NJ: Slack. This book covers a wide range of measures that capture data on such aspects of occupational performance as play, work, activities of daily living, occupational role, and time use. There is also a discussion of qualitative procedures for obtaining data on occupational performance. This text includes information about studies of reliability and validity. Readers should be careful to search for additional publications beyond the publication date of this text.

• The *Buros Mental Measurements Yearbook,* published by the Buros Institute of Mental Measurements, University of Nebraska–Lincoln, provides descriptive information, references, and critical reviews of tests in the areas of personality, achievement, behavior assessment, education, and science.

There are also useful websites for identifying instruments and research on their reliability and validity.

• One such occupational therapy OT site is http://www.cade.uic.edu/moho/. It contains information on a number of instruments related to the Model of Human Occupation. Visitors to the site can learn about the available instruments, view copies of forms, and use a search engine to identify publications on reliability and validity.

• Health and Psychosocial Instruments (HAPI) is a searchable online database that contains research on published and unpublished information-gathering tools that are utilized in health and psychosocial research studies. The site is https://www.ebscohost.com/academic/health-and-psychosocial-instruments-hapi. Information on questionnaires, interview schedules, tests, checklists, rating and other scales, coding schemes, and projective techniques is available from 1985 onward. The database pertains to any medical or medically related condition or treatment outcome. It contains citations to actual test documents, bibliographic citations to journal articles that contain information about specific instruments, and a catalog of commercial test publishers and their available test instruments.

CHAPTER 23

Entering, Storing, and Managing Data

Marcia Finlayson • Toni Van Denend

Learning Outcomes

- List the kinds of information that are typically gathered to monitor and manage the progress of a study.
- Define the basic goal of data management and explain its relevance and importance to research.
- Identify the components of a data management plan.
- Explain the role of a management plan and project timeline in a study.
- Understand the importance of ongoing communication between research team members during the data collection and management process.
- Provide an example of how a coding error might occur during a study and how to prevent such an error from becoming systematically incorporated into a database.

Introduction

The ultimate goal of any research is to produce findings that others can trust and use. This goal is the same regardless of whether the study is quantitative and the findings will be judged on their reliability, validity, objectivity, and generalizability, or whether the study is qualitative and the findings will be judged on their dependability, credibility, neutrality, and transferability (Krefting, 1991). Occupational therapy (OT) researchers should always strive to do rigorous work that will contribute to the advancement of our theories and clinical practices (Kielhofner, Hammel, Finlayson, Helfrich, & Taylor, 2004).

Earlier chapters discussed many different factors that can threaten the quality of the research. Unfortunately, even the best designed study can fail if the research team does not plan for and address issues of data management. Despite many

publications and the wealth of knowledge about how integral data management is to rigorous investigation, its importance is still sometimes underestimated. Many researchers learn about data management by watching their mentors, talking to other researchers, picking up ideas at conferences, and learning from their own mistakes.

This chapter provides a framework for thinking about and planning data management processes and infrastructure. The authors also share some of their own experiences from investigations that they have planned and implemented, and they provide tools and resources that can be used and modified for other studies.

Basic Definitions

For the purposes of this chapter, **data management** is defined as the logistical, reflective, and behind-the-scenes processes and infrastructure that allow a researcher to produce high-quality information to address the study questions and describe how and what has been done during a study accurately and comprehensively.

In the context of data management, **data** refer to all of the pieces of information that are collected from research participants to address a study's questions and all of the information that is gathered to monitor and manage study progress. A few examples of this latter type of information include:

- Recruitment processes and outcomes;
- Progress on data collection, coding, entry, and cleaning;
- Status of data storage and security; and
- Documentation of decisions that will make it easier for the investigator to describe what he or she has done during the course of the study when it is time to disseminate the study findings.

For simplicity and clarity, the term *data* is used to refer to the information collected from

CASE EXAMPLE

Cassidy is an occupational therapy (OT) student in her first year. For her research class, she has been assigned to develop a data management plan for a simple study of the effects of therapeutic horseback riding on the core strength of preadolescent children with autism. Thirty children undertaking 15 weekly sessions of therapeutic horseback riding will be assessed for core strength with a 30-second sit-ups test. Consistent with a within-subjects pretest–posttest design, the children will be assessed before any of the 15 sessions begin (pretest or baseline), and then again after all 15 sessions have been completed (posttest). The number of sit-ups performed in 30 seconds will be counted at two time points: baseline (prior to beginning the therapeutic horseback riding sessions) and posttest (after completing the 15 sessions).

Cassidy begins by creating a project timeline. The lessons are scheduled to begin September 1, and students are taught weekly in six separate groups of five students each. Three groups take their lessons on Saturdays, and three groups take their lessons on Sundays. For her baseline data collection, Cassidy creates a plan to conduct the sit-ups tests on half of the children on Saturday and the other half on Sunday just before their first riding lesson begins. So that she is not overwhelmed by too much work at the end of the 15-week period, Cassidy writes that she will create an anonymous ID variable matched to each child's name and creates a variable within an SPSS database labeled "participant ID." Next, she writes in a data entry plan whereby she enters the number of sit-ups that each child completes for the pretest into an SPSS database under a variable labeled "pretest." After that time, she will create a final, third variable entitled "posttest" where the number of sit-ups will be entered following the test after the 15th lesson. Data will be saved and backed up to two different flash drives. As part of her plan, Cassidy also writes that she will double-check that all data were entered correctly against the data that she records during the actual test, using pencil and paper. Once all data are double-checked, they will, again, be saved and backed up to two different flash drives.

participants, and **project information** is used to refer to the other types of information that a data management system must track.

The Context of Data Management

To begin, it is important to understand the overall context of data management and how it fits within the research process. Figure 23.1 depicts the relationship between data management and research design and illustrates that the ultimate goal of data management is to support the production of findings that are trustworthy and are useful to others. The figure also illustrates that data management is done in conjunction with design. In other words, designs that are truly rigorous must include planning for data management as part of the process, and strong data management systems must take into account the research design (McFadden, LoPresti, Bailey, Clarke, & Wilkins, 1995). These two processes are inseparable in the production

of good-quality data (Nyiendo, Attwood, Llyod, Ganger, & Haas, 2002).

Finally, the figure emphasizes that good-quality data does not automatically mean trustworthy findings that others can use. Selecting the correct analytic techniques for the data that are available and using these techniques appropriately will determine the value of a study's findings. Using techniques appropriately means that a researcher must understand the type of data needed for a given analytic strategy, understand the assumptions of the technique and how these can be determined, and interpret results correctly.

The Importance of Data Management

The larger the project, the more sophisticated the data management plan will be, but all investigators need to plan for and implement a basic system, regardless of the size of their study. Data management is important for:

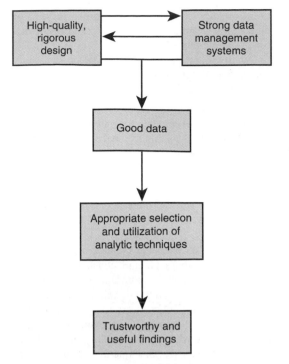

Figure 23.1 The context of data management.

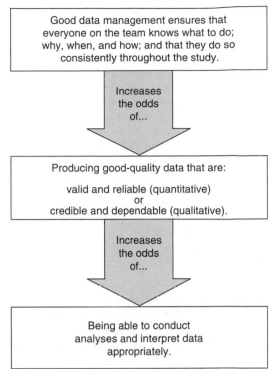

Figure 23.2 The importance of data management.

- Supporting a culture of consistent communication;
- Minimizing data collection and entry errors;
- Facilitating data analysis and interpretation of findings;
- Maximizing data quality by promoting internal validity (credibility) and reliability (dependability) of data;
- Ensuring data security and confidentiality;
- Ensuring compliance with relevant laws;
- Facilitating the preparation of the research report, including the identification of study strengths and limitations; and
- Facilitating data archiving and sharing.

These are summarized in Figure 23.2.

At the most basic level, a data management plan will facilitate and support communication about the research study across members of a project team and between the team and external parties (e.g., participants, funders, colleagues, editors). The plan will offer guidance about how to carry out and document all research-related procedures and their consequences. For example, a data management plan should identify:

- Which members of the research team are responsible for identifying and contacting potential participants,
- What forms are to be used in this process,

- How and where information about new recruits is to be documented, and
- How calculations on response rates are to be summarized.

Documenting the steps and processes of a project makes it easier for all parties involved to be consistent during the course of a research study, regardless of the project's size or the type of research being conducted (e.g., ethnographic, experimental, survey, etc.; Antonakos, Miller, & Caruso, 2002; Gassman, Owen, Kuntz, Martin, & Amoroso, 1995).

Using consistent processes and procedures throughout a project will reduce the likelihood of making errors in the course of data collection and/ or entry of the data into analytic software systems. Minimizing errors at the beginning and throughout a study will reduce problems later in the process that could negatively influence the speed or accuracy of data analysis, limit the types of analyses that are possible, or increase the challenges of preparing the research report (Chan et al., 2013; Hosking, Newhouse, Bagniewska, & Hawkins, 1995; Pogash, Boehmer, Forand, Dyer, & Kunselman, 2001). For example, one of the data management processes used in the *Aging With MS: Unmet*

Needs in the Great Lakes Region Study[1] was a regular team meeting to discuss problems encountered in coding unusual participant responses. During these meetings, the interviewing team and principal investigator discussed the problem, made a coding decision, and then documented that decision for inclusion in the policy and procedure manual. In this way, everyone on the team had access to the decision and was able to code the data in a consistent way if and when the problem occurred again. Without this process, it is likely that unusual responses would not have been consistently coded and would have caused problems later in the analysis phase.

Documentation of policies (rules) and procedures (explanations about how to implement the rules) is a major aspect of a data management plan (Gassman et al., 1995). Documentation for a study should explain:

- How to track what member of the research team has collected what data from which participants,
- When the data were collected,
- If any additional information needs to be collected,
- What the status of the data currently is (e.g., entered or not, where), and
- What data are missing and why. (Antonakos et al., 2002; Chan et al., 2013)

By having all of this information at hand, a data management system facilitates the preparation of a comprehensive and detailed methods section of research and technical reports, as well as other forms of dissemination. Methods that are well documented will be transparent and therefore will be viewed as supporting the internal validity (credibility) and reliability (dependability) of the study.

A strong data management system also ensures that a research team is able to maintain the security of the data collected from participants and demonstrate that guidelines for the protection of human subjects have been followed. It also ensures that the research is in compliance with any other laws that are relevant to the conduct of the research (e.g., Health Insurance Portability and Accountability Act [HIPAA], professional licensing when delivering an intervention, etc.; Hosking et al., 1995; McFadden et al., 1995). It is important to remember that the human subjects committee that approves a study is free to audit the research for compliance at any time. Failing

to follow regulations regarding human subjects or other relevant guidelines or laws could result in a project being closed.

Finally, data management will facilitate study and data archiving that will, in turn, make it easier for a research team to:

- Compare its findings to other similar studies,
- Provide data to students for thesis or dissertation work based on secondary analyses, and
- Share data with other researchers who seek to build on the work that has already occurred.

Being able to explain to others what was done, and how and why, will facilitate later data analyses by members of the team or others who have an interest in the topic.

Failing to address data management in a comprehensive, methodical, and consistent way will result in inconsistencies within and across staff or over time; limit the quality or detail of the methods description in a published article; jeopardize data quality and confidentiality; or, even worse, raise questions about the internal validity or credibility of an entire study. Consequently, data management needs to be included during the initial proposal preparation stages of any research study (see Fig. 23.1). The system needs to be updated as the project evolves so that new issues are addressed and new decisions are documented.

It should be clear at this point that developing a strong data management system involves more than just recording participants' responses to the study questions and measures. It is an administrative process that supports rigorous research and involves:

- Documenting how all forms of data and project information will be collected, handled, stored, and prepared for use;
- Developing tools and systems to operationalize the documentation; and
- Following through on the use of these tools and systems, refining and adding to them as the project evolves over time.

Components of Data Management

Translating the knowledge of why data and project information should be tracked to the actual creation of a data management system is often not straightforward. The process can be significantly complicated by the breadth and depth of what must be monitored, and it will clearly be influenced by the size and scope of the research project,

[1]This project is based on a contract awarded to Dr. Marcia Finlayson by the National Multiple Sclerosis Society through a Health Care Delivery and Policy Research Contract, 2002 to 2005.

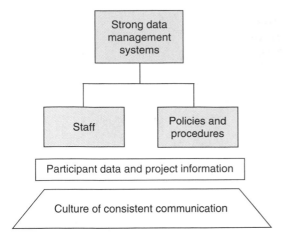

Figure 23.3 Key components of a data management system.

the number of staff involved, and the presence of more than one research site (Gassman et al., 1995; McFadden et al., 1995). Therefore, it can be helpful to think about the components or parts of a data management system when beginning the process. Figure 23.3 illustrates that a strong data management system includes:

• Participant data,
• Project information,
• Processes and infrastructure related to staff, and
• A clearly defined set of policies and procedures.

Furthermore, these components are premised on a foundation of a culture of consistent communication. In the context of data management, consistent communication includes (Gassman et al., 1995; McFadden et al., 1995):

• Verbal and written communication among members of the team (e.g., principal investigator, co-investigators, research assistants, analysts) via team meetings, e-mails, texts, shared, web-based documents, and so forth; and
• Documentation of individual work and decisions (e.g., maintenance of study notebooks, laboratory books).

Written documentation enables the team and others (e.g., funders, collaborators, people using the data for secondary analyses) to track decisions about different aspects of the project easily and to clearly understand the logic behind these decisions. As a project unfolds, documentation will facilitate consistency in how data management problems are resolved (e.g., coding unusual participant responses; Gassman et al., 1995).

Ultimately, without consistent communication, any data management system is at risk of crumbling and therefore compromising both the quality of the data produced and the ability to support the production of trustworthy and useful findings. Later sections of this chapter elaborate on some of the specific tools and strategies that can be used to support the production of good-quality data. We will also point out specific strategies that promote consistent communication.

To summarize this discussion on the components of data management, it is important to think of a data management system as both a product and a dynamic process. When done well, it is the infrastructure that allows the research study to be carried out as planned. When there are problems with data management, even the best designed and funded study can fail to address its intended objectives.

Data Management Issues

Before discussing some of the specific tools that can facilitate data management, a number of issues that need to be considered when developing a data management system will be identified. Some of these issues have already been uncovered in the discussion of the importance and components of data management, for example, specifying the roles and responsibilities of team members, documenting activities, tracking respondents, and so forth. To highlight key issues, see the expanded version of Figure 23.3 shown in Figure 23.4.

This figure illustrates the different types of issues that an investigator needs to consider under both the staff component (e.g., selection of team members) and the policies and procedures component (e.g., data access and security, documentation) of the data management system. Clearly, this figure is not all-inclusive, given the variability across projects, research designs, and populations being studied and the size of different studies. Nevertheless, experience suggests that addressing each of the seven issues included in Figure 23.4 is key to increasing the likelihood of high-quality data management.

The specific tasks that need to be completed to address each of the data management issues identified in Figure 23.4 are outlined in Table 23.1. In addition, an explanation of the importance of doing each of these tasks and when to do them is provided in Table 23.1. A quick scan of the final column of Table 23.1 shows that most of the issues for data management need to be considered during the initial proposal development. This timing is

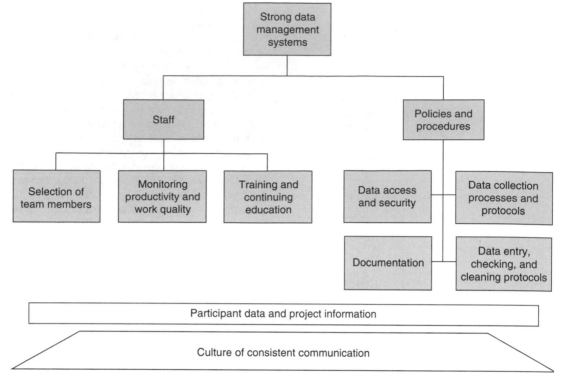

Figure 23.4 Specific issues to be considered in a data management system.

critical because human and financial resources are often required to manage data and project information well (McFadden et al., 1995). Often, new investigators do not fully appreciate the amount of time that is required to manage the everyday administrative aspects of a study, and they fail to incorporate adequate staff time in their project budget. By thinking through data management and carefully analyzing the requirements of the project from beginning to end, an investigator will be in a better position to plan the necessary resources to support project infrastructure (McFadden et al., 1995).

Specific Tools and Resources to Facilitate Data Management

Good data management involves a range of tools and processes that allow the researcher to:

- Track what has been done,
- Track what still needs to be done, and
- Ensure that the final research report and findings will be recognized as products of a rigorous and believable process.

This section includes specific examples of tools that can be used in the process of managing data. Table 23.2 presents the linkages between the tools and resources that are presented in this section and the data management issues from Figure 23.4 and Table 23.1.

These tools and resources are particularly helpful, and their use is supported in the existing literature on data management. What is presented here represents only a sampling of what is possible and does not include all of the different tools that can be used to facilitate data management. The tools described are intended to offer a starting point for those with little or no experience in developing data management systems. Not everything that is presented over the next few pages will be relevant to every project.

Management Plan and Project Timeline

The management plan and project timeline is typically prepared as part of the research proposal. A brief example is provided in Table 23.3. As a data management tool, a **management plan and project timeline** is helpful in identifying the specific tasks that will need to be done over the course

Table 23.1 Data Management Issues, Tasks, Importance, and Timing

Issues to Consider (from Fig. 23.4)	Specific Tasks	Importance	Timing
Staff — Selection of team members	• Determine what skills are needed across the members of the team (e.g., administering specific assessments, delivering interventions, creating data files, entering data, conducting analyses). • Determine the qualifications of individuals who can fulfill these skill requirements. • Clarify the roles, responsibilities, and performance expectations associated with specific jobs on a research team. • Outline reporting and accountability lines, which are important for staff monitoring. • Develop job descriptions. • Use job descriptions to recruit potential team members. • Screen qualifications of potential team members. • Select individuals who have the necessary skills and experience to meet the project needs. • Ensure that members of the research team understand their job descriptions.	• Ensures all aspects of project are being addressed across the members of the team • Enables the principal investigator to put together a team that can meet all of the needs within a project	• Consider during proposal development. • Reconsider and refine at time of project initiation.
Monitoring productivity and work quality	• Track whether staff members are doing the tasks they are assigned, in the way that they were trained. • Monitor staff for ongoing continuing education needs. • Provide opportunities for team members to identify potential problems that may later influence data quality, and solve them before it is too late. • Create and implement systems to address problems in productivity and work quality.	• Ensures that the principal investigator can maintain the rigor of the project	• Consider during proposal development. • Begin and maintain after project is started and staff is hired. • Update as required during project.
Training and continuing education	• Identify project-specific training needs for staff members as a group, as well as individually (e.g., roles and responsibilities, specific job duties, lines of authority and accountability). • Prepare and deliver staff training and continuing education materials. • Develop system to keep staff up to date on the latest developments in the field that may impact a project.	• Enables the principal investigator to contribute to the maturation and sophistication of a team over time	• Consider during proposal development. • Begin and maintain after project is started and staff is hired. • Update as required during project.
Policies and Procedures — Data access and security	• Design and implement a system for assigning ID codes. • Identify who has access to what information (e.g., budgets, participant information, specific data files). • Provide team members with explicit guidelines for: 　○ How and where data and project information are to be stored, 　○ What information is to be password protected (e.g., participant contact information), and 　○ What data needs to be separated (e.g., consent forms from data sheets). • Design and implement a system for conducting data and file backups.	• Ensures compliance with relevant laws, rules, and regulations • Protects participant confidentiality	• Consider at proposal development. • Refine upon human subjects review submission. • Follow-up on project initiation. • Modify as required during project.

Table 23.1 Data Management Issues, Tasks, Importance, and Timing

Issues to Consider (*from Fig. 23.4*)	Specific Tasks	Importance	Timing
Documentation	• Identify what project information must be documented (e.g., recruitment responses, participant attrition and reasons). • Identify where project information is to be documented (e.g., specific files and their locations). • Determine when project information is to be documented (e.g., frequency). • Explain to members of the team the rationale for the documentation.	• Facilitates consistent decision-making • Supports all other aspects of the data collection system • Facilitates report preparation • Ensures compliance with relevant laws, rules, and regulations	• Consider at proposal development. • Begin at project initiation. • Refine and update throughout project.

Data collection processes and protocols	• Explain each of the specific steps to be taken during the data collection, including:
	  ∘ Prepare necessary scripts.
	  ∘ Prepare any anticipated protocols for addressing participants with cognitive impairments, use of proxy respondents, etc.
	  ∘ Prepare any resource materials data collectors will require (e.g., list of relevant phone numbers such as abuse or suicide hotlines).
	• Specify tasks and responsibilities for each member of the team during data collection.
	• Educate team members about how to consistently address challenging situations that may arise during the data collection process (e.g., dealing with participants who disclose abuse; uncovering cognitive impairment that may compromise informed consent).
		• Ensures consistency in data collection, and therefore maximizes data quality
		• Ensures compliance with relevant laws, rules, and regulations
			• Consider at proposal development.
			• Reconsider and refine upon project initiation.
			• Update and refine as new challenges emerge.

Data entry, checking, and cleaning protocols	• Identify each step of the data entry and cleaning process, including:
	  ∘ Who is responsible,
	  ∘ What specific tasks must be completed at what time,
	  ∘ What processes are to be used to confirm data entry, and
	  ∘ How data entry errors are to be documented and resolved.
	• Develop and maintain a code book.
	• Identify timing for data checking and cleaning.
		• Ensures quality data for analysis
		• Saves time at end of project by maintaining data files throughout project
			• Consider at proposal development.
			• Begin at project initiation, in conjunction with decisions about data collection.
			• Refine during data collection, but before data are being entered.

Table 23.2   Examples of Data Management Tools and Their Correspondence With Specific Data Management Issues

Tool, Resource, or Strategy	Data Management Issue Influenced by Tool, Resource, or Strategy	
	Staff	*Policies and Procedures*
Management plan and project timeline	• Monitoring productivity and work quality	• Documentation
Job descriptions	• Selection of team members • Monitoring productivity and work quality	• Data access and security • Data collection processes and protocols • Data entry, checking, and cleaning protocols
Systems to track participants and their data including • Participant identifiers • Master file • ID sheets	• Training • Monitoring productivity and work quality	• Data access and security • Documentation • Data collection processes and protocols
Systems for data entry and confirmation • Protocols for data coding, checking, and cleaning • Codebooks • Development of data collection forms	• Training • Selection of team members • Training • Monitoring productivity and work quality	• Data collection processes and protocols • Data entry and checking processes and protocols • Documentation
Team meetings	• Training • Monitoring productivity and work quality	• Documentation
Backup protocol	• Training	• Documentation • Data access and security

Table 23.3   Sample of a Part of a Management Plan and Project Timeline

Specific Project Tasks	Time Frame	People Responsible	Measure of Task Completion
Activity #2: Conduct focus groups with key informants			
2.1. Work with collaborators to select dates, times, and locations for focus groups	July to August, 2002	PC and RA	Dates and times set
2.2. Work with collaborators and Advisory Group members to identify potential participants for focus groups	July to August, 2002	PI, PC, AG, and RA	Potential participants identified
2.3. Set up office systems to manage focus group documents and data (e.g., master file, logistics task lists, transcription processes, etc.)	July to August, 2002	PI, PC, and RA	Office systems completed
2.4. Contact potential participants to invite participation and provide basic information about the focus group	August to September, 2002	PI, PC, possibly AG	No. of participants contacted

AG = members of advisory group; BM = departmental business manager; PC = project coordinator; PI = principal investigator; RA = research assistant; RS = research specialist; ST = statistician; TR = transcriptionist.

Excerpted from the data management plan for the study: "Aging With MS: Unmet Needs in the Great Lakes Region," Finlayson, principal investigator. Funded by the National Multiple Sclerosis Society, July 2002–June 2005, Contract no. HC0049.

of an entire project and when these tasks need to be completed. Having this information will facilitate the process of identifying the skills and knowledge that will be required of the research team, which will aid in their selection. Later on in the project, the management plan and project timeline will provide guidance for monitoring the productivity and work quality of team members and help in setting goals for data collection and for monitoring its progress.

Job Descriptions

For a research project to operate smoothly, the principal investigator must ensure that the people who are performing the various tasks within the project have the necessary skills and expertise to do so. Specifying these tasks and identifying the necessary qualifications of the individuals who will be performing these tasks are the first steps in developing job descriptions. In large projects when staff members are hired into a specific role, job descriptions facilitate a culture of consistent communication by clearly identifying the roles and responsibilities of each team member. For small projects in which one or two people play multiple roles, job descriptions can ensure that all tasks are addressed and assigned and that each person understands his or her responsibilities. Typical areas to include in a job description are:

• Job title,
• Name and title of direct supervisor,
• Summary of job character and purpose of the position,
• Qualifications and/or specific skills required, and
• Specific list of job duties.

Systems to Track Participants and Their Data

To obtain good-quality data, it is critical that an investigator can track participants throughout the course of a study (Nyiendo et al., 2002; Pogash et al., 2001). This information ensures that all information is collected from participants at the right times, that the data gathered from each participant are handled correctly, and that everyone can be accounted for at the end of the study, including the individuals who were recruited but never actually participated, those who dropped out, or those who were lost to the study (e.g., moved, died, etc.).

In the study *Addressing Concerns About Falling Among Older Adults With Multiple Sclerosis,*[2] the authors explained in detail the process of tracking participants and their data in their policy and procedure manual, including who is responsible to complete which parts of the process, when, and where. Figure 23.5 summarizes the process used, showing the connections between the initial recruitment of a participant and the final data file for analysis.

[2]This project is based on a grant awarded to Dr. Marcia Finlayson and Dr. Elizabeth Peterson by the Retirement Research Foundation, 2004 to 2007.

Figure 23.5 illustrates how a system for tracking participants and their data involves a series of individual tools, all of which are used in concert to achieve the goal of good-quality data. The specific tools and processes within these systems that will be discussed in more detail in this section include developing and assigning participant identifiers, creating and maintaining a master file, and developing and using participant ID sheets.

Developing and Assigning Participant Identifiers

To be able to track participants and their data, it is necessary to be able to link individual data items to the people from whom the data were collected. A participant identifier is a tool critical to this process. A **participant identifier** is a numeric or alphanumeric code (e.g., A-001) that is used in place of the participant's name on all documents pertaining to that individual. In terms of data management, assigning identifiers is more than simply ensuring that participant names are kept confidential, although that is a major reason for using identifiers. The actual process of assigning identifiers can facilitate the data collection and management process by providing a consistent variable that can be used to link files across the study (e.g., master participant list, data file, follow-up files, etc.).

To illustrate how the assignment of identifiers can facilitate data collection, consider the example of the study *Addressing Concerns About Falling Among Older Adults With Multiple Sclerosis* in Box 23.1. In this project, a national sample was used for telephone interviews. To facilitate the interviewing process and reduce the risk that participants would be called at inappropriate times of the day (as a result of differences in time zones), information about the participant's time zone was embedded into the identifier. In addition, because participants were divided into two age groups for sampling, age group was also embedded in the identifier to make it easier to identify how many interviews had been completed in each group.

Identifier information should be maintained in a password-protected file. When working in larger multisite studies, assignment of identifiers must be considered carefully so that when the final data are merged, there is no possibility that identifiers are duplicated. For example, one site may be assigned to use alphanumeric codes starting with the letter A, and the second site may be assigned identifiers starting with the letter B.

For therapists who are conducting research as part of their regular clinical duties, assigning identifiers must be done carefully to ensure that the

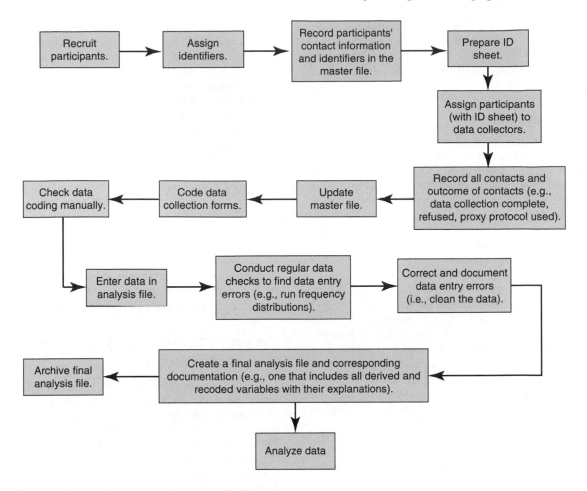

Figure 23.5 Tracking participants and their data.

Box 23.1 Assigning Identifiers—Sample Explanation

The senior research assistant will be responsible for intake, entry, and assigning ID numbers to all eligible respondents.
- ID numbers will be assigned based on time zone and age group.
- Time zone will be the first two digits in the ID code:
  - Eastern Time = ET
  - Central Time = CT
  - Mountain Time = MT
  - Pacific Time = PT
  - Alaska = AT
  - Hawaii = HT

- There are two age groups of interest in this study, 55–64 and 65+. The age groups will be designated as 01 (55–64) and 02 (65+). These will be the second two digits in the ID code.
- The remaining part of the ID code will be the sequential number of the respondent, e.g., 001, 002, 003, etc. Each age group is to have its own sequential numbering starting with 001. Time zone will not be considered in the sequential numbering—only age group.
- A sample ID would therefore be: MT-02-005.

Excerpted from the Policy and procedure manual from the study "Addressing Concerns About Falling Among People Aging With MS" (Finlayson & Peterson, 2004–2007, with funding from the Retirement Research Foundation).

research data and clinical data cannot be confused and inadvertently mixed together. Research data must be kept separate from the medical record and under separate identifiers.

Creating and Maintaining a Master File

When tracking participants and using forms and files to do so, it is important to note that documents containing both the participant's name and identifier should be kept to a minimum because of the sensitivity and confidentiality of these materials. Nevertheless, it is important in most studies to be able to link a participant identifier to information such as name, address, and/or telephone or other means of contact. A master file is one tool to address this data management need.

A basic master file typically contains participant identifying information (e.g., name, contact information) together with the participant identifier code. Because of the sensitivity of this information, this file must be password protected, and access to the file should be restricted to key members of the research team. Master files are usually electronic spreadsheet files. As new participants are recruited into a study, a participant identifier is assigned, and then the master file is updated (see Fig. 23.5). Depending on the project, the master file may also include process-related information, such as how many contacts were attempted with a participant, whether baseline or outcomes measures have been administered, or when follow-up appointments are to be scheduled. It is important to note that this type of information is not data for analysis, but rather data to track the progress of a participant through the study. Data that will be used for analysis are maintained in the analysis file. Personal contact information should never be kept in the analysis file.

Developing and Using Participant ID Sheets

After recruiting participants, assigning identifiers, and adding individuals to the master file, it is very important to do everything possible to maintain participant confidentiality. This typically means that only minimally necessary information about the participant is recorded on other data collection forms. In fact, actual data collection forms should never include the participant's name, but rather only the participant identifier. A key challenge of OT research is that data collectors usually need both the participant identifier as well as contact information, particularly if an intervention or interview

is involved and if the data collector must go out to the participant's home or workplace. Balancing the need to have this information and keeping it confidential can be challenging.

A participant ID sheet is one data management tool that can be used to address this dilemma and ensure that data collectors have the pieces of information they need to maintain their records, and at the same time minimize the number of places where the participant's name and identifier appear together. A sample participant ID sheet is provided in Figure 23.6. A major advantage of an ID sheet is that it can easily be removed from the participants' files when the information it contains is not germane to the activities of the research team. Maintaining clear protocols about how to handle the ID sheet, where it is to be stored, who can have access to it, and when it is to be destroyed is very important. Often, the human subjects' ethics committee will have guidelines about these issues.

Systems for Data Entry and Confirmation

Although data collection is often a major focus during the process of planning a study, it is equally important to consider how to enter and confirm these data after the collection is completed. The issues of data coding, checking, and cleaning are most often discussed in relation to data management, and other authors have described these processes in detail (see Aday & Cornelius, 2006; Hosking et al., 1995; Hulley et al., 2013; McFadden et al., 1995; Pogash et al., 2001; Portney & Watkins, 2009). Given that data coding, checking, and cleaning are process-oriented tasks, most investigators develop protocols to manage them. Therefore, the data management tools are the protocols themselves. In addition to these protocols, other related data management tools and strategies include codebooks and how data collection forms are developed.

Protocols for Data Coding, Checking, and Cleaning

In quantitative research, **data coding** involves translating participant responses into numerical values to facilitate statistical analysis. For variables that are continuous in nature (e.g., age, years since diagnosis), responses are already numerical, so coding simply involves entering a participant's value into the analysis file. For variables that are nominal or ordinal in nature, responses must be assigned a numerical value. For example, consider a survey question that asks participants to reflect

Aging with Multiple Sclerosis Study	

ID Form for Interviewers

Date reply form received:	
Date interview assigned:	
Participant name:	
Participant ID #:	
Participant telephone #:	
# of calls to obtain interview:	
# of calls to complete interview:	
Date interview completed:	
Contact log: Please note when contacts were made with participant (date, time, outcome of contact).	

CONFIDENTIAL

Figure 23.6 Participant ID sheet.

on how they are managing today compared to a year ago. Response options might be either "about the same," "worse," or "better." To be able to use these responses statistically, the answers must be translated into numbers, for example, "about the same" equals 1, "worse" equals 2, and so on. This process is called data coding.

Once data are coded and the values for each response for each participant are entered into the analysis file, the investigator or a designate (e.g., research assistant, statistician) must do the data checking. The term **data checking** primarily relates to quantitative data. Data checking involves running frequency distributions and measures of central tendency and variability on each of the individual variables in the analysis file to check for missing or out-of-range values. If such values are found, it may indicate a data entry error. Potential errors can be checked against raw data and corrected if necessary. The process of correcting data entry errors is referred to as **data cleaning.**

Codebooks

There can be many variables in a project, and keeping track of each of them is critical. Codebooks are one data management tool that can address this need. Codebooks are relevant to both qualitative and quantitative research (MacQueen,

McLellan, Kay, & Milstein, 1998; Nyiendo et al., 2002; Shi, 2007). A codebook can be considered the dictionary for the data set generated by the study. The key contents of a quantitative codebook include the list of variables, their names and labels, and the coding for the different responses. Information in a qualitative code book can include the list of codes, a definition of each code, and a description of when and how to use it.

In quantitative research, a codebook often contains information on the origins of items, how to complete the coding, how to code unusual responses, where individual data files are kept (raw data as well as electronic), who maintains the passwords for the files, and how derived variables were developed. A derived variable is one that is computed using other variables that already exist in the analysis file. An example of a derived variable would be "number of ADL limitations," which could be derived by counting the number of individual ADL items with which each participant identifies requiring assistance.

Development of Data Collection Forms

The key to coding, checking, and cleaning is forethought, careful documentation, and attention to detail. Forms and files need to be linkable, and

---

Box 23.2   Examples of Items From an Interview Guide That Include the Coding for Each Response and the Variable Names That Will Be Used in the Data File

Survey Items and Response Options	Explanation
Would you say that your MS is within the last year (*read all but don't know option*): _____ Stable (1) Msstatus_____ _____ Improving (2) _____ Deteriorating (3) _____ Variable (4) _____ Don't know (888) Thinking about your symptoms and your ability to do everyday activities, how do you think you manage now compared to 1 year ago? (*read all but don't know option*) _____ About the same (1) Ablechg_____ _____ Worse (2) _____ Better (3) _____ Don't know (888)	Both of the survey items that are shown to the left include the response options and the coding for each option (the number in parentheses behind the response). "Msstatus" and "Ablechg" are the variable names that will be used in the data file. The line to the right of these names in the interview guide is used for "coding" after the interview is complete. For example, if a participant responded that in the past year, his or her MS had been "stable," a "1" would be recorded in the line beside "Msstatus"; "1" would also be recorded in the data file for that respondent for this variable.

---

many models exist for achieving linkage (e.g., relational databases, interface files, etc.) (Hulley et al., 2013). A key strategy that can be employed to facilitate linkage and data entry and cleaning is the format and preparation of the data collection forms (Antonakos et al., 2002; Nyiendo et al., 2002; Shi, 2007). For example, all of the interview guides for *Addressing Concerns About Falling Among Older Adults With Multiple Sclerosis* include the data coding for each of the response options (e.g., stable = 1, improving = 2, etc.) for each question right on the data collection form, as illustrated in Box 23.2. In addition, the variable label that is used in the analysis file for the question is included on the data collection form. In Box 23.2, the variable labels are "Msstatus" and "Ablechg." These labels are the ones that appear in the analysis file. The variable labels and codes on the data collection form match the ones in the electronic data file (e.g., SPSS, SAS). Being able to link files and forms together facilitates data management by ensuring that data can be cross-checked, confirmed, and, if necessary, corrected or updated as errors or omissions are found.

In addition, we also include the participant's identifier on each page of each document that is connected to that person, if a paper document is being used. Doing so facilitates data management by ensuring that data collection forms that are unintentionally separated during the data collection process can be reconnected. In recent years, the use of tablets and other mobile technology means that some past issues in paper-based data management are no longer a concern. New issues now include the need for encryption for mobile devices, secure back-ups, and system set-ups that will only allow valid responses to be entered.

Team Meetings

Throughout this chapter, the importance of consistent communication among members of the research team has been emphasized to ensure that data are managed well. One important strategy for facilitating communication is the team meeting. Team meetings are an opportunity for everyone involved in the project to come together to discuss progress, address problems and make decisions to solve them, share achievements, and make joint decisions that influence the project.

To facilitate a culture of consistent communication, everyone on the research team should be included in a team meeting, even if it appears on the surface that the discussion is not directly relevant to his or her duties. Team meetings provide an opportunity for all staff members to see how their own activities and decisions influence the work of others (see Fig. 23.7).

Having an agenda and taking minutes during team meetings is advised, particularly if decisions are made regarding data collection processes, changes to data coding protocols, or other

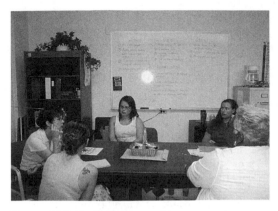

Figure 23.7 Dr. Finlayson and team members review a policy and procedure manual.

important items. In addition, having team meeting minutes can make it easier for an investigator to summarize technical decisions at the end of a project.

Backup Protocols

Nowadays, almost all of the information investigators retain for a research study is saved electronically. For this reason, developing and implementing backup protocols as part of a data management system is essential. There are two basic rules of backups: do them regularly and frequently. One never knows when a file will become corrupted or fall victim to a computer virus or worm, or when the computer hardware might fail. Therefore, planning for and doing backups of all files is an absolute necessity. If data are maintained in the cloud, doing a back-up to an external drive is recommended.

In addition to actually planning for and doing the backups, the protocol should include directions about where the backup files are to be stored (in another location is always best, in case of fire), as well as instructions on how backups can be retrieved if that becomes necessary.

Summary

So far this chapter has described the components of data management, explained why it is important, outlined issues to consider, and described some of the tools and strategies used to address these issues. This last section provides some general tips on data management, including what things to do at different points in the planning process. This latter information elaborates on the information provided in the last column of Table 23.1, presented earlier in this chapter.

Considerations During Proposal Development

As noted earlier, a good data management system will be initiated during the process of preparing a study proposal. At the time of proposal writing, decisions about staffing, project activities and timelines, computers and software, and storage needs (e.g., access to secure online systems) must be made so that a realistic budget can be developed. Realistic budgets support good data management by providing the necessary financial resources to a project. At the time of project planning, the following data management tools and resources will need to be decided upon, developed, or at least initiated:

- Management plan and project timelines,
- Job descriptions,
- Equipment and supply needs (e.g., data management and analysis software, online storage systems), and
- Submissions for human subjects protection (ethics review) and, if necessary, submissions related to the use and protection of personal health information (e.g., Health Insurance Portability and Accountability Act [HIPAA]).

Issues During Project Initiation

The startup phase of any project can be hectic because many different tasks must be completed. In relation to data management, an investigator needs to review all of the materials related to data management developed during the proposal phase of the project and adjust them as necessary. In addition, he or she must:

- Recruit and hire individuals who meet the qualifications of the positions available;
- Train or arrange training for staff on protection of human subjects, use and protection of personal health information (if necessary), and all necessary aspects of their job;
- Decide what policies and procedures will be needed and work with staff to prepare a policy and procedure manual,
- Set up staff monitoring procedures that can be reasonably followed (e.g., weekly team meetings);
- Develop systems to track participant recruitment and outcomes, including how ID numbers will be assigned;
- Review data collection tools and ensure that their design will facilitate accurate data entry;
- Test data entry systems, including data export protocols; and

• Set up and test data storage, security, and backup protocols.

Issues During Data Collection

Many data management problems will first emerge during the actual data collection phase. Some of them will be unexpected, whereas others may have been overlooked in the original planning. During this phase, most of the data management involves following the protocols that were previously set, refining or adding to them as necessary, and documenting all decisions that are made. Specifically, the investigator will need to:

• Document methods and responses to each recruitment strategy;
• Document the outcome for each potential participant—who is in and who is out, including why an individual does not participate or complete the study;
• Update policies and procedures as new situations emerge;
• Maintain and adjust (as necessary) staff monitoring procedures; and
• Document as decisions are made (e.g., how to code unusual responses).

Issues During Data Preparation and Analysis

Once the data collection is completed, data entry will need to begin if the data collection process itself has not used an electronic system (e.g., data entry directly on a tablet). Either way, during the time period in which the data are being prepared for analysis, data management protocols will be in the forefront. The investigator will need to:

• Implement the data checking and cleaning protocols;
• Document corrections made to the data files;
• Document the construction of derived variables;
• Document the process of recoding variables;
• Apply weights to the data, if necessary, and document this process;
• Transfer, if necessary, the data to the analyst; and
• Ensure that all files are securely archived for later use and sharing.

This chapter emphasizes the critical nature of data management and how it influences the quality of the data that a project produces. It also emphasizes that data management involves both the information gathered from participants and the project information that facilitates overall study management. Data management is a complex set of tasks and processes. The key to doing it well is to be logical and methodical and plan for problems before they emerge.

Review Questions

1. What are some common aspects of a data management plan?
2. Why does every research study need a data management plan?
3. What are the purposes of the project timeline and data management plan?
4. What are four ways that members of a research team might maintain ongoing communication during the data collection and management process?
5. How might a coding error occur during a study, and how could you prevent such an error from becoming systematically incorporated into a database?

REFERENCES

Aday, L., & Cornelius, L. (2006). *Designing and conducting health surveys (3rd ed.)*. San Francisco, CA: Jossey-Bass.

Antonakos, C. L., Miller, J. M., & Caruso, C. C. (2002). Critical elements of documentation in data-based research. *Western Journal of Nursing Research, 24*(1), 87–100.

Chan, A.-W., Tetzlaff, J. M., Gøtzsche, P. C., Altman, D. G., Mann, H., Berlin, J. A., . . . Moher, D. (2013). SPIRIT 2013 explanation and elaboration: guidance for protocols of clinical trials. *British Medical Journal, 346,* 7586.

Gassman, J. J., Owen, W. W., Kuntz, T. E., Martin, J. P., & Amoroso, W. P. (1995). Data quality assurance, monitoring and reporting. *Controlled Clinical Trials, 16,* 104S–136S.

Hosking, J. D., Newhouse, M. M., Bagniewska, A., & Hawkins, B. S. (1995). Data collection and transcription. *Controlled Clinical Trials, 16,* 66S–103S.

Hulley, S. B., Cummings, S. R., Browner, W. S., Grady, D. G., & Newman, T. B. (2013). *Designing clinical research* (4th ed.). Philadelphia, PA: Lippincott Williams & Wilkins.

Kielhofner, G., Hammel, J., Finlayson, M., Helfrich, C., & Taylor, R. R. (2004). Documenting outcomes of occupational therapy: The Center for Outcomes Research and Education. *American Journal of Occupational Therapy, 58*(1), 15–23.

Krefting, L. (1991). Rigor in qualitative research: An assessment of trustworthiness. *American Journal of Occupational Therapy, 45,* 214–222.

MacQueen, K. M., McLellan, E., Kay, K., & Milstein, B. (1998). Codebook development for team based qualitative analysis. *Cultural Anthropology Methods, 10*(2), 31–36.

McFadden, E. T., LoPresti, F., Bailey, L. R., Clarke, E., & Wilkins, P. C. (1995). Approaches to data management. *Controlled Clinical Trials, 16,* 30S–65S.

Nyiendo, J., Attwood, M., Llyod, C., Ganger, B., & Haas, M. (2002). Data management in practice-based research.

Journal of Manipulative and Physiological Therapeutics, 25(1), 49–57.

Pogash, R. M., Boehmer, S. J., Forand, P. E., Dyer, A., & Kunselman, S. J. (2001). Data management procedures in the asthma clinical research network. *Controlled Clinical Trials, 22,* 168S–180S.

Portney, L., & Watkins, M. P. (2009). *Foundations of clinical research: Applications to practice* (3rd ed.). Upper Saddle River, NJ: Prentice-Hall.

Shi, L. (2007). *Health services research methods* (2nd ed.). Clifton Park, NY: Thomson Delmar Learning.

CHAPTER 24

Deciding on an Approach to Data Analysis

Renée R. Taylor

Learning Outcomes

- List the two major applications for statistics in occupational therapy.
- Explain the four scales of measurement.
- Understand the components of a standard normal distribution.
- Differentiate descriptive statistics from inferential statistics.
- Name three examples of descriptive statistics.
- Name three examples of inferential statistics.

Introduction

Statistics is a term used to describe how a researcher approaches the manipulation of numbers to answer questions. By definition, **statistics** refer to the means by which data are collected, organized, analyzed, and presented to serve the various objectives of a research study. Statistics may be used to describe features of a single group of clients or to make inferences about an entire population of clients based on the study of a single group of clients. For example, if an occupational therapist wanted to learn about the benefits and drawbacks of constraint-induced therapy in kindergarten-age children with hemiplegia, it would be impossible to study the entire population of all kindergarten-age children with hemiplegia in the world. How would the therapist have the time and money to travel to India to study the children there, let alone to travel to Texas or Connecticut to study the children there? Thus, the researcher has to select a smaller group of kindergarten-age children with hemiplegia to study and make sufficient provisions about the selection of those children such that the smaller group is maximally representative of the larger population of kindergarten-age children with hemiplegia in the world. Thus, statistics helps researchers make conclusions about entire populations based on studying smaller samples from within those populations.

In occupational therapy, statistics are commonly used in two major ways:

1. To describe or summarize the characteristics of a given sample of clients;
2. To test hypotheses that make inferences about the effect of a given treatment approach on client outcomes.

In occupational therapy, many quantitative research studies use statistics in both of these ways. The following Case Example describes one such study.

In this chapter, we present a basic overview that emphasizes the value of learning about statistics as part of the process of being an informed consumer of research. We introduce how statistics are used in research and provide a brief review of the most basic concepts of statistics and their underlying logic. We describe the nature of information that each type of statistic provides and explain how you may use statistical information to guide your decision-making about observations and outcomes in occupational therapy. After reading this chapter, you should have a basic understanding of which kinds of statistics should be utilized to analyze different types of research questions or test hypotheses. Additionally, you should be able to interpret statistical findings in a way that is understandable in terms of study conclusions.

Our intention is not to provide detailed or comprehensive coverage of the topic, and we do not describe any of the mathematics that comprise the formulas from which specific statistical measures and methods are derived. If you are interested in learning about the mathematical foundations of statistics and/or how to conduct statistical analyses for application in research, you may wish to access the wide range of textbooks and coursework resources that best match the level at which you wish to engage in this area. A list of resources from which the content of this chapter is derived is presented in the References section. It is also important to understand that although an occupational therapy (OT) researcher may understand and

CASE EXAMPLE

Jamie manages the rehabilitation unit of a large urban oncology center. During a weekly staff meeting, one of the occupational therapists working in Jamie's unit comments on the extent to which her oncology clients are reporting posttreatment fatigue. Other staff members quickly agree, and one by one they explain how fatigue is the single most debilitating symptom for cancer survivors during rehabilitation. Following an extensive discussion, the unit decides to learn more about how fatigue affects clients and to develop a novel treatment approach that extends current best practice. First, the unit decides to conduct an extensive review of the literature to understand the state of the science and existing knowledge in the topic area.

Based on what was learned from the literature review, the team decides to narrow the type and stage of cancer and treatment level so that the study population and actual sample are clearly defined as stage 1 through 3 breast cancer survivors having completed surgery and radiation therapy. The first research effort undertaken by the team is to collect data that describe beliefs about fatigue duration, fatigue severity, frequency of fatigue (hours per day), and disability consequences of fatigue in this group. Following the collection of these data using valid and reliable assessment tools, the data are analyzed using descriptive statistics (i.e., means of summarizing the characteristics about a single sample of clients, rather than generalizing or making inferences about a larger population of clients from which that sample was derived). This effort represents the first application of statistics in occupational therapy referred to in our introduction (i.e., to describe or summarize the characteristics of a given client population).

The second way in which the team decides to apply statistics is to test the hypothesis that a novel treatment approach they have been using works to reduce fatigue by encouraging engagement in volitionally motivated daily activities (Kielhofner, 2008). This approach consists of interviewing clients to establish volitionally motivated daily activities, to educate clients about why and how engaging in these activities may facilitate their recovery and reduce their fatigue, and to provide a facilitative environment for engagement in these activities. To test the hypothesis that this intervention will work, a group of clients who received this approach will be compared with a group of clients who did not receive this approach on the outcomes of fatigue severity, frequency of fatigue, and disability consequences of fatigue. Inferential statistics will be used to test this hypothesis (inferential statistics are defined as a means of making inferences about a population or larger group of people based upon your sample, which represents a small portion of the larger group). Jamie looks forward to uncovering the findings from this study.

know how to conduct statistical analyses, not all researchers conduct their own statistical analyses on a regular basis, particularly for questions that are at a more advanced level and beyond the scope of this chapter.

Conducting more advanced statistical analyses helps answer more pointed and multifaceted questions, often involving many variables, different levels of analysis, and/or complex relationships between variables. These kinds of analyses require a researcher to have the time necessary to learn the underlying mathematical reasoning and to learn how to operate the computer software that aids in the execution of such analyses. **Biostatisticians** are professionals who are learned in understanding and conducting advanced statistical analyses that concern multiple variables and multiple levels of analysis. Many researchers from a wide range of health-care disciplines rely on biostatisticians to

support them in conducting the more advanced analyses required for many contemporary studies in our field.

Variables

Statistics involve analyzing numeric data that are represented by one or more variables. A **variable** is a means of labeling or giving meaning to a set of characteristics (represented by numbers) that are expected to vary among the clients being studied. For example, sex is a variable because it varies in the general population according to two levels: female and male. Age is another variable that differs among people. Age may be represented by two levels (i.e., young and old) or by many levels (i.e., birth to 122 years of age). In occupational therapy, self-reported pain may be considered a variable because it may range from "no pain" to "extreme pain." Accordingly, ice therapy may be an intervention designed to reduce pain, and it may have three levels (i.e., "no ice therapy" versus "2 minutes of ice therapy" versus "5 minutes of ice therapy").

When two or more variables are measured to test a hypothesis, one variable typically drives the outcome, and the outcome itself is typically measured by another variable. The variable that drives the outcome is referred to as the **independent variable,** and the variable that represents the outcome itself is the **dependent variable** (or **outcome variable**). In our example, the independent variable would be our OT intervention (ice therapy), and the dependent variable would be the target of that intervention (pain).

In statistics, the levels of the two variables of "pain" and "ice therapy" are translated or "coded" in terms of numbers. For example, the variable of "pain" may be represented on a scale of 0 to 10, where 0 = no pain and 10 = severe pain (McCaffery & Beebe, 1993). All of the numbers in between represent gradations of pain in between those anchors. Thus, the variable of pain has 10 levels, using a scale that is anchored by descriptive words. The three levels for the variable of "ice therapy" may be represented as 1 = no ice therapy, 2 = 2 minutes of ice therapy, and 3 = 5 minutes of ice therapy.

Scales of Measurement

In statistics, all variables are expressed numerically according to one of four scales of measurement. A **scale of measurement** explains the rule of logic that defines how numbers are used to describe variation in people, objects, or events. Basic statistical methods describe the following four scales of measurement:

- Nominal
- Ordinal
- Interval
- Ratio

Nominal Scale

A variable that is defined by a **nominal scale** is a scale with two or more categories that represent named classifications and are not ordered in relationship to one another. For example, your client may be categorized in one of the following ways: 1 = inpatient acute orthopedics, 2 = inpatient acute neurorehabilitation, or 3 = inpatient

acute psychiatric care, depending upon the nature of his or her impairment. These categories describe major types of rehabilitation that a client might receive, and clients do not advance up the scale from one category to the next. The value of 2 does not have any significance in relationship to the value of 3 except that it names or encodes a different type of rehabilitation. Moreover, the categories on a nominal scale are mutually exclusive, so one cannot be assigned to more than one category at a time.

A nominal scale is the lowest scale of measurement, and it limits the extent of statistical tests that may be used. Nominal scale data may not be converted to other types of scales, but other types of scales may be converted to nominal scale data. This is because the numbers in a nominal scale are labels, and adding them together or taking their average has no meaning. Nominal scale variables may be further defined as dichotomous or categorical, depending upon how many possible categories exist to define that variable. A **dichotomous scale** variable defines two categories, and a **categorical scale** variable defines more than two. For example, a client may be classified in terms of sex as 1 = female or 2 = male, and sex would be a dichotomous variable. The same client may be classified in terms of current work status, with categorical options of 1 = unemployed, 2 = working part time, 3 = working full time, 4 = attending school, and 5 = volunteer work.

Ordinal Scale

Variables measured according to an **ordinal scale** are also considered to be categorical because the numeric categories that comprise the scale are discrete. In an ordinal scale variable, the numbers representing the different categories are ordered or ranked in a linear way from least to greatest or from greatest to least. Ordinal scales typically consist of a limited number of ordered categories. For example, the clinical outcome of tying shoes may be defined on an ordinal scale from 0 to 3, presented in Box 24.1.

Box 24.1	Clinical Outcome of Tying Shoes Measured on an Ordinal Scale

__0__ not accomplished
__1__ partially accomplished
__2__ fully accomplished

In this example, 0 = not accomplished, 1 = partially accomplished, and 2 = fully accomplished. The categories in an ordinal scale variable are not evenly spaced. For example, how do we know whether the difference between not accomplished and partially accomplished represents the same level of achievement as the difference between partially accomplished and fully accomplished? Let's take another example. If you asked a client to rate his or her fatigue severity on a scale of 1 to 4, where 1 = no fatigue, 2 = minimal fatigue, 3 = moderate fatigue, and 4 = extreme fatigue, how do you know if the difference in experienced fatigue between 1 and 2 is the same as the difference between 3 and 4?

Interval Scale

An **interval scale** is a scale of measurement of data according to which the differences between values can be quantified in absolute but not relative terms and for which any zero is merely arbitrary; for instance, dates are measured on an interval scale because differences can be measured in years. If the categories were evenly spaced, we would refer to that variable as an interval scale variable. An **interval scale variable** defines a scale in which the intervals between values are equivalent. Interval scale variables are also referred to as continuous variables. A **continuous scale variable** may assume any value along a continuum that is defined by a given range. For example, if you are managing a community-based medical clinic in which clients are expected to pay for services based on their income level, it would be important to measure income on an interval scale in terms of dollars earned (i.e., gross annual income of all household members). If one client reports earning $15,000 per year, another reports earning $20,000 per year, and another reports earning $25,000, the difference in the interval of income between the three clients ($5,000) does not vary. Each person makes $5,000 more than the next, and a $5,000 difference remains a $5,000 difference no matter what a client makes.

Data measured according to an interval scale may be converted to an ordinal or nominal scale, if desired. For example, if, as director of the medical clinic, you wanted to show the discount level according to income, you might reclassify annual income in terms of an ordinal scale. An income of $0 to $14,999 might qualify for a level 1 discount (a 40% discount), an income of $15,000 to $29,999 might qualify for a level 2 discount (a $30% discount), and so on.

Ratio Scale

A **ratio scale** is an interval scale in which distances are stated with respect to a rational zero. A ratio scale variable is similar to an interval scale variable in that it is also continuous and may assume any value along a continuum. However, the ratio scale has a zero point which represents true absence of the variable, and an interval scale does not. In an interval scale, zero does not define nonexistence or absence. The measurement of temperature is often invoked as an example of interval measurement, because zero degrees Fahrenheit is represented as negative 17.8 degrees Centigrade, and zero degrees Centigrade is represented as 32 degrees Fahrenheit. Zero is a point on the continuum, but it is not a null value. The difference between 40 and 60 degrees Fahrenheit is the same as the difference between 60 and 80 degrees Fahrenheit, but one cannot say that 80 degrees is twice as hot as 40 degrees because zero does not represent the absence of temperature. A ratio scale, on the other hand, has a true zero value. In occupational therapy, number of falls may be measured on a ratio scale. Having never fallen represents an absence of the variable (equivalent to zero), and someone who has fallen four times has fallen twice as many times as someone who has fallen twice.

Normal Distribution

When you are selecting or designing an OT assessment, being deliberate about your choice of a scale of measurement within that assessment is important. All statistical tests are guided by a specific level of measurement. The type of scale used limits or optimizes the type of statistical test that can be used to answer a research question or test a hypothesis. Interval or ratio scales offer the most flexibility in terms of the range of tests that can be used to answer research questions. An additional benefit to collecting data according to an interval or ratio scale is that interval or ratio scales may always be converted into ordinal or nominal variables to answer simpler questions or to make a point in a more straightforward way. However, variables that begin as nominal or ordinal variables from the point of data collection cannot be converted into interval and ratio variables at a later time. For example, a researcher who designs a questionnaire that asks about age range and offers four ordinal categories (e.g., under 18 years, 19 to 29, 30 to 40, etc.) will never know the exact age of each client. Is a client within the 19 to 29 range 23 years old, 28 years old, or neither? If the researcher wants to

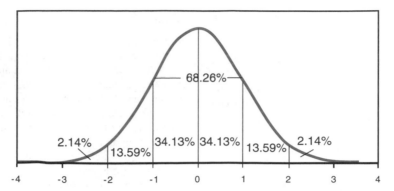

Figure 24.1 Normal standard deviation.

look at the relationship between age and a treatment outcome, he or she may be limited in terms of how she will be able to test that relationship statistically.

Interval and ratio scale data offer a range of values along a broader continuum of choices. These scales introduce a sufficient range of variability necessary for statistical tests that probe inferences about a population (rather than tests that simply describe a single sample of people that were selected from that larger population). Nominal and ordinal scale variables are not normally distributed. Generally, they cannot be used in the same way to answer questions that make inferences about people in the general population.

A **normal distribution** (sometimes referred to as a Gaussian distribution or a bell curve) defines an average or "norm" within a sample of people and describes successive deviations from that norm. For example, tests of cognitive skills, such as the Wechsler Scale of Intelligence for Children (WISC IV; Wechsler, 2004), define the average level of cognitive ability in reference to a full-scale score of 100. The lowest possible score is 40 and the highest 160. Scores below 100 reflect a successively decreasing range of lower and lower levels of cognitive ability. Scores above 100 reflect a successively increasing range of higher and higher levels of cognitive ability. A **standard normal distribution** assumes that the norm (in our case a score of 100) has a zero point and that the deviations from zero occur symmetrically, in units of one standard deviation at both the positive and negative ends of the possible range of choices. In our example of the WISC IV, 100 is equivalent to the zero point. About 68% of people will score within 15 points of 100 in either direction (i.e., a standard deviation of +1 or −1). About 95% of people will score within 30 points of 100

(i.e., two standard deviations of +2 or −2). A final 5% will score at the far ends of the continuum, with less than 2% to 3% scoring above 130 or below 70 (i.e., three or more standard deviations in either direction). Thus, the Wechsler Scale was developed to conform to the requirements for a standard normal distribution. A pictorial example of a standard normal distribution is presented in Figure 24.1.

Earlier in this chapter, we introduced two general applications for statistics in occupational therapy. Statistics may be used to describe or summarize specific characteristics of a given client population, to describe relationships between one set of characteristics and another, and to test hypotheses about the effect of a given treatment approach on outcomes for a client population, for example. In tandem with these applications, there are two major classifications of statistics that may be used to accomplish these goals: descriptive statistics and inferential statistics.

Descriptive Statistics

Descriptive statistics describe or summarize a collection of data. In our case, data generally refer to characteristics of a group of clients who have been selected for a research study. Descriptive statistics are most readily found in the first tables of published peer-reviewed journal articles that present social, demographic, and impairment-related characteristics of the sample that was studied. Variables that reflect social and demographic characteristics include, but are not limited to, average age, sex, race/ethnicity, income level, level of educational attainment, marital status, and parental status. Other sample characteristics that may be described upfront include body mass index or impairment level, for example. Descriptive information about all of these kinds of characteristics allows a researcher to specify the sample under study.

It is important to describe your sample carefully in case another researcher wants to replicate the study and approximate the same characteristics with a different group of people. For example, if you are studying endurance to standing in clients with knee replacement in two different hospitals, it would be important that the average body mass index (BMI) of clients in one hospital does not differ significantly from the average BMI of clients in another hospital. BMI is defined as a client's mass (in pounds) divided by the square of his or her height (in inches), multiplied by 703 (the metric conversion factor). It is important to compare clients across the two hospitals because a client's body mass is likely to affect his or her endurance to standing following surgery. If you are trying to test an intervention that is expected to improve standing endurance in one hospital but not the other, it would be important to make sure that any differences in the average BMI of the clients in the two hospitals did not lead to false conclusions about the effects of the intervention in the hospital in which your intervention is being tested.

After you decide which kinds of characteristics you have selected to describe in your sample, you will need to find a way to summarize those characteristics numerically. Examples of commonly used descriptive statistics include, but are certainly not limited to, frequency distributions, percentage values, measures of central tendency (i.e., mean, median, and mode), and measures of variability. Each of these descriptive statistics is described in the following sections.

Frequency Distributions

A **frequency** (*f*) describes the number of counts within a category. Frequencies are used to summarize nominal and ordinal scale variables. For example, if your sample included 10 people with red hair and 12 with black hair, the frequency of red-haired people would be $f = 10$, and the frequency of black-haired people would be $f = 12$. A **frequency distribution** is a means of describing data in terms of "counts" within each level or category of a variable. Typically summarized in a table, a frequency distribution presents numeric information about the number of times a given event occurs within a fixed range of possibilities. Frequency distributions are used to present nominal (i.e., dichotomous or categorical) scale variables. For example, frequency data for the

dichotomous variable of sex within a total sample of 100 males and females might be presented as follows: *f* males = 45; *f* females = 55. Typically, frequency data are never presented in isolation.

Percentage Values

The total sample size (designated by the symbol *N*) is often included, as is the percentage value for each frequency count. **Percentage values** are calculated by dividing the frequency (or number of counts within a category) by the total number of eligible counts within the sample. Thus, the percentage of males in our sample would be 45/100 = 45%, and the percentage of females would be 55%. A fictitious but typical example of frequency and percentage data describing social-demographic characteristics of a sample of 201 clients with knee replacement is presented in Table 24.1.

Table 24.1 Social-Demographic Characteristics of Knee Replacement Clients (*N* = 201)		
	f	%
Age Range		
40–50	3	1.5
51–61	58	28.9
62–72	70	34.8
73–83	69	34.3
83–93	1	0.5
Sex		
Male	112	55.7
Female	89	44.3
Race/Ethnicity* (*N* = 200)		
African American	16	8.0
Asian/Pacific Islander	3	1.5
Latino	3	1.5
Native American	0	0.0
Mixed Race or Other	13	6.5
White/Caucasian	165	82.5
Income Level		
<$15,000	4	2.0
$15,000–$35,000	15	7.5
$36,000–$56,000	36	17.9
$57,000–$77,000	58	28.9
$78,000–$98,000	61	30.3
>$98,000	27	13.4

*One person did not wish to disclose racial or ethnic information. For this category, the percentage value was calculated based on *N* = 200.

When presenting frequency and percentage data for a sample, it is important to account for missing data and to ensure that the frequency counts within each category tally to a total of 100%. This is referred to as the valid percent because the frequency is divided not by the total sample size but by the size of the sample within the particular category with missing data. When this is not the case, one must disclose how the missing data were treated, as in the Table 24.1 example for the race/ethnicity category.

If we were to describe our sample of clients with knee replacement in the sample or results section of a journal article, we might interpret and present the findings in Table 24.1 in the following descriptive paragraph:

> Our sample is comprised of adults mostly self-identifying as white, with a minority of people identifying as African American, mixed race, Asian/Pacific Islander, or Latino. Most clients in the sample are of middle income and above (i.e., 72.6% with a gross income at or above $57,000 per year). Most are age 62 or above, and there are approximately 10% more males than females."

Measures of Central Tendency

Measures of central tendency define the typical nature of data. Measures of central tendency include the mean, median, and mode. The **mean** *(m)* is the most widely utilized and reliable measure of central tendency. It is another way of defining the average score among all of the scores in your sample. The mean is calculated by dividing the sum of all of the scores (or values) in your sample by the total number of clients (or possibilities) in your sample. For example, the mean BMI among clients with knee replacement in Hospital A is calculated by adding all clients' BMI scores together and dividing by the total number of clients receiving knee replacement in that hospital.

The **median** reflects the middle position in a set of ordered or ranked scores. For example, a data set derived from an assisted care facility contains the following frequency-of-fall scores for seven clients: 1, 1, 2, 2, 3, 4, 5. The median of this set of scores is 2 (there are three scores beneath it and three scores above it). Consider a similar sample of six clients in the community: 2, 3, 3, 4, 5, 6. In this case, the midpoint of this data set is between 3 and 4. Thus, to calculate the median, one takes the average of the two middle scores (i.e., 3 + 4, divided by 2). The median is a more accurate measure of central tendency when you

have extreme values in your data set, because the extreme score will not influence the middle point in the data set. (A mean score pulls the average value toward the extreme score because the size of that extreme score gets added into the total.)

The **mode** is defined as the score that occurs with the highest frequency in your data set. In our assisted care example of frequency-of-fall data we are reminded that our data set contains the following values: 2, 3, 3, 4, 5, 6. Thus, our mode for this data set is 3 because it is the only value that occurs more than once. This data set is further characterized as unimodal because it has only one mode = 3. If there are two modes, the data set is characterized as bimodal, and so on. Certainly, there are distributions that do not have a mode.

Measures of Variability

The most basic measure of variability is **range.** The range defines the difference between the lowest and highest values for a given variable. In our sample of clients with knee replacement, we know that BMI scores range from 19 kg/m^2 (severely underweight) to 42 kg/m^2 (severely overweight). Thus, the BMI range for our subjects is 23 (i.e., $42 - 19 = 23$). This score reflects a tremendous amount of variability in BMI scores. An alternative in many journal articles is to report the upper and lower limits of the range (in our case 19 to 42) to show the upper and lower limits of the data for a given variable.

Variance is defined as the extent to which individual subjects in the sample deviate or drift away from the mean. A sample with a large amount of variance on a given variable is more heterogeneous in terms of that particular variable because the individual scores on that variable vary widely. A sample with a small amount of variance is more homogenous on that variable.

Another means of reporting variability is standard deviation. **Standard deviation** is defined as the average variability of individual scores from the mean. This is the most commonly reported measure of variability, and it is generally reported in parentheses next to the mean, for example: $m = 23.0$ (sd = 3.4) (Note that the numbers for these values were chosen arbitrarily.) The reason standard deviation is reported more often than variance is because it is calculated in terms of the same unit of measurement as the mean.

The standard deviation is always expressed as a positive number. If it is 0, it means there is no variation in the sample with respect to that variable. For example, a sample that included only people with a BMI of 25 would have a standard deviation of 0 for the variable of BMI. All values for the variable of BMI are the same. When the statistic for standard deviation for a given variable is large, it means there is a lot of variability (or heterogeneity) in the sample with respect to that variable. When it is small or closer to 0, it means there is more homogeneity.

Inferential Statistics

In the previous section we covered descriptive statistics, which are used to answer questions that describe the characteristics of a sample. In this section, we describe **inferential statistics,** which are used to test hypotheses (i.e., make inferences) about an entire population based on findings from a single sample thought to adequately represent that population. For example, we cannot study the effects of animal-assisted therapy on all clients in neurorehabilitation, but we can study a representative sample of those clients and then draw conclusions (allowing for a reasonable estimation of error in our conclusions) about the larger population of clients in neurorehabilitation using animal-assisted therapy.

The *p* Value

Inferential statistics are built on the concept of probability. **Probability** refers to the likelihood that a predicted outcome or event will actually occur, or the degree to which an event will occur in a series of observations. For example, an occupational therapist studying the use of therapy dogs to increase mobility on neurorehabilitation units in the southern United States concludes that 70% of clients improve their mobility when walking in the unit with a therapy dog. Thus, there is a 70% probability that clients encouraged to walk with therapy dogs will improve their mobility. This is not the same as concluding that every client has a 70% chance of improvement when walking with a therapy dog. Thirty percent of clients will not show improvement, and some may even show decline. Whether an individual client in the general population of clients in neurorehabilitation belongs to the 30% category or to the 70% category is not known.

In this example, the notion of probability was used to describe the likelihood that observations of clients using dogs in the southern United States will reflect observations of clients using dogs in the entire population (e.g., how well our sample data estimate the population parameter). Probability also defines the extent to which the improvement observed in our study of southern clients would represent true improvement in the larger population, or if these improvements could have happened by chance. The extent to which an observed difference (or improvement) occurs by chance is referred to as **sampling error.**

In statistics, the probability of true difference or improvement is represented as a *p* value. The *p* **value** is used as a cutoff point to determine the extent to which a conclusion about a sample reflects a true difference within the larger population, versus the conclusion being due to error or chance. Typically, OT researchers set the *p* value at 0.05 or 0.01. A value of $p \leq 0.05$ suggests that there is a 5% probability that a conclusion is due to sampling error or chance. A value of $p \leq 0.01$ is more conservative, suggesting that there is a 1% probability that a conclusion is due to sampling error or chance. **Statistical significance** is determined by a finding from a statistical test meeting the probability cutoff of $p \leq 0.05$ or $p \leq 0.01$.

Hypothesis Testing

Inferential statistics are used to answer questions about relationships between variables within and between groups of clients. These questions are generally posed in terms of **hypotheses,** or probability-based statements about the relationship between variables. **Hypothesis testing** defines the process by which outcomes or significant differences found in a study reflect true outcomes or are due to chance or error. Hypothesis testing is focused on whether there is enough strength of evidence to be able to reject the conclusion that the observed outcomes or differences are due to error or chance. The symbol for a null hypothesis is H^0. A **null hypothesis** states that an observed difference or outcome is due to chance. The point of hypothesis testing is to be able to reject the null hypothesis. The **alternative hypothesis** (designated as H^1 and also referred to as the **research hypothesis**) specifies a relationship between variables that is not due to chance. This relationship may be directional or nondirectional. For example, a directional research hypothesis might state the following:

> H^1: A daily 3-week stretching protocol will lead to significantly lower self-ratings of pain during and immediately following the treatment period.

Sometimes researchers present the research hypothesis in terms of a question:

> Will a 3-week stretching protocol practiced daily lead to decreased pain during and immediately following the treatment period?

A nondirectional research hypothesis might state the following:

H²: There will be a significant association between fatigue and pain scores in a sample of adults diagnosed with fibromyalgia syndrome.

In the first hypothesis, we see that the independent variable is the stretching intervention and the dependent variable is pain. For this reason, a statistical test that tests a directional relationship between variables would be appropriate. In the second hypothesis, fatigue and pain scores are interchangeable, and so a statistical test that probes nondirectional relationships would be appropriate. Typically, a researcher's goal is to show statistical evidence in favor of the research hypothesis and to reject the null hypothesis. As noted earlier, a researcher is permitted to reject the null hypothesis when a statistical finding reaches significance as designated by a p or alpha level, denoting the chance of this being an erroneous finding as either 5% or 1%, depending on how conservative you wish to be in asserting your conclusions (e.g., $p \leq 0.05$ or $p \leq 0.01$).

Commonly Used Inferential Statistical Tests

Inferential statistical tests can be further broken down into two major categories: parametric statistics and nonparametric statistics. Inferential statistics are used to infer a particular conclusion or outcome from the data.

Parametric Statistics

Parametric statistics is a branch of statistics that assumes that sample data come from a population that follows a probability distribution based on a fixed set of parameters. This is the most commonly used classification of statistical tests. Many researchers prefer to use them because they allow researchers to be more confident about their conclusions, and there are a wider range of choices of tests available. Parametric statistical tests may be used provided that the following criteria are met:

- The dependent variable(s) being measured are continuous (i.e., use an interval or ratio scale); and
- The sample size is large enough ($N > 30$) so that assumptions about normality and variance are likely to be met.

Usually, when these two criteria are met, the sample approximates a normal distribution (discussed earlier in the chapter), and homogeneity of variance is assumed (i.e., the variance of the dependent variable is the same across all levels of the independent variable).

When selecting a statistical test, another important consideration to bear in mind is whether the variables being compared are from the same sample group or whether they are from two (or more) different sample groups. When a statistical test is being performed on variables from the same sample group, it is referred to as a **related-samples** test. Other names that are sometimes used in the literature to describe related-samples tests include **correlated-samples** tests, **paired-samples** tests, **within-subjects** tests, and **dependent-samples** tests. When a statistical test is being performed on variables from two or more different sample groups, it is classified as an **independent-samples** test. Another way of referring to an independent-samples test is a **between-subjects** test.

In our case example at the beginning of the chapter, a hypothesis that an intervention designed for clients with breast cancer would serve to reduce fatigue was tested. A group of clients receiving the intervention were compared with a group of clients not receiving the intervention (a control group). Therefore, the statistical tests that would be used for these comparisons would be independent-samples tests. If a comparison had been made within the same group of women (for example, if the women were tested according to a pretest–posttest design in which fatigue levels were measured before and after the intervention), then the test would have been referred to as a related-samples test (or a within-subjects test).

Examples of the most commonly used univariate parametric statistical tests for independent and related samples are presented in Table 24.2.

Pearson Correlation Test

Correlation defines the extent to which two (or more) variables are associated with each other without making any implications that one has caused the other to occur. For example, height and weight tend to be correlated, but that relationship is not always causal (being taller does not always cause weight gain, and weight gain does not cause one to be taller). A **Pearson correlation test** (formally named the Pearson product moment correlation) is the most commonly used measure of association in statistics. According to this test, the strength of the association between two variables is represented as an r-value and ranges from $r = -1$

Table 24.2 Univariate Parametric Statistical Tests

Name of Test	Test Purpose	Variables Measured
Pearson correlation	Measuring the degree and direction	Two continuous variables of association between two variables
Independent-samples *t*-test	Comparing means from two groups	One two-level independent variable (e.g., group assignment) and one continuous dependent variable
Paired-samples *t*-test	Comparing means from the same group	Paired continuous variables from different time points (e.g., pretest and posttest measures of the same variable)
One-way ANOVA	Comparing means from three or more groups	One independent variable with three or more levels and one continuous dependent variable

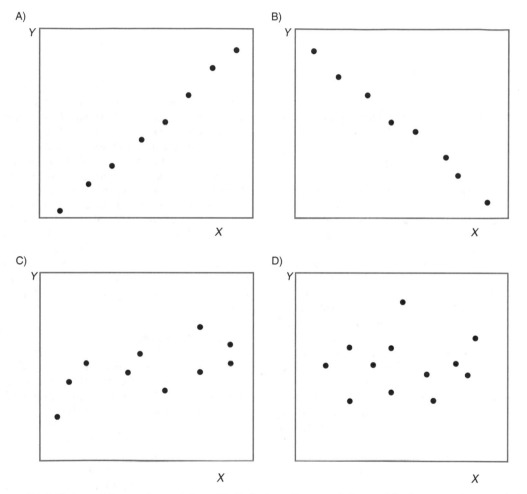

Figure 24.2 Various patterns of correlation. (A) Perfect positive correlation. (B) Perfect negative correlation ($r = -1.0$). (C) Matrix correlation ($r = .60$). (D) No correlation ($r = 0$).

to +1. A correlation of 1 in either direction (positive or negative) reflects a perfect (strongest) association. A perfect positive relationship of $r = +1$ means that the two variables increase or decrease in tandem.

For example, in Figure 24.2A, as the variable along the *x*-axis increases, the variable along the *y*-axis increases. A perfect negative relationship of $r = -1$ means that as one variable increases, the other variable decreases. In Figure 24.2B, as the variable along the *x*-axis increases, the variable along the *y*-axis decreases. In Figure 24.2C, a moderate positive relationship is shown at $r = 0.60$ because the data points plotted on the graph reflect a general trend toward increasing values on the x-axis as we see increasing values on the y-axis. Figure 24.2D shows no relationship at $r = 0$, or what is referred to as a zero correlation, because the pattern of data between the $-x$ and y-axes appears random.

Correlation coefficients are generally interpreted as follows:

- $r = 0$ to ± 0.20 suggests a negligible relationship between the two variables.
- $r = \pm0.20$ to ± 0.40 suggests a low correlation.
- $r = \pm0.40$ to ± 0.60 suggests a moderate correlation.
- $r = \pm0.60$ to ± 0.80 suggests a high correlation.
- $r = \pm0.80$ to ± 1.00 suggests a very strong relationship.

In our fictitious example of clients with knee replacement, let's say we want to explore whether there is a relationship between BMI and number of days of adherence to a recommended pre-operative exercise program.

Independent-Samples t-Test

Independent-samples t-tests compare the means from two independent groups or samples. The statistic that reflects whether the two means from the two different samples are equal or different is denoted as t. In this test, the t statistic is generally reported with degrees of freedom (df) in addition to its significance value (e.g., $p \leq 0.05$ or $p \leq 0.01$). **Degrees of freedom** refer to the number of independent observations in a sample, subtracting the number of parameters that must be estimated from the sample data. Additionally, the means of the two groups are reported along with the standard deviation for each mean. Let's take our fictitious Case Example from the beginning of the chapter. We will use an independent-samples t-test to test the hypothesis that an intervention designed for clients with breast cancer would serve to reduce fatigue. A group of 120 clients receiving the intervention were compared with a group of 128 clients not receiving the intervention (a control group) for a total sample size of 248 clients. Findings as they might be presented for reporting are presented in Table 24.3.

Paired-Samples t-Test

Paired-samples t-tests compare the means from a single group of clients, typically at two points in time. As in the independent-samples test, the statistic that reflects whether the two means from the two measurements are equal or different is

Table 24.3 Independent t-Test Findings for a Fatigue Intervention for Clients With Breast Cancer ($N = 248$)

Group	Mean (Std. Deviation)	t	df	p
Intervention group	4.98 (3.42)			
Control group	9.23 (3.12)			
		7.98	246	0.00

In this case, findings suggest that clients in the intervention group reported significantly lower levels of fatigue ($m = 4.98$) as compared with controls ($m = 9.23$) ($t = 7.98$ [246] $p < 0.01$).

denoted as t. Similarly, the t-statistic is generally reported with degrees of freedom (df) in addition to its significance value (e.g., $p \leq 0.05$ or $p \leq 0.01$). Additionally, the means of the two measurements are reported along with the standard deviation for each mean. Taking our prior fictitious example about fatigue in patients with breast cancer, let's imagine that we wanted to test the hypothesis that our intervention was so powerful that fatigue scores continued to decrease over time in the intervention group. Our group of 120 clients receiving the intervention is measured immediately following the intervention (time 1) and 1 year later (time 2). Findings as they might be presented for reporting are presented in Table 24.4.

One-Way ANOVA

A **one-way analysis of variance (ANOVA)** allows you to test differences between three or more means (or levels) of a single independent variable. If there had been three groups of women compared in terms of the outcome of fatigue in our breast cancer study (i.e., one group receiving the intervention, one group receiving a placebo intervention, and one control group receiving usual care), then we would have used a one-way ANOVA to test differences in fatigue scores among the three groups. In a one-way ANOVA, scores for each level of the independent variable on some anticipated outcome are reflected as values for the dependent variable. The term *one-way* refers to the fact that this test allows you to test only a single independent variable. The statistic that reflects whether the means from the different levels are equal or different is denoted as F. This statistic is generally reported with degrees of freedom (df)

Table 24.4 Paired *t*-Test Findings for a 1-Year Follow-Up Study of a Fatigue Intervention for Clients With Breast Cancer (*N* = 120)

Measurement	Mean (Std. Deviation)	*t*	df	*p*
Time 1	4.98 (3.42)			
Time 2	2.23 (0.92)			
		6.08	119	0.00

In this case, findings suggest that clients continued to report significantly lower levels of fatigue 1 year after intervention (*m* = 4.98 vs. 2.23) (*t* = 6.08 [119] *p* < 0.01).

in addition to its significance value (e.g., $p \leq 0.05$ or $p \leq 0.01$). Additionally, the means of the measurements are reported along with their standard deviations.

Nonparametric Statistics

Nonparametric statistics and statistical tests are used when assumptions about normality and homogeneity of variance are not met. Generally, this is the case when

- The dependent variable(s) is nominal or ordinal and
- The sample size is small ($N < 30$).

Coverage of nonparametric statistical tests is beyond the scope of this chapter. Readers seeking a more detailed and comprehensive description of nonparametric statistics and other parametric statistical tests are encouraged to engage in further study and to consult the list of references at the end of this chapter.

Summary

In this chapter, we describe the two major applications for statistics: to portray descriptive information about the characteristics of our clients and to test research questions and hypotheses. We explain the role of variables in statistical testing and describe the four scales of measurement, including each of their strengths and limitations. We explain the standard normal distribution and how assumptions about normality guide the use of parametric statistical testing. We explain the differences and uses of descriptive versus inferential statistics and provide examples of commonly used tests within these two major classifications.

Review Questions

1. What are the two major applications for statistics in occupational therapy?
2. What are the strengths and limitations for each of the four scales of measurement?
3. What are the components of a standard normal distribution?
4. What types of research questions are addressed by descriptive statistics?
5. What types of research questions are addressed by inferential statistics?

REFERENCES

Kielhofner, G. (2008). *Model of Human Occupation: Theory and application* (4th ed.). Philadelphia, PA: Lippincott, Williams, & Wilkins.

McCaffery, M., & Beebe, A. (1993). *Pain: Clinical manual for nursing practice.* Baltimore, MD: V.V. Mosby Company.

Wechsler, D. (2004). *The Wechsler intelligence scale for children—fourth edition.* London, England: Pearson Assessment.

Meta-Analysis

Kenneth J. Ottenbacher • Patricia Heyn • Beatriz C. Abreu

Learning Outcomes

- Define meta-analysis.
- Identify the steps involved in conducting a meta-analysis.
- Evaluate the various approaches to defining effect size in meta-analysis.
- Provide an example of a meta-analysis relevant to occupational therapy.
- Explain the advantages and disadvantages of meta-analysis as a research method in occupational therapy.

Introduction

The dramatic expansion of research in health care over the past 30 years is well documented (Institute of Medicine, 2001). Primary studies published in the health-care research literature routinely recommend further investigation of topics so that the findings can be corroborated. These calls for additional research are based on the belief that scientific knowledge should be cumulative. Ideally, cumulative scientific findings lead to valid knowledge that can be integrated into practice to improve health-related outcomes. In the current climate of accountability and evidence-based practice, this cumulative approach to determining scientific knowledge is extremely powerful (Abreu, 2010). A **meta-analysis** is a comprehensive study that summarizes the findings of several individual studies to answer scientific (and clinical) questions. This summary includes statistical data that reflect a best estimate of the cumulative evidence for the explanation of a mechanism or outcome in occupational therapy.

The Importance of Meta-Analysis

Meta-analytic studies are important to occupational therapy, and to health care in general, because they represent the highest level of evidence in support of a phenomenon or outcome. Evidence-based practice emerged in the 1990s and continues to provide a strong incentive for increased research designed to refine and guide practice in clinical fields, including occupational therapy (Evidence-Based Medicine Working Group, 1992; Tickle-Degnen, 1998). The focus of evidence-based practice over the past 20 years has been to develop strategies to translate research findings into information that can be used to justify and improve clinical decision-making (Straus, Glasziou, Richardson, & Haynes, 2010).

A sophisticated system of evaluating quantitative studies has been established to identify those investigations that provide the best evidence for determining treatment effectiveness. The system is often referred to as "levels of evidence," and it provides a hierarchy of research designs and grades of evidence. Figure 25.2 includes an overview of the levels-of-evidence hierarchy currently used by the Centre for Evidence-Based Medicine (Straus et al., 2010; University Health Network, 2004). Inspection of the figure indicates that the strongest level of evidence is a systematic review or meta-analysis of randomized trials. The terms *meta-analysis* and *systematic review* are often used interchangeably, but there is an important difference. A **systematic review** summarizes the findings of multiple studies on a given topic but does not need to contain a *statistical* synthesis of the results from the included studies. This might be impossible if the designs of the studies are too different for a statistical average of their results to be meaningful, or if the outcomes measured are not sufficiently similar, or if the studies reviewed are qualitative in nature. If the results of the individual studies are statistically combined to produce an overall quantitative outcome, this is usually called a meta-analysis. The remainder of this chapter describes the procedures used to conduct a meta-analysis. These same procedures, with the exception of computing a common statistical metric (effect size), are used to conduct a systematic review. Therefore, they can be taken

CASE EXAMPLE

Isabel is an occupational therapy (OT) fieldwork student who is new to the field of neurorehabilitation. For her level II fieldwork placement, she is assigned to work on a rehabilitation unit at a remote rural hospital. Because she is nervous about what to expect, she decides to access the intranet of her university's library and conduct a literature review regarding the effectiveness of stroke rehabilitation programs. She comes across a meta-analysis published in *Neurology* titled "The Results of Clinical Trials in Stroke Rehabilitation Research" (Ottenbacher & Jannell, 1993). This meta-analysis involved 36 clinical trials examining stroke rehabilitation and included a total of 3,717 patients. The overall quantitative results suggested that the average patient in the treatment group receiving a focused program of stroke rehabilitation had a better outcome than 65.5% of the patients in the control groups not receiving rehabilitation (*d*-index of 0.40).

All primary research studies included in the meta-analysis involved a comparison between a group of persons who received a focused program of rehabilitation following a stroke and a group that received standard medical care on a neurological or medical unit within the hospital. The outcome measures in this meta-analysis were categorized as activities of daily living (ADLs), visual/perceptual, language/cognition, length of stay, motor/reflex, and other. The consistency and accuracy of the coding for all study characteristics were examined by having three raters independently review and complete the coding form for 20 randomly selected studies. The intraclass correlation coefficient values ranged from 0.77 to 1.00, indicating good to excellent agreement for the items on the coding form used in the analysis.

The meta-analysis found the largest effect size (*d*-index) for measures labeled as ADL and the smallest average effect size for language/cognition measures. An important variation in study results was found related to the type of research design. The type of research design was coded in each study as experimental, quasi-experimental, or pre-experimental. There was a significant difference in the average effect size (*d*-index) based on whether the outcome measure was blindly recorded. Blind recording means that the persons collecting the outcome information did not know if the individual subject was a member of the treatment or control group. The impact of blind recording, however, was only found for research designs in which subjects were not randomly assigned to a treatment or control group (pre- and quasi-experimental designs). Figure 25.1 displays the interaction between research design and how the outcome measures were recorded.

In contrast to the narrative literature reviews published in 1989 (Dobkin, 1989; Reding & McDowell, 1989) that reported conflicting findings regarding the effectiveness of stroke

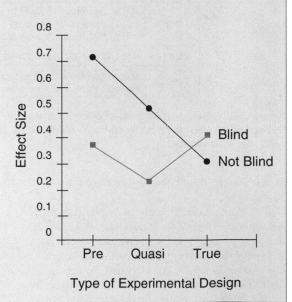

Figure 25.1 Interaction between type of research design and method of recording outcome measure (blind versus not blind). *(Reprinted with permission from Ottenbacher, K. J., & Jannell, S. J. [1993]. The results of clinical trials in stroke rehabilitation research. Neurology, 50, 37–44.)*

(case study continues on page 344)

rehabilitation programs, the stroke rehabilitation meta-analysis illustrates how quantitative reviewing procedures can produce consensus by systematically combining the results of multiple studies. This meta-analysis also illustrates how study design characteristics can be examined in unique ways not possible in a single or primary research investigation. The meta-analysis on stroke rehabilitation outcomes found an interaction between blind recording of the outcome measures and type of study design. This information is important to the interpretation of existing research investigations in this area, but it is also important to researchers planning future studies.

Isabel reflected on these findings and applied them during her rural fieldwork II experience. Knowing that ADL gains were anticipated to come more readily during rehabilitation than cognitive and language gains, she was able to put her experiences with clients into better perspective.

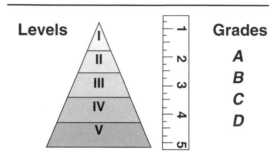

Evidence-based practice research design rating system

Levels of Evidence Based on Research Design	
Level 1	a. Systematic review (meta-analyses) of randomized trials with narrow confidence intervals b. Individual randomized trial with narrow confidence intervals
Level 2	a. Systematic review (meta-analyses) of homogenous cohort studies b. Individual cohort studies and low-quality randomized trials (e.g., trials with <80% follow-up)
Level 3	a. Systematic review (meta-analyses) of homogenous case-control studies b. Individual case-control studies
Level 4	Case series and poor-quality cohort and case-control studies
Level 5	Expert opinion without explicit critical appraisal or based in physiological or bench research

Figure 25.2 Description of levels-of-evidence hierarchy used in evidence-based clinical medicine. Developed by Centre for Evidence-Based Medicine (http://www.cebm.net/). Not all grades are shown for each level of evidence.

as relevant to the review of qualitative research publications.

There are several systems for defining the strongest or best evidence for integrating research findings with clinical practice. Some disciplines, such as nursing, have developed variations of the levels-of-evidence hierarchy currently used by the Centre for Evidence-Based Medicine. The vast majority of the different levels-of-evidence frameworks used in health-care research rate meta-analyses or systematic reviews as providing the best or highest level of research evidence.

Why are the results from meta-analyses studies considered the highest level of evidence in making evidence-based decisions to improve clinical practice? Traditional quantitative studies are based on a model of hypothesis testing using statistical tests. The results of these tests provide estimates of the probability that a research hypothesis is valid and should be supported. Whenever a researcher conducts a statistical test and makes a decision about whether to accept or reject the null hypothesis, there is a chance of making an error. In a typical research study, the investigator may report a statistical value followed by $p < .05$. This means the researcher has found a statistically significant result and will reject the null hypothesis and accept the research hypothesis (i.e., that there is a difference between the groups or conditions compared). In making this decision, the researcher is usually correct, but there is also a probability of being wrong. The probability of being wrong in this case is 5% ($p < .05$). The fact that even the best controlled and most rigorously conducted study may come to an incorrect conclusion (type I or type II error) is why replication and corroboration of research findings are so important.

The details of statistical hypothesis testing are not the topic of this chapter and are discussed elsewhere in this text. The important point is that evidence from one study is not sufficient to draw conclusions about the outcomes of a health intervention. To determine the effectiveness of a treatment, or the validity of a scientific finding, multiple studies are required that address the same research question and produce consistent findings. Meta-analysis is a systematic method of combining the results of multiple individual research studies to answer a scientific question. The ability to obtain a statistical consensus across many studies is why meta-analysis produces the highest level or best evidence in making evidence-based decisions.

The capacity to synthesize multiple research studies is at the heart of the evidence-based practice movement and philosophy. **Narrative reviews** of aggregated investigations have traditionally been used to synthesize information from individual quantitative research studies. These narrative reviews have been shown to be biased and subjective, and they often lead to conflicting conclusions (Glass, McGaw, & Smith, 1981; Whitehead, 2002). For example, two narrative reviews were published in *Neurology* in 1989 examining the effectiveness of stroke rehabilitation programs. One paper was titled "Focused Stroke Rehabilitation Programs Improve Outcomes" (Reding & McDowell, 1989), and the second article was titled "Focused Stroke Rehabilitation Programs Do Not Improve Outcomes" (Dobkin, 1989). Both papers were written by respected researchers and appeared in a prestigious journal. From the titles, there was a clear difference in the conclusions. These two narrative reviews generated confusion rather than consensus.

The subjective and biased outcomes of narrative reviews led to the development of methodologies and techniques in the 1970s to systematically integrate findings from many individual research studies (Glass et al., 1981; Rosenthal, 1978). The procedures associated with meta-analysis are designed to treat the review process as a unique type of research endeavor that produces an objective quantitative synthesis of research results (Cooper, Hedges, & Valentine, 2009; Lipsey & Wilson, 2001). The procedures provide a mechanism for investigating variation in study characteristics such as sampling, design procedures, and type and number of dependent and independent variables (Cooper, 2010). Variance in these variables is then related to study outcome. This type of comparison is not possible in traditional literature reviews based on narrative descriptions of published studies. Figure 25.3 presents a comparison of the characteristics of narrative reviews of the research literature and meta-analysis.

Cooper and Cooper (1989) argue that integrating separate research projects involves scientific inference. They have conceptualized meta-analysis as a unique type of research endeavor with a series of distinct steps. In the remainder of this chapter we present the steps involved in conducting a meta-analysis and the advantages and disadvantages of meta-analysis as a research method in occupational therapy.

Steps in Meta-Analysis

Meta-analysis typically follows the same steps used in a primary research design. The investigator first defines the research question or problem, the inclusion criteria, the selection method, and the data collection process. Sample selection in meta-analysis consists of applying procedures for locating studies that meet the specified criteria for inclusion. Data are collected from studies in two ways:

- Major study features are coded according to the objectives of the review, and
- Study outcomes are transformed to a common metric called an effect size, so that they can be compared.

Effect size (ES) is the name given to a family of indices that measure the magnitude of a treatment effect. Unlike significance tests, these indices are independent of sample size. They are calculated by taking the difference between control and experimental group means and dividing that difference by the standard deviation of the scores of both groups combined. It is also called delta or *d*.

Contrasting Approaches to Summarizing Information from Individual Research Studies

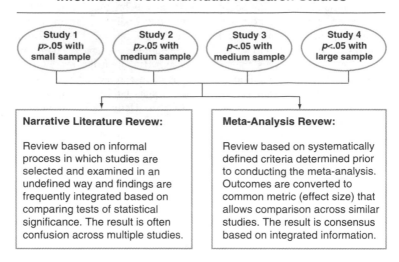

Figure 25.3 Schematic diagram of meta-analysis process including comparison of narrative review and meta-analysis methods.

The procedures necessary to conduct a meta-analysis study are summarized in Table 25.1.

Problem Formation

The first task in any research endeavor is to identify the focus or formulate the problem to be studied. In its most basic form, the research problem includes definitions of relevant variables and a rationale for relating the variables to one another. Two levels of definition are commonly associated with variables included in the problem formation step; these levels are conceptual and operational.

The independent variable or treatment must first be defined conceptually. Both primary researchers and research reviewers must choose a conceptual definition and a degree of abstractness for variables contained in the problem. The conceptual definitions employed by reviewers using quantitative methods tend to be rather broad to include all relevant instances of a particular construct. For instance, in the example described earlier the problem question might be stated as: "Do rehabilitation programs improve functional outcomes for persons who have had a stroke?"

After the variables have been identified conceptually, they must be linked to empirical reality. This is accomplished by the formulation of an operational definition that relates the concept under study to concrete events. The operational definition allows the investigator to determine whether a concept is present in a particular situation.

Primary research usually involves only one or two operational definitions of the same construct. In contrast, meta-analysis reviews may involve many empirical versions of a concept. For instance, in a meta-analysis of sensory integration, the variable "sensory integration therapy" may be operationalized in a number of ways across the studies that are reviewed.

As a consequence of the variety of operational definitions of a construct, the evidence retrieved by reviewers typically contains more method-generated variance than evidence collected as primary data. The fact that a particular concept or construct may be operationally defined in a variety of ways across different studies is referred to as **operational multiplicity.** The presence of multiple operationalizations in a meta-analysis represents an important source of variance. Two reviewers using an identical label for a construct may employ different operational definitions. For example, in a meta-analysis on the effectiveness of rehabilitation for stroke described earlier, the authors looked at the impact of rehabilitation programs for stroke on functional outcomes. Functional outcomes were operationally defined as measures of ADLs, length of stay (LOS), language/cognitive tests, and motor/reflex tests. Other investigators have included physiological measures such as muscle strength, sensation, and/or proprioception as functional outcomes. A meta-analysis that operationally defines functional outcomes as only ADLs will produce different results than a meta-analysis

Table 25.1 Steps Involved in Planning, Conducting, and Reporting a Meta-Analysis Review of Published Research

1. Problem formulation	A topic that can be addressed by meta-analysis is selected. followed by a formulation of a research question relevant to the topic of interest. It includes identification of the problem and formation of the research questions.
2. Data collection	A comprehensive, sensitive, and extensive search strategy is developed to compile possible reports. Key words and variables determine sources of potentially relevant reports. The inclusion criteria are defined and eligibility criteria are set for the meta-analysis. Construct definitions are used to distinguish relevant from irrelevant studies.
3. Data evaluation and coding	Includes three areas: 1. *Study Quality Assessment:* Assessment of the methodological quality and validity of the studies. 2. *Data Identification and Quantification:* Outcome variables are identified and extracted into a coding system. Group's contrasts and effect-size calculations are performed. 3. *Characteristics of Interest:* General information regarding study/trial design should be standardized into a coding system for further analysis, such as treatments and sample characteristics.
4. Analysis and interpretation	It includes two areas: 1. *Statistical Procedures:* Compiling the data for quantitative synthesis and summary effect sizes by using appropriate methods and effects models (random or fixed) should be clearly stated. Effect models should explore the sources of variation if variability is present (e.g., differences in study quality, participants, treatments, or outcomes). 2. *Interpretation of Results*: Translating the results with caution and reanalyzing the data due to the robustness or uncertainty of results is desired. Results could be uncertain due to imperfections in original study reports or missing data.
5. Reporting results	Key aspects of all of the previous stages should be clearly stated in the final report to allow replication and critical appraisal of the meta-analysis. The process of reporting should be rigorous and explicit. Methodological limitations of both original studies and the meta-analysis should be highlighted, and any recommendations should be followed by practical and evidence-based advice. A proposal for future research should be included.

that operationally defines functional outcomes as including measures of ADLs, LOS, and language/cognitive and motor/reflex tests.

In the problem formation stage, it is important for the researcher to provide a clearly stated research question. This question must include detailed operational descriptions of how the concepts will be defined. This, in turn, determines which studies will be included in the meta-analysis.

Data Collection

Research reviewers have multiple methods at their disposal to identify and retrieve research studies relevant to the research problem or question. Most evidence today is accessed via different health-related search engines on the Internet. Many search engines are freely available to the public through a general search, whereas others are available through a university or health-care system library intranet system. The computer search is a time-saving technique that allows the reviewer to exhaustively scan several retrieval sources at a rapid rate. The fact that different electronic resources contain different journals and document indicators or descriptors is a limitation of online databases. **Bibliographic searches** using the same terms as descriptors or keywords may produce different results depending on the database searched.

A related retrieval approach is to employ a descendency search using the *Science* or *Social Science Citation Indexes* (Web of Science). A **descendency search** uses author names and highly similar study topics to build a compendium of related studies. Because the citation indexes are primarily organized by author (not topic), they are most useful when particular investigators or research papers are closely associated with an area of investigation. In contrast to the descendency approach, a reviewer may employ the **ancestry method,** in which the reviewer retrieves information by tracking citations from one study or research report to another. Most reviewers are aware of several studies related to their problem before they formally begin the literature search. These studies provide bibliographies that cite earlier research reports that may be related to the topic under study. The most informal method of retrieving research reports occurs when researchers who are working in a particular area exchange digital reprints and other study information (Crane, 1969).

The investigator conducting a meta-analysis samples completed studies. Reviewers may attempt to retrieve an entire population of studies rather than draw a representative sample of the studies on a particular topic. The multiple methods of study retrieval may affect the results of various reviews. Research reports available may differ from one source to another. Two reviewers who use different retrieval techniques to locate studies may end up with different sets of research reports and potentially different evidence. Diversity in information retrieval methods represents a procedural variation that may affect review conclusions. Therefore, reviewers should specify the various retrieval sources or methods they employed just as primary researchers would report the procedures used to select subjects to include in their sample.

Data Evaluation and Coding

Each research report retrieved is examined carefully to determine whether it meets certain predetermined criteria. These criteria are formulated to eliminate studies not related to the problem under investigation or not meeting particular operational parameters.

Reviewers may differ in the identification of criteria for evaluating the relevancy of a particular research report. For instance, some reviewers may decide to include only studies published in peer-reviewed journals. Other investigators may attempt to be more inclusive and obtain research reports presented at professional meetings or in nonpublished sources such as master's theses or doctoral dissertations.

Decisions about which studies to include depend upon:

• The availability of research reports,
• How many studies there are in total,
• How many studies are published,
• The frequency and quality of research designs used, and
• The research question that is being examined.

In making decisions regarding which studies to include, two important questions must be addressed:

• What are the criteria for choosing studies?
• What are the implications for a particular selection strategy?

An area that requires special attention in making an evaluation decision is the type of research design used in the study (Lipsey & Wilson, 2001).

There is considerable disagreement in the literature on meta-analysis regarding this issue. One approach widely used in the biomedical research literature is to include only reports published in peer-reviewed journals that are based on randomized clinical trials (RCTs). The argument supporting this approach is that these studies use designs that reduce bias and have the greatest ability to ensure that any effects are the result of the treatment (independent variable) as opposed to some uncontrolled or unknown factors (Light & Pillemer, 1984). In addition, studies appearing in scientific journals have undergone a rigorous review process, and this helps ensure the validity and accuracy of the findings.

In contrast, Glass and colleagues (1981) suggest that all potentially relevant studies be included in the meta-analysis and that no prior judgments about the quality of a study design be made. They argue that the question of study "quality" and how quality variables affect the outcome of a study can be addressed using the appropriate quantitative reviewing methodology. Previous research has reported mixed results regarding the impact of study design on outcomes. In some research areas, the design is associated with a higher probability of achieving a positive or negative outcome (Colditz, Miller, & Mosteller, 1989). Generally, the poorer or lower-level designs (see Fig. 25.1) are associated with a higher likelihood of a positive outcome. Other studies have found no relationship between design characteristics, such as random assignment of subjects, and study outcome (Concato, Shah, & Horwitz, 2000). The researcher conducting a meta-analysis must make a decision regarding which approach to use in evaluating whether to include a study in the final group of articles to be examined.

Once the evaluation decisions have been clearly specified, information is extracted from the individual studies. In a primary research study, data are collected from the individual subjects participating in the investigation. In a meta-analysis, information is gathered by coding the characteristics of the individual studies. Systematic coding frames are developed to record information and outcomes from each individual study. An example of a coding frame used in a meta-analysis examining the effects of exercise programs on physical, behavioral, and social outcomes in older adults with dementia or Alzheimer's disease (Heyn, Abreu, & Ottenbacher, 2004) is shown in Figure 25.4.

The accuracy and reliability of the coding process and information recorded on the coding frame must be determined. This is accomplished by having more than one rater record information

UTMB/TLC Interventions Trial Quality Form
Systematic Review of Exercise Training & Physical Activity for Elderly People with
Dementia and Cognitive Impairments

SINGLE STUDY QUALITY SCORE

Rater Name: _____ Date _____

Study Author and Year:_____

Study Title:_____

Recommendation for analysis: ☐ Yes   ☐ No   ☐ Unclear

IVS: ☐ 3 ☐ 2 ☐ 1   EVS: ☐ 3 ☐ 2 ☐ 1

Study Quality Points (%)
____ ≥22 points (≥95%) = Very High
____ 19–21 points (81–95%) = High
____ 16–18 points (70–81%) = Medium
____ ≤15 points (≤69%) = Low

Grade of Evidence
__A   __B   __C   __D   __E
Level of Evidence
__1   __2   __3   __4   __5
__a   __b   __c

A. Descriptions	Yes	No	Unclear	
• Was the study population well described (time, place, and person)?	1. ☐	☐	☐	
Was the intervention well described (what, how, who, where)?	2. ☐	☐	☐	Total
	+ ___ 2	– ___ 2	0 ___ 2	___ 2
Comments:				

B. Sampling	Yes	No	Unclear	
• Did the authors specify the sampling frame or universe of selection for the study population?	3. ☐	☐	☐	
• Did the authors specify the screening criteria for study eligibility (MMSE of † 25; or CI descriptions as stated by primary study author)?	4. ☐	☐	☐	
• Was the population that served as the unit of analysis the entire eligible population?	5. ☐	☐	☐	
• Are there other selection bias issues not otherwise addressed (high refusal, inappropriate control, restricted sampling)?	6. ☐	☐	☐	Total
	+ ___ 4	– ___ 4	0 ___ 4	___ 4
Comments:				

C. Measurement	Yes	No	Unclear	
• Did the authors attempt to measure exposure to the intervention?	7. ☐	☐	☐	
• Was the exposure variable:				
- Valid (Cronbach's alpha)?	8. ☐	☐	☐	
- Reliable (consistent, reproducible, interrater, ICC, kappa)?	9. ☐	☐	☐	
• Were the outcome and other independent (or predictor) variables:				
- Valid?	10. ☐	☐	☐	
- Reliable (consistent & reproducible)?	11. ☐	☐	☐	Total
	+ ___ 5	– ___ 5	0 ___ 5	___ 5
Comments:				

D. Data Analysis	Yes	No	Unclear	
• Did the authors conduct appropriate statistical testing by:				
- Conducting statistical testing (when appropriate)?	12. ☐	☐	☐	
- Reporting which statistical tests were used?	13. ☐	☐	☐	
- Controlling for design effects in the statistical model?	14. ☐	☐	☐	
- Controlling for repeated measures in populations that were followed over time?	15. ☐	☐	☐	
- Controlling for differential exposure to the intervention?	16. ☐	☐	☐	

(continued)

Figure 25.4 An example of a coding frame used in a recent meta-analysis examining the effects of exercise programs on physical, behavioral, and social outcomes in older adults with dementia or Alzheimer's disease. *(Heyn, Abreu, & Ottenbacher, 2004).*

• Using a model designed to handle multi-level data when they included group-level and individual co-variates in the model? • Are there other problems with the data analysis? Describe.	17. ☐ 18. ☐	☐ ☐	☐ ☐	 Total
	+ ___ 7	− ___ 7	0 ___ 7	___ 7
Comments:				

E. Interpretation of Results	Yes	No	Unclear	
• Did at least 80% of enrolled participants complete the study?	19. ☐	☐	☐	
• Did the authors assess the confounding variables? - Whether the units of analyses were comparable prior to exposure to the intervention (report *p* values and ICC for demographic age and gender)?	20. ☐	☐	☐	
- Correct for controllable variables or institute study procedures to limit bias appropriately (e.g., randomization, restriction, matching, stratification, or statistical adjustment)?	21. ☐	☐	☐	Totals
	+ ___ 3	− ___ 3	0 ___ 3	___ 3
Comments:				

F. Reporting of Biases or Confounders	Yes	No		
• Check yes if authors reported all or most potential biases or unmeasured/contextual confounders.	22. ☐	☐	☐	
	+ ___ 1	− ___ 1	0 ___ 1	___ 1
Comments:				

				Total
				22

22A. Grade for Internal Validity

	Definition (after Portney & Watkins, 2015)
Internal Validity	Represents the degree of confidence that the results of a study can be attributed to the intervention rather than to flaws in the research design (confidence in the relationship between the independent and dependent variables). Nine areas that can lower the confidence are as follows: selection, history, maturation, repeated testing, instrumentation, regression to the mean, experimental mortality, selection–maturation interaction, and experimenter bias. A variable is an observed and measurable characteristic or concept: the independent variable is the causal intervention or manipulation, and the dependent variable is the outcome measure.
3	High internal validity: no alternate explanation for outcome.
2	Moderate internal validity: attempt to control for lack of randomization.
1	Low internal validity: 2 or more serious alternative explanations for outcome.

Internal Validity Score (IVS): _____

22B. Grade for External Validity

	Definition (after Portney & Watkins, 2015)
Internal Validity	Refers to the degree to which the findings of the study are useful and generalized outside the experimental participants, setting, and times. It is the heterogeneity of the sample that allows you to generalize well. (i.e., age range, one gender, a specific diagnosis, one level of function).
a (3)	**High external validity: S's represent population – AND – treatments represent current practice.** If the participants, settings, and times are all varied the level is High.
b (2)	**Moderate external validity: between high and low.** If two of the three (participants, settings, or times) are varied the level is Moderate.
c (1)	**Low external validity: heterogeneous sample without being able to understand whether effects were similar for all diagnoses – OR – treatment does not represent current practice.** If only one of the three (participants, settings, or times) is varied, the level is Low.

External Validity Score (EVS): _____

Figure 25.4 *Continued*

Confounders for Internal Validity
(From the First Measure to the Second Measure)

1. **History:** The potential effect that participation in specific events may be responsible for change in the outcome (dependent) variable. (e.g., participation in other therapies, or global event such as state law mandating specific behaviors)

2. **Maturation:** The potential effect that passage of time affecting subjects or measures may be responsible for change in the outcome (dependent) variable (e.g., growing older, stronger, healthier, more experienced, weaker, tired, or bored)

3. **Attrition:** The potential effect that (also called experimental mortality) the loss of study subjects by dropout or death may be responsible for changing the randomness; also called experimental mortality (e.g., group with unequal variances)

4. **Testing:** The potential effect that the pretest or repeated measure may be responsible for a change in the outcome (dependent) variable. (e.g., coordination tests may be reactive measures)

5. **Instrumentation:** The potential effect (nonreliable testing) that the calibration, observer, or tester experience and skill may be responsible for the change in the outcome (dependent) variable

6. **Statistical regression:** The potential effect of a (nonreliable) test to tend to extreme scores on pretest to regress toward the mean of the posttest and be responsible for the change in the outcome

7. **Selection:** The potential effect that the difference between the groups (control vs. treatment) cannot be balanced out

8. **Interaction:** The potential effect that the interaction between any combination of selection, maturation, history, and/or instrumentation may be responsible for the change in the outcomes

9. **Treatment:** The potential effect that ambiguity of cause–effect, diffusion of treatment, imitation of treatment, compensatory equalization of treatments, or compensatory rivalry and resentful demoralization of participants receiving less desirable treatment causes the differences in outcomes

10. **Experimental Bias:** The potential effect that the experimenter's or subject's expectation or best presentation is not representative of natural behavior

Grade of Recommendation	Level of Evidence	Therapy/Prevention, Etiology/Harm
A	1a	SR (with homogeneity) of RCTs
	1b	Individual RCT (with narrow confidence interval)
	1c	All or none
B	2a	SR (with homogeneity) of cohort studies
	2b	Individual cohort study (including low-quality RCT; e.g., <80% follow-up)
	2c	Outcomes research
C	3a	SR (with homogeneity) of case-control studies
	3b	Individual case-control study
D	4	Case series (and poor-quality cohort and case-control studies)
E	5	Expert opinion without explicit critical appraisal, or based on physiology, bench research, or first principles

Figure 25.4 *Continued*

from the study and then comparing their independent ratings.

The reliability and accuracy of collecting information from the primary studies included in a meta-analysis is improved when the definitions for treatments, outcomes, study design, subject characteristics, and other variables are clearly and completely described.

Another potential problem in extracting information from studies is coder bias. Strategies have been developed to help reduce coder bias, including training and pilot testing the coding forms. One method to reduce bias is to have examiners code the introduction, demographics, and methodology sections of the article without knowledge of the findings. The results and discussion sections of the article are rated independently so that they will not be influenced by the knowledge of the study design and type of subjects participating or by knowledge of the investigators or institution where the research was conducted. A comprehensive discussion regarding how to evaluate coding decisions and reduce error and bias is available in the literature (Orwin, 2009; Stock, 2009).

Analysis and Interpretation

The traditional criterion for gauging the importance of quantitative research findings is statistical significance. Significance testing is strongly influenced by the size of the sample, and various authorities have questioned its continued use in empirical research (Carver, 1978). Significance testing, which compares an observed relation to the chance of no relation, becomes less informative as evidence supporting a phenomenon accumulates (Hunter & Schmidt, 2009).

The question turns from whether a treatment effect exists to how much of an effect exists. Effect-size measures can play an important role in determining the degree to which a treatment exerts an influence on different outcomes. As noted earlier, the use of a summary statistical measure such as an effect size is what distinguishes meta-analysis from systematic reviews.

Two primary methods were originally advocated to statistically integrate results across multiple studies:

- Combining probabilities by adding z-scores and
- Explaining variation in study-effect sizes.

The technique of combining probabilities, referred to as the Stouffer method, is easy to compute when probability levels are reported. However, the method of combining probabilities has two major inadequacies:

- Studies with significant p-levels are more likely to be published than are studies with nonsignificant p-levels.
- The technique does not tap the wealth of information contained in the variation of results found in multiple studies.

As a consequence, the method of combining probabilities is rarely used in current meta-analysis investigations.

Quantitative procedures capable of uncovering systematic variation in study outcomes were pioneered by Cohen (1988). He defines an effect size measure as the "degree to which the null hypothesis is false." Cohen developed and cataloged effect-size measures appropriate for use with most types of research design and statistical analysis. Three types of effect sizes are used in most meta-analyses conducted in OT research:

- The standardized mean difference,
- The odds ratio, and
- The correlation coefficient.

Table 25.2 contains a brief description of each of these measures of effect size.

There are other types of effect size measures available to investigators conducting a meta-analysis, and these effect sizes are described in many excellent publications available on meta-analysis (Cooper et al., 2009; Petitti, 2000). The standardized mean difference, or d-index, is among the most widely used effect-size measures in meta-analysis studies reported in occupational therapy. For example, Vargas and Camilli (1999) used d-indexes to compare the effects of sensory integration therapy to conditions in which the subjects either received no therapy or a comparison therapy. The d-index is a number that tells how far apart two group means are in terms of their common standard deviation. If a d-index equals 0.3, it indicates that 3/10 of a standard deviation separates the average person in the two groups being compared. This effect size transforms the results from any two-group comparison into a standardized metric, regardless of the original measurement scales.

The d-index can be computed from t- and F-ratios when means and standard deviations are not reported in an article. Friedman (1968) has provided formulas and a rationale for transforming t- and F-values to d-indexes. In cases where t- and F-ratios are not reported, they may be estimated from the significance level and sample size. When nonparametric statistics or percentiles are reported, effect sizes can be computed using procedures described by Glass and others (Glass et al., 1981; Hedges & Olkin, 1985).

Table 25.2 Description of Effect-Size Measures Commonly Used in Occupational Therapy Meta-Analysis Studies

Effect Size	Formula	Description	Range
d-Index	$\overline{ES} = \dfrac{\overline{X}_{G1} - \overline{X}_{G2}}{S_{pooled}}$	The d-index represents a standardized group contrast on a *continuous* measure. It is commonly used for designs where two groups or conditions are compared. X represents the mean of groups, and S_{pooled} is the pooled standard deviation (some situations use control-group standard deviation). Sometimes referred to as g.	0.20–0.49 = small 0.50–0.79 = medium >0.80 = large
Odds ratio*	$\overline{ES} = \dfrac{ad}{bc}$	The odds ratio is based on a 2 × 2 contingency table, such as the one following this table. The odds ratio is the odds of success in the treatment group relative to the odds of success in the control group.	1.50–2.49 = small 2.50–4.29 = medium >4.30 = large
r-index	$\overline{ES} = r$	Represents the strength of association between two continuous measures. Generally reported directly as r (the Pearson product moment coefficient).	0.10–0.24 = small 0.25–0.39 = medium >0.40 = large

* 2 × 2 table used to compute odds ratio:

	Frequencies	
	Success	Failure
Treatment group	a	b
Control group	c	d

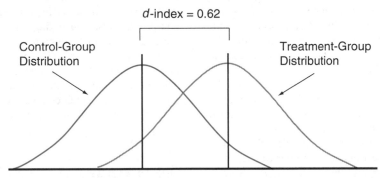

d-index = 0.62

Control-Group Distribution   Treatment-Group Distribution

Figure 25.5 Overlapping distributions of effect sizes from the control group and treatment group. The U_3 associated with a d-index of 0.62 is 0.73. The U_3 value indicates that the average performance of subjects in the higher-meaned (treatment) groups is "better" than 73% of the subjects in the lower-meaned (control or comparison) groups not receiving the intervention. Data are from a meta-analysis examining the effects of exercise on older adults with cognitive impairment and dementia (Heyn, Abreu & Ottenbacher, 2004) in which 2,020 subjects participated in 30 trials evaluating exercise in persons 65 years and older with cognitive impairment. The overall mean effect size (d-index) between exercise and nonexercise groups for all outcomes was 0.62 (95% confidence interval [CI], 0.55–0.70).

Cohen (1988) presents several measures of distribution overlap meant to enhance the interpretability of effect size indexes. The overlap measure most often employed in meta-analysis is called U^3. The U^3 value indicates the percentage of the population with the smaller mean (generally control groups) that is exceeded by the average person in the population with the higher mean (generally treatment groups). Figure 25.5 presents the overlapping distributions for two groups of subjects being compared in a meta-analysis investigation. The U^3 associated with a d-index of 0.30 is 61.8. This means that the average performance of subjects in the higher-meaned (treatment) groups is "better" than 61.8% of the subjects in the lower-meaned (control or comparison) groups not receiving the particular intervention or independent variable.

Once the type of effect size to be used has been determined, there are several other analysis concerns that the investigator must address. One of the most important is dealing with potential sampling bias and error in the studies examined.

It is generally accepted that effect sizes should be weighted based on the number of participants included in the individual study. This is because large samples will produce more accurate population estimates. For example, a d-index or r-value based on a sample of 500 subjects will give a more precise estimate of the true population effect size than a sample of 50 subjects. Effect sizes from the studies included in the meta-analysis should reflect this fact. Various sample-size weighting systems have been developed for different effect-size measures.

Another sampling-related concern is the degree of variability present in the sample of effect-size values included in the meta-analysis study. This is tested by what is called a homogeneity analysis. The sample of effect-size values generated by a meta-analysis will vary due to normal sampling error. The researcher wants to know if the amount of variability in the effect sizes is greater than would be expected by chance (sampling error). The homogeneity analysis asks the question: Is the observed variance in effect sizes significantly different from that expected by sampling error? If the answer is "No," then some statisticians would argue that the analysis should stop because sampling error is the simplest explanation for why effect sizes differ. If the answer is "Yes," that is, the variance in effect size values is larger than would be expected from sampling error, then the investigator begins to examine whether study characteristics, such as research design, are associated with differences in effect sizes. The sophistication of statistical procedures to examine this variation has increased dramatically over the past two decades and is beyond the scope of this introductory chapter. Information on statistical methods used in meta-analysis to test the homogeneity of effect sizes is provided in a number of excellent sources (Cooper et al., 2009; Hedges & Olkin, 1985).

Reporting Results

Cooper and Cooper (1989) observed that reviewers using traditional narrative methods have no formal guidelines describing how to structure the final report of their findings (see Fig. 25.3). Narrative reviewers have traditionally followed informal guidelines provided by previous reviews on the same or related topics. In most cases, the reviewer chooses a format that is convenient for the particular review problem. Cooper and Cooper (1989) proposed that reviewers employing quantitative methods report their results using a format similar to that employed by investigators conducting

primary research studies. The results of a meta-analysis should include the following sections:

• Introduction,
• Methods,
• Results, and
• Discussion.

In the introduction, the investigator identifies the problem under review and discusses the results of previous research and traditional literature reviews. The need for a meta-analysis is established in the introduction. The methods section describes the procedures the reviewer used to retrieve research reports and the sources searched. Information on the number of studies selected, criteria used for inclusion, and coding of studies (i.e., what information was extracted from each research report) is also included in this section of the meta-analysis. The results section includes the findings of the quantitative synthesis and should contain information on the type of effect size used, how it was computed, the basic unit of analysis, and the actual statistical outcomes. Finally, the discussion section allows the reviewer to summarize the findings, compare them to previous narrative reviews and primary research studies, and suggest areas in need of further investigation.

Table 25.3 lists a number of meta-analyses that have been published on topics directly relevant to occupational therapy. These studies provide examples of how to conduct and report the findings of meta-analyses in the professional and research literature.

Advantages and Limitations of Meta-Analysis

Light and Pillemer (1984) have identified four specific advantages in the use of meta-analysis to integrate studies:

1. Increased statistical power,
2. Obtaining an estimate of the magnitude of experimental effects,
3. Greater insight into the nature of relationships among variables, and
4. The ability to objectively explore contradictions in a group of studies.

Statistical power is related to the sensitivity or ability of a study to find a true difference between groups (treatment and control groups) when a difference actually exists. Statistical power is directly influenced by sample size; the larger the sample

Table 25.3 Meta-Analysis Articles Related to Occupational Therapy

Year	Author(s)	Topic
1985	Ottenbacher & Peterson	Vestibular stimulation research
1986	Cusick	Research in occupational therapy
1993	Ottenbacher & Jannell	Clinical trials in stroke
1996	Carlson et al.	Occupational therapy for older patients
1997	Lin, Wu, Tickle-Degnen, & Coster	Occupational embedded exercise
1998	Wu	Context and cerebrovascular accident (CVA)
1998	Tickle-Degnen	Collaborative treatment
1999	Vargas & Camilli	Sensory integration treatment
2000	Sudsawad	Kinesthetic training and handwriting in children
2000	Dennis & Rebeiro	Occupational therapy and mental health
2002	Horowitz	Geriatric rehabilitation
2002	Reid, Laliberte-Rudman, & Hebert	Seated mobility devices and performance of users and caregivers
2002	Trombly & Ma	Occupational therapy for stroke, part 1
2002	Ma & Trombly	Occupational therapy for stroke, part 2
2002	Deane et al.	Paramedical therapies and Parkinson's disease
2002	Steultjens et al.	Occupational therapy for rheumatoid arthritis
2003	Mulligan	Sensory integration and children
2003	Handy et al.	Upper limb function after stroke
2003a	Steultjens et al.	Occupational therapy for persons with multiple sclerosis (MS)
2003b	Steultjens et al.	Occupational therapy for stroke (cognition)
2004	Steultjens et al.	Occupational therapy for children with cerebral palsy (CP)
2004	Kielhofner, Hammel, Finlayson, Helfrich, & Taylor	Outcomes research
2007	Legg et al.	Occupation therapy for activities of daily living (ADLs) in persons with stroke
2008	Clemson et al.	Environmental intervention to prevent falls
2011	Zadnikar & Kastrin	Hippotherapy and postural control in children with CP
2012	Kim, Yoo, Jung, Park, & Park	Occupational therapy for persons with dementia
2013	Smits-Engelsman et al.	Motor performance in children with developmental coordination disorder
2013	Blikman et al.	Energy conservation and fatigue in MS
2015	Leong, Carter, & Stephenson	Sensory integration for developmental and learning disabilities
2015	Lockwood, Taylor, & Harding	Home assessment and return to the community

size, the greater the statistical power when all other factors remain the same. Statistical power is also associated with type II errors. A type II error occurs when a researcher mistakenly rejects a null hypothesis (indicating no difference between groups) although a difference actually does exist.

Meta-analysis increases statistical power by increasing the sample size used in making comparisons between groups. For example, in the meta-analysis examining the effectiveness of stroke rehabilitation, the combined sample size for the 36 studies was 3,717. This sample size is much larger than the sample size included in any individual primary research study and ensures that the

results generated from the meta-analysis will not be a type II error.

The second advantage is the ability to determine the magnitude of a treatment effect. This advantage is related to the distinction between findings that are statistically significant versus findings that are clinically or practically important. Statistical significance is an all-or-none determination based on a probability level, usually $p < .05$. Effect sizes, in contrast, allow for a range of interpretations. The interpretations require judgments on the part of the researcher or reader. As implied earlier, statistical significance is closely related to sample size, such that with large sample sizes

small differences between groups may be statistically significant. These small differences may have
limited practical importance. In contrast, large differences that are practically important may not be
statistically significant if the sample size is small.

Measures of effect size provide a more direct
indication of treatment impact. Effect size measures can be converted to percent differences using
indexes such as the U^3 value described earlier. For
example, the d-index of 0.40 reported for the stroke
rehabilitation meta-analysis described earlier can
be converted to a U^3 value of 65.5% (Cohen,
1988). This U^3 value means that the average person
in the treatment groups receiving stroke rehabilitation did 15.5% better than the average person
in the control or comparison group who received
standard medical care. Using this information,
the reader is able to make a judgment regarding
whether a 15.5% increase in performance is clinically or practically important.

The third advantage of meta-analysis is the
ability to better understand the relationship
between study subject characteristics and study
outcome. Because multiple studies are included
in a meta-analysis, there is greater variability in
study design and subject characteristics than is
found in an individual primary research study.
This variability allows the researcher conducting
a meta-analysis to examine questions that cannot
be asked in a primary study. The meta-analysis on
stroke rehabilitation provides an example of such
a question. As noted in the previous section, an
interaction was found between the type of research
design (pre-experimental, quasi-experimental, and
true experimental) and how the outcome measures
were recorded (blind recording versus not blind)
(see Fig. 25.1). This relationship could not have
been found in a primary research study.

The final advantage is the potential to explore
contradictions across a series of primary research
studies. Meta-analysis allows the investigator to
systematically examine moderating or confounding variables that may explain contradictory outcomes in primary studies. For example, if age is
a variable that impacts the outcome of interest so
that a treatment is more likely to work for subjects older than 60 years of age than for those
younger than age 60, this can be detected in a
meta-analysis; a meta-analysis may help explain
why previous studies including younger subjects
produce results different from or contradictory to
studies using the same treatment but that include
older subjects.

Meta-analysis procedures also have limitations that must be recognized and acknowledged.
Meta-analysis methods contain aspects of both art

and science, as does all research. The science is
revealed in the systematic application and definition of a research approach related to literature
reviewing. The art refers to the judgments that
need to be made in the application of the procedures. Like all research methods, meta-analysis
involves assumptions that must be made explicit,
and if these assumptions are not clear to the user
or reader, misleading conclusions may occur.
Box 25.1 describes how meta-analysis is now
being applied to qualitative research in addition to
quantitative research.

The ability of meta-analysis procedures to test
certain interactions or relationships contained
within aggregated studies does not mean that all
problems of conceptualization or methodological
artifact can be resolved in this manner. As in evaluating a single study, alternate conceptualizations
of included treatment variables may rival the one
offered. In addition, some readers may judge that
the quantitative synthesis of results from multiple
studies may create an illusion of statistical objectivity that is not justified by the data obtained from
the review. Related to the issue of statistical precision is the fact that multiple hypotheses tests may
be included in a single research report, and effect
sizes generated from these multiple hypotheses
are not independent data points. This introduces
the problem of nonindependence, which may
affect the results of inferential statistical procedures used to analyze the data. The role of inferential statistical procedures in the data analysis
stage of meta-analysis is controversial and beyond
the scope of this introductory chapter (Lipsey &
Wilson, 2001).

Summary

Meta-analysis offers researchers a powerful means
of summarizing aggregate data in a systematic
way. To conduct a meta-analysis, the researcher
must first define the research question or problem,
then the inclusion criteria, the sample selection
method, and the data collection process.

In spite of the limitations and challenges cited
earlier, meta-analysis represents a significant
advance over the traditional narrative methods of
reviewing quantitative research. Meta-analysis is
particularly relevant to disciplines such as occupational therapy that are in the early stages of
developing theory and research to support clinical
practice. The use of meta-analysis represents an
important shift in scientific thinking in which the
literature review is conceptualized as a form of
scientific inquiry in its own right. The continued
evolution and application of meta-analysis should

Box 25.1   Qualitative Methods and Meta-Analysis

Researchers using qualitative methods have proposed applying the concepts associated with systematic reviews to synthesize findings from multiple qualitative studies (Paterson, Thorne, Canam, & Jillings, 2001). Upshur (2001) suggested that there are two different definitions of evidence from the qualitative perspective. The first narrative evidence he describes as primarily Qualitative/Personal and the second as Qualitative/General. Qualitative/Personal evidence is concrete, particular, and historical, whereas Qualitative/General evidence is historical and social.

Occupational therapists have embraced qualitative methodologies in search of a better understanding of the social and personal aspects of health care (Clark, 1993; Krefting & Krefting, 1991); in conducting individual studies, however, we were unable to find examples of systematic reviews of qualitative research in the occupational therapy literature. Examples do exist in the broader health-care literature (Clemmens, 2003; McCormick, Rodney, & Varcoe, 2003; Sandelowski, Lambe & Barroso, 2004; Varcoe, Rodney, & McCormick, 2003).

Qualitative systematic reviews are a new research methodology, and the procedures and technology are not well developed (Schreiber, Crooks, & Stern, 1997). Qualitative research has informed health-care practitioners for decades; it deepens our understanding of human experience and of phenomena that illustrate that experience (Morse, 1997). Standards for assessing the rigor of qualitative research methods for conducting and disseminating systematic reviews need to be developed and tested (Davies & Dodd, 2002; Whittemore, Chase, & Mandle, 2001). There is also a lack of agreement regarding how to assess the quality and usefulness of qualitative studies for evidence-based practice (Marks, 1999; Morse, 1997; Morse, Swanson, & Kuzel, 2001; Paterson et al., 2001).

Practitioners traditionally combine the art and science of occupational therapy to determine the quality of clinical care. This integrative perspective requires the use of qualitative studies to improve our understanding of occupational therapy and occupational science (Giacomini, 2001). The contributions to occupational therapy evidence are complemented by both methodologies; they both can enhance client and caretaker empowerment and the quality of occupational therapy and occupational science. One of the challenges facing researchers in occupational therapy is to collectively integrate the information from multiple qualitative investigations.

help researchers establish a scientifically respected foundation for evidence-based practice in occupational therapy.

Review Questions

1. What are the role and purpose of meta-analysis in OT research and practice?
2. What are the steps involved in conducting a meta-analysis?
3. What are the various approaches to defining effect size in meta-analysis?
4. What are the advantages and disadvantages of meta-analysis as a research method in occupational therapy?

REFERENCES

Abreu, B. C. (2010). Evidence-based practice. In G. L. McCormack, E. Jaffe, & M. Goodman-Lavey (Eds.), *The occupational therapy manager* (5th ed., pp. 351–373). Bethesda, MD: AOTA Press.

Blikman, L. J., Huisstede, B. M., Kooijmans, H., Stam, H. J., Bussmann, J. B., & van Meeteren, J. (2013). Effectiveness of energy conservation treatment in reducing fatigue in multiple sclerosis: A systematic review and meta-analysis. *Archives of Physical Medicine and Rehabilitation, 94*(7), 1360–1376.

Carlson, M., Fanchiang, S. P., Zemke, R., & Clark, F. (1996). A meta-analysis of the effectiveness of occupational therapy for older persons. *American Journal of Occupational Therapy, 50*, 89–98.

Carver, R. P. (1978). The case against statistical significance testing. *Harvard Educational Review, 48*, 378–399.

Clark, F. (1993). Occupation embedded in a real life: Interweaving occupational science and occupational therapy. 1993 Eleanor Clarke Slagle Lecture. *American Journal of Occupational Therapy, 47*(12), 1067–1078.

Clemmens, D. (2003). Adolescent motherhood: A metasynthesis of qualitative studies. *The American Journal of Maternal/Child Nursing, 28*(2), 93–99.

Clemson, L., Mackenzie, L., Ballinger, C., Close, J. C. T., & Cumming, R. C. (2008). Environmental interventions to prevent falls in community-dwelling older people: A meta-analysis of randomized trials. *Journal of Aging and Health, 20*(8), 954–971.

Cohen, J. (1988). *Statistical power analysis for the behavioral sciences* (2nd ed.). Hillsdale, NJ: Lawrence Erlbaum Associates.

Colditz, G. A., Miller, J. N., & Mosteller, F. (1989). How study design affects outcomes in comparisons of therapy. Part 1: Medical. *Statistics in Medicine, 8*, 441–454.

Concato, J., Shah, N., & Horwitz, R. I. (2000). Randomized, controlled trials, observational studies, and the hierarchy of research designs. *New England Journal of Medicine, 342*, 1887–1892.

Cooper H. M. (2010). *Research synthesis and meta-analysis: A step-by-step approach* (4th ed). Thousand Oaks, CA: Sage.

Cooper, H. M., & Cooper, H. M. (1989). *Integrating research: A guide for literature reviews*. Newbury Park, CA: Sage.

Cooper, H. M., Hedges, L. V., & Valentine, J. C. (2009). *The handbook of research synthesis* (2nd ed.). New York, NY: Russell Sage Foundation.

Crane, D. (1969). Social structure in a group of scientists: A test of the invisible college hypothesis. *American Sociological Review, 34,* 335–352.

Cusick, A. (1986). Research in occupational therapy: Meta-analysis. *Australian Occupational Therapy Journal, 33,* 142–147.

Davies, D., & Dodd, J. (2002). Qualitative research and the question of rigor. *Qualitative Health Research, 12*(2), 279–289.

Deane, K. H., Ellis-Hill, C., Jones, D., Whurr, R., Ben Shlomo, Y., Playford, E. D., & Clarke, C. E. (2002). Systematic review of paramedical therapies for Parkinson's disease. *Movement Disorders, 17,* 984–991.

Dennis, D. M., & Rebeiro, K. L. (2000). Occupational therapy in pediatric mental health: Do we practice what we preach? *Occupational Therapy in Mental Health, 16,* 5–25.

Dobkin, B. H. (1989). Focused stroke rehabilitation programs do not improve outcome. *Archives of Neurology, 46,* 701–703.

Evidence-Based Medicine Working Group. (1992). Evidence-based medicine: A new approach to teaching the practice of medicine. *Journal of the American Medical Association, 268,* 2420–2425.

Friedman, H. (1968). Magnitude of experimental effect and a table for its rapid estimation. *Psychological Bulletin, 70,* 245–251.

Giacomini, M. K. (2001). The rocky road: Qualitative research as evidence. *ACP Journal Club, 134*(1), A11–A13.

Glass, G. V., McGaw, B., & Smith, M. L. (1981). *Meta-analysis in social research.* Beverly Hills, CA: Sage.

Handy, J., Salinas, S., Blanchard, S. A., & Aitken, M. J. (2003). Meta-analysis examining the effectiveness of electrical stimulation in improving functional use of the upper limb in stroke patients. *Physical and Occupational Therapy in Geriatrics, 21,* 67–78.

Hedges, L. V., & Olkin, I. (1985). *Statistical methods for meta-analysis.* Orlando, FL: Academic Press.

Heyn, P., Abreu, B. C., & Ottenbacher, K. J. (2004). The effects of exercise training on elderly persons with cognitive impairment and dementia: A meta-analysis. *Archives of Physical Medicine and Rehabilitation, 85,* 1694–1704.

Horowitz, B. P. (2002). Rehabilitation utilization in New York state: Implications for geriatric rehabilitation in 2015. *Topics in Geriatric Rehabilitation, 17,* 78–89.

Hunter, J. E., & Schmidt, F. L. (2009). Correcting for sources of artificial variation across studies. In H. M. Cooper & L. V. Hedges (Eds.), *The handbook of research synthesis* (pp. 323–336). New York, NY: Russell Sage Foundation.

Institute of Medicine. (2001). *Crossing the quality chasm: A new health system for the 21st century.* Washington, DC: National Academy Press.

Kielhofner, G., Hammel, J., Finlayson, M., Helfrich, C., & Taylor, R. R. (2004). Documenting outcomes of occupational therapy: The center for outcomes research and education. *American Journal of Occupational Therapy, 58,* 15–23.

Kim, S-Y., Yoo, E-Y., Jung, M-Y., Park, S. H., & Park, J-H. (2012). A systematic review of the effects of occupational therapy for persons with dementia: A meta-analysis of randomized controlled trials. *NeuroRehabilitation, 31,* 107–115.

Krefting, L., & Krefting, D. (1991). Leisure activities after a stroke: An ethnographic approach. *American Journal of Occupational Therapy, 45*(5), 429–436.

Legg, L., Drummond, A., Leonardi-Bee, J., Gladman, J. R., Corr, S., Donkervoort, M., . . . Langhorne, P. (2007). Occupational therapy for patients with problems in personal activities of daily living after stroke: Systematic review of randomised trials. *British Medical Journal, 335,* 922–925.

Leong, H. M., Carter, M., & Stephenson, J. R. (2015). Meta-analysis of research on sensory integration therapy for individuals with developmental and learning disabilities. *Journal of Developmental and Physical Disabilities, 27*(2), 183–206.

Light, R. J., & Pillemer, D. B. (1984). *Summing up: The science of reviewing research.* Cambridge, MA: Harvard University Press.

Lin, K., Wu, C., Tickle-Degnen, L., & Coster, W. (1997). Enhancing occupational performance through occupationally embedded exercise: A meta-analytic review. *Occupational Therapy Journal of Research, 17,* 25–47.

Lipsey, M. W., & Wilson, D. B. (2001). *Practical meta-analysis* (vol. 49). Thousand Oaks, CA: Sage.

Lockwood, K. J., Taylor, N. F., & Harding, K. E. (2015). Pre-discharge home assessment visits in assisting patients' return to community living: A systematic review and meta-analysis. *Journal of Rehabilitation Medicine, 47,* 289–299.

Ma, H. I., & Trombly, C. A. (2002). A synthesis of the effects of occupational therapy for persons with stroke. Part II: Remediation of impairments. *American Journal of Occupational Therapy, 56,* 260–274.

Marks, S. (1999). Qualitative studies. In A. McKibbon (with A. Eady & S. Marks), (Eds.), *PDQ evidence-based principles and practice* (pp. 187–204). Hamilton, Ontario: B. C. Decker.

McCormick, J., Rodney, P., & Varcoe, C. (2003). Reinterpretations across studies: An approach to meta-analysis. *Qualitative Health Research, 13*(7), 933–944.

Morse, J. M. (Ed.). (1997). *Completing a qualitative project: Details and dialogue.* Thousand Oaks, CA: Sage.

Morse, J. M., Swanson, J. M., & Kuzel, A. J. (2001). *The nature of qualitative evidence.* Thousand Oaks, CA: Sage.

Mulligan, S. (2003). Examination of the evidence for occupational therapy using a sensory integration framework with children: Part one. *Sensory Integration Special Interest Section Quarterly, 26,* 1–4.

Orwin, R. G. (2009). Evaluating coding decisions. In H. M. Cooper & L. V. Hedges (Eds.), *The handbook of research synthesis* (pp. 139–162). New York, NY: Russell Sage Foundation.

Ottenbacher, K. J., & Jannell, S. (1993). The results of clinical trials in stroke rehabilitation research. *Archives of Neurology, 50,* 37–44.

Ottenbacher, K. J., & Petersen, P. (1985). A meta-analysis of applied vestibular stimulation research. *Physical and Occupational Therapy in Pediatrics, 5,* 119–134.

Paterson, B. L., Thorne, S. E., Canam, C., & Jillings, C. (2001). *Meta-study of qualitative health research: A practical guide to meta-analysis and meta-synthesis* (vol. 3). Thousand Oaks, CA: Sage.

Petitti, D. B. (2000). *Meta-analysis, decision analysis, and cost-effectiveness analysis: Methods for quantitative synthesis in medicine.* New York, NY: Oxford University Press.

Portney, L.G. & Watkins, M.P. (2015). *Foundations of Clinical Research,* (3rd ed.). Philadelphia: FA Davis.

Reding, M. J., & McDowell, F. H. (1989). Focused stroke rehabilitation programs improve outcome. *Archives of Neurology, 46,* 700–701.

Reid, D., Laliberte-Rudman, D., & Hebert, D. (2002). Impact of wheeled seated mobility devices on adult users' and their caregivers' occupational performance: A critical literature review. *Canadian Journal of Occupational Therapy, 69,* 261–280.

Rosenthal, R. (1978). Combining results of independent studies. *Psychological Bulletin, 85,* 185–193.

Sandelowski, M., Lambe, C., & Barroso, J. (2004). Stigma in HIV-positive women. *Journal of Nursing Scholarship, 36*(2), 122–128.

Schreiber, R., Crooks, D., & Stern, P. N. (1997). Qualitative meta-analysis. In J. M. Morse (Ed.), *Completing a qualitative project: Details and dialogue* (pp. 311–326). Thousand Oaks, CA: Sage.

Smits-Engelsman, C. M., Blank, R., Van Der Kaay, A. C., Mosterd-Van Der Meijs, R., Vlugt-Van Den Brand, E., Polatajko, H. J., & Wilson, P. H. (2013). Efficacy of interventions to improve motor performance in children with developmental coordination disorder: A combined systematic review and meta-analysis. *Developmental Medicine and Child Neurology, 55*(3), 229–237.

Steultjens, E. M., Dekker, J., Bouter, L. M., Cardol, M., van de Nes, J. C., & van den Ende, C. H. (2003a). Occupational therapy for multiple sclerosis. *Cochrane Database Systematic Reviews,* CD003608.

Steultjens, E. M., Dekker, J., Bouter, L. M., van de Nes, J. C., Cup, E. H., & van den Ende, C. H. (2003b). Occupational therapy for stroke patients: A systematic review. *Stroke, 34,* 676–687.

Steultjens, E. M., Dekker, J., Bouter, L. M., van de Nes, J. C., Lambregts, B. L., & van den Ende, C. H. (2004). Occupational therapy for children with cerebral palsy: A systematic review. *Clinical Rehabilitation, 18,* 1–14.

Steultjens, E. M., Dekker, J., Bouter, L. M., van Schaardenburg, D., van Kuyk, M. A., & van den Ende, C. H. (2002). Occupational therapy for rheumatoid arthritis: A systematic review. *Arthritis Rheumatism, 47,* 672–685.

Stock, W. A. (2009). Systematic coding for research synthesis. In H. M. Cooper & L. V. Hedges (Eds.), *The handbook of research synthesis* (pp. 125–138). New York, NY: Russell Sage Foundation.

Straus, S., Glasziou, P., Richardson W. S., & Haynes, R. B. (2010). *Evidence-based medicine: How to practice it* (4th ed.). Edinburgh, Scotland: Churchill Livingstone.

Sudsawad, P. (2000). The effect of kinesthetic training on handwriting performance in grade one children with handwriting difficulties [Dissertation Abstract: 2000-95010-344]. *Dissertation Abstracts International: Section B: The Sciences & Engineering, 60*(11-B), 5472.

Tickle-Degnen, L. (1998). Communicating with clients about treatment outcomes: The use of meta-analytic evidence in collaborative treatment planning. *American Journal of Occupational Therapy, 52,* 526–530.

Trombly, C. A., & Ma, H. I. (2002). A synthesis of the effects of occupational therapy for persons with stroke, Part I: Restoration of roles, tasks, and activities. *American Journal of Occupational Therapy, 56,* 250–259.

University Health Network. (2004). *Centre for Evidence-Based Medicine.* Retrieved from http://www.cebm.utoronto.ca/

Upshur, R. E. G. (2001). The status of qualitative research as evidence. In J. M. Morse, J. M. Swanson & A. J. Kuzel (Eds.), *The nature of qualitative evidence* (pp. 5–26). Thousand Oaks, CA: Sage.

Varcoe, C., Rodney, P., & McCormick, J. (2003). Health care relationships in context: An analysis of three ethnographies. *Qualitative Health Research, 13*(7), 957–973.

Vargas, S., & Camilli, G. (1999). A meta-analysis of research on sensory integration treatment. *American Journal of Occupational Therapy, 53,* 189–198.

Whitehead, A. (2002). *Meta-analysis of controlled clinical trials.* Chichester, England: John Wiley & Sons.

Whittemore, R., Chase, S. K., & Mandle, C. L. (2001). Validity in qualitative research. *Qualitative Health Research, 11*(4), 522–537.

Wu, C. Y. (1998). Effects of context on movement kinematics in adults with and without cerebral vascular accident [Dissertation Abstract: 1998-95002-215]. *Dissertation Abstracts International: Section B: The Sciences & Engineering, 58*(7-B), 3593.

Zadnikar, M., & Kastrin, A. J. (2011). Effects of hippotherapy and therapeutic horseback riding on postural control or balance in children with cerebral palsy: A meta-analysis. *Developmental Medicine and Child Neurology, 53*(8), 684–691.

CHAPTER 26

Single-Subject Research

Jean Crosetto Deitz

Learning Outcomes

- Describe single-subject research and its advantages.
- Evaluate the four central design approaches to single-subject research in terms of validity and ethical issues.
- Describe three common types of multiple-baseline designs.
- Identify the considerations in data analysis and reporting for single-subject research.
- Explain how variables are defined and data are collected in single-subject research.
- Understand the importance of socially validating findings from single-subject research.
- Describe the limits of generalization in single-subject research.

Introduction

Single-subject research defines a group of related methodological approaches that involve in-depth analyses of the behaviors of a single research subject or of a relatively small group of subjects that is considered collectively, with the subjects serving as their own controls. Research questions are often derived from clinical practice. In turn, it finds its greatest utility in terms of illuminating clinical concepts and providing data to validate new and existing conceptual practice models (Backman, Harris, Chisholm, & Monette, 1997).

A therapist working in a technology center wanted to know if her client, an individual with a high-level spinal cord injury, would be more successful in terms of text entry using system A as opposed to system B. A second therapist, working with four individuals who were institutionalized with chronic depression, wanted to know if these individuals would initiate conversation more in their group therapy session if it followed a pet therapy session. These examples characterize the types of questions that therapists continually ask, and both of these questions can be addressed using single-subject research methods.

Single-subject research, sometimes referred to as single-system research, is based on within-subject performance. Each participant serves as his or her own control and there are repeated measurements over time of the same dependent variable or variables. Also, while other factors are held constant, there is systematic application, withdrawal, and sometimes variation of the intervention (independent variable).

Single-subject research methods are useful for answering questions regarding the effectiveness of specific interventions for specific individuals by providing experimental control and by contributing to clear and precise clinical documentation. They are especially suited to occupational therapy (OT) research because groups of persons with similar characteristics are not required, and thus these methods are appropriate for use when the therapist has one or, at most, a few clients with whom a particular intervention is employed. They are also appropriate in situations in which the therapist is working with an individual with a low-incidence diagnosis or impairment. A further advantage of single-subject research is that it does not require the withholding of treatment from a no-treatment control group. Because each participant serves as his or her own control, the treatment typically is withheld from the participant for one or more periods of time, and then it is instituted or reinstituted. Also, because only one or a small number of individuals are studied, the financial and time demands are realistic for practice settings. Even though only one or a small number of individuals are studied, the findings from single-subject research can be used to inform practice and to justify and inform larger-scale investigations (Ottenbacher, 1990). Information learned in the process of single-subject research can be used in designing more costly group experimental studies involving numerous participants and multiple sites, as shown in the following Case Example.

CASE EXAMPLE

An interdisciplinary group wanted to know if the use of therapy balls as classroom seating devices affected the behavior of students with attention deficit-hyperactivity disorder (ADHD) (Schilling, Washington, Billingsley, & Deitz, 2003). Their first research question was, "What effect does using therapy balls as chairs have on in-seat behavior?" (Schilling et al., 2003, p. 535). The convenience sample for the study consisted of three children (two males and one female) with ADHD and average intelligence. The three children were from the same fourth-grade public school classroom, and during language arts, all demonstrated out-of-seat behavior requiring repeated teacher verbal and/or physical prompts (Fig. 26.1).

The dependent variable, in-seat behavior, was measured by a rater who scored the participants as displaying either out-of-seat or in-seat behavior following each 10-second observation (Schilling et al., 2003). Each participant was observed for five 2-minute periods during language arts, for a total of 60 observations per session. Data systematically were collected for in-seat behavior for each of the participants individually. During language arts, the three participants and all other class members experienced (1) a series of days during which chairs were used for seating (first baseline phase); (2) a 1-week novelty period during which balls were used for seating; (3) a series of days during which balls were used for seating (first intervention phase); (4) a series of days during which chairs were used for seating (second baseline phase); and (5) last, a series of days during which balls were used for seating (second intervention phase). Throughout the study, efforts were made to hold all factors constant that could potentially have influenced the results of the study. For example, the teacher was the same each day; data were collected at the same time each day; and, throughout the duration of the study, each participant's medication for ADHD was held constant in terms of type and dosage.

Throughout all baseline and intervention phases, even though all of the children in the classroom participated in the intervention, data were collected only for the three children with ADHD. Data were graphed and examined for each of the three participants individually. Refer to Figure 26.2 for an example of graphed data for the percentage of intervals seated for Emily (pseudonym). It indicates that Emily displayed in-seat behavior in a higher percentage of intervals when using the therapy ball for seating during language arts than when using a chair for seating. For Emily, confidence in the effect of the intervention is supported because her in-seat behavior increased immediately following institution of the intervention, dropped markedly when the intervention was removed, then increased again when the intervention was reinstituted. The graphs for the other two participants were similar to the graph depicted in Figure 26.2, thus providing additional support for the use of therapy balls for classroom seating for fourth-grade students with ADHD. Studies such as the one just described support evidence-based practice.

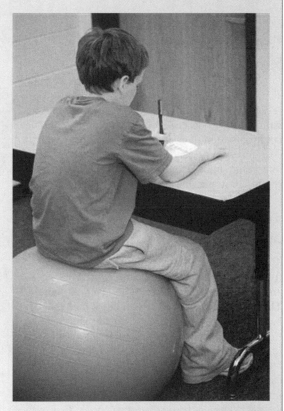

Figure 26.1   A study participant is observed working while using a therapy ball as a chair.

(case study continues on page 362)

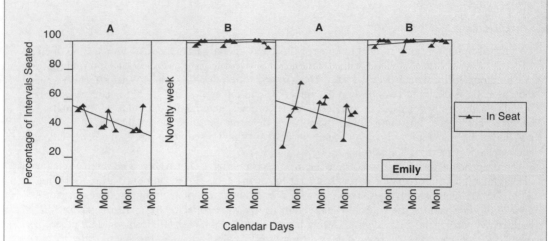

Figure 26.2 Graph of Emily's in-seat behavior. Connected data points represent consecutive days within the same week. Variability in the number of data points was the result of a nonschool day or absence from class. The A sections show baseline data (Emily sitting in a chair), and the B sections show intervention data (Emily sitting on a therapy ball). *(Copyright 2003 by the American Occupational Therapy Association, Inc. Reprinted with permission.)*

Common Single-Subject Research Designs

There are nine common types of single-subject research designs, all based on the *A–B* design, which will be described in this section. A simple notation system is used for single-subject research designs: *A* represents baseline, *B* represents the intervention phase, and *C* and all other letters represent additional interventions or conditions.

The *A–B* Design and Variations

The design upon which all others are built is the *A–B* **design,** where *A* indicates a baseline phase and *B* indicates a treatment (or intervention) phase. This can be exemplified by looking at both the first baseline phase (*A*) and the treatment phase (*B*) in Figure 26.2 in our Case Example discussing the therapy ball study. This displays the data for Emily for the percentage of intervals seated. The vertical axis of the graph indicates the percentage of intervals seated, and the horizontal axis indicates the days. During the first baseline phase (*A*), Emily experienced 12 days of sitting on classroom chairs as usual, and data were systematically kept on percentage of intervals seated. Note that Emily's percentages of intervals seated were consistently

below 60%. Following the novelty week, phase *B* (intervention) was started, and Emily used the therapy ball for seating during language arts. Note that the percentage of intervals seated increased substantially during the treatment phase. If the study had stopped after data were collected for only a baseline phase and an intervention phase, this would have been an *A–B* design.

A common variation of the *A–B* design is the *A–B–C* **successive intervention design.** With this design, a second intervention is introduced in the *C* phase. For example, the therapist studying the effects of the alternative seating devices might have chosen to introduce the therapy ball for seating in the *B* phase and an air cushion for seating in the *C* phase in an attempt to see if one device was more effective than the other.

Another variation of the *A–B* design is the *A–B–C* changing-criterion design, which is characterized by having three or more phases, with the criterion for success changing sequentially from one intervention phase to the next. This design is suited to interventions that are modified in a stepwise manner because the criterion for success is changed incrementally with each successive intervention phase (Hartmann & Hall, 1976). It is appropriate for situations in which the goal is stepwise increases in accuracy (e.g., quality of letters written), frequency (e.g., number of repetitions completed), duration (e.g., length of exercise session), latency (e.g., time it takes to begin to respond after a question is asked), and magnitude (e.g., pounds of weight lifted) (Hartmann & Hall, 1976). Consider a client who seldom or never exercises and is enrolled in a health promotion program because of health concerns. The baseline phase (A) might involve recording the number of continuous minutes the individual walks on a treadmill at 1.5 miles per hour. During the first intervention phase (B), the criterion for success might be 30 continuous minutes of treadmill walking at 1.5 miles per hour; during the second intervention phase (C), the criterion for success might be 30 continuous minutes of treadmill walking at 2.0 miles per hour; and during the third intervention phase (D), the criterion for success might be 30 continuous minutes of treadmill walking at 2.5 miles per hour. This could continue until the desired rate of walking was achieved. The changing criterion design also is useful in situations in which stepwise decreases in specific behaviors are desired.

With both the A–B and A–B–C designs, no causal statements can be made. In the therapy ball study, if data had been collected only for an initial baseline phase and a treatment phase (see Fig. 26.2), the therapist would not have known if some factor other than the introduction of the therapy ball for classroom seating resulted in Emily's increase in in-seat behavior. For example, at the beginning of the intervention phase, the language arts assignments might have changed to a topic of greater interest to Emily and that change, rather than the therapy ball, might have influenced Emily's in-seat behavior. Therefore, this design is subject to threats to internal validity.

Withdrawal Designs

The **A–B–A or withdrawal design** has stronger internal validity than the A–B and A–B–C designs. This design consists of a minimum of three phases: baseline (A), intervention (B), and baseline (A) or, conversely, B–A–B. However, it can extend to include more phases, with the **A–B–A–B design** being one of the most common. In this design, the baseline and intervention phases reverse twice so that subjects are exposed to both conditions twice. The A–B–A–B design has ethical appeal in situations in which the intervention is effective because you do not end by withdrawing the intervention. Withdrawal designs are exemplified by the therapy ball study described earlier in which the therapy ball for seating was removed after the intervention phase and data were again collected under baseline conditions, and then the intervention was reinstituted (see Fig. 26.2). Because this design involves a return to baseline, it is most appropriate for behaviors that are reversible (likely to return to the original baseline levels when the intervention is withdrawn). This is a true experimental design in the sense that causal inferences can be made related to the participant or participants studied. For example, in the therapy ball study, because the percentage of in-seat behavior increased during the intervention phase and then returned to the original baseline levels during the second baseline phase and then increased when the intervention was reinstituted, it is possible to say that the use of the therapy ball likely resulted in an increase of in-seat behavior for Emily during language arts.

Multiple-Baseline Designs

Multiple-baseline designs, the next category of designs, require repeated measures of at least three baseline conditions that typically are implemented concurrently, with each successive baseline being longer than the previous one. Multiple-baseline designs can be across behaviors, across participants, or across settings.

Multiple-Baseline Design Across Behaviors

In a **multiple-baseline design across behaviors,** the same treatment variable is applied sequentially to separate behaviors in a single participant. Consider the hypothetical example of an adult with dementia who frequently displays three antisocial behaviors: swearing, door slamming, and screaming. The therapist is interested in knowing whether or not her use of systematic behavioral reminders is successful in reducing or eliminating the frequency of occurrence of these behaviors. For 5 days, during a 2-hour socialization group the researcher collects baseline data on these behaviors, making no change in intervention (Fig. 26.3). On the sixth day, the researcher introduces the systematic behavioral reminders, thus starting the treatment phase (B) for the first behavior (swearing). The researcher makes no change in the treatment program for door slamming and screaming. These two behaviors remain in baseline (A). After 10 days the researcher initiates the same intervention for door slamming, and, after 15 days, she initiates this same intervention for screaming. If the researcher can demonstrate a change across all three behaviors following the institution of the intervention, this provides support for the effectiveness of the intervention in decreasing antisocial behaviors in the adult studied. This exemplifies a multiple-baseline design across behaviors.

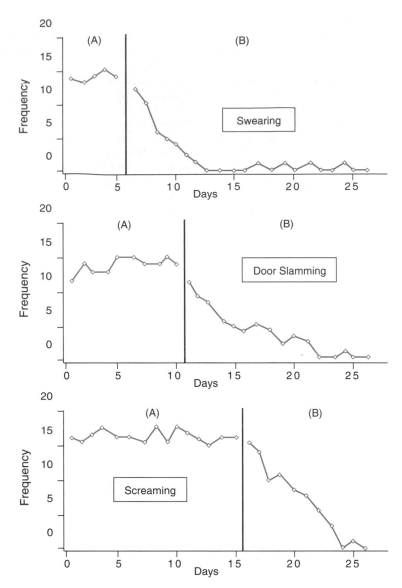

Figure 26.3 Multiple-baseline design across behaviors—example of graphed data for patient with dementia who showed antisocial behaviors of swearing, door slamming, and screaming. The (A) sections show the baseline data; the (B) sections show postintervention data.

Multiple-Baseline Design Across Participants

With a **multiple-baseline design across partici-pants,** one behavior is treated sequentially across matched participants. For example, if an occupa-tional therapist has three male clients with limited grip strength, the therapist might institute a squeeze ball for the first man on the 8th day, for the second man on the 16th day, and for the third man on the 26th day to compare grip strength before and after

therapy. Figure 26.4 displays hypothetical data for such a study.

A variation of the multiple-baseline design across participants is the **nonconcurrent multiple-baseline design across individuals** (Watson & Workman, 1981), whereby different individu-als are studied at different times, a feature that makes it ideal for clinical settings where it often is impractical to start multiple clients in a study simultaneously. With this design, the researcher predetermines the length of time for each baseline

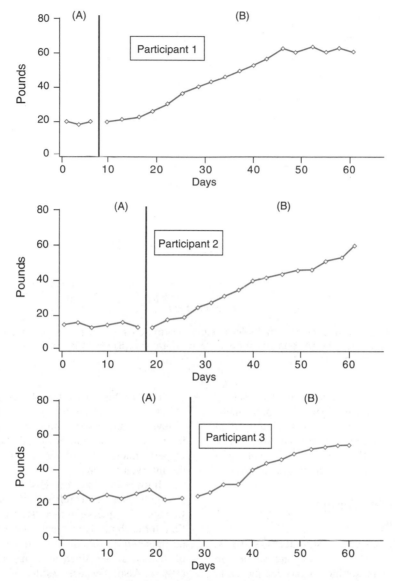

Figure 26.4 Multiple-baseline design across participants—example of graphed data for three men with limited grip strength. The (A) sections show baseline data; the (B) sections show postintervention data.

period and randomly assigns these to participants as they become available. For example, in a non-concurrent multiple-baseline design across the three men with limited grip strength, the researcher might choose baseline lengths of 6 days, 10 days, and 13 days. The first participant might start a squeeze ball exercise regime on April 1, the second might start on April 13, and the last might start on April 26. For each of the three participants, the researcher would randomly select one of the baseline lengths to see if a stable pattern emerges. For example, the researcher might select the man

with the April 13 start date and begin measuring his grip strength for a fixed amount of time. If his baseline data (i.e., grip strength measurements) does not achieve stability within the predetermined time frame, the man with the April 13 start date would be eliminated. He would not be replaced by a new participant. See Figure 26.5 for a graphic display of this hypothetical data. Because baseline data collection typically is continued until a stable pattern emerges, Watson and Workman (1981) recommend dropping a participant if his or her baseline data do not achieve stability within the

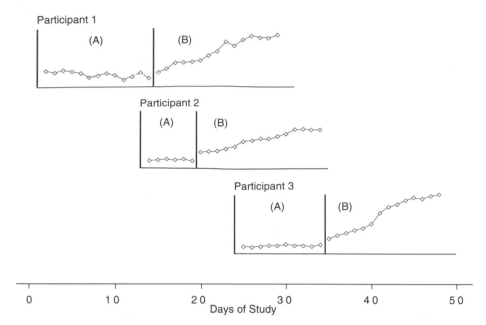

Figure 26.5   Nonconcurrent multiple-baseline design across participants—example of graphed data. The (A) sections show baseline data; the (B) sections show postintervention data.

predetermined time for the participant's baseline. Because each of the participants in a nonconcurrent multiple baseline study starts the intervention at a different randomly determined time, some control is provided for other variables that could result in desired changes in the target behavior.

Multiple-Baseline Design Across Settings

With a **multiple-baseline design across settings,** the same behavior or behaviors are studied in several independent settings. Consider the child with autism who is in an inclusive school setting. This child repeatedly interrupts. He does this in the classroom, in the cafeteria, and on the playground. The therapist collects baseline data in all three settings for 5 days. Then, she implements a reward program based on the principles of operant conditioning in which the child earns points for every interaction that does not involve interrupting others in the classroom (the first setting), while simultaneously continuing to collect baseline data in the other two settings. After 3 more days, she introduces the intervention in the second setting (the cafeteria), while continuing to collect baseline data in the third setting. Last, after 3 more days, she introduces the intervention in the third setting (the playground). Refer to Figure 26.6 for a graph of hypothetical data.

With multiple-baseline designs, intervention effectiveness is demonstrated if a desired change in level, trend, or variability occurs only when the intervention is introduced. In addition, the change in performance should be maintained throughout the intervention phase.

Multiple-baseline designs have three major strengths. The first relates to internal validity. Because the intervention is started at a different time for each individual, behavior, or setting, these designs help to rule out the internal validity threat of history, as described by Campbell and Stanley (1963). Also, because results of research using these designs can show that change is effected in multiple individuals, behaviors, or settings, support is provided for the demonstration of causal relationships. The second strength of multiple-baseline designs is that they require no reversal or withdrawal of the intervention, a characteristic that makes them appealing and practical for research when discontinuing therapy is contraindicated. The third strength of multiple-baseline designs is that they are useful when behaviors are not likely to be reversible. Often, therapists expect that an intervention will cause a difference that will be maintained even when the intervention is withdrawn. For example, once a therapist has taught a client who has had a spinal cord injury to dress independently, the therapist expects the client will be able to dress independently, even when

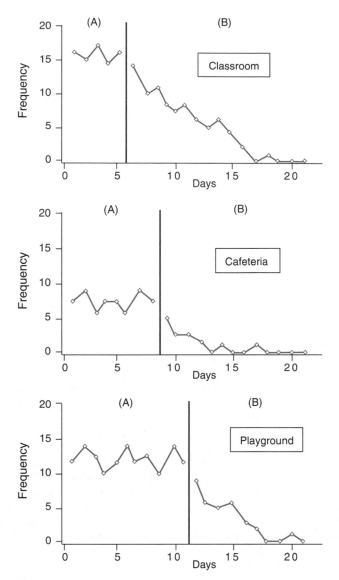

Figure 26.6   Multiple-baseline design across settings—example of graphed data. The (A) sections show baseline data; the (B) sections show postintervention data.

therapy is withdrawn. This makes it inappropriate to use the withdrawal design discussed earlier, because with this design, intervention effectiveness is demonstrated when the behavior returns to the original baseline level following withdrawal of the intervention.

The primary weakness of multiple-baseline designs is that they require more data collection time because of the staggered starting times for the intervention phases. Because of this, some behaviors or participants are required to remain in the baseline phase for long periods of time, which may prove to be problematic. For example, in the first hypothetical study involving an adult with dementia (see Fig. 26.3), the last behavior (screaming) was allowed to continue for 15 days prior to the institution of the intervention.

Alternating-Treatments Design

The **alternating-treatments design** and/or minor variations of it also have been termed the multielement baseline design, the randomization design, and the multiple schedule design (Barlow & Hersen, 2008). These designs can be used to

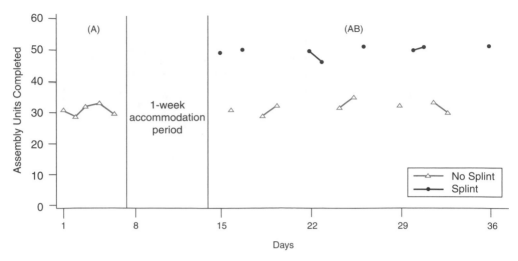

Figure 26.7   Alternating-treatments design—example of graphed data.

compare the effects of intervention and no intervention, or they can be used to compare the effects of two or more distinct interventions. This can extend to comparing the effectiveness of two or more different therapists or the effectiveness of providing a specific intervention at one time of day versus another. In all cases, these designs involve the fast alternation of two or more different interventions or conditions. Although they typically have a baseline phase, it is not essential. These designs are not appropriate when behavior is expected to take time to change, when effects are expected to be cumulative, or when multiple-treatment interference is anticipated.

Alternating-treatments designs are useful in situations when change is expected in the dependent variable over time because of factors such as a disease process (e.g., rheumatoid arthritis) or a natural recovery process (e.g., strokes, burns). With other designs, such factors could result in changes in the dependent variable that could compromise interpretation of study results. However, with the alternating-treatments design, effects from these changes largely are controlled because each intervention is instituted within a short period of time, typically 1 or 2 days.

Because alternating-treatments designs require interventions that will produce immediate and distinct changes in behavior, they are suited to independent variables that can be instituted and removed quickly and whose effects typically are immediate. Thus, they are suited to studying the effects of independent variables such as splints, orthoses, positioning devices, and assistive technology.

For example, a woman's productivity on an assembly line is compromised because of arthritis. The therapist wants to know if use of a specific splint will result in an increase in productivity. The independent variable is the splint, and the dependent variable is the number of assembly units completed per hour. See Figure 26.7 for a graph of hypothetical data, noting that data for both the intervention and nonintervention conditions are plotted on the same graph.

During the first phase of the study, baseline data on the number of assembly units completed per hour were collected for five sessions. The woman did not wear the splint during this phase. Phase 2 began after the woman wore the splint for a 1-week accommodation period. During the 16 days of phase 2, the order of the two conditions (with and without splint) was counterbalanced by random assignment without replacement. Therefore, for 8 of the 16 days in phase 2, the woman wore the splint at work; for the other 8 days she did not use the splint. In both conditions, data were systematically collected on the number of assembly units completed per hour. As depicted in the graph, the woman's work productivity improved, thereby providing support for the use of the splint in the work setting for this woman.

This design also has been used when studying the effects of interventions on dependent variables such as self-report measures, overt behavior exhibited during specific interventions, and exercise repetitions. For example, Melchert-McKearnan, Deitz, Engel, and White (2000) studied the effects of play activities versus rote exercise for children during the acute phase following burn injuries. Outcome measures were the number of repetitions of therapeutic exercise completed, number and type of overt distress behaviors displayed, scores on self-report scales of pain intensity, and self-report of overall enjoyment of the activity. The alternating-treatments design was chosen for this study because it was expected that there would be changes in the children as a result of the recovery process, and it was expected that the effect of the intervention on each of the outcome variables would be immediate.

The alternating-treatments design has three primary strengths. First, it does not require a lengthy withdrawal of the intervention, which may result in a reversal of therapeutic gain. Second, it often requires less time for a comparison to be made because a second baseline is not required. Third, with this design, it is possible to proceed without a formal baseline phase. This is useful in situations where there is no practical or meaningful baseline condition or where ethically it is difficult to justify baseline data collection.

The primary weakness of the alternating-treatments design stems from its vulnerability to a validity threat relating to the influence of an intervention on an adjacent intervention (multiple-treatment interference). As a partial control for this threat, all variables that could potentially influence the results of the study should be counterbalanced. For example, if a therapist was trying to determine which of two electric feeders was best for his client relative to time to complete a meal, and feeder A always was used at lunch and feeder B always was used at dinner, it might be that the client did more poorly with feeder B because he strained his neck when using feeder A at lunch, and this influenced his use of feeder B. Randomizing the order of use of the feeders, although it would not eliminate order effects, would allow for order effects to be identified if they did exist (Hains & Baer, 1989).

Other Variations

The research designs described are only a sample of the possibilities. The literature is replete with creative examples of design variations. For example, Wacker and colleagues (1990) advocated for the sequential alternating-treatments design, a combination of the alternating-treatments and multiple-baseline designs, and others have suggested extending the withdrawal design to include more phases and multiple-intervention conditions (e.g., A–B–A–C–A–D–A–C–A–D–A–B–A).

Definition of Variables and Collection of Data

Similar to group research, dependent variables have to be operationally defined, and data collection methods that are replicable and reliable must be used. In addition to using physiological measures (e.g., oxygen saturation), strength or endurance measures (e.g., pounds of grip strength, time spent exercising at a given level), frequency measures (e.g., number of bites of food taken without spilling during a meal), and self-report measures (e.g., level of pain, level of satisfaction), interval-recording techniques often are used. There are three common interval-recording techniques: momentary time sampling, partial-interval recording, and whole-interval recording (Harrop & Daniels, 1986; Richards, Taylor, & Ramasamy, 2013). With momentary time sampling, a response is recorded if it occurs precisely at a predetermined moment. For example, consider a study in which in-seat behavior is the dependent variable. Using momentary time sampling, a data collector, listening to a tape of beeps recorded at 5-second intervals, would record whether or not the child was displaying in-seat behavior at the moment of each beep. By contrast, with partial-interval recording, a response is scored if the behavior occurs in any part of the interval. For example, in the previous example, the child would be scored as "in seat" if she was in her seat during the first 2 seconds of the 5-second interval and out of her seat during the last 3 seconds of that interval. With whole-interval recording, the child would have to be in her seat during the full 5-second interval to be scored as "in seat."

Typically, with interval-recording techniques, either the data collector uses headphones to hear a tape of beeps recorded at regular intervals, such as every 30 or 60 seconds, or uses videos of recorded sessions with beeps superimposed on the tapes. The data collector typically records responses on a recording mechanism such as the digital questionnaire presented in Figure 26.8, which was designed for use for 10 minutes of data collection with 20-second intervals. For each interval, the researcher indicates whether the child was displaying either "in-seat" or "out-of-seat." This approach of making the same mark (clicking in the bubble) regardless of whether "in seat" or "out of seat" is scored is important in situations where two data collectors, in close proximity, must collect data simultaneously for reliability checks. Otherwise, the subtle sounds of writing an "I" or an "O," for

	First 20 Seconds		Second 20 Seconds		Third 20 Seconds	
	In Seat	Out of Seat	In Seat	Out of Seat	In Seat	Out of Seat
Minute 1	O	O	O	O	O	O
Minute 2	O	O	O	O	O	O
Minute 3	O	O	O	O	O	O
Minute 4	O	O	O	O	O	O
Minute 5	O	O	O	O	O	O
Minute 6	O	O	O	O	O	O
Minute 7	O	O	O	O	O	O
Minute 8	O	O	O	O	O	O
Minute 9	O	O	O	O	O	O
Minute 10	O	O	O	O	O	O

Figure 26.8   Sample recording sheet for interval recording (momentary time sampling, whole-interval recording, or partial-interval recording).

example, might inadvertently provide a cue to the other data collector, possibly biasing results.

Data Reporting and Analysis

Data Graphs

Typically, with single-subject research, data for each variable for each participant or system are graphed with the dependent variable on the y-axis and time (e.g., days, weeks) on the x-axis. Vertical lines indicate phase changes, and lines connect data points reflecting consecutive days. See Figure 26.2 for an example. When graphing data for one variable for more than one participant, the scale for each graph should be the same to facilitate comparisons across graphs. For example, if one participant's data ranged from 3 to 29 and another's ranged from 20 to 58, both graphs should start at 0 and extend to at least 60. This facilitates visual comparison across participants. Carr and Burkholder (1998) described the process for creating graphs for single-subject research using Microsoft Excel.

Researchers graph data either within an equal-interval graph or using a standard behavior chart. The primary benefit of the former is that it is easily understood. Benefits of the standard behavior chart are that behaviors with extremely high or low rates can be recorded on the chart, and the graph progresses in semilog units, thus facilitating the estimation of linear trends in the data (Carr & Williams, 1982).

Phase Lengths

Although the researcher estimates phase lengths prior to implementation of the study, typically the actual length of each phase is determined during the course of the study, with data collection within a phase continuing until a clear pattern emerges. In determining estimates for phase lengths prior to study implementation, several factors should be taken into account. First, the researcher should decide whether or not he or she intends to use statistical analyses because these often necessitate a specified minimum number of data points in each condition to meet the required assumptions for their use. Second, in situations where change is expected due to factors such as development or a disease process, the researcher should consider making the lengths of baseline and intervention phases comparable. This facilitates the visual analyses of the resulting data. Third, the researcher should consider the variability in the expected data and the magnitude of the expected change. In cases where high variability and/or small (but important) changes are expected, longer phases are advised.

Visual Analysis

Visual analysis of graphically presented data to infer conclusions about cause and effect involves looking for a change in level, trend, or variability between phases when treatment is instituted or withdrawn (Ottenbacher & York, 1984; Wolery & Harris, 1982). See Figure 26.9 for potential patterns of data reflecting no change and change.

In some cases, incorporating additional descriptive information into graphs can be used to augment

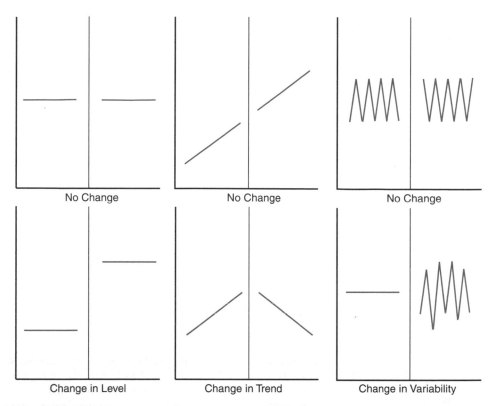

Figure 26.9   Patterns of data reflecting no change and change.

visual data analyses. For example, the split-middle technique can be used to describe data and predict outcomes given the rate of change. The accuracy of these predictions depends on the number of data points on which the prediction is based and on how far into the future a prediction is being made. The split-middle technique also can be used to facilitate the examination and comparison of trends in two or more phases.

Using the split-middle technique, once data for a phase are plotted on a graph, a celeration line reflecting the direction and rate of change is determined. For details concerning the process for using the split-middle technique and creating celeration lines, refer to Kazdin (2010), Barlow and Hersen (2008), or Ottenbacher (1986). Although these strategies typically are used to facilitate visual analyses, statistical change can be evaluated by applying a binomial test to determine whether or not a significant proportion of data points in an intervention phase fall above or below the celeration line projected from baseline. For computational details, refer to the writings of White (1972), Barlow and Hersen (2008), or Ottenbacher (1986).

Another example of descriptive information that can be incorporated into graphs to augment visual analyses is the use of a dashed line across each phase demarcating the mean for that phase. Although useful in some situations, this approach can contribute to misinterpretations of the data when the data reflect either an upward or downward trend, when there are few data points within a phase, and when data points within a phase are highly variable. For example, relative to the former, it is possible to have similar means in adjacent A and B phases, thus suggesting no effect from the intervention. However, if there was a steady increase in an undesirable behavior (upward trend) in the A phase and a steady decrease in the undesirable behavior (downward trend) in the B phase, comparison of the means could lead to the erroneous conclusion of no difference between the two phases. See Figure 26.10 for a hypothetical example.

Statistical Significance

If the researcher using single-subject methods plans to determine statistical significance for a study to supplement visual analysis, the researcher needs to design the study to meet the necessary assumptions. One of the best and most underutilized statistical tests appropriate for use in single-subject research is the randomization test (Edgington, 1980, 2007;

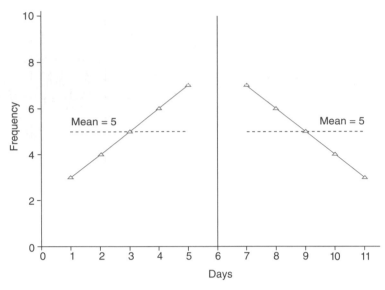

Figure 26.10   Example of misleading use of comparison of means across phases.

Onghena & Edgington, 1994; Todman & Dugard, 2001; Wampold & Worsham, 1986). It is a conservative way to evaluate shifts in time-series data and is ideal because it is robust in showing serial dependency (i.e., correlation among successive responses in one individual) and systematic trends in the data, and it does not require a normal distribution. It focuses exclusively on the data available, evaluating the probability of the actual outcome when compared to the set of all possible outcomes. If a researcher plans to use randomization tests to analyze data from single-subject research, it is important that the researcher randomly assign experimental conditions (Edgington, 1980, 2007). In doing this, the researcher should consider the need to control for systematic trends over the course of the study that may be attributable to developmental or recovery processes.

Incorporation of Social Validation Procedures Into the Design

According to Schwartz and Baer (1991), the purpose of assessing social validity is to evaluate the acceptability or viability of an intervention. Typically this is accomplished through use of one or more questionnaires directed to the research participants and others in their environments (e.g., family members, teachers). Social validation is important because it is possible for an intervention

to result in desirable changes in the dependent variable but still be identified by research participants or other stakeholders as being unacceptable. For example, results from a research study may indicate that use of a specific type of splint decreases daily reports of pain and increases range of motion. However, in a social validation questionnaire, the research participant may indicate that the splint limits function and is cosmetically unacceptable and therefore would not be chosen for use.

Social validation procedures were used in the therapy ball study described in the Case Example at the beginning of this chapter (Schilling et al., 2003). Social validation involved three steps. First, the target children and all other children in the class and the teacher filled out social validity questionnaires. Second, at the conclusion of the study, all were instructed to write about what they "liked" and "didn't like" about using therapy balls for classroom seating. Last, evidence of social validity was obtained by observing the teacher's choices following the completion of the study. She continued to use therapy balls for seating for the children with ADHD, and she ordered additional balls for other students, thus supporting the social validity of the intervention.

The Issue of Generality

Although a well-designed and implemented single-subject study completed with one individual has strong internal validity, it is weak relative to external validity. Thus, although we may have confidence in the findings for the individual studied, we do not know the extent to which these findings generalize to other comparable individuals. Generality in single-subject research is achieved only through replication with other individuals, in other settings, and with other therapists. For example, in the therapy ball study described previously, two other children, in addition to Emily, were studied. Because results for all three children were similar, some support is provided for the generality of the findings. Additional replications by other researchers, in other settings, and with different children would further increase generality if comparable outcomes continued to be achieved.

Kazdin (2010) distinguished between direct replication that involves systematically applying the same procedures across different, but similar, individuals and systematic replication that involves repeating the study with systematic variations. An example of the latter would be to design and conduct a replication study using different types of participants (e.g., children with autism instead of children with ADHD). Ideally, in a systematic replication study, only one variable is changed at a time. Systematic replications expand understanding regarding with whom and under what conditions the intervention is effective.

Summary

Single-subject research methods are useful in addressing many important questions related to the extent to which different intervention strategies are successful with different clients. These methods are congruent with responsible OT practice in that they emphasize clearly articulating desired outcomes, defining intervention and measurement strategies, and collecting data in a reliable manner, over time. Both the process and the products of single-subject research support evidence-based practice.

Review Questions

1. How are variables defined in single-subject research?
2. What are the four most common design approaches to single-subject research?
3. What are the advantages and limitations of using single-subject research?
4. Provide an example of the use of a multiple-baseline design. When might this design approach be relevant to answering a question emerging from practice?
5. How are data typically analyzed and reported in a single-subject research study?
6. Why is it important to socially validate findings from single-subject research?
7. Why is single-subject research limited in terms of generalization?

REFERENCES

Backman, C., Harris, S. R., Chisholm, J., & Monette, A. D. (1997). Single-subject research in rehabilitation: A review of studies using AB, withdrawal, multiple baseline, and alternating treatments designs. *Archives of Physical Medicine and Rehabilitation, 78,* 1145–1153.

Barlow, D. H., & Hersen, M. (2008). *Single case experimental designs strategies for studying behavior change* (3rd ed.). New York, NY: Pergamon Press.

Campbell, D., & Stanley, J. (1963). *Experimental and quasi-experimental designs for research.* Chicago, IL: Rand McNally.

Carr, B. S., & Williams, M. (1982). Analysis of therapeutic techniques through use of the standard behavior chart. *Physical Therapy, 52,* 177–183.

Carr, J. E., & Burkholder, E. O. (1998). Creating single-subject design graphs with Microsoft Excel. *Journal of Applied Behavior Analysis, 31,* 245–251.

Edgington, E. S. (1980). Random assignment and statistical tests for one-subject experiments. *Behavioral Assessment, 2,* 19–28.

Edgington, E. S. (2007). Single subject randomization tests. In E. S. Edgington (Ed.), *Randomization tests* (4th ed.). New York, NY: Chapman and Hall.

Hains, H., & Baer, D. M. (1989). Interaction effects in multielement designs: Inevitable, desirable, and ignorable. *Journal of Applied Behavior Analysis, 22,* 57–69.

Harrop, A., & Daniels, M. (1986). Methods of time sampling: A reappraisal of momentary time sampling and interval recording. *Journal of Applied Behavior Analysis, 19,* 73–77.

Hartmann, D. P., & Hall, R. V. (1976). The changing criterion design. *Journal of Applied Behavior Analysis, 9,* 527–532.

Kazdin, A. E. (2010). *Single-case research designs: Methods for clinical and applied settings* (2nd ed). New York, NY: Oxford University Press.

Melchert-McKearnan, K., Deitz, J., Engel, J., & White, O. (2000). Children with burn injuries; Purposeful activity versus rote exercise. *American Journal of Occupational Therapy, 54,* 381–390.

Onghena, P., & Edgington, E. S. (1994). Randomization tests for restricted alternating treatments designs. *Behaviour Research & Therapy, 32,* 783–786.

Ottenbacher, K. (1986). *Evaluating clinical change: Strategies for occupational and physical therapists.* Baltimore, MD: Williams & Wilkins.

Ottenbacher, K. (1990). Clinically relevant designs for rehabilitation research: The idiographic model. *American Journal of Physical Medicine & Rehabilitation, 69,* 286–292.

Ottenbacher, K., & York, J. (1984). Strategies for evaluating clinical change: Implications for practice and research. *American Journal of Occupational Therapy, 38,* 647–659.

Richards, S. B., Taylor, R. L., & Ramasamy, R. (2013). *Single subject research: Applications in educational and clinical settings* (2nd ed). Belmont, CA: Wadsworth.

Schilling, D. L., Washington, K., Billingsley, F., & Deitz, J. (2003). Classroom seating for children with attention deficit hyperactivity disorder: Therapy balls versus chairs. *American Journal of Occupational Therapy, 57,* 534–541.

Schwartz, I. S., & Baer, D. M. (1991). Social validity assessments: Is current practice state of the art? *Journal of Applied Behavior Analysis, 24,* 189–204.

Todman, J. B., & Dugard, P. (2001). *Single-case and small-n experimental designs: A practical guide to randomization tests.* Mahwah, NJ: Lawrence Erlbaum Associates.

Wacker, D., McMahon, C., Steege, M., Berg, W., Sasso, G., & Melloy, K. (1990). Applications of a sequential alternating treatments design. *Journal of Applied Behavior Analysis, 23,* 333–339.

Wampold, B. E., & Worsham, N. L. (1986). Randomization tests for multiple-baseline designs. *Behavioral Assessment, 8,* 135–143.

Watson, P. J., & Workman, E. A. (1981). The non-concurrent multiple baseline across-individuals design: An extension of the traditional multiple baseline design. *Journal of Behavior Therapy and Experimental Psychiatry, 12,* 257–259.

White, O. R. (1972). *A manual for the calculation and use of the median slope—a technique of progress estimation and prediction in the single case.* Eugene, OR: University of Oregon, Regional Resource Center for Handicapped Children.

Wolery, M., & Harris, S. (1982). Interpreting results of single-subject research designs. *Physical Therapy, 62,* 445–452.

CHAPTER 27

Survey Research

Kirsty Forsyth • Frederick J. Kviz

Learning Outcomes

- Describe survey research, including its major components and advantages.
- Understand the role of response bias in survey research.
- Weigh the advantages and disadvantages of the different approaches to data collection in survey research.
- Discuss the four steps involved in building a survey questionnaire or interview.
- Describe the survey implementation process.
- List ways to increase survey response rates.
- Explain how to prepare survey results for statistical analysis.

Introduction

Survey research is a method of inquiry characterized by collecting data using structured questions to elicit self-reported information from a sample of people (Aday & Cornelius, 2006; DePoy & Gitlin, 2010). Surveys are characterized by these key dimensions:

- Identifying the population of interest and appropriately sampling that population,
- Identifying the research aims and question and generating survey questions to systematically gather the necessary information, and
- Developing statistical estimates that can be generalized to the population under study.

The main advantages of survey research are that investigators can reach a large number of **respondents** (people responding to the survey) with relatively minimal expenditure, collect data on numerous variables, and perform statistical manipulation during data analysis that permits multiple uses of the data set (Rea & Parker, 2005).

There are two main factors that can influence the rigor of survey research (Fowler, 2008). The first is potential **nonresponse bias** (i.e., respondents selected for the sample who elect not to respond). These second is potential **response bias,** which may result from factors such as:

- Respondents being unable to recall information accurately,
- Respondents interpreting the meaning of a question differently than the meaning intended by the researcher, or
- Response choices that do not accurately express respondents' experiences or opinions.

When designing survey research, investigators must take care to reduce these two forms of bias as much as possible, as discussed throughout the chapter.

Another important consideration in survey research is governmental regulations affecting the privacy of patients. This varies, of course, by country. In the United States the Health Insurance Portability and Accountability Act (HIPAA) privacy rule has requirements that must be followed in medical research. Medical research that falls under HIPAA regulations must conform to these rules. Although these rules govern all forms of research involving patients, they can have particular implications for survey research. A useful source of information on how HIPAA regulations affect research is the National Institutes of Health website: http://privacyruleandresearch.nih.gov/.

The types of surveys used to collect data include self-administered questionnaires, telephone interviews, and face-to-face interviews. Self-administered questionnaires may be mailed, administered online, or distributed and collected at convenient points of contact, such as in schools, workplaces, clinics, or hospitals. This chapter focuses on:

- How to choose the specific survey data gathering method,
- How to build the questionnaire/interview,
- How to administer the survey (including sampling), and
- Preparation for data analysis.

CASE EXAMPLE

Dr. Cussil is an occupational therapy (OT) researcher who has been studying improvements and deficiencies in health-care communication for over a decade. Thus far, she has been successful in using research approaches that capture clients' perspectives regarding the strengths of their relationships with their therapists and the positive aspects of therapeutic communication. Dr. Cussil's main frustration is that she has found it difficult to accurately represent clients' perspectives regarding the degree and nature of their dissatisfaction within their relationships with their therapists. She has found a halo effect, in which clients tend to overreport the strengths within their relationships with their therapists, and they tend to underreport the weaknesses and communication mistakes their therapists make. When sharing her frustration with a colleague at an OT conference, her colleague suggests a survey research approach with an anonymous sample. Her colleague speculates that one reason clients may be reluctant to report negative aspects about their relationships with their therapists is that they may feel grateful or indebted to them for helping them with their rehabilitation goals. Alternatively, they may be concerned that, despite all reassurance to the contrary, the findings could hurt the feelings of their therapists or affect their own ability to receive care within the setting. An anonymous survey research approach would allow clients to depersonalize their experiences in therapy and report their feelings more honestly.

To accomplish this aim, Dr. Cussil requests to purchase a random sample of 1,000 member names with corresponding surface mail addresses from a national self-help organization for individuals recovering from stroke. In this case, she chooses surface mail over e-mail to increase visibility for her study and to maximize the perception of confidentiality among respondents. In its efforts to support research, this organization customarily obtains permission from the 40,000 individuals in its membership base to be included on invitation e-mail lists for the purposes of anticipated participation in research. Dr. Cussil then designs a consent process and creates a survey questionnaire. The consent process describes the provisions for protecting confidentiality. The survey questionnaire contains detailed, probing questions about both optimal and less-than-optimal approaches to communication. To encourage high response rates, Dr. Cussil makes sure that the introduction and consent for the questionnaire emphasize the importance of communication in health care. The study design mandates up to four separate mailings of the questionnaire to each member, separated by 2 weeks each, with the mailings stopping upon return of the survey by mail.

After 8 weeks, the study closes to accrual, and Dr. Cussil is pleased to have received 673 surveys out of 1,000 invited members. This marks an 67.3% response rate, which is adequate for further analysis of the findings.

Choosing Data Gathering Methods

As noted in the preceding section, survey research uses questionnaires (administered directly, by mail, or electronically) and interviews (telephone, cell phone, or face to face) to collect data. Quantitative survey interviews are quite distinct from interviews used in qualitative studies. In a survey, the interview questions are fixed, and the interviewer seeks to administer the interview in an objective manner following the interview protocol.

When choosing a survey data gathering method, the advantages and disadvantages of each method need to be considered. These are discussed in the following subsections and illustrated in Table 27.1.

Mailed Questionnaires

Traditionally, the most common method of collecting survey data has involved the dissemination of printed questionnaires through the mail to a sample of respondents (Fig. 27.1). Respondents are asked to complete the questionnaire on their own and return it to the researchers. One advantage of the mailed questionnaire over interviews is that the questionnaire can be completed at the respondent's convenience with no time constraint. Finally, because there is no personal contact with an interviewer, respondent anonymity may be better preserved, and potential interviewer bias is not a factor (Rea & Parker, 2005).

A potential disadvantage of all questionnaires is that they require literacy skills. When studying

Table 27.1 Advantages and Disadvantages of Different Methods of Data Collection in Survey Research

Type of Survey	Advantages	Disadvantages
Questionnaires	• Relatively low cost. • Respondent anonymity may be better preserved. • Interviewer bias is not a factor.	• Response rate tends to be lower. • Any confusion about the question cannot be clarified. • Requires literacy skills.
Mailed questionnaires	• Can be completed at the respondent's convenience. • No time constraint.	• Can be time consuming. • Many follow-ups may be required.
Directly administered questionnaires	• Take less time. • No mailing costs.	• Limits sampling strategies. • Less flexibility in time frame.
Online questionnaires	• Fast. • Web-based. • Administration can incorporate features that paper questionnaires cannot. • Data can be directly imported for analysis.	• Only people with computers or computer skill can be contacted. • Raises concerns over privacy and anonymity.
Interviews	• Greater flexibility to probe for more detail and administer more complex questionnaires. • Ensure the integrity of the questionnaire.	• Expensive (personnel and training costs).
Telephone interviews	• Potentially short data collection period. • Usually cost less. • Afford more perceived anonymity. • Easier to sample a large geographical area.	• Less interviewer control. • Limited ability to support questionnaires with visual aids. • Only people with telephones can be contacted. • Opportunity to establish credibility is more limited.
Face-to-face interviews	• Ideal for contacting hard-to-reach populations. • Reduce/eliminate missing data.	• Cost of travel. • Longer data collection period. • Interviewer can be a source of bias. • Concerns about personal safety of the interviewers and lack of respondent anonymity.

certain disadvantaged or intellectually impaired populations, researchers may have to deal with a lack of or limited literacy. Moreover, the lack of interaction with the respondent means that any parts of the questionnaire that are misunderstood for any reason cannot be clarified by the data collector.

A specific disadvantage of mailed questionnaires is that the response rates tend to be lower than that for interview methods. Moreover, many follow-ups (repeated mailings of the questionnaire) may be required to obtain an acceptable response rate. In addition, mailing and return of questionnaires, along with any necessary follow-ups to secure sufficient respondents, can be time consuming (Abramson & Abramson, 1999). Mail surveys usually take 3 to 4 months for respondents to complete and return the questionnaires in response to the three mailings (initial plus two

follow-ups) that are typically required. Later in the chapter, strategies for follow-up are discussed in more detail.

Directly Administered Questionnaires

Directly administered questionnaires are given to participants in person at an opportune moment when the researcher has a captive audience. For example, a researcher might distribute questionnaires to patients at a monthly networking and educational gathering for patients at an outpatient rehabilitation center. Directly administered questionnaires have the same advantages as mailed questionnaires, with the exception that the investigator may ask for the questionnaire to be completed within a given time frame. Direct administration of questionnaires has the additional advantage that

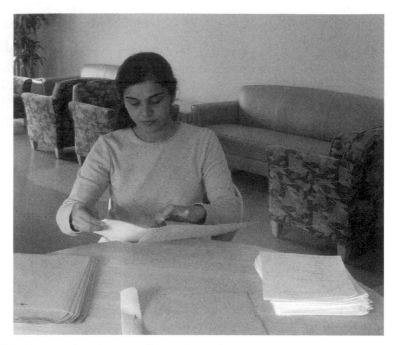

Figure 27.1   A research assistant stuffs envelopes in preparation for a mailed survey.

it does not take the long period of time required for mailed surveys. Finally, it is the least costly survey method.

The major disadvantage of direct administration is sampling. Because direct administration requires a clustering of respondents in a specific physical setting, the usual strategies for obtaining a representative sample are not possible. Thus, directly administered questionnaires are most useful when the setting where the data are collected is the focus of the study and/or the persons in that setting are the population of interest. However, this is often not the case. Consequently, surveys done through direct administration are limited in their generalizability. Direct administration of questionnaires is most often used to pilot (and thus refine) the questionnaire, or to collect pilot data for a larger study that will use appropriate sampling strategies.

Electronic Questionnaires

Electronic (e.g., e-mail, Web-based, and app-based) methods of administering questionnaires are being used at an increasing rate. There are two main methods of electronic administration. The first is an e-mail survey. In this method, the questionnaire is contained in the body of the e-mail or in a document that is sent with the e-mail as an attachment. The respondent is requested to complete the survey

and return it (as an e-mail or an attached completed document, depending on how the survey was sent). The second method is when a survey is accessed through a secure, password-protected portal on the World Wide Web. Respondents are sent a request to complete the survey by e-mail with a link to the URL for the survey. The survey may be provided in html format online, or as an app-based version for smartphone use.

Online questionnaires are used to increase the speed and sophistication of delivery as well as efficiency of processing the data once received. Additionally, online questionnaires have control features that mailed surveys do not. For example, computer programs that support online questionnaires can prevent a respondent from skipping certain questions by not advancing to the next question or page of the survey until a response is designated. Another feature offered by online questionnaires are skip patterns that hide certain questions from respondents when the respondent answers in such a way that would make a subsequent question nonapplicable. Additionally, online questionnaires often offer superior graphics that allow respondents to respond using visual probes rather than relying on a simple numeric ordinal scale with descriptive words as anchors.

The advantages of both means of online administration are that they are fast. The Web-based administration has the potential to incorporate features not available on a printed questionnaire such as pull-down menus and checkboxes. An additional benefit of the Web-based survey is that data can typically be exported directly to a statistical analysis package, bypassing the need to do manual data entry.

The main disadvantage of this method of questionnaire administration is that it requires, minimally, access to and knowledge of computer use on the part of the respondent. In the case of Web-based administration, somewhat more skill on the part of the respondent and substantial technological skill on the part of the researcher are required. For these reasons, there can be particular problems of sampling or nonresponse bias. There can also be substantial concerns about the privacy and anonymity of the respondent.

Telephone Interviews

Some surveys collect data through interviews conducted via telephone or cellular phone by trained interviewers (Fig. 27.2). Telephone interviews have the advantage of allowing the researcher to ensure that the respondent is attending to the survey and understanding the questions. Like many electronic survey options, interviewers can also maintain the integrity of the ordering of the questions (whereas someone completing a surface-mailed questionnaire may not complete it in sequence, resulting in bias).

A unique advantage of telephone interviews is a potentially short data collection period. In some situations, data can be gathered and processed within several days. Although they are more expensive than mailed questionnaires (i.e., they involve personnel and training costs), telephone interviews usually cost less and afford more perceived anonymity than face-to-face interviews. In particular, telephone interviews (along with mailed questionnaires) offer an advantage over face-to-face interviews when the sample is distributed over a large geographical area (Rea & Parker, 2005).

A disadvantage of phone interviews is that the interviewer has less control than in a face-to-face interview. The interviewer's opportunity to establish credibility is more limited over the phone. Moreover, respondents can put down the phone at any time. A disadvantage that affects sampling is that only people with telephones can be contacted. Thus, in some studies, constituents of the population of interest may be missed. Finally, there is limited ability to support questionnaires with visual aids that can clarify questions in the interview (Abramson & Abramson, 1999).

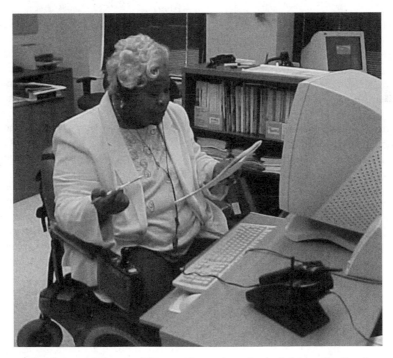

Figure 27.2 Phone interviews are a frequently used method of data collection in research.

Face-to-Face Interviews

Survey data can be collected in person by trained interviewers. These interviews are typically conducted at the respondent's residence. However, other sites, such as schools, workplaces, or clinics, may also be used. This method has many of the same strengths as phone interviews. Face-to-face interviews are ideal for contacting hard-to-reach populations—for example, homeless or incarcerated criminal offenders—and they are usually completed with little or no missing data.

Some disadvantages of face-to-face interviews are the high costs (for travel as well as personnel and training) and the time involved in traveling and performing the data collection. Despite the potential advantages of face-to-face interviews, the interviewer can also be a source of bias. For example, the face-to-face encounter may influence the respondent to seek approval from the interviewer. Moreover, sex, age, or cultural differences may bias the respondent. Finally, face-to-face interviews can raise concerns about the personal safety of the interviewers and lack of anonymity for the respondent (Abramson & Abramson, 1999).

Selecting and Combining Data Collection Methods in Surveys

There are multiple considerations in making a decision about which data collection method to use in survey research. In the end, the investigator must select the method that best suits the research question, the population under study, and the available resources and constraints for the study. In some studies, a combination of methods may be used to lower costs and improve data quality. For example, telephone interviews may be conducted with persons who do not respond to a mailed questionnaire. Or, a respondent to a face-to-face interview may be asked to complete and return by mail a self-administered questionnaire that requires consulting household records or other household/family members (Hoyle, Harris, & Judd, 2002; Siemiatycki, 1979).

Building the Questionnaire/ Interview

At the heart of the survey process is development of the questionnaire or **interview schedule** (the written form or guide to be used by the interviewer). Many of the principles for constructing the survey data collection method are the same whether it is a questionnaire or an interview. Therefore, the following discussion pertains to both unless specific points are made about one or the other. The usual steps in building an interview or questionnaire are:

1. Defining and clarifying the survey variables,
2. Formulating the questions,
3. Formatting the questionnaire or interview schedule, and
4. Piloting and revising the questionnaire/interview schedule.

These steps are discussed in the following subsections.

Defining and Clarifying Survey Variables

The first step in building the survey is to identify key variables to be measured. This can be done through a review of the literature and/or interacting with the target population (e.g., via focus groups or unstructured interviews) to gain a full understanding of the issues to be studied. There is not an ideal number of variables for a survey study. The rule "as many as necessary and as few as possible" is sound advice so as to minimize respondent burden and survey costs (Abramson & Abramson, 1999).

The variables chosen for a survey study depend on the aim and research question(s) of the study. Some survey research aims primarily to describe particular phenomena. For example, the periodic survey conducted by the National Board for Certification in Occupational Therapy (NBCOT) in the United States (NBCOT, 2013) aims to characterize the practice of occupational therapists in order to guide the development of the certification examination. This survey is guided by questions concerning areas of practice, diagnoses seen, the types of interventions conducted, and so on.

Other surveys aim to determine whether relationships exist between variables. In this case, the study questions will ask whether and how variables under study correlate, or whether a number of variables can be shown to account for variability in a selected variable.

Each of the variables should be clearly defined both conceptually and operationally. Part of the process of clarifying each variable is identifying the appropriate level of data desired (i.e., nominal, ordinal, ratio, interval, as discussed in Chapter 24) and the corresponding format for collecting that level of data. For example, in the NBCOT 2013 survey, most of the variables were nominal, such as the variable that referred to the type of setting in which one is employed. The same type of information might also have been asked in order to obtain ordinal data. For instance:

How frequently do you work in a pediatric setting?

Never.. 0
Rarely 1
Often 2
Always 3

Determining the variables under study and the level of data to be collected is a critical step. It not only affects the overall quality of the study but also determines the type of analysis that can be carried out with the data. Hence, when doing this step, investigators should anticipate the statistical analyses they plan to undertake.

Formulating Questions

Once the variables have been identified, questions are formulated to elicit data on those variables. For a complex variable, it may be necessary to develop several questions. Moreover, when several questions are asked about a variable in order to form a scale, the variable can be captured with greater reliability and validity (see Chapter 21). Questions should:

• Have face validity, that is, they should reflect what the investigator wants to know and be obvious in meaning for the respondents;
• Ask about things for which the respondent can be expected to know the answer; and
• Be clear and unambiguous, be user-friendly, and not be offensive (Bradburn, Sudman, & Wansik, 2004).

Questions must not contain assumptions that might confuse a respondent or introduce potential bias. For example, the question, "What was your experience of occupational therapy during your last hospital admission?" assumes that the respondent recalls which of the services received during the hospitalization were occupational therapy.

Complex and lengthy sentences are particularly likely to be misunderstood by respondents. Thus, questions should be short and simple (Converse & Presser, 1986). Questions that have two components should be avoided; the following is an example of such a question: "Recalling how many times you came to occupational therapy, do you think it was adequate?" Breaking these double-barreled questions into separate questions would be more straightforward. For instance:

> "How many times did you come to occupational therapy?"
> followed by
> "Do you think that was adequate?"

Sometimes a filter question is employed to find out if the respondent has knowledge/experience of an issue before asking him or her to answer more specific questions about the issue (Hoyle et al., 2002). For example,

> "Do you remember receiving occupational therapy during your hospitalization?"

If the respondent answers "yes" to this question, then it would be appropriate to ask about the experience of occupational therapy. If not, then there is no point in asking further about occupational therapy.

Questions may be asked in two general forms: closed questions or open questions. A closed question provides specific response choices and therefore allows for more uniformity in response and simplifies the analysis. The following is an example of a closed question:

> Which of the following factors is the most important in your documentation?
> Identification of client's occupational needs .. 1
> Communication to the interdisciplinary team 2
> Capturing the client's narrative 3

Also, by presenting response choices, the researcher is providing the same frame of reference to all respondents. Closed questions provide options to be considered and therefore can act as a memory prompt (Hoyle et al., 2002). There is, however, concern that they may force people to choose among alternatives that are predetermined by the researcher instead of answering in their own words (Converse & Presser, 1986).

The following is an example of an open question:

> What factors influence the content of your documentation?

Open-ended questions, such as this one, are useful for eliciting a more detailed narrative response. Although answers to this type of open-ended question may provide rich information, they may also be challenging to categorize for analysis (Converse & Presser, 1986).

Investigators sometimes use open-ended questions initially with a small pilot study sample of the population to generate the closed questions for the main survey (Schuman & Presser, 1996). This approach helps to generate closed questions with options that are understandable to the respondents.

Often researchers use both types of questions in a survey. A common approach is to give some response choices and then provide an "other (please specify)" category. For example:

> Which of the following do you use to assess a client's occupational participation?
>
> Formal outcome measure................................1
> Informal interview with the client 2
> Informal observation of the client 3
> Other 4
> Please specify_____

Formatting the Questionnaire

The design of the questionnaire needs to allow for making the task of reading questions, following instructions, and recording answers as easy as possible. This section should be read with Figures 27.3 and 27.4 in mind. Mailed questionnaires must be clear and attractive to complete. They require formatting that ensures ease of use and accuracy of response. With telephone and face-to-face

SPN_____{Private}
Interviewer ID_____

ROYAL INFIRMARY OCCUPATIONAL THERAPY PROGRAM FOLLOW-UP
(Telephone interview)

Hello, my name is _____, and I'm calling from the Royal Infirmary occupational therapy department. May I please speak with _____? We are interviewing previous clients of the Royal Infirmary occupational therapy service to learn more about how occupational therapy can help people to get back to doing everyday activities following discharge from the Royal Infirmary. We are calling you because the occupational therapy records show that you have difficulty doing everyday activities, and we would like to ask you some questions about your clinic experiences, health, and everyday activities.

Time interview began: _____ : _____ *(use 24-hour clock)*

1. In general, how would you describe your health at this time? Would you say it is. . .

    Very poor, ...1
    Poor, ...2
    Good, or 3
    Very good 4
    Don't know 8

2. Compared to other people <u>about your age</u>, how would you describe your health in general? Would you say it is. . .

    Worse than average, ...1
    About average, or 2
    Better than average 3
    Don't know 8

3. If 1 is not important and 5 is very important, how important is it for someone <u>your age</u> to be able to do everyday activities independently?

Not Important				Very Important	*Don't know*
1	2	3	4	5	8

Figure 27.3 Format of a telephone survey.

SPN_____{Private}

**ROYAL INFIRMARY OCCUPATIONAL THERAPY SERVICE
SURVEY OF HEALTH AND EVERYDAY ACTIVITY BEHAVIOR**

*Please circle one response code number according to your answer
except where instructed otherwise.*

1.   In general, how would you describe your health at this time?

Very poor, ... 1
Poor, ... 2
Good, or... 3
Very good 4

2.   Compared to other people <u>about your age</u>, how would you describe your
health in general?

Worse than average, ... 1
About average, or 2
Better than average 3

3.   What was your <u>main</u> reason for attending occupational therapy?

Difficulty doing self-care 1
Difficulty doing work tasks 2
Difficulty doing leisure activities 3
Other (*Please specify*) 4
_____

4.   Do you feel satisfied with your occupational therapy experience?

Yes...............................1   *(SKIP to Q.30)*
No................................2

Figure 27.4   Format of a mailed survey.

interviews, more weight is given to formatting the written questionnaire for interviewer convenience and to allow the interviewer to easily record the responses. Sometimes for telephone interviews, the interviewer may use a computer-based questionnaire that allows the data to be entered directly to the computer. This method avoids the extra step of data entry that occurs when responses are recorded by the interviewer on paper.

Formatting Principles

There are a number of overall formatting principles that should guide questionnaire construction (Box 27.1). The first is to develop a clear, attractive front cover. It should contain the title of the study, directions for completion of the survey, and the name of the financial sponsor and/or institution of the principal investigator.

Respondents are more likely to trust a known institution rather than a named individual whom they do not know. Adding a picture or illustration can be informative and add interest. The back cover of the questionnaire should not have any questions on it. It should contain only an invitation for further comments, a statement of thanks, instructions for returning the completed questionnaire, and a mailing address for the survey.

Having an uncluttered appearance to the survey is paramount. Using extra paper is preferable to condensing the questionnaire into fewer pages, which can lead to confusion and errors (Salant & Dillman, 1994). For clarity of reading, 12-point type in a standard font (e.g., Arial or Times New Roman) is preferable. For a questionnaire that will be mailed to respondents who may have lowered vision, such as elderly persons, a larger type size, such as 14 point, should be used.

Thorough instructions must be provided so that it is clear how the interviewer or respondent should indicate his or her response to a question (e.g., "circle the number of your answer"). Directions for completing the questionnaire should be distinguished from the questions by using special typographic formatting for emphasis, such as italics, bold, parentheses, or brackets. Caution is urged when using all capital letters; this format is difficult to read when applied to more than a few words. There need to be very clear instructions about negotiating "skip patterns" in situations where a certain subset of questions may not apply to some respondents (e.g., because they apply only to one sex or a particular age group). Question 4

in Figure 27.4 illustrates how a skip pattern can be indicated in a questionnaire.

Each question should be assigned a number sequentially throughout the questionnaire. The questions should be written out in full rather than using a one-word variable label, for example, "What is your age?" rather than, "Age?" The questions should all start at the left margin. All response choices should be indented and all start at the same place. Leader dots can be helpful for visually linking the response choices with the numerical codes. All the parts of the same question and its response choices should be on the same page, never split between two pages. Response categories should be presented in a vertical list format rather than a horizontal format (Bradburn et al., 2004). Each response choice should be assigned a numerical code that will be circled by the respondent or interviewer to record each response. These numerical codes are likely to yield fewer mistakes than using checkboxes when coding and processing the completed questionnaire for data entry.

Creating a vertical flow by aligning response codes along the right-hand margin helps to reduce the number of errors. Vertical flow and a generous use of spacing and indentation give the survey an uncluttered, user-friendly appearance. For a series of items that share the same root question and the same response choices, an efficient format is illustrated by question 19 in Figure 27.5.

Sequencing Questions

The sequence of questions is also important. Every questionnaire should start with a few easy questions that have obvious relevance to the topic of the survey. Following these few introductory questions, the main study questions are presented. Usually issues related to a respondent's beliefs,

---

BOX 27.1   General Principles of Survey Formatting

- The front cover should be clear and attractive.
- The back cover of the questionnaire should not have any questions.
- The survey should have an uncluttered appearance.
- A 12-point type font is preferable.
- Questions need sequentially assigned numbers.
- Clear instructions need to be provided.
- Questions need to be written out in full rather than one word.
- The questions should all start at the left margin.
- All the parts of a question should be on the same page.
- Response categories should have a vertical response format.
- Response choices should have a numerical code to be circled.
- Space generously to avoid a cluttered look.

---

19. What kind of occupational therapist support would you find helpful?

	Very helpful	Somewhat helpful	Not at all helpful	Don't know
a. Self-help materials..................	1	2	3	8
b. A lifestyle class......................	1	2	3	8
c. An activity support group........	1	2	3	8
d. One-to-one activity coaching..	1	2	3	8
e. Something else (*specify*).......	1	2	3	8

Figure 27.5   A sample question from an occupational therapy survey.

behaviors, and attitudes are explored related to the study topic. Topically related subjects should be clustered together.

Some respondents regard questions about their demographic background as invasive, and the relevance of such questions to the study topic is often not apparent if they are asked early in a questionnaire. Therefore, questions about the respondent's demographic background are often placed at the end of the questionnaire, except where it is necessary to screen a respondent's eligibility to answer a particular group of subsequent questions (e.g., only questions about recent therapy outcomes would be asked of respondents who have received therapy recently).

It is helpful to have smooth transitions between topics. This may be achieved by presenting questions in a chronological order when appropriate, by using section headings, or by inserting a brief statement introducing a group of questions about a new topic. This is especially important for sensitive questions that may provoke embarrassment, be viewed as private or personal, or ask about illegal behaviors. Respondents will be more likely to respond to such questions if there is an appropriate context given for the questions and the respondent can see the relevance of the questions to the study purpose. For example, when asking about use of illegal drugs, the survey might include the following statement:

> The next questions refer to your experiences with the use of alcohol and street drugs.

Within a topical area of the survey, the questions should be sequenced in a logical order. The "funnel" principle, which is used frequently, starts with general questions followed by ones that become increasingly more specific (Hoyle et al., 2002). It is also important to avoid a potential question-sequence effect (Tourangeau & Rasinski, 1988). That is, one should avoid asking a question sequence in which a previous question will likely bias the response to the next question.

For example, in a survey to parents about equipment and services that are needed within a school system, the following set of questions might be biased toward prompting parents to choose sensory-based equipment, causing a question-sequence effect:

1) Please select the kind of sensory equipment that would best fit your child's needs.
   a. Sensory equipment for tactile input
   b. Sensory equipment for vestibular input
   c. Sensory equipment for proprioceptive input
   d. Sensory equipment for oral input
   e. Sensory equipment for soothing auditory input
2) Please list the equipment you believe is most important for our therapists to use to address your child's educational needs: _____
_____

From this example, it is clear that Question 1 might bias the types of responses parents provide to the open-ended question (Question 2). Question 1 did not ask about other types of educational equipment or technologies that might be relevant to a child's education. It only asked about sensory equipment, thus prompting a potential bias in parents' responses to Question 2.

Formatting Questions for Different Scales

By their nature, nominal and ordinal scales have finite categories. For example, a question using a nominal scale is:

> What is your sex?
> Male..1
> Female 2

The respondent can respond only by choosing one of the two finite categories.

Nominal categories may be randomly listed to eliminate the possibility of any sequencing effect. Other alternatives for nominal categories are to list them in descending order, starting with the ones that are likely to be chosen most frequently, or to list them alphabetically.

An ordinal scale asks the respondent to choose one of a number of finite categories. The following is an example of an ordinal scale that asks the respondent to choose one of three ratings on an ordinal scale of importance:

> How important is your relationship with your client to the outcomes of therapy?
> Not so important 1
> Important..2
> Extremely important.......................................3

Ordinal responses should be listed in logical order. Listing ordinal responses from lowest to highest (as in the previous example) not only makes them clearer, but also avoids the need to reverse the coding scheme for the analysis.

Responses to an interval scale may be assigned to an infinite number of possible points or to specified ranges. Deciding on categories for interval scales involves judgment. For example, if asking respondents about their age, it is generally fine to ask how many years old someone is, because people can easily retrieve their age from memory.

12. The following are some statements about how occupational therapists might deal with clients who are having difficulty doing everyday activities. For each statement, please indicate if you strongly disagree, disagree, agree, or strongly agree.

	Strongly Disagree	Disagree	Agree	Strongly Agree
a. My occupational therapist should <u>advise</u> me how to engage in daily activity.........	1	2	3	4
b. My occupational therapist should <u>teach</u> me how to engage in daily activity.........	1	2	3	4

Figure 27.6   An example of Likert scales from a survey of occupational therapy practice.

However, if the question is about income, people may have more difficulty recalling the exact amount, and thus the use of ranges, such as $30,000 to $35,000, may be preferable. The decision about using actual amounts versus ranges depends on consideration of this factor along with how important it is to have exact information versus information characterized by a range. When using ranges, use boundaries that conform to traditional rounded breaking points. For example, in asking for years of experience it is better to ask: "0–4 years, 5–9 years" rather than "0–4.5 years, 4.6–9.5 years."

Scaled response mechanisms, such as Likert scales, have response choices to elicit opinions. Likert scales are bipolar, ranging from the most negative point at one end of a continuum to the most positive point at the opposite end, for example, using an "agree/disagree" continuum. The questions should be focused on one issue or domain. The response choices should be balanced, with an equal number of similar points ranging from low to high, for example, "strongly agree," "agree," "disagree," and "strongly disagree" (see Fig. 27.6, question 12).

Piloting the Questionnaire

Piloting the questionnaire is essential before the main study. By doing a pilot study, an investigator can find out whether respondents can reasonably understand and respond to the questions. Piloting can also determine in an interview-based survey whether the interviewers will be able to convey the questioning format as it is written.

Within a pilot study, investigators can gather data to evaluate the intended survey instrument. Three of the most common ways of gathering such

data are focus groups, field pretesting, and individual interviews (Presser et al., 2004). They are discussed in the following subsections.

Focus Groups

Every researcher's views can be widened by systematic discussions within a focus group (Stewart, Shamdasani, & Rook, 2007). **Focus groups** ordinarily involve a small group of persons who represent the range of characteristics expected in the study sample. The investigator guides the group through a discussion that aims to elicit every member's opinion.

Focus groups can be used during the initial planning of the investigation to help define the key study. They can also be used to evaluate the questions once they have been developed into the questionnaire. Focus groups can provide information about the complexity of what is being asked and how people understand the terms in the questionnaire. In some instances, focus groups can involve a question-by-question review of the questionnaire.

Field Pretesting

For telephone or face-to-face interviews, investigators ordinarily will conduct a small number of interviews (usually about 15 to 30) with people who are similar to those who will be respondents in the planned survey. For mailed questionnaires, respondents who are from the study population are asked to complete the questionnaire. There can be some debriefing questions at the end of the questionnaire asking for feedback on such factors as what was unclear or confusing. Field pretests also provide critical information on the practical aspects of administering the survey tool that allows unforeseen problems to be addressed before doing the larger study. A valuable tool for assessing these aspects is to conduct a debriefing interview with pretest interviewers.

Debriefing Interview

A debriefing interview with respondents about their understanding of questions can be helpful (Lessler, Tourangeau, & Salter, 1989). The focus of the interview is to find out the respondent's reactions to the questions. The debriefing interview involves three steps:

1. Asking the questions or providing the questionnaire,
2. Allowing the respondent to answer the questionnaire or interview, and
3. Asking the respondent what was going through his or her mind during the process.

An investigator may also ask respondents to:

• Paraphrase their understanding of the questions,
• Define the terms used in the interview, and/or
• Identify any confusion or concern.

Debriefing interviews are very helpful in identifying how the respondent experiences the questionnaire or interview process and whether anything needs to be changed to improve the accuracy of the data they yield.

Implementing a Survey Study

The procedures used in implementing a survey study will have a large impact on the rigor of the investigation (Fowler, 2008). Three key factors that influence study rigor are sampling, response rates, and how the survey is carried out. Each is discussed in the following sections.

Sampling Strategies

As noted at the beginning of this chapter, most survey data are collected from a sample of a relatively small number of members of a target population. These sample data are used to make estimates of the target population's characteristics (parameters). A census is a special case in which survey methods are used to collect data from or about every member of a population, that is, a 100% sample.

The main reason for collecting data from a sample instead of from an entire population is that it is much less expensive. Also, when available funding is fixed, resources can be allocated to collect information about more variables than would be possible in a survey of the entire population. Another important reason for sampling is that it usually reduces the data collection period, making the study findings available for dissemination and application much sooner. Finally, in cases in which gaining access to population members requires special strategies (e.g., negotiating access to worksites, or screening randomly composed numbers for a telephone interview survey), the strategy can be done more effectively and efficiently with a sample than with the entire population.

Some survey samples are selected by nonprobability methods (e.g., selecting respondents who are convenient or who have volunteered). Selecting a sample using such procedures, which depend on subjective judgments (by the respondents or by the researcher) about who should be included, may result in a sample that constitutes an unrepresentative (biased) population subgroup. Although such a sample may be useful for an exploratory or pilot study about a new topic or new population, great caution must be exercised in generalizing from a nonprobability sample to a target population. There are no systematic methods to account for possible selection bias. Also, standard statistical methods (e.g., confidence intervals) that are based on a random sampling theoretical model cannot be applied appropriately to data from a nonprobability sample.

Consequently, a hallmark of a well-designed survey study is that the respondents are selected randomly from the target population. Random (probability) sampling, in conjunction with good questionnaire design and data collection procedures, provides the foundation on which reliable estimates of population characteristics may be derived from sample data.

In random sampling, the selection of each respondent is independent of the selection of any and all others. Thus, for example, a person would not be included automatically in a sample because someone else in his or her household (e.g., spouse) is selected. Each population member has a unique, independent chance of being selected. That chance must be greater than zero, and it must be known or it must be possible to calculate it. Although it often is desirable that the probability of selection is the same for each population member, this is not an essential aspect of random sampling. In cases in which the probability of selection varies (e.g., in a disproportionate stratified sampling design), the researcher must calculate weights to adjust for this in the analysis.

The basic model underlying sampling theory and inferential statistics is simple random sampling with replacement (i.e., returning the respondent selected to the population after sampling so that he or she has an equal chance of being selected subsequently) (Cochran, 1977). In common survey practice, however, it is not practical or desirable to collect data from the same population members more than once. Therefore, virtually all survey samples are selected without replacement. The first step in selecting any random sample is to obtain or compile a list of all (or as near as possible) of the members of the target population (e.g., all the members of the British College of Occupational Therapists). This list is called the sampling frame. In simple random sampling without replacement, every element (population member) on the frame is assigned a unique number from 1 to N (N = the number of elements). Then n (n = the desired sample size) elements are identified to be in the sample by referring to a random number source (such as a random number table, or a random number generator on a calculator or computer), from which the researcher selects n unique numbers corresponding to elements on the sampling frame. When sampling without replacement, once an element's number is selected, it is set aside and not used again; that is, it is ignored if it is derived more than once from the random number source.

In many cases, the sampling process is greatly simplified by using systematic random selection, which is used commonly in survey research (Levy & Lemeshow, 2008). Again, every element on the frame is assigned a unique number from 1 to N. Next, a selection interval (k) is calculated by dividing the population size by the sample size: $k = N/n$. For example, to select a sample of 200 elements from a population of 1,600, $k = 1,600/200 = 8$. Then, after selecting a random starting point in the interval from 1 to k (1 to 8 in this example), the researcher selects that first element from the sampling frame and every k element thereafter. Thus, if the random starting point is 4, using a selection interval = 8, the sample will consist of elements on the sampling frame that previously were assigned the numbers 4, 12, 20, 28 ... 1,596 (Fig. 27.7).

Before using systematic random selection, however, the sampling frame must be assessed for any preexisting periodic arrangement of elements that might coincide with the selection interval. This is because a random procedure is used only once, when the first selection point is identified. Thereafter, all the other elements selected in the sample are identified by their relative position on the sampling frame. For example, if for some reason every

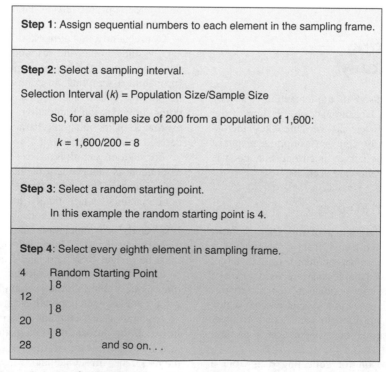

Figure 27.7 The steps for systematic random selection.

eighth person listed on the sampling frame in our example (starting with person number 4) happens to be a certain sex or in a certain occupational category, the sample may be biased. Fortunately, in most studies potential periodicity bias may be avoided effectively by first arranging the sampling frame in a random or nearly random order, usually alphabetically by surname.

A stratified random sample may be selected using information that is already available about the population members to divide them into subgroups (strata) that are of special interest for the study purpose. For example, a sample of occupational therapists might be stratified according to length of employment, which would be available from employee records. Then a separate random sample would be selected from within each of the length of employment strata. For example, three samples might be selected, one each from among those employed less than 1 year, 1 to 4 years, and 5 years or longer. The main advantages of stratification are that it ensures that each subgroup will be included appropriately in the sample, and there will be more stability (less sampling error) across all possible samples of the same size. Both of these aspects contribute toward obtaining more precise estimates of population parameters from the sample statistics. Several strategies may be used to decide how to construct strata and to determine the number of elements to select from each stratum. In some cases, stratification involves giving population members unequal probabilities of selection. Accordingly, the researcher must adjust for this in the analysis by weighting the data (Cochran, 1977).

Response Rate

An important aspect of the quality of the data collected from a representative sample is how successful a survey is in obtaining cooperation from the persons selected into the sample. As noted at the beginning of the chapter, failure to collect data from a high percentage of the sample is a major source of potential survey error, called nonresponse bias. In addition to the degree of nonparticipation, nonresponse bias depends on the extent to which nonrespondents differ systematically from respondents in terms of their characteristics on key variables under study (Fowler, 2008; Groves, 2004; Kviz, 2015). In such cases, the absence of nonrespondents from the analysis may cause survey estimates of population parameters to be lower or higher than their true value. For example, if persons who engage in risky behaviors are less willing than others to participate in a survey about

health risks, then the estimates of the prevalence of those behaviors based on data from the survey sample will be too low.

Availability is another source of nonresponse, especially in telephone and face-to-face interview surveys. If the data collection times are within working times, then it will be challenging to gather data on a working population. Less educated people and those older than 65 years of age are less willing to be interviewed in a random-digit telephone procedure (Groves & Couper, 1998). Even with a relatively high response rate, there still is a potential for nonresponse bias if the reason for nonresponse is related strongly to the survey topic. Therefore, it is important that efforts are put into reducing nonresponse and/or comparing any systematic difference between respondents and nonrespondents.

Reducing nonresponse rates in telephone and face-to-face interview surveys involves ensuring access and gaining cooperation (Groves & Couper, 1998). Access can be increased by making multiple calls and by ensuring these happen at varied times, including evenings and weekends. An average of 10 calls is usually made before deciding that the person being called is a nonrespondent. Having interviewers who have flexible schedules and can make appointments at the respondents' convenience enhances access to the sample. Cooperation can be elicited by an advanced letter clearly stating the purpose of the study and the content of the interview. Being clear at the start of the interview of the purpose of the questions and reassuring the respondents their information is important to the outcome of the research will support cooperation. Training interviewers who understand the importance of good response rates and who can handle challenging questions with sensitivity is essential.

Reducing nonresponse in a mailed survey involves developing a well-presented questionnaire and sending multiple mailings to nonrespondents. Three mailings of the questionnaire and a cover letter are recommended, with the mailings about 1 month apart (Dillman, 2007). If questionnaires are mailed to a general population without appropriate follow-up techniques, the response rate is likely to be less than 50% (Edwards et al., 2002; Heberlein & Baumgartner, 1978).

The response rate is an important mechanism for assessing the potential for nonresponse bias. In general, the response rate is calculated as the number of sample members from whom a completed questionnaire is collected, divided by the number of sample members who are eligible to participate in a particular survey, expressed as a percentage (Kviz, 1977). However, special considerations often must be taken into account depending on various aspects of any particular survey. Although there still is no generally accepted standard for computing response rates, many survey professionals have adapted the guidelines set forth by the American Association for Public Opinion Research (2015), which are available from the organization's website along with a response rate calculator that may be downloaded free at http://www.aapor.org.

Response rates vary widely across the various survey data collection modes, and even across studies using the same mode. In general, response rates are highest and quite similar for the two interview survey methods, with response rates tending to be about 5% higher for face-to-face interviews than for telephone interviews. Response rates generally are lower for mailed questionnaires (Aday & Cornelius, 2006). A review by Goyder (1985) found that response rates for mailed questionnaires using the strategies we recommend here range from about 30% to as high as 80% or higher, with the range of 60% to 70% being regarded by some survey experts as a realistic average expectation for a well-implemented mail survey. Response rates for "typical" face-to-face interview surveys range from about 70% to 90% or higher (Goyder, 1985). Blair, Czaja, and Blair (2014) suggest the following response rates may be expected for most typical surveys: 65% to 95% for face-to-face interviews, 60% to 90% for telephone interviews, and 45% to 75% for mailed questionnaires.

There is no agreed-upon standard minimum for an acceptable response rate. Some have suggested 50% to 60% as adequate (Rea & Parker, 2005), whereas others have suggested above 70% is acceptable (Fowler, 2008). Of course, as discussed earlier, in addition to the response rate, any assessment of potential nonresponse bias must consider whether and to what extent nonrespondents are likely to differ from respondents in terms of key variables under study. However, even with a 90% response rate there may be some nonresponse bias.

Carrying Out the Survey

Face-to-face interviews afford the opportunity for an advance letter that informs the potential respondent of the details of the study. Telephone random digit dialing is always a cold contact. However, other telephone surveys may afford the opportunity to send a letter prior to the call to increase response rates. Mail surveys can send an advance letter explaining that a questionnaire will be mailed to respondents shortly. Cover letters are critical to response rates of mailed surveys

(Salant & Dillman, 1994). It is the only opportunity the researcher has to anticipate and deal with the respondents' questions and concerns about participating in the survey. The cover letter should be printed on letterhead stationery and have the mailing date and the name and address of the anticipated respondent. It should include at a minimum why the study is important, why the respondent's answers are important, assurance of confidentiality of their answers, and whom to contact if they have questions about the survey. The letter should conclude with a thank you and be signed with an original signature whenever possible.

Telephone and face-to-face interviews obtain higher cooperation rates in the evenings and weekends, which is when most respondents are likely to be available for interview (Weeks, Kulka, & Pierson, 1987). Interview schedules need to be developed to reflect when the sample can be accessed. Interviewers generally are instructed to let a phone ring up to 10 rings to allow respondents sufficient time to pick up the phone. Leaving a message on an answering machine or voice-mail system usually is not advised unless this will be the last attempt to contact a respondent. It is best for the interviewer to make direct contact. Few respondents return a call in response to a message left by an interviewer.

All forms of survey need appropriate follow-up procedures to maximize response rates. The majority of face-to-face interviews are carried out within six contact attempts (Kalsbeek, Botman, Massey, & Lui, 1994). The number of follow-ups is dependent on cost. A careful cost–benefit analysis should be completed before deciding how many repeat calls the interviewers make before assigning a nonresponse status to a sample unit.

It is more cost effective to complete contacts to nonrespondents in telephone interview surveys. If there is a busy signal, for example, it has been recommended to call back a maximum of three times, 3 minutes apart (Survey Research Laboratory, 1987). When the sample is selected from a list, a minimum of 10 callbacks at different times on different days is usually completed for nonrespondents. When working with a random-digit-dialing sample, where there is a chance for more nonresidential telephone numbers to be included in the sample, most survey research organizations attempt a minimum of about 15 calls.

Mailed surveys require a systematic approach to administration to ensure acceptable response rates (Table 27.2). Follow-up mailings to everyone in the sample (even those who have responded) are not efficient and may confuse or irritate those who have already responded. Targeted repeated

Table 27.2 Procedure for Administration of Mailed Surveys

Time Frame	Action
Before survey is sent	Mail a personalized, advanced letter to everyone in the sample.
Round 1	**Mail a personalized cover letter with more detail of the study, the questionnaire, and a stamped self-addressed return envelope.**
4–8 days later	Send a follow-up postcard or letter to thank everyone who has responded and ask those who have not done so to respond.
Round 2 4 weeks after first questionnaire was sent	**To nonrespondents, send a new personalized cover letter, replacement questionnaire, and stamped self-addressed envelope.**
Round 3 8 weeks after first questionnaire was sent out	**To nonrespondents, send a new personalized cover letter, replacement questionnaire, and stamped self-addressed envelope.**
End data collection 12 weeks after first questionnaire was sent out	

administrations can be achieved if there is a way of identifying those who have not responded. This can be achieved if a sample point number (SPN) is placed at the top right-hand corner of the questionnaire. This number corresponds to the respondent's entry in the sampling frame, which should be kept in a locked physical file and/or in a password-protected computer file to protect respondent confidentiality. It is good practice to tell people what the number is used for in the cover letter. If it is important that the respondent not be identifiable even to the researcher, then a postcard procedure can be employed (Fowler, 2008), whereby a postcard bearing the respondent's SPN is enclosed with the questionnaire along with a request for the respondent to mail it separately when he or she mails back the completed questionnaire. The text of the postcard states, "Dear researcher, I am sending this postcard at the same time that I am sending my completed questionnaire. Because the questionnaire is completely anonymous [the SPN is not recorded on the questionnaire in this case], this will let you know I have returned my questionnaire." This procedure maintains anonymity while enabling the researcher to track who has responded to the survey. Whatever procedure is used, it must be approved by an ethical board that judges the procedure to be warranted in light of the potential respondents' rights to consent and to confidentiality.

Preparing for Data Analysis

The formal process of gathering survey data was outlined earlier. The data this process generates must now be presented in an understandable format. During the planning stage of the research, the researcher should know how the data will be analyzed to meet the objectives of the study. This process of thinking forward to the analysis phase early on can often identify and allow correction of gaps in the data that will be obtained through the questionnaire.

Survey data are usually entered into a computer data file for statistical analysis. Each statistical program has different criteria in how the data should be formatted. To facilitate computer processing and analysis, codes must be assigned to all responses on a completed questionnaire. There should be clear rules as to which numbers are assigned to which answers on the survey. A code book should be developed that clearly indicates which codes are reflective of which questionnaire answers and in which column the questionnaire can be found in the electronic data set (Fig. 27.8).

If the coding is complex, detailed coding instructions will need to be developed. These need to be clear to ensure coding reliability. Codes need to be assigned to missing data to identify whether the respondent refused to answer a question, left a response blank inadvertently, a question was not applicable to the respondent, or the respondent did not know the information requested by a question. Codes need to be generated for open questions, or for "other" choices, where the responses are not predictable. The researcher identifies categories that emerge as themes in the answers to the open question.

Quality control procedures include having trained coders independently check each coder's

Variables in Export Sequence

Column Location   Content of Column

1-3:   subject identifier (001-999) (3 numeric code)

4-6:   repeat code (001-999) (3 numeric code)

7-8:   translation used (1 character code/1 numeric code)
                    missing data: 09

9-11:   country in which data was collected code (3 character
                    code) missing data: 009

12-13:   age (2 numeric code)
                    missing data: 99

14:                 gender (M or F)
                    missing data: 9

15-17:   nationality (3 character code)
                    missing data: 009

18:                 ethnicity (single numeric code)
                    missing data: 9

19:                 years of education (single numeric code)
                    missing data: 9

20-21:   degree earned (2 character code)
                    missing data: 09

22-23:   employment status (2 character code)
                    missing data: 09

24-25:   living situation (2 character code)
                    missing data: 09

26:                 independence in occupational behavior (1 character
                    code) missing data: 9

27-28:   major disabling condition category (2 character code)
                    missing data: 09

29-32:   specific major disabling condition (4 numeric code)
                    missing data: 0009

Figure 27.8   An example of the demographic information section of a code book.

work, and coders should write notes about codes of which they are not sure so that they can be checked by the supervisor. Other quality control methods include using a well-developed interface between the computer and the data entry personnel. Computer programs (e.g., ACCESS, SPSS, SAS, Epi-Info) now can develop data entry screens to ease the process of entering data. These programs can be set to accept only a certain range of codes in a particular field, thereby reducing error codes in a field. The data can be entered twice in two different files, and then the files can be correlated to identify potential errors in data entry. This can be expensive, and therefore a 10% random sample can be entered in twice to check accuracy. The rate of error from data entry should be less than 1% (Fowler, 2008). Survey researchers are increasingly exploring effective ways of collecting survey data using electronic approaches and the Internet (Dillman, 2007).

Summary

Surveys allow for the systematic collection of information from a sample of people to generate an understanding of the population from which the sample was drawn. Completing a rigorous survey study requires careful attention to building the survey, administering the survey, and processing the data. If these procedures are followed, the summary statistics can be generalized to the population under study, which is the aim of survey research.

Review Questions

1. What is one type of research question that is better answered by survey research than by another approach?
2. What are the steps involved in constructing a survey questionnaire or interview?
3. What are the three approaches to pilot testing a questionnaire?
4. When implementing a survey study, what are the three considerations that influence rigor?

REFERENCES

Abramson, J., & Abramson, Z. (1999). *Survey methods in community medicine* (5th ed.). New York, NY: Churchill Livingstone.

Aday, L., & Cornelius, L. J. (2006). *Designing and conducting health surveys: A comprehensive guide* (3rd ed). San Francisco, CA: Jossey-Bass.

American Association for Public Opinion Research. (2015). *Standard definitions: Final dispositions of case codes and outcome rates for surveys* (8th ed). Retrieved from https://www.esomar.org/knowledge-and-standards/research-resources/aapor-standard-definitions.php

Blair, J., Czaja, R., & Blair, J. (2014). *Designing surveys: A guide to decisions and procedures.* Thousand Oaks, CA: Sage.

Bradburn, N. M., Sudman, S., & Wansik, B. (2004). *Asking questions.* San Francisco, CA: Jossey-Bass.

Cochran, W. G. (1977). *Sampling techniques* (3rd ed). New York, NY: John Wiley & Sons.

Converse, J., & Presser, S. (1986). *Survey questions: Handcrafting the standardized questionnaire* (2nd ed.). Beverly Hills, CA: Sage.

DePoy, E., & Gitlin, L. (2010). *Introduction to research: Understanding and applying multiple strategies* (4th ed). St. Louis, MO: Mosby.

Dillman, D. A. (2007). *Mail and Internet surveys: The tailored design method* (2nd ed) New York, NY: John Wiley & Sons.

Edwards, P., Roberts, I., Clarke, M., DiGuiseppi, C., Pratap, S., Wentz, R., . . . Kwan, I. (2002). Increasing response rates to postal questionnaires: Systematic review. *British Medical Journal, 324*(7347), 1183–1191.

Fowler, F. (2008). *Survey research methods. Applied social research methods series* (Vol. 1, 4th ed) Thousand Oaks, CA: Sage.

Goyder, J. (1985). Face-to-face interviews and mailed questionnaires: The net difference in response rate. *Public Opinion Quarterly, 49*(2), 234–252.

Groves, R., & Couper, M. (1998). *Nonresponse in household interview surveys.* New York, NY: John Wiley & Sons.

Groves, R. M. (2004). *Survey errors and survey costs.* New York, NY: John Wiley & Sons.

Heberlein, T., & Baumgartner, R. (1978). Factors affecting response rates to mailed questionnaires: A quantitative analysis of the published literature. *American Sociological Review, 43,* 447–462.

Hoyle, R. H., Harris, M. J., & Judd, C. M. (2002). *Research methods in social relations* (7th ed.). Pacific Grove, CA: Wadsworth.

Kalsbeek, W., Botman, S., Massey, J., & Lui, P. (1994). Cost efficiency and the number of allowable call attempts in the National Health Interview Survey. *Journal of Official Statistics, 10,* 133–152.

Kviz, F. J. (1977). Toward a standard definition of response rate. *Public Opinion Quarterly, 41,* 265–267.

Kviz, F. J. (2015). Nonresponse. Wiley StatsRef: Statistics Reference Online: 1–8.

Lessler, J., Tourangeau, R., & Salter, W. (1989). Questionnaire design research in the cognitive research laboratory. *Vital and Health Statistics* (Series 6, No. 1; DHHS Publication No. PHS-89-1076). Washington, DC: Government Printing Office.

Levy, P. S., & Lemeshow, S. (2008). *Sampling of populations: Methods and applications* (4th ed). New York, NY: John Wiley & Sons.

National Board for Certification in Occupational Therapy. (2013). *2012 practice analysis of the occupational therapist registered.* Gaithersburg, MD: Author.

Presser, S., Couper, M. P., Lessler, J. T., Martin, E., Martin, J., Rothgeb, J. M., et al. (2004). Methods for testing and evaluating survey questions. *Public Opinion Quarterly, 68,* 109–130.

Rea, L., & Parker, R. (2005). *Designing and conducting survey research: A comprehensive guide* (3rd ed). San Francisco, CA: Jossey-Bass.

Salant, P., & Dillman, D. (1994). *How to conduct your own survey.* New York, NY: John Wiley & Sons.

Schuman, H., & Presser, S. (1996). *Questions and answers in attitudes surveys.* Thousand Oaks, CA: Sage.

Siemiatycki, J. (1979). A comparison of mail, telephone, and home interview strategies for household surveys. *American Journal of Public Health, 69*(3), 238–245.

Stewart, D., Shamdasani, P., & Rook, D. W. (2007). *Focus groups: Theory and practice* (2nd ed.). Thousand Oaks, CA: Sage.

Survey Research Laboratory, University of Illinois. (1987). *Chicago area general population survey on AIDS (SRL No. 606), interviewer manual.* Chicago, IL: Author.

Tourangeau, R., & Rasinski, K. (1988). Cognitive processes underlying context effects in attitude measurement. *Psychological Bulletin, 103,* 299–314.

Weeks, M., Kulka, R., & Pierson, S. (1987). Optimal call scheduling for a telephone survey. *Public Opinion Quarterly, 51,* 540–549.

Resources

Websites

American Association for Public Opinion Research—"Best Practices for Survey and Public Opinion Research": http://www.aapor.org/Standards-Ethics/Best-Practices .aspx

American Association for Public Opinion Research—"Code of Professional Ethics and Practices": http://www.aapor.org/Standards-Ethics/AAPOR-Code-of-Ethics.aspx

American Association for Public Opinion Research—"Response Rate Calculator": https://www.google.com/webhp?sourceid=chrome-instant&ion=1&espv=2&es_th=1&ie=UTF-8#q=aapor%20response%20rate%20calculator&es_th=1

American Statistical Association, Survey Research Methods Section—Proceedings: http://www.amstat.org/sections/srms/Proceedings/

Online proceedings of the American Statistical Association Survey Research Methods Section from 1978 to present. Also includes papers from the Joint Statistical Meetings and some papers from the American Association of Public Opinion Research meetings. More than 3,000 papers in all.

Sage Publications—*The Survey Kit* (2nd ed): https://us.sagepub.com/en-us/nam/the-survey-kit/book225666
A collection of brief, applied books by various authors about survey research methods.

U.S. Office of Management and Budget—"Revisions to the Standards for the Classification of Federal Data on Race and Ethnicity" (October 30, 1997): https://www.whitehouse.gov/omb/fedreg_1997standards

Articles

Couper, M. P., Traugott, M. W., & Lamias, M. J. (2001). Web survey design and administration. *Public Opinion Quarterly, 65,* 230–253.

Schaeffer, N. C., & Presser, S. (2003). The science of asking questions. *Annual Review of Sociology, 29,* 65–88.

Schwarz, N. (1999). Self-reports: How the questions shape the answers. *American Psychologist, 54*(2), 93–105.

Books

Couper, M. P., & Nicholls, II, W. L. (1998). The history and development of computer assisted survey information collection methods. In M. P. Couper, R. P. Baker, J. Bethlehem, C. Z. F. Clark, J. Martin, W. L. Nicholls II, . . . O'Reilly, M. (Eds.), *Computer assisted survey information collection* (pp. 1–21). New York, NY: John Wiley & Sons.

DeVellis, R. F. (2003). *Scale development: Theory and applications.* Newbury Park, CA: Sage.

Fink, A. (1995). *How to ask survey questions.* Thousand Oaks, CA: Sage.

Fowler, F. J., Jr. (1998). Design and evaluation of survey questions. In L. Bickman & D. J. Rog (Eds.), *Handbook of applied social research methods* (pp. 343–374). Thousand Oaks, CA: Sage.

Harkness, J. A., van de Vijver, F. J. R., & Mohler, P. P. (2002). *Cross-cultural survey methods.* San Francisco, CA: Jossey–Bass.

Presser, S., Rothgeb, J. M., Couper, M. P., Lessler, J. T., Martin, E., Martin, J., . . . Singer, E. (Eds.). (2004). *Methods for testing and evaluating survey questionnaires.* New York, NY: John Wiley & Sons.

Schwarz, N., & Sudman, S. (Eds.) (1996). *Answering questions: Methodology for determining cognitive and communicative processes in survey research.* San Francisco, CA: Jossey-Bass.

Sudman, S., Bradburn, N. M., & Schwarz, N. (1996). *Thinking about answers: The application of cognitive processes to survey methodology.* San Francisco, CA: Jossey-Bass.

Tourangeau, R., Rips, L. J., & Rasinski, K. (2000). *The psychology of survey response.* New York, NY: Cambridge University Press.

Willis, G. B. (2005). *Cognitive interviewing: A tool for improving questionnaire design.* Thousand Oaks, CA: Sage.

*Note: Many universities have expertise in survey design and can be consulted when creating a survey.

CHAPTER 28

Needs Assessment Research

Marcia Finlayson

Learning Outcomes

- Describe the four dimensions across which needs assessments vary in occupational therapy.
- Explain the different ideological perspectives by which client need may be defined in occupational therapy.
- Differentiate between normative, expressed/felt, and comparative need (from the perspective of an occupational therapy researcher).
- Discuss social and political variables that play a role in determining the value for and potential contributions of a needs assessment.
- Articulate common data collection approaches in needs assessment research.
- Understand five of the most widely used approaches to conducting a needs assessment.

To succeed in these broader types of activities, OT practitioners and researchers must have a basic but solid grounding in the theories and methods of needs assessment. This foundation must include the knowledge and skills that are necessary to conduct high-quality needs assessments and the ability to work with others to translate findings into action. Therefore, the objectives of this chapter are to:

- Provide a theoretical overview of the concept of need,
- Examine the processes and dimensions of a needs assessment,
- Describe and compare models and approaches to needs assessment,
- Evaluate methods commonly used in needs assessments, and
- Outline how needs can be translated into actions for solutions.

Introduction

Every day, occupational therapists are faced with determining whether an individual client has a problem or set of problems that could be remediated through occupational therapy (OT) services and, if so, which intervention would be the most appropriate to apply. Consequently, practitioners are well versed in how to assess the needs of individual clients, translate these needs into intervention goals, assess progress toward goals, and determine when discharge should occur. Equally important is the process of **needs assessment,** which involves identifying the needs of broader groups of people in order to develop or modify services, programs, and policies and their respective goals. This process is a requirement for occupational therapists who are developing new areas of practice, expanding services within existing settings, examining ways to allocate limited resources to best meet the needs of a particular client base, or trying to advocate for policy changes that will affect entire populations.

What Is a Needs Assessment?

The term needs assessment is commonly used and seemingly easy to understand. At the most basic level, it refers to the process of determining what a group of individuals, an organization, a community, or a population requires to achieve some basic standard or to improve its current situation. Altschuld and Kumar (2010) describe a needs assessment as "the process of identifying needs, prioritizing them, making needs-based decisions, allocating resources, and implementing actions in organizations to resolve problems underlying important needs" (p. 20). Consequently, a needs assessment is simultaneously a form of applied research and a political process (Martí-Costa & Serrano-García, 1983; Minkler, 2012). Needs assessments vary across four dimensions: the sophistication of the project design, the level of involvement of the stakeholders, the project's political orientation, and the scope of the issue being addressed (see Fig. 28.1).

CASE EXAMPLE

Asia, an OT researcher known for her work and publications involving hunger and poverty within densely populated urban areas, receives an e mail from the director a food pantry. The director of the food pantry requests that a needs assessment be conducted in order to identify the strengths of the individuals served by the pantry as well as the social, financial, and geographical barriers they face. Because Asia's research is grounded in theories of community psychology and participatory research, she decides to apply a concerns report methods survey approach to better understand the individuals served by the pantry.

Asia's first step in carrying out this process is to conduct a series of focus groups with the individuals served. She arranges her schedule so that she is available during times when there is likely to be a critical mass of people coming to the pantry. During the focus group, Asia obtains informed consent, collects contact information for each person, and asks them a series of questions to better understand their values, concerns, and priorities regarding their access to food. Asia then uses the findings from the focus group to construct the following survey:

Sample Statements From a Concerns Report Method Survey
I have access to transportation for shopping.

How important is this to you personally?
    Very important _____ Somewhat important _____ Not important _____
How satisfied are you with your own situation?
    Very satisfied _____ Somewhat satisfied_____ Not satisfied _____

I am able to shop independently.

How important is this to you personally?
    Very important _____ Somewhat important _____ Not important _____
How satisfied are you with your own situation?
    Very satisfied _____ Somewhat satisfied_____ Not satisfied _____

I am able to prepare nutritious meals independently.

How important is this to you personally?
    Very important _____ Somewhat important _____ Not important _____
How satisfied are you with your own situation?
    Very satisfied _____ Somewhat satisfied_____ Not satisfied _____

I am aware of community programs that provide nutritious meals.

How important is this to you personally?
    Very important _____ Somewhat important _____ Not important _____
How satisfied are you with your own situation?
    Very satisfied _____ Somewhat satisfied_____ Not satisfied _____

In constructing the survey, Asia was careful to ensure that each item had an importance dimension and a satisfaction dimension. Asia then used the contact information provided by the focus-group members as a starting point for a broader-based administration of this survey to the community within a 10-mile radius surrounding the food pantry.

Dimension 1: Sophistication of the Project Design

As a form of applied research, needs assessments range in quality and rigor, just like any other form of research. This variability is reflected in the first dimension of a needs assessment: the sophistication of the project design. To accurately inform judgments about policies and programs, and ultimately the allocation of resources, the ideal needs assessment is one that is rigorously designed. This means that it takes into account all of the key components of a high-quality study—clearly defined questions that are grounded in theory, appropriate

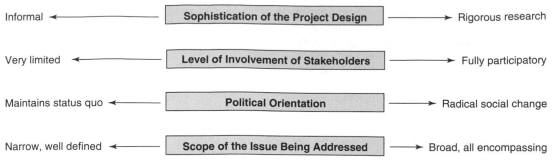

Figure 28.1 Dimensions of a needs assessment.

sampling, psychometrically sound data collection tools and processes, and correctly applied analytic strategies. As previous authors have noted, needs assessments should be systemic, empirically based, outcome oriented, and focused on solving real-world problems through the application of a variety of research methodologies and methods (Altschuld & Kumar, 2010).

Often, though, the term *needs assessment* is used loosely for projects that are little more than informal questioning of convenient individuals with little to no rigor or possibility of replication.

As a political process, needs assessments are value laden, focus on collectives rather than individuals, and raise awareness of everyday problems and their causes. They seek to mobilize communities into action in order to influence and inform policymaking, infrastructure changes, and human and financial resource management and distribution (Martí-Costa & Serrano-García, 1983). Through these processes, the ultimate goal of a needs assessment is to gather meaningful data to inform actions that build on community strengths and remediate any problems that are uncovered (Kretzmann & McKnight, 1993; Witkin & Altschuld, 1995). As such, two additional dimensions of a needs assessment are the level of involvement of stakeholders and the project's political orientation.

Dimension 2: Level of Involvement of Stakeholders

Stakeholders are the individuals, organizations, and policymakers who have a role in defining the issues and/or addressing the concerns that arise from the needs assessment process. Witkin and Altschuld (1995) conceptualize stakeholders at three levels—individuals who are receiving services, the providers of services, and organizations as a whole. An example of these different levels may include older adults who have experienced a stroke, the occupational therapists who provide

services to these individuals, and the hospital that employs the therapists. It is important to realize that stakeholders can also include individuals and organizations associated with the individuals in each of these three levels. For example, additional stakeholders could include families, friends, other professionals providing services (e.g., physical therapy, social work), organizations to which clients are referred on discharge (e.g., home care, stroke support group), and insurance companies.

A needs assessment that is fully participatory would seek input and direction from all three levels of stakeholders at all points during the assessment process (e.g., setting the question, determining the methods, collecting data, etc.). This type of needs assessment would draw on the principles of community building (Minkler, 2012) and participatory action research (Reason & Bradbury-Huang, 2013). (See Chapter 29.) Involvement of stakeholders in the needs assessment process is critical to increase the odds that the stakeholders will embrace and utilize the findings in a way that moves the organization forward (Green & Mercer, 2001). At the opposite end of the continuum are the needs assessments that do not actively involve stakeholders. In these types of needs assessments, an external needs assessor is brought in to act as an expert consultant who designs and implements the project, analyzes the findings, and presents recommendations to the contracting group.

Dimension 3: Political Orientation

The political orientation of a needs assessment will to a large extent depend on who initiated the process. Some needs assessments are initiated by organizations in order to maintain the status quo or, alternatively, to justify a decision that has already been made (Martí-Costa & Serrano-García, 1983; Witkin & Altschuld, 1995). For example, hospital administrators may conduct a needs assessment that recommends a new computerized documentation system or a different staffing configuration on the rehabilitation units to improve patient care. Although these infrastructure changes may benefit patients indirectly, they often do not emerge from the issues and concerns of patients themselves.

At the opposite end of the continuum are needs assessments that are initiated for the purposes of raising awareness of the issues within a community and for promoting community building and social change. For example, a needs assessment of older adults who have experienced a stroke and are being discharged back to the community may uncover issues and concerns related to housing accessibility, lack of social support, and inadequate outpatient follow-up. By documenting these issues and sharing findings with the community, a needs assessment team can provide empirical data to support social change efforts such as mobilizing community volunteers, changing discharge policies, or developing a fund to subsidize home modifications for older adults who require home modifications after a catastrophic health event.

Dimension 4: The Scope of the Issue Being Addressed

A final dimension of a needs assessment reflects the scope of the issue or problem being addressed. Many needs assessments are narrow and well defined in their orientation, for example, determining the recreational needs of teenage members of a specific community center. Other needs assessments are much broader in their orientation, for example, determining the needs of individuals in the United States who are newly diagnosed with multiple sclerosis.

What Is It That We Are Assessing?

At the heart of the needs assessment process is the concept of need. *Need* is a vague term that is poorly understood and rarely defined in the research literature. Nevertheless, defining and operationalizing need is critical to conducting a needs assessment that is rigorous and can produce findings that have utility for informing political action. Within many disciplines, need is essentially viewed as a discrepancy between what an individual's or group's present situation or status is and what is desired (Reviere et al., 1996; Witkin & Altschuld, 1995). But the definition raises two key questions: What is desirable? Who defines desirable?

Trying to answer these questions illustrates the complexity of defining and then trying to assess need. Authors from the disciplines of psychology, sociology, philosophy, and political science (Bradshaw, 1972; Dill, 1983; Doyal & Gough, 1991; Maslow, 1954; Thomson, 1987) suggest that the concept of need is complex because of the different ways the term is used (as a noun and as a verb), the extent to which need is value laden, and because of its links to ideas about what is moral and good. For example, the term *need* is used to describe basic physiological drives, goals that are sought after (ends), as well as the strategies to achieve those goals (solutions) (Dill, 1983; Doyal & Gough, 1991). Furthermore, need can be conceptualized at both an individual level as well as a collective one. These ideas are explored in the following sections.

Need as a Physiological Drive

As a basic physiological drive, need is a "motivational force instigated by a state of disequilibrium or tension set up in an organism because of a particular lack" (Thomson, 1987, p. 13). Defining needs as drives is illustrated in the classic hierarchy described by Maslow (1954), which suggests that humans are motivated to first address physiological needs for food and water, then safety and security, and finally to belong, to develop self-esteem, and to seek self-actualization. Examples of needs as drives can be illustrated in the following statements: "I need a glass of water," "I need a house," or "I need to participate in meaningful activity." Note that in all of these statements the term *need* is used as a verb and "points to what is required or desired to fill the discrepancy—solutions, a means to an end" (Witkin & Altschuld, 1995, p. 9). Yet, the discrepancy itself is not explicit, nor is the specific end (e.g., becoming hydrated, having shelter, being engaged in an occupation).

Need as a Solution

Although need as a drive is not the perspective used for the majority of needs assessments that are conducted by occupational therapists, using the term *need* as a verb and conceptualizing need as a solution is very common. Consider, for example, the situation of a community mental health agency that is examining life skills programming for its clients. Staff members set off to conduct a needs assessment to help its board of directors determine whether clients need more occupational therapists within the scope of the agency's service package. What is missing in this scenario is an explicit indication of what the actual goal might be and a willingness to explore solutions other than more occupational therapists.

Presumably, the goal of this needs assessment would be improved ability of the agency's clients to manage in the community independently. Unfortunately, by framing the needs assessment from a solution orientation (i.e., do clients need more occupational therapists?), it is unlikely that other options to achieve this goal will be identified. If alternatives are not identified, the board of directors cannot consider them in their decision-making and resource-allocation decisions.

For this reason, Altschuld and Witkin (1999) argue against conceptualizing needs as solutions because such an approach fails to identify the underlying issues and concerns, thereby limiting the opportunity to explore and examine a range of possible solutions. Yet, many needs assessments completed within health and social services conceptualize need in this way. A classic example of this type of needs assessment is the survey that provides respondents with a list of services, and then asks them to review the list and check off what they "need." Such an approach risks the possibility of identifying "needs" that do not address the underlying issue.

Need as Relative to the Assessor

In addition to conceptualizing needs as either goals or solutions, it is also possible to consider needs relative to the assessor and the method of determining the need. The classic typology presented by Bradshaw (1972) is an example of conceptualizing needs from these perspectives. Bradshaw discusses four types of needs: normative, felt, expressed, and comparative. Table 28.1 provides definitions and examples of these types of needs, as well as related terms that have been used by other authors.

Normative Need

Normative need is defined by professionals and experts rather than by members of the community themselves. Consequently, a needs assessment that uses a normative needs perspective would have little to no involvement of the stakeholders. In addition, defining needs using this approach is highly subject to the cultural and value biases of the expert and can vary greatly across experts. For example, when asked to identify the needs of young men in a homeless shelter, an occupational therapist may identify needs related to their roles and habits. For the same group of young men, a

Table 28.1 Bradshaw's Categories of Need

Bradshaw's Need Categories	Explanation/Illustration
Normative need	Expert definitions
Expressed need	Refers to demand for a service as measured by actual use as well as requests for services (e.g., waiting lists).
Felt need	Want
Comparative need	Need based on comparisons to and equity with others. For example, group A receives a service, but group B does not, even though the groups are equivalent on key characteristics. Therefore, group B is determined to be in need of the service.

social worker may identify needs related to communication and social interactions. A drug and alcohol counselor may identify the primary need of these young men as substance abuse rehabilitation. As a result, using a normative perspective means that the needs assessor must be vigilant about the reliability of the data collection tools and processes so that the findings can be replicated.

Expressed and Felt Need

In comparison, individuals themselves determine expressed need and felt need. **Felt need** refers to want, with or without actions to obtain that which is wanted. **Expressed need** refers to demand for a service, either through current use or waiting lists. The problem with both felt and expressed need is twofold. First, both frame needs in terms of solutions—a problem that has already been discussed earlier in this section. Second, these ways of defining need cannot account for people who do not know about a service—one cannot want something of which one is unaware. Expressed need is further problematic because there are often individuals who want a service, but who do not request it because they know it is not physically or financially accessible, or because they are simply tired of fighting the system. Consider, for example, individuals who have been consistently refused third-party funding for assistive technology and simply give up asking for it. Both felt need and expressed need focus on the solution, and not necessarily the underlying issue or concern.

Comparative Need

Conceptualizing need from a comparative perspective is relatively common in public health and in the health and social services. Consider the situation in which a group of older adults living in one seniors' apartment complex (baseline group) is compared to a group of older adults living in another complex (comparison group). If the comparison group does not have the same programs and services as the baseline group, members of the comparison group are determined to have need. Through this approach, need is framed in terms of solutions (i.e., the programs and services provided), which is problematic because it carries with it important assumptions that are often difficult to test. Specifically, taking a **comparative need approach** assumes that those in the baseline group actually need the programs and services that their complex provides and that they are receiving them in the correct amount. It further assumes that all of the baseline group's needs are actually being met and that the programs that are being provided are the best solution to the underlying problem.

Identifying Needs as a Political Process

At the beginning of this chapter, needs assessment was described as both a form of applied research and as a political process. Regardless of whether need is viewed as a goal or a solution, it is value laden and culturally influenced. As such, it is affected by sociopolitical factors that are operating within the organization, community, or region in which the needs assessment is being conducted. Sociopolitical factors encompass basic beliefs about what is moral or good, overriding political philosophies, and the nature and operations of systems that are either leading the needs assessment efforts or will respond to the findings (Dill, 1983; Doyal & Gough, 1991; Shi & Singh, 2014). As such, the process, measures, outcomes, and actions of a given needs assessment are fundamentally linked to either the principles and values of the marketplace (e.g., a needs assessment to determine whether to expand a private practice rehabilitation clinic) or to a commitment to the social good (e.g., a needs assessment to determine the accessibility of public housing in an urban center) (Shi & Singh, 2014).

Although the majority of needs assessments will have a primary link to one of these positions, a needs assessment may also have secondary goals and objectives in the other. For example, a health management organization may conduct a needs assessment in a rural area to determine the demand for an assistive technology clinic and the economic viability of developing one. This needs assessment would be linked primarily to the principles and values of the marketplace and the organization's need to be economically successful. Nevertheless, it may also be linked to a secondary understanding that access to assistive technologies is not equitably distributed between rural and urban areas, and that the health and quality of life of individuals with a wide range of disabilities may be negatively influenced by the lack of such a program.

Needs Assessment Grounded in a Marketplace Philosophy

Needs assessments that are grounded in a marketplace philosophy equate need with demand and define needs in terms of solutions. In other words, they take both a felt needs and an expressed needs conceptualization that focus primarily on the individuals. Individual preferences and autonomy are viewed as key to determining need (Shi & Singh, 2014). Although there is room within a marketplace philosophy of needs assessments for expert definitions of needs (i.e., normative needs), it could be argued that this approach would focus more on the needs of the organization that would deliver the service rather than the individual receiving it.

Using the marketplace philosophy, needs can best be met through the free market and through a conservative approach to the development and maintenance of health and social service policies. Services that are provided as a result of the needs assessment are viewed as an economic good and are distributed based on people's ability to pay, either independently or through various types of insurance (Shi & Singh, 2014).

Needs Assessment Grounded in a Philosophy of the Social Good

Alternatively, needs assessments that are grounded in a philosophy of the social good equate need with disparities across groups and inequities of service supply and access, and they focus on the collective rather than the individual (Shi & Singh, 2014). As such, needs assessments grounded in this way have the potential to address underlying problems and issues, as well as identify potential solutions. Two types of need are key to this perspective: normative need and comparative need. From the perspective of the social good, the purpose of conducting needs assessments is to identify areas that need to be remediated to improve the standard of living and/or quality of life of the collective and to determine how to allocate services fairly.

The provision of services to address the identified needs is seen as a social good (if one person is better off, everyone is better off) and generally involves governmental intervention, whether at the community, county, state, regional, or national level. The products of these types of needs assessments guide actions that emphasize equity and ensure that some basic set of standards is met. Actions to remediate these needs are more likely to be met through liberal or democratic policies and social advocacy and action movements (Shi & Singh, 2014). Consequently, needs assessments grounded in this philosophy are more consistent with ones that are participatory in orientation and are directed at social change (see Fig. 28.1).

Why Try to Measure Need?

These discussions suggest that need is ultimately "created" by the people and organizations that are conducting needs assessments, particularly when needs are conceptualized as solutions. The question then becomes: Why try to measure need? As a number of authors have pointed out, needs assessment is one of many potential tools in the processes of strategic and ongoing planning, quality improvement, and outcomes management. Ultimately, the results of needs assessments allow decision makers to justify expenditures to develop new services or to refocus, modify, or eliminate existing services.

In summary, the concept of need is complex and multilayered. The term *need* is used in different ways, and these ways influence the processes and outcomes of a needs assessment. In addition, the conceptualization of needs is influenced by values, culture, politics, and ideas about what is moral and good. Although the idea of "needs assessment" is seemingly easy to understand, this theoretical overview suggests that it is much more complex than many people realize. It would be easy to become mired in these theoretical perspectives and be unable to move forward to assess the needs of a group of individuals, an organization, a community, or a population. Instead, the intention of this overview is to highlight the importance of being clear on what is being assessed and to provide potential frameworks within which current or future needs assessors can consider their work.

Models for Approaching Needs Assessments

Although the definitions of need are multifold, and the philosophical basis for doing needs assessments varies, the actual process of needs assessment is

systematic. Over the years, a number of models or approaches to needs assessments have been presented in the literature. Five important approaches are:

1. Logic models,
2. Three-phase model,
3. Concerns report method,
4. Participatory approaches, and
5. Community-building approaches.

The key features of these models are summarized in Table 28.2.

Logic Models

Logic models, first defined by Weiss (1972), are typically presented in graphical or figure form. The visual image portrays relationships between resources (inputs), activities, outputs (deliverables), and outcomes (impacts), which are used for program planning or program evaluation. Resources are defined as any type of human, monetary, or material effort that is needed to facilitate the program. Activities define the functionality of the program, or how it operates to produce the outputs and outcomes. Outputs represent the nature, quality, and quantity of deliverable objects produced by the program. Outcomes define the broader improvements, changes, or social and physical benefits resulting from the program.

Logic models were originally developed as a tool to facilitate program planning and evaluation. Although logic models continue to be primarily used for these purposes, they also have great utility for the process of planning a needs assessment (Rush & Ogborne, 1991). Figure 28.2 presents a logic model that was developed by a group of students at the University of Illinois at Chicago for a needs assessment they conducted for a local suburban department of public health. Although a logic model does not identify the philosophical stance of the needs assessment or point to particular types of methods, it does offer a concrete way of communicating the work of a needs assessment team to people outside of the immediate group. It is also an excellent tool to keep a needs assessment focused on the long-term goal of the project and how the information that is being gathered will be used.

Three-Phase Model

The **three-phase model** is another tool that can be used to facilitate the planning of a needs assessment. This model was originally described by Witkin and Altschuld (1995) and then updated by Altschuld and Kumar (2010). The model fundamentally operates as a checklist of steps and

Table 28.2 Comparison of Key Features of Different Models and Approaches to Needs Assessment

	Logic Model	Three-Phase Model	Concerns Report Method	Participatory Approach	Community Building
Is there a clearly defined philosophical or theoretical stance?	No	No	Yes	Yes	Yes
Is it apparent what research approach fits with this model (i.e., qualitative, quantitative, or mixed)?	No	No	Yes	Yes	No
Are the specific research methods fitting with this model defined?	No	No	Yes	No	No
Is it clear within this model what tasks are done in what order, by whom, and so forth? In other words, does it have a defined structure?	Somewhat	Yes	Somewhat	No	No
Is it clear how a needs assessor would move through the process of a needs assessment based on this model?	Somewhat	Yes	Yes	Yes	Somewhat
Would the use of this model be resource intensive?	No	Maybe—depends on the issues and the community	Maybe—depends on the issues and the community	Yes	Yes
What is the expected outcome of a needs assessment using this model?	Planning tool	Action plans	Task forces that develop solutions to community concerns	Stronger community with ownership over issues	Stronger community with ownership over issues

activities that must be achieved over the following stages of a needs assessment:

1. Preassessment
2. Assessment
3. Postassessment

The first phase of this model is preassessment, during which a planning group is established and the purpose of the needs assessment is defined. Preliminary data from existing sources is gathered in order to determine if it is necessary to carry on to a full needs assessment process. The preassessment phase is an opportunity for the needs assessment team to learn about the community and its social and political context. This phase of the needs assessment process is fully described by Altschuld and Eastmond (2010). The second phase

of this model is called the assessment phase. Using information obtained during the preassessment, the members of the needs assessment team determine the plan and implement the data collection process identify and prioritize discrepancies, and begin to, analyze potential causes of needs. Potential strategies to address needs are identified. This phase of the needs assessment process is fully described by Altschuld (2010). The final phase of this model is the postassessment phase, during which needs are translated into priorities for action, potential solutions are identified and compared, the needs assessment process is evaluated, and results are communicated. This phase of the needs assessment process is fully described by Altschuld and White (2010). Like the logic model, the three-phase model is a structural and planning tool that does not have

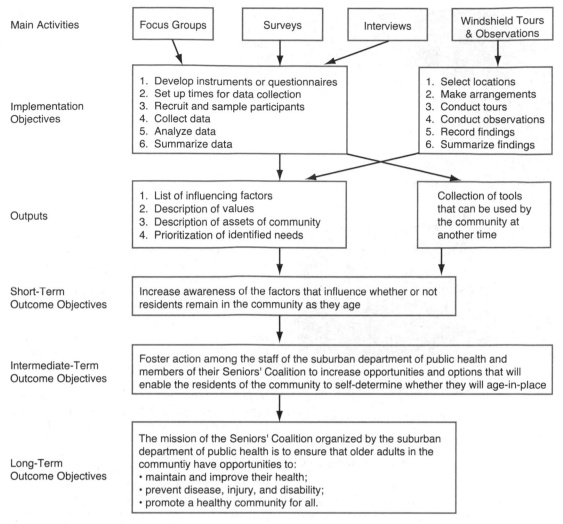

Figure 28.2 Sample logic model.

a clear philosophical or theoretical stance, nor does it identify particular methods of data collection.

Concerns Report Method

In comparison to the logic model and the three-phase model, the **concerns report method** has a clear grounding in theories of empowerment, self-help, and community development (Ludwig-Beymer, Blankemeier, Casas-Byots, & Suarez-Balcazar, 1996; Schriner & Fawcett, 1988). This grounding leads to a participatory action research approach to needs assessments that uses this model. Methodologically, the concerns report method draws on focus groups, survey research, and analytic strategies that originate in discrepancy modeling (Ludwig-Beymer et al., 1996). Through the use of the concerns report method, communities work

with the needs assessment team to identify community strengths as well as issues and concerns. Strengths are then built upon to address the issues and concerns. The basic steps of the concerns report method are as follows:

- Focus groups are conducted to identify community values, concerns, and priorities (Fig. 28.3);
- Findings from the focus groups are used to develop a structured survey in which each item has an importance dimension and a satisfaction dimension;
- The survey is administered to members of the community;
- Data are analyzed;
- Results are shared with the community through public meetings;
- During the public meetings, community members discuss ways to preserve and enhance

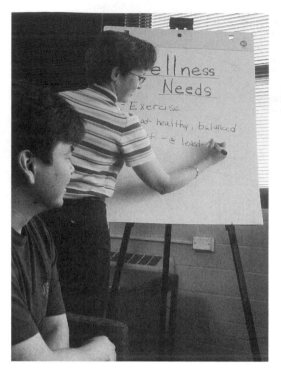

Figure 28.3 Dr. Finlayson conducts a focus group to identify student wellness needs.

community strengths and address issues and concerns;
- Action committees are established; and
- A final report is disseminated throughout the community.

One of the interesting and unique features of the concerns report method is the survey and how the way it is structured produces a prioritization of community needs. The Case Example at the beginning of this chapter provides examples of statements from a concerns report method survey that focused on identifying the issues and concerns of older adults related to food acquisition and preparation. From the results of these surveys, a needs index is calculated for each statement, as follows:

- The proportion of respondents who state that an item is very important is calculated,
- The proportion of respondents who state that they are very satisfied with the item is calculated, and
- Need index = proportion very important—proportion very satisfied.

Through this strategy, the needs assessment team is able to provide the community with a list of issues in order of priority. The range of scores on the need index can range from +100, which indicates a very high need (i.e., the issue is very important

to everyone, but no one is very satisfied), to −100, which indicates a very low need or, alternatively, a community strength (i.e., the issue is very important, yet everyone is very satisfied). A score of zero on this score range indicates that needs are being addressed (i.e., there is a balance).

Participatory and Community-Building Approaches

Both community-building and participatory approaches to needs assessment focus on social change, and they draw from practices of community development and participatory action research. Both approaches are based in critical social theory, and therefore both focus on the critical examination of rules, habits, traditions, and beliefs about an issue and how these factors affect social relationships and structures (Lindsey & McGuinness, 1998; Lindsay, Shields, & Stajduhar, 1999; Wallerstein & Duran, 2003). In both of these approaches to needs assessment, the key is community involvement and community ownership over the entire process.

In **participatory approaches** to needs assessment, the underlying assumption is that knowledge is power, and that knowledge development within a community will lead to social action (Lindsay et al., 1999; Lindsey & McGuinness, 1998; Wallerstein & Duran, 2003). Therefore, participatory approaches to needs assessment link social science to social activism, and they link research, action, and education into a single project. For the purposes of a needs assessment, participatory approaches provide significant theoretical guidance in terms of process. For example, using a participatory approach will require active involvement of the stakeholders in all aspects of the research process and associated decision-making. Developing effective partnerships will be key, and the primary needs assessor will take the role of facilitator and technician. Beyond these theoretical and process guides, taking a participatory approach does not dictate the use of specific methods during the needs assessment process.

In **community-building approaches** to needs assessment, the focus is on the community and on fostering development of a collective to promote social change. Raising critical consciousness and promoting reflection are key to the use of a community-building approach to needs assessment. There are four aspects or components to this model of needs assessment: citizen action, voluntary participation and collaborative problem solving, empowerment, and holistic community-wide outcomes (Wallerstein & Duran, 2003). Like the participatory approach to needs assessment, the community-building approach provides strong theoretical and process guidance, but it does not dictate the use of particular methods.

Advantages and Disadvantages of the Models

Through this review of models and approaches to needs assessment, it should be apparent that this is an area of research that requires further methodological and conceptual clarity. Each of these models and approaches offers advantages and disadvantages, and these are summarized in Table 28.3. Logic models and the three-phase models are really structural and organizational in nature, providing guidance for process but little else. Community-building and participatory approaches provide theoretical guidance and therefore a philosophical stance to guide the needs assessment process. They do not provide guidance for the step-by-step activities of a needs assessment, nor the methods that can and should be used. The concerns report method falls in between these

two extremes. It has a clear structure and a step-by-step process about what activities to complete in which order. It also has a clear theoretical orientation that can guide the process conceptually. Ultimately, mixing and matching these models and approaches may have the greatest utility for a needs assessment team. For example, using the three-phase model together with a community-building approach would provide guidance to a needs assessment team in terms of theory as well as step-by-step activities.

Common Data Collection Methods for Needs Assessment

Up to this point in the chapter, variability in needs assessments and how they are designed has been the message. Yet, one factor that high-quality needs assessments have in common is that multiple and mixed methods are used to collect the data simply because of the multi-dimensional aspects of need. It is this feature of needs assessment—multiple and mixed methods—that make this form of applied research unique as well as exciting and

Table 28.3 Advantages and Disadvantages of the Different Models and Approaches to Needs Assessment

	Advantages of Using This Model	Disadvantages of Using This Model
Logic model	• Tool that can assist with planning • Promotes communication among stakeholders • Keeps the project focused on the long-term outcome	• Provides no theoretical guidance • Provides no guidance about methods
Three-phase model	• Clearly defined, step-by-step process • Good for novices who need checklist formats to guide them through the needs assessment process • Emphasizes use of a needs assessment advisory committee	• Provides no theoretical guidance • Provides no guidance about methods
Concerns report method	• Clearly defined, step-by-step process • Clearly defined guiding theory • Clearly defined methods • Role of community explicit	• May be time and resource intensive, depending on the community
Participatory approach	• Clearly defined guiding theory • Role of community explicit • Community controls process • Involving community members in the research process increases the likelihood of ownership over findings	• Time and resource intensive • Provides no guidance about methods • May require needs assessor to train community members in research processes
Community building approach	• Clearly defined guiding theory • Role of community explicit • Community controls process • Typically involves multiple constituencies (e.g., business, social services, government, etc.)	• Time and resource intensive • Provides no guidance about methods • Involvement of multiple constituencies is likely to require specialized and experienced facilitators to negotiate multiple viewpoints.

challenging. Using multiple methods means that the research team often must be larger and more diverse to ensure that adequate expertise is available for designing and analyzing the data from each method. It also means that preparing the findings and making recommendations may become more complicated, particularly when trying to integrate qualitative and quantitative data and data from different methods that may contradict each other. These challenges can often be overcome by revisiting the stakeholders, refocusing on the values of the community, and being clear about the scope and purpose of what is and can be addressed.

Table 28.4 summarizes the most commonly used methods in needs assessments, as well as their advantages and disadvantages. Because many of these methods are discussed in other chapters in this book, they are not discussed here. Instead, Table 28.4 provides a cross-reference to other chapters that address the method. In addition, references are provided at the end of the chapter for readers who wish to learn more about the particular methods described in the table.

Preparing Needs Assessment Findings, Developing Recommendations, and Taking Action

Previously in this chapter, needs assessment was described as both applied research and a political

process. Although early needs assessments were often simply a list of problems, needs assessments have evolved (Reviere et al., 1996). Needs assessors have a responsibility to translate their findings into recommendations that the community can consider for action. Typically, recommendations to address the identified needs fall into one of three categories (Carter, 1996):

• Development of a new policy or program;
• Modification of an existing policy or program; or
• Modification to the delivery processes of an existing program or policy (e.g., eligibility criteria, staffing, funding, etc.).

To prepare recommendations that a community can use, it is critical that the needs assessor understands his or her audience. This understanding includes issues such as what audience members want to know, what they value and think is important, what they have the ability to change/influence, and how they prefer to acquire information. Needs assessors who engage the community members in their work should be able to develop a strong sense of the audience for the needs assessment findings and recommendations. Developing recommendations that can be used by the community can be facilitated in a number of ways, as explained in the next section.

Developing Recommendations

First, the needs assessor can draft and share findings as the needs assessment is being conducted

Table 28.4 Commonly Used Methods in Needs Assessments

	Advantages	Disadvantages	Chapters in Which Method Is Discussed
Self-administered surveys (mail or in-person)	• Can be longer (people can be interrupted and return later) • Nonthreatening for sensitive information • Don't have to hire or train interviewers • Potential for broader coverage of population • Medium length of data collection period	• Low response rates generally, particularly for mail-outs • Biased against people with low literacy levels or visual impairments • Usually have to do a lot of data cleaning and editing • Don't know who really filled out survey • Questions must be simple (e.g., generally avoid skip patterns).	27
Interviewer-administered surveys (telephone or face to face)	• Consistent data across all subjects • Enables statistical analysis • Relatively quick method, generally speaking	• Must train interviewers extensively for good reliability • Don't get participant's own words • Choices may not fit participant's experiences.	17, 27

Table 28.4 Commonly Used Methods in Needs Assessments—cont'd

	Advantages	Disadvantages	Chapters in Which Method Is Discussed
Semistructured and open-ended interviews (including key-informant interviews)	• Good when the researcher knows little about the topic • Allows the researcher to obtain "natural wording" • Provides the participant with the opportunity for self-expression • Enables the researcher to identify relevant variables from the participant's perspective	• The quality of data is dependent on the quality of the interviewer. • Interviewer ability to listen and probe • Interviewer ability to guide the discussion without controlling it • Interviewer ability to cover all topics • Sensitive topics are difficult to address, risk of obtaining socially acceptable responses only. • Time consuming • Challenging to analyze	17
Focus groups	• Provide data from a group of people more quickly and less expensively than one-on-one interviews • The researcher can directly interact with participants. • Allow for clarification, follow-up questions, and nonverbal cues • Obtain respondents' own words • Allow respondents to react and build on the responses of other people • Can be used with children • Can be used with people with low literacy levels	• Need to think carefully about sampling and focus-group member mix • Responses of participants are not independent of one another. • Results can be biased by a dominant or opinionated member. • Summarization of results can be challenging if the group members have very divergent opinions. • Moderator can bias results.	17
Nominal group technique	• Focuses on identifying priorities quickly • Accommodates stakeholders with different levels of power in the same group • Good for setting priorities for action	• Not a brainstorming technique, so issues become very focused very quickly. • Must get participants together	28
Secondary data (e.g., administrative records, census figures, social indicators)	• Provides a broader perspective and larger sample sizes • Can provide contextual information that other methods cannot • Good for determining the size and scope of a problem	• Often requires sophisticated statistical knowledge • Access can sometimes be problematic (e.g., Health Insurance Portability and Accountability Act [HIPAA], cost to buy data). • The quality of findings is dependent on the quality of the original data collection procedures.	17
Observation, including windshield tours	• See community in its natural form • Permits descriptions of people, behaviors, settings, and person–environment fit • Can be qualitative or quantitative • Can accommodate different levels of participation	• Requires good training and data management • Analysis can be challenging. • Researchers who are external to the environment may have inadequate knowledge to interpret observations accurately.	17

and seek feedback and interpretation from key stakeholders as the project proceeds. Taking this action has a number of benefits. First, it provides these individuals with the opportunity to become familiar with the findings and begin to think about possible solutions to the issues being addressed. It may make it easier for some individuals and organizations to be open to radical changes if they have an opportunity to contemplate the findings well before the final report is disseminated.

Engaging stakeholders in the process of determining priorities for action can also facilitate the development of recommendations. Most needs assessments uncover more problems and concerns than can be reasonably addressed. Therefore, setting priorities for action is critical. Many strategies can be used to set priorities, for example, simple rank ordering based on the frequency with which a need was identified during the data collection process (e.g., results of a concerns report survey) [Altschuld & White, 2010]).

Two criteria for setting priorities have been defined in the needs assessment literature: importance and feasibility. The importance of a need can be considered in a number of ways, as outlined by Witkin and Altschuld (1995). Important needs are ones that:

- Are experienced by greater numbers of people;
- If addressed, would contribute to the mission and goals of the community;
- Are immediate in nature, and cannot be resolved by time; and
- If resolved, would have additional benefits in other areas.

Feasibility concerns the extent to which addressing the identified needs is possible. Factors that play a role in feasibility include current knowledge, the availability of human and financial resources, and the commitment of the stakeholders to make changes to their operations (e.g., change policies, develop programs, change resource allocations). For occupational therapists, evidence-based practice plays a large role in determining feasibility—what evidence exists that the needs can be addressed effectively?

To evaluate the importance and feasibility of a list of needs identified through the needs assessment data collection, one can use the Q-sort methodology or other methods to rank order items (Chinnis, Paulson, & Davis, 2001; McKeown & Thomas, 2013). Ultimately, the goal is to identify and address the needs that are both high in importance and highly feasible. For these needs, one then moves to consider potential solutions. As already noted, recommending solutions to the identified needs may take the form of suggesting modifications to existing programs or policies or the development of new ones.

The key to these final steps of the needs assessment process is to engage community members and listen to what they value. It is also critical to be open to a range of possible solutions and to work with the community to explore what might be possible. Various brainstorming techniques, such as town hall meetings and the nominal group technique (Delbecq, Van deVen & Gustafson, 1986), can be used to facilitate the discussion of possible solutions. Town hall meetings in particular are useful for obtaining commitment from stakeholders to take action on the findings of the project and to engage community members in the process of enacting solutions.

Summary

The objectives of this chapter were to provide a theoretical overview of the concept of need, examine the processes and dimensions of a needs assessment, describe and compare models and approaches to needs assessment, evaluate methods commonly used in needs assessments, and outline how needs can be translated into actions for solutions. The foundation presented here, in addition to some extra reading on methods, should give readers a better and stronger understanding of the needs assessment process and its importance in occupational therapy research and practice. To close this chapter and summarize its important points, here is a list of proposed criteria for a good-quality needs assessment:

- Develop a clear conceptualization of need, focusing on the underlying issue rather than the potential solution.
- Ground the needs assessment in a clear philosophical and theoretical stance.
- Actively involve stakeholders.
- Design a rigorous project.
- Use multiple data collection methods.
- Make recommendations based on empirical evidence.
- Ensure that plans are put in place to address the needs that are uncovered.

Review Questions

1. What are two contrasting examples of how needs assessments vary in rigor and approach?
2. What are three ideological perspectives by which client need may be defined in occupational therapy?

3. What social and political variables must be considered when deciding upon an approach to needs assessment?
4. What are some of the common data collection approaches in needs assessment research?
5. What are five of the most widely used approaches to conducting a needs assessment?

REFERENCES

Altschuld, J. W. (2010). *Needs assessment: Phase II, collecting data*. Needs Assessment Kit 3. Thousand Oaks, CA: SAGE.

Altschuld, J. W., & Eastmond, J. N. (2010). *Needs assessment: Phase I, getting started*. Needs Assessment Kit 2. Thousand Oaks, CA: SAGE.

Altschuld, J. W., & Kumar, D. D. (2010). *Needs assessment: An overview*. Thousand Oaks, CA: Sage.

Altschuld, J. W., & White, J. L. (2010). *Needs assessment: Analysis and prioritization*. Needs Assessment Kit 5. Thousand Oaks, CA: SAGE.

Altschuld, J. W., & Witkin, B. R. (1999). Setting needs-based priorities. In J. W. Altschuld & B. R. Witkin, *From needs assessment to action: Transforming needs into solution strategies* (pp. 99–132). Thousand Oaks, CA: Sage.

Bradshaw, J. L. (1972). A taxonomy of social need. In G. McLachlan (Ed.), *Problems and progress in medical care: Essays on current research* (pp. 71–82). London, England: Oxford University Press.

Carter, C. (1996). Using and communicating findings. In R. Reviere, S. Berkowitz, C. C. Carter, & C. G. Ferguson (Eds.), *Needs assessment: A creative and practical guide for social scientists* (pp. 185–201). Washington, DC: Taylor & Francis.

Chinnis, A. S., Paulson, D. J., & Davis, S. M. (2001). Using Q methodology to assess the needs of emergency medicine support staff employees. *Journal of Emergency Medicine, 20*(2), 197–203.

Delbecq, A. L., Van deVen, A. H., & Gustafson, D. H. (1986). *Group techniques for program planning: A guide to nominal group and Delphi processes*. Middleton, WI: Green Briar Press.

Dill, A. (1983). Defining needs, defining systems: A critical analysis. *The Gerontologist, 33*(4), 453–460.

Doyal, L., & Gough, I. (1991). *A theory of human need*. New York, NY: Guilford Press.

Green, L. W., & Mercer, S. L. (2001). Can public health researchers and agencies reconcile the push from funding bodies and the pull from communities? *American Journal of Public Health, 91*(12), 1926–1929.

Kretzmann, J., & McKnight, J. (1993). *Building communities from the inside out: A path toward finding and mobilizing a community's assets*. Chicago, IL: ACTA Publications.

Lindsey, E., & McGuinness, L. (1998). Significant elements of community involvement in participatory action research: Evidence from a community project. *Journal of Advanced Nursing, 28*(5), 1106–1114.

Lindsey, E., Shields, L., & Stajduhar, K. (1999). Creating effective nursing partnerships: Relating community development to participatory action research. *Journal of Advanced Nursing, 29*(5), 1238–1245.

Ludwig-Beymer, P., Blankemeier, J. R., Casas-Byots, C., & Suarez-Balcazar, Y. (1996). Community assessment in a suburban Hispanic community: A description of method. *Journal of Transcultural Nursing, 8*(1), 19–27.

Martí-Costa, S., & Serrano-García, I. (1983). Needs assessment and community development: An ideological perspective. *Prevention in Human Services, 2*(4), 75–88.

Maslow, A. H. (1954). *Motivation and personality*. New York, NY: Harper & Row.

McKeown, B., & Thomas, D. (2013). *Q methodology* (2nd ed.). Thousand Oaks, CA: Sage.

Minkler, M. (Ed.). (2012). *Community organizing and community building for health*. New Brunswick, NJ: Rutgers University Press.

Reason, P., & Bradbury-Huang, H. (Eds.). (2013). *The Sage handbook of action research: Participatory inquiry and practice* (2nd ed). Thousand Oaks, CA: Sage.

Reviere, R., Berkowitz, S., Carter, C. C., & Ferguson, C. G. (1996). *Needs assessment: A creative and practical guide for social scientists*. Washington, DC: Taylor & Francis.

Rush, B., & Ogborne, A. (1991). Program logic models: Expanding their role and structure for program planning and evaluation. *The Canadian Journal of Program Evaluation, 6*(2), 95–106.

Schriner, K. F., & Fawcett, S. B. (1988). Development and validation of the community concerns report method. *Journal of Community Psychology, 16,* 306–316.

Shi, L., & Singh, D.A. (2014). *Delivering health care in America: A systems approach* (6th ed.), Sudbury, MA: Jones & Bartlett.

Thomson, G. (1987). *Needs*. London, England: Routledge & Kegan Paul.

Wallerstein, N., & Duran, B. (2003). The conceptual, historical and practice roots of community based participatory research and related participatory traditions. In M. Minkler & N. Wallerstein (Eds.), *Community based participatory research for health* (pp. 27–52). San Francisco, CA: Jossey Bass.

Weiss, C. H. (1972). *Evaluation research: Methods for assessing program effectiveness*. Englewood Cliffs, NJ: Prentice-Hall, Inc.

Witkin, B. R., & Altschuld, J. W. (1995). *Planning and conducting needs assessments: A practical guide*. Thousand Oaks, CA: Sage.

RESOURCES

Fowler, F. J., Jr. (2013). *Survey research methods* (5th ed.). Thousand Oaks, CA: Sage.

Gilmore, G. D. (2011). *Needs and capacity assessment strategies for health education and health promotion* (4th ed.). Mississagua, Canada: Jones and Bartlett.

Gubrium, J. F., Holstein, J. A., Marvasti, A. B., & McKinney, K. D. (Eds.). (2012). *The SAGE handbook of interview research: The complexity of the craft.* Thousand Oaks, CA: Sage.

Krueger, R. A., & Casey, M. A. (2014). *Focus groups: A practical guide for applied research* (5th ed.). Thousand Oaks, CA: Sage.

Work Group for Community Health and Development. (2007). Assessing community needs and resources. Community Tool Box. Univ. of Kansas. Retrieved from http://ctb.ku.edu/en/table-of-contents

CHAPTER 29

Program Evaluation Research

Brent Braveman • Yolanda Suarez-Balcazar • Gary Kielhofner • Renée R. Taylor

Learning Outcomes

■ Understand the range of activities that comprise program evaluation.

■ Discuss the necessary steps in program development.

■ Apply the theoretical concept of the scholarship of practice to research in program evaluation.

■ Differentiate formative from summative evaluation.

■ List commonly utilized research designs and approaches used in program evaluation.

Introduction

Program evaluation defines a range of systematic approaches to using data to answer important process- and outcomes-related questions about occupational therapy (OT) services and programs. Historically, program evaluation emerged as a means of assessing the impact of programs, examining if programs are implemented as planned, assessing the intended (and unintended) processes and outcomes of community-based programs, and addressing social problems. Private and public granting agencies, insurance providers, and other health-care funding networks prioritize the need for data concerning the quality, extent, and nature of programmatic outcomes.

This chapter explores the integration between research and the development and evaluation of OT programs. Examples are presented throughout this chapter to illustrate this integration and to highlight the relationship between the research methodologies presented in this book, evidence based on research, and the processes of developing and evaluating programs of service.

The Relationship Between Program Development and Program Evaluation

Program development defines the systematic design, planning, and implementation of new services, innovations, or initiatives. It may range from relatively simple ventures such as implementing a standard approach to care in a given setting to complex endeavors such as creating interventions for populations facing new conditions and significant challenges. For example, program development occurs when the administrator of a rehabilitation center decides to develop and introduce a new approach (e.g., sensory integration) into an existing program of OT pediatric services. Another example of program development would include an occupational therapist who collaborates with a local YWCA to design services for women and children who have self-identified as being survivors of domestic violence.

Regardless of the level of complexity, the integration of research methods into the program development process can foster success. Integrating research methods into program development may:

• Provide formative data that shape what services are provided and how they are delivered;
• Increase the likelihood that services will be used, sustained over time, and designed to meet the needs of participants; and
• Provide evidence of the assumptions that support the program components.

Program evaluation is a process that documents the impact of a newly developed or existing intervention or program of services. Impact can be assessed using outcome data (indicators of change). Similar to program development, approaches to program evaluation range in complexity. They may involve evaluation of a single aspect of an intervention or program with a limited number of clients or evaluation of multiple related interventions with a large population in order to establish their effectiveness.

In some circumstances, program development and program evaluation are taken on as separate activities in isolation of one another. For example, this might occur when an evaluation of outcomes is requested of a program of OT services that has been in existence for a long period of time. Other circumstances might call for the development of

CASE EXAMPLE

Dr. Needling serves as associate professor of occupational therapy at a large public research university. The university boasts a central mission of service and outreach to its local community, which consists primarily of agricultural workers. Dr. Needling leads an elective interdisciplinary course within the college titled "Community Practicum." In this course, subgroups of first-year students are assigned to evaluate the services provided to the workers by local community-based organizations. This year, Dr. Needling decides to center the course on a farm workers' health center that provides various basic services, including family planning, prenatal/postpartum care, pediatric care, diagnosis of acute and chronic illnesses, immunizations, home-based rehabilitation, and health education. Yukiko, a student in the course, decides to lead the subgroup focusing on home-based rehabilitation. This is a small unit within the health center consisting of a single occupational therapist and a single physical therapist who provide a range of general physical rehabilitation and neurorehabilitation services to adult and older adult farm workers and their family members.

Yukiko and her classmates decide on an approach to the program evaluation of these services that will be feasible to complete within a single semester and minimally intrusive to the agency (and the occupational therapist) providing the services. Because the rehabilitation program is already in progress, Yukiko decides that there is no need to cover the steps involved in program development, including a needs assessment and program planning. Instead, she decides to begin by gathering an understanding of the overall implementation of the program using formative evaluation. She proceeds by posing the following questions to the therapists:

- How many hours of rehabilitation services are provided on a daily, weekly, monthly, and annual basis?
- How many clients are served on a daily, weekly, monthly, and annual basis?
- What referral problems are being addressed by the service and at what frequency?
- How many of these hours are delivered on site versus at home?
- What are the difficulties encountered by the therapists in providing rehabilitation services (on site, at home, and in general)?
- What facilitators to service provision (on site, at home, and in general) do the therapists report?
- How is feedback concerning service delivery being collected from clients (informally, formally, not at all)?
- What are clients reporting about their experiences with rehabilitation services (informally, formally)?

Because Yukiko and her classmates are only at the clinic for a semester, she does not conduct a summative evaluation to assess service outcomes. However, she does recommend that students in the next class conduct a single-group evaluation design in which return to prior occupation and duration of return to prior occupation are the major outcomes. Yukiko does report the findings of her formative evaluation to the clinic leadership and staff. They are presented in Table 29.1.

---

a new program or intervention. In these cases, program development is often accompanied by **formative evaluation** (ongoing evaluation and refinement of the process of service implementation) and followed by a **summative evaluation** (evaluation of the ultimate outcomes or effectiveness of the program). In this chapter, program development and program evaluation are treated as coexisting along a continuum that includes program development, formative evaluation, and summative evaluation. This approach of undertaking program development and program evaluation simultaneously is widely supported as the

preferred approach by different fields, including the health and social sciences.

A Scholarship of Practice

Regardless of how familiar or complex an intervention is, the process of developing and evaluating a program of service can be made easier if it is guided by sound principles that connect theory and research (both methods and the resulting evidence) to practice. The relationship between theory, research, and practice has been described as a scholarship of practice (Crist & Kielhofner,

Table 29.1 Formative Evaluation Findings

Average Hours of Rehabilitation Service	7/day, 35/week, 105/month, 1,680/year
Average Number of Clients Served	13/day, 65/week, 195/month, 3,120/year
Reasons for Referral	Knee replacement 580 Hip replacement 230 Stroke and other cardio 410 Developmental disability 185 Cancer 670 Mental health and behavioral 1,045
Location of Service Delivery	On site = 701 Home = 971
Difficulties	On site: client attendance; limited space; clinic noise; inflexible hours Home: lack of equipment; distractions; confidentiality; sanitary problems General: client overload; low wages; outdated equipment; technology infrastructure
Facilitators	On site: safety and hygiene; ethical leadership at clinic Home: help of family General: public support for clinic
Feedback From Clients	Collected via a suggestions box at the clinic and through word of mouth • Need more time with therapist • Clinic temperature too cold in winter • Therapists often late to home visits • Therapists who appear tired/overworked

2005; Hammel, Finlayson, Kielhofner, Helfrich, & Peterson, 2002; Kielhofner, 2005).The **scholarship of practice** offers a bidirectional conceptual framework that envisions a process in which theoretical concepts and empirical knowledge resulting from research inform practice, and problems raised by practice inform questions to be addressed through research and further theoretical development. Maintaining a discourse between theory, practice, and research is an ideal framework for program development because programs translate theory into services, and research can guide the process and demonstrate its impact.

For example, Braveman and Kielhofner (2005) describe the use of theory and research evidence to develop OT programming focused on preparing persons living with HIV/AIDS to return to employment in a community-based setting in which occupational therapy previously had not been provided. Similarly, Fisher and Braveman (2005) describe the use of methods commonly used in research, such as interviews and focus groups, to collect and organize data, information, and other forms of evidence to help with the processes of needs assessment, program planning, and program evaluation.

As noted earlier, the range of program development efforts and the resulting need to evaluate services can vary widely in complexity. Although less complex efforts may require less sophisticated evaluation approaches, the amount and usefulness of the resulting evidence are also limited. Naturally, more complex program development efforts require more sophisticated evaluation approaches, and these approaches may result in a greater amount of evidence with broader applications.

In research and in program development and evaluation, there is always a trade-off between the investment of time and effort and the value of the results. Figure 29.1 presents a continuum of research and evaluation approaches and the advantages and disadvantages that come with expending less or more time and effort. The key is to match the approach and level of effort with the desired outcome and the needs of your situation. The left side of the figure represents low-complexity programs, such as the implementation of an established approach to care in a familiar setting with a limited population (e.g., developing a cardiac rehabilitation protocol for a new cardiology program in a general hospital). The right side of the figure represents high-complexity programs, such as a two-site randomized controlled trial that examined the efficacy of an energy-conservation education program for people with multiple sclerosis (Mathiowetz, Finlayson, Matuska, Chen, & Lou, 2005).

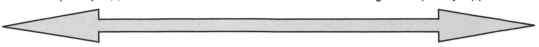

- Few resources needed
  - Lower time investment
  - Lower cost
- Less sophisticated research skills needed

- Considerable resources needed
  - Higher time investment
  - Higher cost
- More sophisticated research skills needed

Low-Complexity Approaches   High-Complexity Approaches

- Low generalizability
- Narrower yield of data
- Greater threat to validity and reliability of results

- High generalizability
- Broader yield of data
- Less threat to validity and reliability of results

Figure 29.1   A continuum of research and evaluation approaches.

Using Research to Guide Program Development

The primary tenets of both evidence-based practice and of a scholarship of practice are that the most effective programs are designed using the best available evidence. Although other forms of evidence, such as the testimony of experts, clinical guidelines provided by professional groups, information from Internet sites, and even one's own clinical experience, are valid and sometimes the only evidence available, the strongest evidence is obtained through the application of sound research strategies, tools, and methodologies. Such strategies, tools, and methodologies are described throughout the other chapters of this book. Although these approaches are used to carry out research to develop or validate the theories that guide programming, many of the same strategies, tools, and methodologies may also be used to collect and synthesize data, information, and other forms of evidence *during* the program development process. In other words, rather than associating a strategy, tool, or methodology just with the generation of knowledge, one should realize that all of these also assist with the application of knowledge.

The Process of Program Development

The process of program development may be conceptualized as a series of four steps, as listed here and shown in Figure 29.2:

1. Needs assessment,
2. Program planning,
3. Program implementation, and
4. Program evaluation. (Calley, 2011).

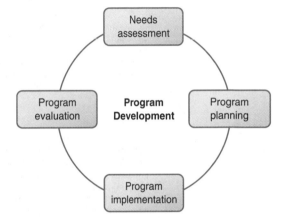

Figure 29.2   The four steps of program development.

Table 29.2 lists each of these four steps across the top of the table. In addition, common research strategies, tools, and methodologies are listed along the left side of the table. Each cell of the table provides an example of how the strategy, tool, or methodology could be applied in the process of developing a new program or service. The strategies, tools, and methods presented in Table 29.2 are not an exhaustive list; rather, they represent a sampling of such approaches. Next, each of the four steps of program development is described in more depth, and additional examples of the use of research strategies, tools, and methodology in the program development process are provided.

Needs Assessment

The first step in developing a program of service is to determine the needs of the target population that the program addresses. **Needs assessment** is a systematic set of procedures undertaken to make

Table 29.2 Sample Applications of Research Strategies, Tools, and Methodologies Within the Steps of Program Development

Research Strategy, Tool, or Methodology	Needs Assessment	Program Planning	Program Implementation	Program Evaluation
Questionnaires and surveys	Identify desires and needs of target populations and customers internal and external to an organization.	Determine customer preferences, validate perception of needs, and gather data to plan for personnel, equipment, and other programmatic needs.	Monitor and improve staff satisfaction, identify opportunities for continuous quality improvement efforts, and facilitate communication with key stakeholders.	Gather information during formative and summative evaluation of customer satisfaction and assessment of outcomes.
Record reviews	Gather demographic data and rates of incidence, prevalence, and service utilization.	Establish baseline benchmarks for productivity and financial monitoring as well as assessment of outcomes.	Determine levels of productivity, determine compliance with accreditation or other standards, and collect trend data to help plan for financial management and budgeting.	Gather necessary data for participation in database benchmarking of customer satisfaction, financial performance, or outcomes.
Interviews or focus groups	Identify needs and desires of stakeholders internal and external to the organization.	Garner support of key stakeholders, identify roadblocks to success, validate the focus of your product or service, and collect information on program competitors.	Plan and conduct human resource functions, including performance appraisal and staff development.	Explore critical incidents to learn about cases in which customer expectations or outcomes were either surpassed or not met.
Observation	Visit existing programs to learn about space needs and space design, work flow, and customer expectations.	Ensure compliance with accreditation and safety standards and gather information to help plan continuous quality improvement and other evaluation systems.	Become more familiar with the challenges and obstacles faced by staff in service delivery and communicate a desire for open communication.	Carry out human resource functions, including assessment of competency or performance appraisal.

decisions about program improvements (Altschuld & Kumar, 2010). As noted in Chapter 28, it is a process of determining what a group of persons, a community, or a population requires in order to achieve some basic standard or to improve their current situation. The needs assessment process can range from simple to complex depending on the characteristics of those who will receive services and the scope of planned services. In more complicated examples, determining the needs of a target population may in fact be the *focus* of

a research effort (Altschuld & Kumar, 2010). In most cases of program development, however, previous research is combined with the results of a needs assessment to guide the choice of conceptual practice models and other elements of an intervention designed to respond to identified needs.

Strategies for needs assessment should be chosen based on ease of use, resources available, and the results they produce. Research strategies and tools such as questionnaires, surveys, or reviews of records may help you obtain specific information about the needs of a target population, such as demographic characteristics and services already utilized. For example, an occupational therapist interested in developing OT services for a client population not yet served (e.g., adults with sensory impairment who reside in an underserved urban neighborhood) might begin by initiating a relatively simple needs assessment. This needs assessment might involve reviewing existing information on the prevalence of individuals with sensory impairment in the neighborhood served by the medical center and information about sensory impairment services offered by other medical centers or community-based organizations within the same neighborhood.

Other situations might require a more systematic approach to needs assessment. For example, once preliminary data are obtained, the same administrator might gain access to the clients with sensory impairment and survey them directly to assess the likelihood that they would use OT services. Such quantitative strategies can assist one to begin to understand how the target population may be similar to or different from previously researched populations. Interviews or focus groups may generate deeper insights on the needs of the target population, such as perceived barriers to accessing services or desired outcomes of services. Qualitative strategies such as focus groups can also be useful. Scholars have also advocated for participatory and mixed-methods methodologies to engage in systematic assessment of community needs (Suarez-Balcazar & Balcazar, 2016).

Program Planning

The same strategies (and sometimes the same tools or assessments) used to assess the needs of a target population can be adapted and used to guide program planning. **Program planning** involves determining the type of service to be provided, enumerating resources needed to provide the services, characterizing the population, and identifying how the services/program will be delivered.

Continuing with the example of using an evidence-based approach to plan a new program of services for adults with sensory impairment, program planning would follow the comprehensive needs assessment described in the preceding section and in Chapter 28. Following the needs assessment, the act of program planning might involve creating a spreadsheet in which the collected information about the needs of the population and the information about other existing services within the community would be analyzed, compared, and discussed. In addition, findings

from a literature review of any existing outcomes research on the efficacy of various approaches to occupational therapy with individuals with various types of sensory impairment would be summarized, added to the spreadsheet, and compared to guide the development of a conceptual model of care.

Many resources are available to help OT practitioners become skilled at finding, evaluating, and integrating evidence into their practice (Braveman, 2005; Law & McDermid, 2013). Questionnaires or surveys may assess how potential users view planned services and the extent to which they intend to use a service if it is offered. Quantitative data gained during these efforts can also help with planning for personnel, equipment, and space needs because they may provide information related to the potential volume and intensity of service utilization.

Qualitative methods, including interviews, focus groups, and observations, can assist with planning a program by uncovering potential roadblocks to the program's success. Such strategies may also be useful in learning information about existing services or competitors and why members of your target population might choose to use your service rather than another option. As one approaches the step of program implementation, these strategies also assist with planning management and human resource functions such as systems for continuous quality improvement, the assessment of competencies, and the development of job descriptions.

A tool that is often used in program planning is the logic model (Frechtling, 2007). A logic model is a tool that describes the program components specifying what needs to be measured and why. A logic model can be utilized for the purpose of program planning (see page 421 for a description of the logic model).

Program Implementation

Program implementation involves the actual delivery of the program or services. Data collection is used during program implementation to document when the service was provided, how many hours of service were provided, who provided the service, what type of service was provided, and how many clients were served.

Maintaining an activity log will help the occupational therapist generate a record of program implementation. Both quantitative and qualitative approaches can be used to collect and analyze data, information, and other forms of evidence from various sources for ongoing program evaluation. The output of these efforts may be used for functions such as monitoring and improving customer and staff satisfaction, planning and conducting human resource functions such as performance appraisals and staff development, or in continuous quality improvement efforts.

Unfortunately, once program implementation begins, the evidence-based strategies used in program planning often lapse. However, the relationship between research and the development, implementation, and evaluation of programs of service should be both reciprocal and continuous. Practitioners should continuously raise questions that may be answered by researchers. Researchers should continuously provide new evidence that should be evaluated by practitioners to improve programs of service. To enable this process of continuous relationship between scholarship and practice, ongoing, systematic, and consistent record keeping and data collection is critical.

Program Evaluation

The fourth step of the program development process is program evaluation. Although this step is listed last, program evaluation is actually a continuous process that is integrated throughout the planning and implementation of a program of service. In this section, the different types of program evaluation, the different methodological strategies used to evaluate OT interventions, and a framework that includes practical steps to conduct program evaluation are introduced.

Program evaluation is the use of tools, methods, and skills to determine whether a human service or program is meeting the needs of participants, if the program is offered as planned, and if it is having the desired impact on the lives of participants (Posavac, 2011; Stufflebeam, 2001). Program evaluation implies a process that contributes to the provision of quality services (Posavac, 2011) and to decisions about improving a program or intervention (Fawcett et al., 1996; Suarez-Balcazar & Harper, 2003).

The need for program evaluation has grown quite rapidly during the last 20 years (Fetterman, Kaftarian, & Wandersman, 2015). The demand for community-based services has come with an increased demand from funders of agencies and organizations to conduct evaluations of their interventions and programs, especially in times of budget cuts. Philanthropic entities as well as private and public sources of funding are requesting program evaluations. It is now a common practice among funding agencies to make financial support of community programs and services contingent on evaluation of such initiatives. Program

evaluation provides information about human services and interventions in ways that such information can be used to improve services, policies, or practices (Posavac, 2011).

Human services staff and professionals deem the evaluation of their initiatives to be both a necessity and a challenge (Connell & Kubisch, 1998; Suarez-Balcazar, Taylor-Ritzler, & Morales-Curtin, 2015). Finding the appropriate measurement tools and specifying the right indicators can be challenging (Flora & Grosso, 1999; Suarez-Balcazar, Orellana-Damacela, Portillo, Sharma, & Lanum, 2003). Nevertheless, professionals are now under pressure to engage in practice supported by evidence.

Program evaluation supports evidence-based practice. By documenting the impact of IT interventions, practitioners will be engaging in practice supported by evidence. Evaluation theory is rooted in outcomes-based evidence models, which have gained much attention in OT literature and have major implications for research and practice (Calley, 2011).

Strategies for Program Evaluation

Program evaluation is comprised of two central components: formative evaluation and summative evaluation. Briefly, formative evaluation comprises an assessment of the process of implementing a program, and summative evaluation represents an assessment of program outcomes. Scientific research strategies must be used to assess the outcomes of any evaluation, and so formal research designs and methodologies are generally employed during the stage of summative evaluation.

Formative Evaluation

Formative evaluation occurs during the initial steps of planning and implementing a program and reports process information. It is used to assess the extent to which actual programming matches that which was planned and the extent to which programming and services address the identified needs of the target population. Formative evaluation often focuses on the process of documenting the delivering of services. The evaluation of process is designed to examine how a program or intervention is being implemented; it helps verify program implementation (Rossi, Lipsey, & Freeman, 2004). Therefore, by using process information, the evaluation can improve not only the plan for services but also the implementation and delivery of programs. When information is gathered to document the implementation and delivery of a program, the purpose of the evaluation is then formative evaluation.

More specifically, formative evaluation, or the evaluation of process, answers questions about the program such as, *Is the program or intervention being implemented as planned?* For instance, an OT intervention designed to teach self-advocacy skills to family members of children with disabilities may ask the following questions to respond to process evaluation: Do the parents' needs for advocacy training match what they are being taught? How is the intervention being implemented? How many parents have been trained? What specific advocacy training strategies and topics are being covered? Is the training going as planned?

Keeping detailed records of program implementation allows for the documentation of process. Often the information collected is reported in terms of outputs about program descriptors, such as the following:

- How many training sessions were implemented?
- How many parents were trained?
- What do parents say about the program?

Monitoring the implementation of a program is also a part of formative evaluation. This is the most common practice in terms of evaluation. For the most part, all human services document their programs by maintaining records of the services they provide and participants served. In fact, before conducting an outcomes evaluation, monitoring the program allows for an actual record of the program itself and of the population being served.

Another example of formative evaluation involves conducting weekly staff meetings to determine whether a given program of services is being delivered as it was originally designed and intended. Meetings might determine whether the intended content of services is being delivered, whether services are being delivered at the anticipated rate, whether the anticipated numbers of clients are utilizing the services, and how staff are experiencing the process of service delivery. Asking clients to complete weekly feedback forms that reflect how they are experiencing the OT services offered is another example of a type of formative evaluation. One uses process information to report on a formative evaluation.

Summative Evaluation

Summative evaluation is also an ongoing process but typically focuses on the outcomes or effectiveness of service delivery. Summative evaluation provides information about the extent to which a program achieves the objectives for which it was developed. As with the other steps described, both quantitative and qualitative data and information may be gathered using strategies, tools, or methodologies that match the evaluation question and the resources available for evaluation. One example of a summative evaluation involves collecting data from clients with hand injuries on functional outcomes following a course of therapy.

Evaluation of outcomes documents the impact the program or intervention is having on participants' attitudes, knowledge, skills, abilities/competencies, and/or conditions. The data collected through summative evaluation should help assess the merit of a program or select among interventions.

Outcome evaluation answers questions such as the following:

- Which intervention is most effective in producing changes in participants' skills (when comparing more than one intervention)?
- Did the attitudes of participants change as a result of the program?
- Did participants' behaviors or skills/competencies change as a result of the intervention?
- Did participants' knowledge change as a result of the intervention?
- Which intervention produced the most impact on participants?
- Did participants' conditions change as a result of the intervention?

Researchers have also classified outcomes in terms of short-term outcomes, intermediate outcomes, and long-term outcomes (Frechtling, 2007). Short-term outcomes are changes in participants' knowledge and/or attitudes, intermediate outcomes are changes in participants' behavior, and long-term outcomes are changes in participants' skills/competencies and/or condition. For instance, an OT intervention designed to increase the job-related skills and employment status of individuals with disabilities may document the following:

- Short-term outcomes: Did participants' knowledge of employment resources change as a function of the training?
- Intermediate outcomes: Did participants' job-seeking skills (e.g., writing a resume, preparing for an interview) change as a function of the intervention?
- Long-term outcomes: How many participants found jobs and maintained them at 3 months, 6 months, and 12 months after training?

To evaluate the impact of an intervention, researchers need to rely on scientific methods of inquiry. The next section provides an overview of research methods used in evaluation, from the least sophisticated design to the most sophisticated design.

Scientific Research Strategies in Program Evaluation

The type of strategy used to assess the outcome of an intervention and the success of the program depends on many factors, including the evaluation information needs of different stakeholders; the resources available for the evaluation, timeline, and deadlines imposed by stakeholders; the type of program being evaluated; and the timing of the evaluation. The evaluation of outcomes may go from the least sophisticated design, such as a single-group evaluation design, to the most complex, such as an experimental group evaluation design.

This section briefly overviews designs that can be used for program evaluation. Table 29.3 displays a summary of the characteristics and advantages and disadvantages of each of the designs and methodological strategies available for evaluating OT programs and interventions.

Single-Group Evaluation Design

According to Posavac (2010), the simplest form of summative evaluation is the **single-group design,** which includes one observation after the intervention has taken place. For instance, in the example of a job training program for people with disabilities, the single-group evaluation design may answer the following question: How many individuals with disabilities who completed training are employed at 6 months after training? Or in the example of family members learning advocacy skills, outcome evaluation may answer the following question: How many individuals acquire advocacy skills?

Although this design might be an easy way for human service professionals to evaluate the program, it does not answer the questions of whether participants' knowledge or skill would have changed if no intervention was provided. Also, the degree of change cannot be assessed because of the lack of a premeasure or baseline.

Pretest–Posttest Design

The **pretest-posttest design** implies an observation before and after the intervention has taken

place. This design will help answer the question of whether participants improved or changed while receiving the intervention. For instance, in the example of an advocacy skills training program for families of children with disabilities, the occupational therapist could assess the level of advocacy skills and knowledge of disability rights using a validated instrument before and after training. Posavac (2011) advises that when there are clear standards for the outcome of a human service program and no participants drop out of the program, the pretest–posttest design is an alternative that is inexpensive and simple, and it might provide enough information for human service staff.

Quasi-Experimental Approaches to Evaluation

Quasi-experimental designs, according to Posavac (2011), lend insight into the following questions:

- Does the cause precede the effect?
- Does the cause covary with the effect?

These designs also allow alternative explanations of the observed effects to be ruled out. Within quasi-experimental designs, one might use a time-series design in which data are collected several times across a period of time. This design allows for control of some alterative explanations for the observed effects, such as maturation (Campbell & Stanley, 1963). Another potential design is the **nonequivalent control-group design.** In this design, more than one comparable group is observed, at least one of which does not receive the intervention. Another possibility is to combine designs such as the time-series and the nonequivalent control design.

Qualitative Strategies in Program Evaluation

Evaluators often rely on the use of qualitative research strategies as a complement or an alternative to quantitative methods. **Qualitative research methods** may be the most appropriate program evaluation methods when:

- The program has complex and multifaceted goals,
- The program uses empowerment and/or participatory strategies,
- There is a strong need to be culturally sensitive to participants, and
- There may be different desires or conflicts of interest that exist among key stakeholders. (Posavac, 2011; Suarez-Balcazar et al., 2003)

Table 29.3 Program Evaluation Designs: From the Least Sophisticated to the Most Sophisticated

Design	Characteristics	Advantages	Disadvantages
Qualitative strategies	Examples: Focus groups, interviews, public forums, participant observation	• Rich narrative information from the perspective of participants based on their personal experience • Help to understand the intervention • Help to interpret quantitative data • Culturally sensitive to some populations	• Difficult to identify outcome indicators • Difficult to generalize to other similar populations • Difficult to establish cause–effect relationships
Post-measure design only	One systematic observation/assessment after the intervention	• Simplest form of evaluation • Useful to follow up on simple, discrete behaviors (e.g., how many people have jobs after 6 months of completing training)	• Does not show change over time • Difficult to generalize to other similar populations (threats to external validity) • Difficult to establish cause–effect relationships (threats to internal validity)
Pre–post measure	Observation/assessment both before and after the intervention	• Simple form of evaluation, appropriate for simple, inexpensive, and standard interventions • Identifies change over time	• Difficult to generalize to other similar populations (threats to external validity) • Difficult to establish cause–effect relationships (threats to internal validity)
Quasi-experimental designs Time series Nonequivalent comparison group	Collection of data across several time intervals on a single unit of behavior. Comparison of two groups that have not been selected randomly and are nonequivalent but somehow similar	• Controls for some internal validity threats (maturation) • Used by behavior analysts • Allows for comparing the target group with a nontreated control group	• Not appropriate for complex behaviors • Groups are nonequivalent, which threatens external validity.
Experimental design	Participants selected randomly and assigned to control and experimental group	• Allows for cause–effect relationships • Control for treats to internal and external validity	• Is expensive and complex • Random assignment to groups not as feasible in applied settings

Qualitative strategies include observational methods, such as participant observation and direct observation, and other strategies, such as interviews with key stakeholders, focus groups, and public forums. Qualitative strategies, for the most part, provide rich narrative information from the perspective of those who experience the program or intervention. Program evaluators recommend combining strategies, qualitative and quantitative, and using multiple informants. Different stakeholders (e.g., participants, significant others, and program staff) can provide useful and relevant information about a program.

Planning and Conducting an Evaluation

A framework for conducting a program evaluation includes the following four phases:

1. Planning the evaluation,
2. Developing a program logic model,
3. Selecting the methodology and data collection procedures, and
4. Reporting and utilizing research findings (Suarez-Balcazar et al., 2003).

See Figure 29.3 for the phases of an evaluation.

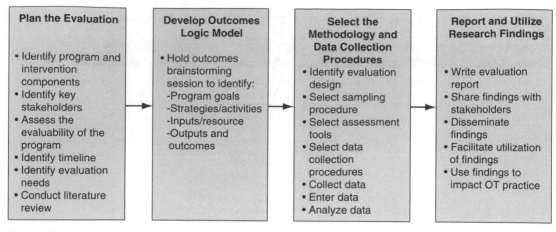

Figure 29.3   Program evaluation phases.

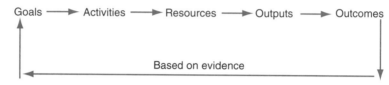

Figure 29.4   Development of a logic model.

Phase I: Planning the Evaluation

The planning of the evaluation should begin at the same time that the program is being developed and planned. This is critical because the use of some evaluation designs requires collecting information about participants and about the program at the onset of the program. During this phase, the evaluation team needs to clarify the following:

- The program/intervention to be evaluated,
- Stakeholders who need to be involved,
- Information needs of different stakeholders,
- Timeline for the evaluation, and
- Resources needed.

It is also important to discuss roles and expectations and to identify evaluation questions of interest to different stakeholders as well as how the data gathered are going to be utilized.

Phase II: Developing an Outcomes Logic Model

A program logic model is a visual representation of the link between program goals, inputs, activities, outputs, outcomes, and impact (Frechtling,

2007). A program logic model is usually developed in an outcomes brainstorming session that fosters critical thinking and self-determination about the program or service (Fetterman, Kaftarian, & Wandersman, 2015; Garcia-Iriarte, Suarez-Balcazar, & Taylor-Ritzler, 2011).

A number of outcome models, also referred to as program logic models, have been proposed in the evaluation of human service programs and interventions. Among these frameworks are the following: the Milstein and Chapel (2015) model of change; the Linney and Wandersman (1996) prevention plus model; and the Connell and Kubisch (1998) and Weiss (1995) theory-of-change approach.

A number of current outcomes models highlight the connection between program goals, inputs, activities, outputs, and outcomes. Within these models, program goals are specific statements of who the target population is and what the program is intended to achieve; inputs are defined as program resources and context. Activities and outputs include the program components and strategies that take place, whereas outcome evaluation involves measuring changes in participants' knowledge, skills and behaviors, and/or attitudes, or changes in community conditions (Fig. 29.4).

Phase III: Selecting the Methodology and Data Collection Procedures

During the third phase, the evaluation design that is most suitable to the problem and intervention being evaluated must be selected. In addition, important decisions about sampling, assessment tools, and methods to measure relevant outcome indicators need to be considered. These important decisions are followed by data collection and data analysis. Most commonly, the sampling, assessment tools, and data collection strategies depend on the design selected. In this decision-making process, one needs to keep in mind what is feasible, measurable, realistic, objective, and reliable.

Evaluation experts have called for the use of multiple levels of analysis and multiple measures in the evaluation of human services. Those supporting a more participatory and empowering approach to evaluation have also recommended using both qualitative and quantitative strategies (Fetterman et al., 2015; Suarez-Balcazar et al., 2015) and that the unit of analysis include the individual and community conditions (Hollister & Hill, 1995).

The selection of a methodology is dependent on the program to be evaluated and the population being served. It is critical that tools and methods selected be culturally sensitive to the population of interest (Marín, 1993). For instance, researchers have asserted that ethnic minority individuals— African Americans and Hispanics—are more likely to respond to one-on-one interviews and focus groups than to mail surveys (Suarez-Balcazar et al., 2003). Similar strategies have been reported as successful ways to collect information from people with disabilities.

Phase IV: Reporting and Utilizing Research Findings

During this phase, a report needs to be produced based on the data analysis conducted. Once an evaluation report is developed, the findings are disseminated among different stakeholders. The findings must be interpreted carefully because decisions are likely to be made based on the evaluation findings. The use of an experimental design calls for stronger recommendations, however, whereas a nonexperimental design may yield weak results about key outcome indicators. Qualitative methods may yield interesting and rich subjective comments from participants about the program.

Kloos, Hill, Thomas, Wandersman, and Elias (2011) consider effective communication of findings imperative, given the potential impact of the findings on community members and agencies' subsequent actions in their communities. However, working together with agency staff, other health professionals, and diverse stakeholders in interpreting and reporting findings can minimize the challenges (Harper & Salina, 2000).

Maximizing the use of evaluation information is a crucial component of any evaluation effort. Currently, there is an emphasis in the evaluation field on assessing the impact of the evaluation process on the agencies (Royce, Thyer, & Padgett, 2016). This is a reaction to the fact that evaluation results have sometimes been ignored by stakeholders (Royce et al., 2016). Several authors have reported that participatory and empowerment approaches to evaluation increase the likelihood of the stakeholders using the information generated by the evaluation (Fetterman, Kaftarian, & Wandersman, 2015). This increase occurs due to:
- A sense of ownership of the evaluation,
- Credibility and trust in the process, and
- Increase in capacity to engage in evaluation-related activities and a more thorough cognitive processing of the information (Suarez-Balcazar, et al., 2015; Wandersman et al., 2004).

Utilization should be a focus of the evaluation throughout the entire process. At the beginning of the evaluation process, all stakeholders invested in the evaluation should be asked to consider ways in which they would use the evaluation information. During the planning and data collection phase, stakeholders should be included in the decision-making process and should be kept informed of the preliminary information to ensure utilization. Evaluation utilization should be prompted through a thorough discussion of findings.

Summary

This chapter describes general approaches to developing and evaluating occupational therapy programs of service. A four-step process for program development is described, and the phases of program evaluation are explored in further detail. Throughout the chapter, the value of integrating research strategies, methodologies, and findings into program development and program evaluation (e.g., an evidence-based approach) is emphasized. Examples of the types of services that might be developed, implemented, and evaluated by occupational therapy personnel are provided to reinforce that these efforts may occur across a continuum of complexity and effort. Regardless of the level of complexity, the tools, methodologies, and approaches covered in other chapters of this book may be utilized to foster success in program development and evaluation endeavors.

Review Questions

1. What types of research activities comprise program evaluation research?
2. Why is a needs assessment important to program development?
3. What is the scholarship-of-practice approach, and why is it important in program evaluation research?
4. What are the steps involved in conducting a program evaluation?
5. What design approach(es) would you recommend in program evaluation research? Justify your answer.

REFERENCES

Altschuld, J. W., & Kumar, D. D. (2010). *Needs assessment: An overview, volume 1.* Thousand Oaks, CA: Sage.

Braveman, B. (2005). *Leading and managing occupational therapy services: An evidence-based approach.* Philadelphia, PA: F.A. Davis.

Braveman, B., & Kielhofner, G. (2005). Developing evidence-based occupational therapy programming. In B. Braveman (Ed.), *Leading and managing occupational therapy services: An evidence-based approach* (pp. 215–244). Philadelphia, PA: F.A. Davis.

Calley, N. G. (2011). *Program development in the 21st century: An evidence-based approach to design, implementation, and evaluation.* Thousand Oaks, CA: Sage.

Campbell, D. T., & Stanley, J. C. (1963). *Experimental and quasi-experimental designs for research.* Chicago, IL: Rand-McNally.

Connell, J., & Kubisch, A. C. (1998). Applying a theory of change approach to the evaluation of comprehensive community initiatives: Progress, prospects, and problems. In K. Fulbright-Anderson, A. C. Kubisch, & J. P. Connell (Eds.), *New approaches to evaluating community initiatives* (pp. 15–44). New York, NY: Aspen Institute.

Crist, P., & Kielhofner, G. (2005). *The scholarship of practice: Academic and practice collaborations for promoting occupational therapy.* Binghamton, NY: Hayworth Press.

Fawcett, S. B., Paine-Andrews, A., Francisco, V. T., Schultz, J. A., Richter, K. P., Lewis, R. K., ... Fisher, J.L. (1996). Empowering community health initiatives through evaluation. In D. Fetterman, S. Kaftarian, & A. Wandersman (Eds.), *Empowerment evaluation: Knowledge and tools for self-assessment and accountability* (pp. 256–276). Thousand Oaks, CA: Sage.

Fetterman, D. M., Kaftarian, S., & Wandersman, A. (Eds.). (2015). *Empowerment evaluation: Knowledge and tools for self-assessment and accountability* (2nd ed.). Los Angeles, CA: Sage.

Fisher, G. S., & Braveman, B. (2005). Understanding health systems. In B. Braveman (Ed.), *Leading and managing occupational therapy services: An evidence-based approach* (pp. 23–52). Philadelphia, PA: F.A. Davis.

Flora, C., & Grosso, C. (1999). Mapping work and outcomes: Participatory evaluation of the farm preservation advocacy network. *Sociological Practice: A Journal of Clinical and Applied Sociology, 1*(2), 133–155.

Frechtling, J. A. (2007). *Logic modeling methods in program evaluation.* San Francisco, CA: Jossey-Bass.

Garcia-Iriarte, E., Suarez-Balcazar, Y., & Taylor-Ritzler, T. (2011). A catalyst for change approach to evaluation capacity. *American Journal of Evaluation, 32*(2), 168–182.

Hammel, J., Finlayson, M., Kielhofner, G., Helfrich, C., & Peterson, E. (2002). Educating scholars of practice: An approach to preparing tomorrow's researchers. *Occupational Therapy in Health Care, 15,* 157–176.

Harper, G. W., & Salina, D. (2000). Building collaborative partnerships to improve community-based HIV prevention research: The university-CBO collaborative (UCCP) model. *Journal of Prevention and Intervention in the Community, 19,* 1–20.

Hollister, R. G., & Hill, J. (1995). Problems in the evaluation of community-wide initiatives. In J. Connell, A. Kubisch, L. Schorr, & C. Weiss (Eds.), *New approaches to evaluating community initiatives: Concepts, methods, & contexts* (pp. 127–172). Washington, DC: Aspen Institute.

Kielhofner, G. (2005). Scholarship and practice: Bridging the divide. *American Journal of Occupational Therapy, 59,* 231–239.

Kloos, B., Hill, J., Thomas, E., Wandersman, A., & Elias, M. J. (2011). *Community psychology: Linking individuals and communities* (3rd ed.). Belmont, CA: Wadsworth/Thomson Learning.

Law, M., & McDermid, J. (2013). *Evidence-based rehabilitation: A guide to practice* (3rd ed.). Thorofare, NJ: Slack.

Linney, J. A., & Wandersman, A. (1996). Empowering community groups with evaluation skills: The prevention plus III model. In D. Fetterman, S. Kaftarian & A. Wandersman (Eds.), *Empowerment evaluation: Knowledge and tools for self-assessment and accountability* (pp. 256–276). Thousand Oaks, CA: Sage Publications.

Marín, G. (1993). Defining culturally appropriate community interventions: Hispanics as a case study. *Journal of Community Psychology, 21,* 149–161.

Mathiowetz, V., Finlayson, M., Matuska, K., Chen, H. Y., & Lou, P. (2005). Randomized controlled trial of an energy conservation course for persons with multiple sclerosis. *Multiple Sclerosis, 11*(5), 592–601.

Milstein, B., & Chapel, T. (2015). *Developing a logic model or theory of change. Community tool box* (Chapter 2, section 1). Retrieved from http://ctb.ku.edu/en/table-of-contents/overview/models-for-community-health-and-development/logic-model-development/main

Posavac, E. J. (2011). *Program evaluation: Methods and case studies* (8th ed.). New York, NY: Routledge.

Posavac, E.J. (2010). *Program Evaluation: Methods and Case Studies, 8th Edition.* New York, NY: Routledge.

Rossi, P., Lipsey, M., & Freeman, H. (2004). *Evaluation: A systematic approach* (7th ed.). Thousand Oaks, Sage Publications.

Royce, D., Thyer, B. A., & Padgett, D. K. (2016). *Program evaluation: An introduction to an evidence-based approach* (6th ed.). Boston, MA: Cengage.

Stufflebeam, D. L. (2001). *Evaluation models. New directions for program evaluation (no. 89).* San Francisco, CA: Jossey-Bass.

Suarez-Balcazar, Y., & Balcazar, F. (2016). Functional analysis of community concerns: A participatory action approach. In L. Jason & D. Glenwick (Eds.), *Handbook of methodological approaches to community-based research.* Oxford University Press.

Suarez-Balcazar, Y., & Harper, G. W. (Eds.). (2003). *Empowerment and participatory evaluation of community interventions: Multiple benefits.* New York, NY: The Haworth Press.

Suarez-Balcazar, Y., Orellana-Damacela, L., Portillo, N., Sharma, A., & Lanum, M. (2003). Implementing an outcomes model in the participatory evaluation of community initiatives. In Y. Suarez-Balcazar & G. W. Harper (Eds.), *Empowerment and participatory evaluation of community interventions: Multiple benefits* (pp. 5–20). New York, NY: The Haworth Press.

Suarez-Balcazar, Y., Taylor-Ritzler, T., & Morales-Curtin, G. (2015). Building evaluation capacity to engage in empowerment evaluation. In D. Fetterman, S. Kaftarian, & A. Wandersman (Eds.), *Empowerment evaluation* (2nd ed.). Los Angeles: Sage Publications.

Wandersman, A., Keener, D., Snell-Johns, J., Miller, R., Flaspohler, P., Livet-Dye, M.,...Robinson, L. (2004). Empowerment evaluation: Principles and action. In L. Jason, K. Keys, Y. Suarez-Balcazar, R. Taylor, M. Davis, J. Durlak, & D. Isenberg (Eds.), *Participatory community research: Theories and methods in action* (pp. 139–156). Washington, DC: American Psychological Association.

Weiss, C. H. (1995). Nothing as practical as good theory: Exploring theory-based evaluation for comprehensive community initiatives for children and families. In J. P. Connell, A. Kubisch, L. Schorr, & C. H. Weiss (Eds.), *New approaches to evaluating community initiatives: Concepts, methods, and contexts* (pp. 65–92). Washington, DC: Aspen Institute.

RESOURCES

American Evaluation Association: http://www.eval.org/
Information about evaluation practices, methods, and uses through application and exploration of program evaluation.
American Occupational Therapy Association (AOTA)— Evidence-Based Practice Project: http://www.aota.org
Occupational Therapy Critically Appraised topics: http://www.otcats.com
OTSeeker: http://www.otseeker.com/

CHAPTER 30

Participatory Research Approaches

Renée R. Taylor • Yolanda Suarez-Balcazar • Kirsty Forsyth • Gary Kielhofner

Learning Outcomes

- Define the research–practice gap in occupational therapy.
- Differentiate participatory research from applied clinical research and other forms of research.
- Understand the limitations of traditional approaches that prompt the need for participatory research.
- Describe key attitudes and interpersonal behaviors that are essential for engaging in participatory research.
- Discuss some of the practical challenges in conducting participatory research.

Introduction

Participatory research is an inductive approach to research that strives to address the problems, goals, and agendas of **stakeholders** (e.g., clients) by conforming to their worldviews and local ways of engaging in occupations, thereby empowering them to take a leadership role in research. A stakeholder is an individual (or group of individuals) who has something to gain or lose from the project, inquiry, or intervention being conducted. Participatory approaches to research have been applied by investigators to address a number of health issues, ranging from macro-level community needs to specific needs of disabled clients for resource acquisition and empowerment (Balcazar, Taylor, et al., 2004).

Recently, participatory approaches have been discussed and used in occupational therapy (Scaffa & Reitz, 2014). This chapter overviews participatory research and discusses its rationale, principles, procedures, and steps. In addition, it illustrates how participatory research can be used within occupational therapy.

The Need for Participatory Research in Occupational Therapy

The need for participatory research in occupational therapy is indicated by two important

---

CASE EXAMPLE

Renuka is a student in a course on community-based approaches to occupational therapy. Her main assignment for the semester is to gain entry into a community-based agency where occupational therapy (OT) services may be needed. Renuka decides to create a relationship with the local Center for Independent Living, where adolescents and adults with a range of disabilities congregate to work together, share information, and promote legal advocacy and social change for people with disabilities.

Due to a lack of preparation and experience with participatory research methods, Renuka has not taken enough time to ask important questions about the organization or to conduct formal and informal research on the agency's mission, vision, and activities. As a consequence, Renuka's relationship with the agency does not begin in an optimal way. For example, Renuka enters the agency with customary questions about the services provided, populations served, equipment available, and service-delivery outcomes. From the beginning of the conversation with the center director, it is clear to Renuka that she has asked a number of wrong questions. The director briskly informs her that the center does not *serve* its members but instead strives to *empower* its members to serve themselves through self-advocacy. The director reminds Renuka that the agency does not refer to its members as a *population that is served* because he finds this language dehumanizing. Renuka acknowledges that she has more reading and learning to do and that she is eager to return to the agency once she feels more prepared. Renuka's first plan is to learn more about participatory research.

Because participatory research involves bringing together people with quite different backgrounds and perspectives, interactions can readily involve mistrust and misunderstanding. A productive dialogue requires finding common ground between what are often the disparate perspectives of researchers and practitioners.

Knowing that genuine dialogue requires a number of communication skills, Renuka reviews the range of interpersonal approaches she might use to bridge this gap. These include:

- Hearing the perspectives of the director and staff in a nonjudgmental way,
- Being willing to change her perspective on what people with disabilities may want when interacting with an occupational therapist,
- Working toward a common language with the staff and members of the agency,
- Confronting legitimate disagreements over what is most important,
- Negotiating and compromising,
- Using a two-way communication style,
- Having an attitude of being as ready to learn as to teach,
- Recognizing that others have important knowledge to contribute, and
- Being ready to acknowledge diversity of opinions.

Participatory research often challenges investigators to share power in unaccustomed ways. Conversely, it asks therapists and clients to take on responsibilities for and control over matters for which they ordinarily have little or no involvement or influence. As a result, all those involved in participatory research have to constantly reflect on their own attitudes and behaviors with reference to issues of power. This is not necessarily an easy task because often researchers are the ones who come in with the resources and funding and the aura of expertise of research, and therapists and/or clients can be readily intimidated. Among other things, true power sharing requires:

- Shared responsibility, voice, and decision-making about all aspects of the investigation;
- Respect and acknowledgement of the unique expertise and insights of all those involved,
- Willingness to step outside their usual roles and responsibilities;
- Identification and remediation of sources of power imbalance, such as money and access to technology; and
- Sharing resources (e.g., paying for a staff time to devote to the project, providing participants with stipends).

After reading and learning about participatory approaches, Renuka decides to spend a significant amount of time at the center. The director informs Renuka that if she is going to continue to work with the agency, she would do well to talk with the staff members and learn about issues of disability rights and social justice. As Renuka embarks on her discovery, she begins to understand that the people involved with the agency are not clients of the agency, and they certainly are not patients. They do not need to be fixed, rehabilitated, helped, or otherwise made to feel like medical objects under social scrutiny and judgment. Instead, members of the center could benefit from access to knowledge about how to change social and physical barriers to employment, transportation, and housing. Members would benefit from having an advocate and ally who understands discrimination and can produce research and other scholarly work that ultimately leads to increased opportunities for equality and access to the everyday aspects of life and the environment to which all human beings are entitled.

By the end of the semester, it is clear that Renuka has not learned nearly enough about people with disabilities or about centers for independent living to argue that she has gained entry into a community-based agency. However, by approaching the director, staff, and members of the agency with an open attitude and a willingness to strive to gain a better understanding of how disability is socially and publicly defined, she has taken an important step in terms of learning about what participatory research involves.

circumstances. The first is the gap that often exists between research and practice in occupational therapy. The second is the growing call for clients' voices in shaping the aims and content of occupational therapy services they receive.

The Research–Practice Gap

There can be a significant gap between what research suggests and what actually occurs in professional practice (Kielhofner, 2005b). Although many factors contribute to this gap, a key factor is how the knowledge that is supposed to guide practice is created (Schon, 1983). Traditionally, academics who create theory and evidence for practice are isolated from practice settings and practitioners (Peloquin & Abreu, 1996; Thompson, 2001). As a result, they may not be aware of important circumstances and constraints faced by the practitioners who are expected to use that research (Higgs & Titchen, 2001). Even when conducting applied research studies in occupational therapy, academics have largely conceived and executed the research, with practitioners mostly filling secondary roles as consultants, advisors, service providers, or data collectors.

Not surprisingly, practitioners have expressed concerns that research findings lack relevance to clinical situations, address irrelevant topics, and fail to present findings so as to facilitate application (Creek & Ilott, 2002; Dubouloz, Egan, Vallerand, & von Zweck, 1999; Dysart & Tomlin, 2002; Metcalfe et al., 2001; Sudsawad, 2003). Even when practitioners indicate that they believe that research holds value for practice, they report substantial difficulty integrating it into their practice (Dubouloz et al., 1999; McCluskey, 2003; McCluskey & Cusick, 2002). Ultimately, the difficulties of applying research in practice can be linked to the fact that practitioners ordinarily have little influence over what gets studied and how it is studied.

The Need for Consumer Voice

Within occupational therapy, the concept of client-centered practice makes the important point that individual clients should have a voice in determining their services (Law, 1998). However, outside the field, disability scholars and activists are calling for more. They argue that the disability community should have a voice in the development and validation of services they receive (Fawcett, Seekins, Whang-Ramos, Muiu, & Suarez-Balcazar, 1987). This call suggests that occupational therapy needs to go beyond client-centered practice to embrace

a disability community-centered practice that is informed by the collective experiences and perspectives of disabled consumers of our services (Kielhofner, 2005a).

Scholars from disability studies argue that the experience of living with a disability is, in part, a function of social oppression, discrimination, and exclusion, and that individuals with disabilities have been exploited, oppressed, ridiculed, excluded, and disadvantaged by society (Fine & Asch, 1990; Hahn, 1990; Katz, Hass, & Bailey, 1988; Meyerson, 1990; Oliver, 1990). Moreover, they argue that rehabilitation services, including occupational therapy, have the potential to be oppressive, stigmatizing, and largely irrelevant to the needs of individuals with disabilities (Kielhofner, 2005a). This situation exists, in part, because of the lack of control given to the consumer in deciding what services are needed and how they should be provided (Charlton, 1998). Frequently, disabled consumers observe that their individual and collective voices are missing from the discussion of how occupational therapy construes disability and how to improve the services provided (Kielhofner, 2009).

The Promise of Participatory Research in Addressing These Needs

Participatory research is predicated on the belief that research should be committed to solving practical problems, and, to that end, should involve stakeholders as equal partners in the research process. In occupational therapy, stakeholders are the therapists who deliver, the clients who receive, and the communities or groups that are affected by OT services. Hence, participatory research is well suited to address the need for greater practitioner and client voice in developing and studying OT service. As such, it promises to contribute knowledge that practitioners can readily use and that consumers will find relevant to their needs.

Definitions and Approach of Participatory Research

Participatory research is an approach to doing research that embraces certain values, perspectives, principles, and processes outlined in this chapter. Many researchers integrate qualitative research methods into participatory research. However, participatory research is also compatible with rigorous experimental designs (Taylor, Braveman, & Hammel, 2004). Participatory research often uses a combination of quantitative and qualitative strategies. For example, data collection in a study may combine standardized measures along with interviewing key informants and conducting focus groups and public forums. Moreover, participatory research is compatible not only with exploratory and case study designs but also with quasi-experimental and experimental designs.

Participatory research can take many forms, but the following are four key characteristics:

1. Participatory research is conducted in the setting or type of setting where the knowledge to be generated is expected to have relevance. In occupational therapy this means that participatory research takes place in practice contexts.
2. Participatory research involves innovation and experimentation that allows inquiry to generate new or modified services and examine how they work. Consequently, participatory research typically combines an ongoing and reflective process of initial investigation, ongoing input from the stakeholders, changes and modifications in the services, and examination of the impact of those changes. This process is used to continuously improve services in concert with gathering evidence about their impact (Reason & Bradbury, 2013).
3. Participatory research seeks to empower stakeholders by allowing them to shape the research agenda so that their needs remain the focus of the research process. By definition, participatory research aims to achieve practical outcomes as they are defined by therapists, clients, and other stakeholders, rather than simply to address problems conceptualized by the researcher (Freire, 1970; Park, 1999). In participatory research, stakeholders engage in many or all aspects of the research process (Park, 1999).
4. Participatory research brings stakeholders into a mutual dialogue and cooperation with investigators to address issues of relevance to those involved. The researcher's role in participatory research is to become an intimate knower and facilitator of the research process (Balcazar, Garate-Serafini, & Keys, 2004).

General Principles for Implementing Participatory Research in Occupational Therapy

Because participatory research takes place in practice settings and must be responsive to the circumstance of those settings and to the stakeholders who are involved, it requires considerable flexibility on the part of the researcher. Consequently, there is no single or fixed way to conduct participatory research. Nonetheless, scholars have suggested general principles for this type of inquiry (Balcazar, Keys, Kaplan, & Suarez-Balcazar, 1998; Nyden, Figert, Shibley, & Burrows, 1997; Selener, 1997). Building on their recommendations, we offer the following key principles that should shape participatory research in occupational therapy.

Stakeholders Must Be Recognized as Having the Capacity to Participate Fully in the Research Process

In participatory research, researchers must recognize stakeholders' capacity to be involved in research. This recognition begins with acknowledging the kind of expertise that stakeholders bring to the research process. For instance, practitioners bring their accumulated experience in day-to-day practice as well as their local knowledge of the context under study. Consumers bring their intimate knowledge of the problems they face in everyday life as well as their own desires and aims for improving their lives. Ultimately, in participatory research, stakeholders must be viewed as co-researchers working in partnership with the investigators.

Participatory Research Should Empower Everyone Involved

Everyone involved in participatory research has their own agenda. Researchers typically want to create new knowledge, generate publications, meet the expectations of funders, and provide practical and research opportunities for students. Practitioners typically want to increase their skills, provide better services, and have evidence to support what they do. Consumers want to improve their quality of life and have more control over their own lives. Participatory research is most successful when all partners are empowered to address their agendas as much as possible (Fig. 30.1). Moreover, when there are conflicting agendas, a process of negotiation must occur and result in a fair compromise.

Elden and Levin (1991) argue that participatory research empowers those involved in three ways:

- First, specific insights, new understandings, and new possibilities for addressing issues are

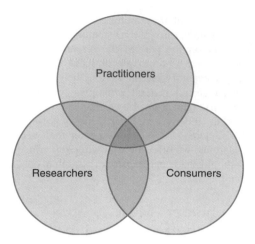

Figure 30.1   Partnerships in participatory research

generated, empowering those involved in the process of discovery.

* Second, those who engage in participatory research learn how to learn. This aspect is especially beneficial to practitioners or consumers who may feel insecure about themselves and their own knowledge.
* Third, participatory research is empowering because it often leads those involved to change their own circumstances.

True empowerment occurs when stakeholders are increasingly able to sustain what they learned to do through the research process to address new needs and barriers that occur in the future.

Participatory Research Should Involve a Dialogical Process Among Constituents That Leads to Critical Awareness

Dialogue gives researchers a more accurate understanding and appreciation of practice settings and consumers' lives. Conversely, it gives practitioners and clients an understanding of how inquiry works and can address practical problems with which they are concerned. Beyond the learning that occurs with the exchange of information, dialogue can also lead those involved to reflect on their own assumptions, attitudes, knowledge, and behavior in a critical way that leads to new awareness.

The dialogue between practitioners, consumers, and researchers is facilitated by using strategies such as listening sessions, focus groups, public forums, and constant ongoing team meetings in which all stakeholders are involved. When implemented in this way, participatory research can be a transformative and liberating process of mutual discovery.

The Research Agenda Is Shaped by the Researchers, Practitioners, and Consumers, and It Aims to Address Local Social Issues

Participatory research works best when the agendas of all those involved are openly discussed and addressed. Participatory research means that stakeholders other than the researchers are involved to some significant extent in helping to identify what gets studied, how questions are formulated, what kinds of data will be collected, and how data will be analyzed, shared, and used to make change. Involving practitioners and clients in these decisions often requires a great deal of discussion and negotiation between the stakeholders and the researchers. In traditional OT scholarship, the research agenda is formulated by the researchers based on personal research agendas (i.e., the desire to prove or disprove an existing theory). In participatory research, the researcher's agenda is important, but it must be balanced with the agendas of stakeholders such as the therapists or consumers (see Fig. 30.1).

Participatory Research Generates Knowledge That Is Intended to Be Used

Utilization of findings to either inform or shape services, practices, and policies is a key feature of participatory research. Moreover, participatory research often involves an ongoing cycle of research informing practice and practice informing research. Thus, scientific knowledge and practical knowledge mutually inform each other.

In participatory research, practical real-world utility is considered, along with empirical rigor, as a hallmark of good research (Higgs & Titchen, 2001). Participatory research recognizes that genuine knowledge arises out of efforts to achieve desired changes or solve problems in a particular context (Bradbury & Reason, 2013; David, Zakus, & Lysack, 1998). Participatory research projects are interested in practical outcomes at the local level. In the case of occupational therapy, they ask such questions as: What are the specific changes in practice and its impact resulting from the research process?

Inserting Stakeholders' Voices Into the Research Process

As we have noted, participatory research aims to give stakeholders a genuine role in the research process so that their perspectives and needs are addressed. A key challenge of participatory research is to find ways in which practitioners and consumers have a true voice in shaping the questions, methods, and outcomes of the research process (Boyce & Lysack, 2000; Taylor et al., 2004). The appropriate approach to involving stakeholders in the research process depends on many factors. These factors include:

- The aims and scope of the research,
- Organizational and contextual policies,
- The culture of those involved,
- Available resources,
- The level of readiness and desire of stakeholders for participation, and
- The collaborative attitude and approach taken by the researchers.

Approaches to Practitioner and Consumer Participation in Research

The particular form that the participatory research process actually takes depends on the context of the research. An important factor to consider is the degree of power or control that the stakeholders have over the research process. Danley and Langer-Ellison (1999) have created a handbook that may be downloaded from the Web free of charge at: http://cpr.bu.edu/store/books/handbook-participatory-action-researchers. They suggest that we can think of a continuum of power held by stakeholders that spans from little power to full power or control. At the low end of the spectrum are advisory committees, which are sometimes called participatory. The reality in such research is that stakeholders have some involvement but ultimately very little power or authority over the research project.

On the other end of the continuum are projects in which participants have full control over the research process, including hiring and firing authority over the professional researchers. Midpoints on the continuum include hybrid projects in which stakeholders have a high degree of control over the research process, but researchers are responsible to outside funding agencies and thus retain decision-making authority over some areas. For example,

Whyte's (1991) approach involves stakeholders in the research process "from the initial design of the project through data gathering and analysis, to the final conclusions and actions arising out of the research" (p. 7). In this approach, stakeholders become actively involved in the quest for information and ideas to guide their future actions.

Schema for Ensuring Participation

Table 30.1 was derived from a schema proposed by Danley and Langer-Ellison (1999) and revised by Balcazar, Garate-Serafini, et al. (2004). This version, which is an adaptation to OT research, provides a means of conceptualizing the extent of stakeholder involvement in the clinical research process. Practitioners' and consumers' roles are classified on the basis of three criteria: the degree of control that participants have over the research process (Litvak, Frieden, Dresden, & Doe, 1997), the extent of collaborative decision-making between stakeholder participants and professional researchers (Turnbull & Friesen, 1997), and the levels of input from and commitment of participants to the research process (Gordon, 1997).

This schema can be useful in evaluating how "participatory" a research project is. It is important to note that one end of the continuum is not automatically superior to the other. Rather, the continuum should be seen as a structure for thinking about the amount of stakeholder involvement the researcher is willing to negotiate, how much is good for the project, and how much is allowed by funders and other organizational constituencies that affect the research resources and implementation.

Knowledge Creation and Evaluation in Participatory Research

Within participatory research, knowledge is redefined and judged in ways that go beyond the traditional focus on propositional, rationally deduced forms of knowledge and the processes for ensuring rigor of such knowledge. There is a new emphasis on alternative epistemologies that recognize, for example, the importance of experiential and procedural knowledge (Bradbury & Reason, 2013; Maxwell, 1992). This means that participatory research values the kind of knowledge that is generated among the participants in the study (i.e., what they have experienced and what they have learned to do). In this same vein, Selener

Table 30.1 The Continuum of Stakeholder Involvement in Participatory Research Implementation

Level of Participation	Degree of Control Influence	Typical Amount/Type of Collaboration	Degree of Commitment/ Ownership
Nonparticipatory	Practitioners and clients have no control or influence on the research process.	Serve as implementers or recipients of services studied or as participants in the study	None
Low	Practitioner and/or client opinions and feedback are considered and used by researchers at the latter's discretion.	Serve as advisors to the research project Provide feedback in pilot studies or discuss implications of findings at the advisory board meeting	Minimal commitment and ownership
Medium	Practitioners and/or clients, and/or representatives of consumer groups, participate in research meetings and in aspects of the research implementation.	Provide ongoing advice, review, and consultation. Participate in discussions leading to decisions about the research	Multiple commitments to and partial ownership of the research process
High	Practitioners, clients, and/or representatives of consumer groups function as equal partners with researchers in making all decisions about the research.	Full partners in making key research decisions	Full commitment to and equal ownership of the research process with the researchers
Very high	Practitioners, clients, and/or consumer groups lead the research, with researchers assisting them.	Research leaders	Full commitment and complete ownership of the research process

(1997) suggests that feeling and acting are ways of knowing that should also emerge from research. He argues that traditional scientific methods rely exclusively on cognitive activities as a source of knowledge. Participatory researchers typically embrace the idea that reflection and action are important to the research process.

Using Dialogue to Access Subjective Knowledge

Participatory research also values the stakeholders' knowledge and experiences as important resources. Such subjective knowledge is viewed as a necessary part of the process of understanding any situation. Elden and Levin (1991) argue that those inside a particular context get to know more about it and have more ways of making sense of their world than would be possible for any outsider to appreciate. The best way to access such knowledge is through dialogue, allowing individuals to share their views in a free and supportive process. In this way, stakeholders' perspectives can define:

- What issues are important,
- How problems can be framed and defined,
- What strategies work in the community, and
- The local challenges and barriers to change.

This kind of local knowledge is critical to the success of participatory research and is included whether the primary research design is qualitative or quantitative. In qualitative participatory studies, the subjective experiences of stakeholders are used throughout. In quantitative participatory studies, subjective knowledge and experiences may be used at critical points (e.g., when deciding on the content of services to be studied or when interpreting the findings)

A Framework for Knowledge Generation in Participatory Research

One challenge of participatory research is how to balance traditional concerns for developing rigorous generalizable knowledge with concerns of solving real-world problems and empowering stakeholders in the research context (Kielhofner, 2005b). According to Elden and Levin (1991), participatory research involves coming to understand a particular situation by working with those within it to develop, test, and enhance knowledge that improves people's lives. In this approach researchers are interested in generating knowledge that helps people learn how to better control their circumstances. This approach implies a cycle of knowledge generation in which theory shapes practice and practice shapes theory (see Fig. 30.2). Theory that is generated or enriched through participatory research builds on knowledge that accumulates as people work together to improve understanding of a particular situation (Park, 1993).

Senge and Scharmer (2001) express a similar view of participatory research, proposing that it involves "a knowledge-creating system." We have adapted their ideas to discuss a general model of participatory research for occupational therapy. In our model, researchers, practitioners, and consumers work together as part of what Senge and Scharmer (2001) call a "continuing cycle of creating theory, tools and practical know-how" (p. 238). They further engage in three interacting domains of activity (illustrated in Fig. 30.2):

• Discovery and understanding of concepts and data whose relevance transcends the particular situation—that is, knowledge that is generalizable. This knowledge is generally the primary objective of the researcher.
• Creation of practical knowledge and capacity-building, which enhances practitioners' and clients' awareness and capabilities. Practical knowledge emphasizes utilization and usefulness of the knowledge generated in addressing

social issues of importance to consumers. Capacity building is also critical in this model because it speaks for one of the essences of participatory research, and that is increasing skills, knowledge, and capabilities of participants to address their own concerns. This kind of knowledge is local and personal because it involves such things as enhancing the practical know-how of OT practitioners and empowering clients with knowledge of how to manage their circumstances.
• Practice innovation, which involves creating new possibilities and means for achieving them. Such knowledge can involve rethinking practice aims or methods. It involves creating or improving practical tools and approaches that work out in a particular situation but that are irrelevant to other, similar situations. Practice innovation often aims at creating tools that not only work in the situation at hand, but that can also be used in other practice situations.

These three components of knowledge creation are collectively addressed within a single community of people working together. As a result, concepts, evidence, and practice innovations are created at the same time that practitioners' knowledge of and use of these resources is increased.

In this knowledge-creating system, practitioners and clients are centrally involved along with researchers in the process of creating knowledge. Conversely, researchers join practitioners and consumers in solving practice problems and innovating in practice. Furthermore, in a knowledge-creating system there is no artificial division between creating and assessing knowledge on the one hand and applying it on the other. Finally, all stakeholders are involved in co-generative learning in which

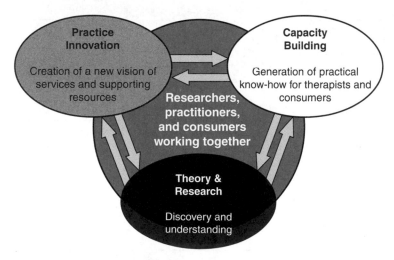

Figure 30.2 A knowledge-creating system.

their initial perspectives are altered or replaced through dialogue and co-discovery (Elden & Levin, 1991).

The Steps of Participatory Research in Occupational Therapy

Discussions of the process of participatory research have been offered in the literature (Balcazar, Keys, & Suarez-Balcazar, 2001; Fawcett et al., 2003; Selener, 1997; Suarez-Balcazar & Harper, 2004; Taylor et al., 2004). Based on these ideas, we propose here a framework for the process of participatory research in occupational therapy. According to this framework, participatory research involves six steps, as depicted in Figure 30.3. These steps, discussed next, are part of an ongoing cycle of discovery, change-making, and evaluation of change. Although the research ordinarily begins with the first step, it can begin at any stage and may involve implementing elements of different stages simultaneously. It is important to recognize that before participatory research begins and throughout its implementation, there is a process of entry and building trust wherein the researcher establishes and maintains a true partnership with the stakeholders.

Furthermore, as illustrated in Figure 30.3, the phases of participatory research are not linear. In fact, they are interactive and mutually informing. Often, stages will be combined and implemented simultaneously or iterated in small cycles. For example, it is common that phase 5 and phase 6 are interwoven. When this is the case, the research involves a reflection–action–reflection cycle (Freire, 1970) in which ongoing understanding of new problems and action to address those problems continues as knowledge is generated in the research process (Park, 1999).

Phase 1: Delineating the Problem Through Critical Reflection and Analysis

In traditional research, problems to be investigated are most often identified from careful study of the literature. In participatory research, delineating the problem to be studied also involves careful attention to how stakeholders define the problem locally and to the larger context that may be influencing the problem. Moreover, the problem to be addressed will emerge out of the practice context. In this phase it is important to ask the following questions:

* How does the literature shed light on the problem?
* How do different stakeholders view the problem?

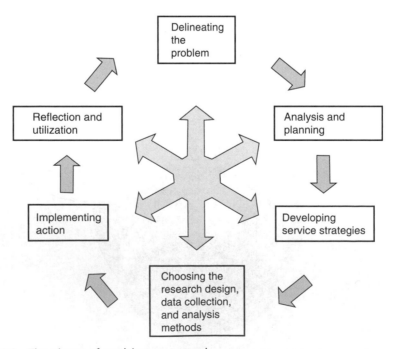

Figure 30.3   The phases of participatory research.

- What are contextual and environmental factors affecting the problem?
- When all these dimensions are considered together, how do they frame the problem?

In participatory research, researchers and stakeholders engage in ongoing reflection aimed at achieving a critical awareness of the problem. Without critical reflection, research can move forward to solve a problem before it is fully defined and its multiple dimensions are fully understood. Participatory research seeks to confront and address the full complexity of any problem rather than trying to isolate and study only one aspect. In this way, participatory research is more likely to generate solutions that actually work in the real-life situation. Often, given the cyclical nature of participatory research, the problem may be redefined as the research unfolds.

Phase 2: Analyzing and Planning the Participatory Research

Careful and critical analysis of the problem sets a foundation for the next step of the process, planning the research. This step involves selecting the research questions or hypotheses that will be answered or tested in the research. Because of the previous step, the research questions or hypotheses will not be grounded only in preexisting empirical and theoretical knowledge. They will also reflect key stakeholders' perspectives on what they need to understand or know. In this phase, it is important to consider the following kinds of questions:

- Given the dimensions of the problem, what do we need to know to understand or address the problem?
- What kinds of information do we want to generate about the problem and how the solutions work?
- How would the information that is generated be used?

Because stakeholders are involved along with researchers, the questions generated will have not only theoretical but also utilitarian ends. Information is sought not only to create understanding of what is being studied but also to achieve workable solutions to local problems.

Phase 3: Developing Service Strategies

The third phase involves an analysis of potential service strategies that can be implemented to understand and address the problem and its dimensions. In occupational therapy these strategies can include such diverse things as modifying or generating a new assessment or intervention, developing a program to meet an unmet need, promoting organizational change that affects health-care delivery for a client group, or engaging in advocacy efforts to change insurance legislation to affect a consumer group. Depending on the context, choosing or implementing a solution may require systematic deliberations, complex negotiations, and even struggles between different perspectives or with existing power structures.

In this phase it is important to consider the following questions:

- What are potential strategies to address the problem?
- Are the strategies appropriate given the situation and perspectives of the stakeholders involved?
- What are the anticipated likely consequences of applying the proposed strategies or ways of addressing the problem?

In answering these questions, the researchers and stakeholders work together to integrate existing scientific knowledge with local knowledge.

Phase 4: Choosing the Research Design and Data Collection and Analysis Methods

After strategies for addressing the problem have been chosen, the researcher and stakeholders engage in choosing the research design and the approach to data collection and analysis. Once again, these methods must fit the interests of stakeholders and available resources (Fawcett et al., 2003; Park, 1999). In participatory research, investigators and stakeholders often participate equally in data collection, data analysis, and decisions as to how the success of a given strategy will be judged. By shaping such data analysis, stakeholders have an important role in determining what conclusions will be drawn from the research. In this phase it is important to consider the following questions:

- Are the design, the methods for gathering data, and the kind of data collected appropriate for evaluating the strategies?
- Are the design, the methods for gathering data, and the kind of data collected appropriate to the context and the concerns of stakeholders?
- Will the design, data collection, and analysis provide information that is both credible in the scientific community and relevant to making future decisions in the research setting?

This phase requires achieving an important balance between scientific and practical concerns. The design and data will not only address concerns of a larger scholarly community but also provide information about whether a local problem has been effectively addressed.

Phase 5: Implementing Action

A key element of participatory research is that it involves action. Participatory research in occupational therapy will involve implementing the strategies that have been designed to address the problem. As noted earlier, these strategies can range from fairly minor modifications of services to new programs of services to large-scale changes in service delivery. Whatever the action being implemented, a key feature is that this action is undertaken in a reflective way. This means that the following kinds of questions are typically asked:

- Are the service strategies working as anticipated?
- What unexpected problems or barriers have emerged?
- Have efforts to implement the innovations in service been successful? Have they created new complications?

Depending on the design of the research, answers to these types of questions may be used to modify the services on an ongoing basis, or they will be used to provide critical information about how the service strategies work.

Phase 6: Reflection and Utilization

In the sixth phase, researchers and stakeholders reflect on the strategies implemented in the research and the results they have achieved as indicated by the data collected and by their experiences in the process. During this phase, questions such as the following are asked:

- What do the findings mean?
- What are their implications for future action in this setting?
- How can we use the results to improve services, programs, and practice in general?
- How can the knowledge be disseminated to others?
- What new questions or problems have emerged from taking action?

By addressing such questions, the research team is accountable for ensuring that the research findings can be used locally and broadly within the profession to improve OT practice.

Challenges of Conducting Participatory Research

Like all forms of research, participatory research has its own unique challenges. Two of the most challenging aspects of participatory research are creating a dialogue and sharing power. Participatory research inevitably involves the following elements (Balcazar et al., 2001; Prilleltensky and Nelson, 2002; Riger, 2001; Suarez-Balcazar et al., 2004):

- Working together with others who share different views;
- Taking on nontraditional roles;
- "Thinking outside the box" of traditional, discipline-defined research;
- Balancing power, control, and resources; and
- Breaking from traditional researcher–participant relationships.

For this reason, participatory research can be, at its extremes, both frustrating and exhilarating. It requires a serious commitment to the underlying vision of why participatory research is important for the field and careful attention to the guidelines and procedures we have outlined in this chapter.

Summary

This chapter overviews the rationale and need for participatory research in the context of occupational therapy and discusses its underlying epistemological assumptions. It also suggests ways to think about the extent of participation by stakeholders, it offers principles, and it offers a model to guide participatory research. In addition, this chapter notes some of the challenges involved in participatory research.

Participatory research protects the voice of consumers and clients and provides a venue for researchers and practitioners to work together and advance both scholarship and practice. Moreover, its emphasis on innovation and reflection makes it particularly suited to achieve creative new approaches to service. Consequently, participatory research has a unique role in advancing OT practice.

Review Questions

1. Do you think there is a research–practice gap in occupational therapy? Justify your answer.

2. How does participatory research differ from applied clinical research and other forms of research in occupational therapy?
3. What limitations of traditional approaches prompt the need for participatory research?
4. What are the key attitudes and interpersonal behaviors that are essential for engaging in participatory research?
5. What are some of the practical challenges in conducting participatory research?

REFERENCES

Balcazar, F. E., Garate-Serafini, T. J., & Keys, C. B. (2004). The need for action when conducting intervention research: The multiple roles of community psychologists. *American Journal of Community Psychology, 33*(3–4), 243–252.

Balcazar, F. E., Keys, C. B., Kaplan, D. L., & Suarez-Balcazar, Y. (1998). Participatory action research and people with disabilities: Principles and challenges. *Canadian Journal of Rehabilitation, 12,* 105–112.

Balcazar, F. E., Keys, C. B., & Suarez-Balcazar, Y. (2001). Empowering Latinos with disabilities to address issues of independent living and disability rights: A capacity-building approach. *Journal of Prevention and Intervention in the Community, 21*(2), 53–70.

Balcazar, F. E., Taylor, R. R., Kielhofner, G. W., Tamley, K., Benziger, T., Carlin, N., Johnson, S., Suarez-Balcazar, Y., Taylor, R.R., . . . Davis, M.I. (2004). Participatory action research: General principles and a study with a chronic health condition. In L. A. Jason, C. B. Keys, et al. (Eds.), *Participatory community research: Theories and methods in action* (pp. 17–35). Washington, DC: American Psychological Association.

Boyce, W., & Lysack, C. (2000). Community participation: Uncovering its meanings in CBR. In M. Thomas & M. J. Thomas (Eds.), *Selected readings in community based rehabilitation: CBR in transition* (Series 1, pp. 42–54). Bangalore: Asia Pacific Disability Rehabilitation Journal.

Bradbury, H., & Reason, P. (2013). Conclusion: Broadening the bandwidth of validity: Issues and choice-points for improving the quality of action research. In P. Reason & H. Bradbury (Eds.), *Handbook of action research: Participative inquiry and practice* (2nd ed., pp. 447–455). London, England: Sage.

Charlton, J. I. (1998). *Nothing about us without us.* Los Angeles, CA: University of California Press.

Creek, J., & Ilott, I. (2002). *Scoping study of occupational therapy research and development activity in Scotland, Northern Ireland and Wales. Executive summary.* London, England: College of Occupational Therapists.

Danley, K., & Langer-Ellison, M. (1999). *A handbook for participatory action researchers.* Boston, MA: Center for Psychiatric Rehabilitation, Boston University. Retrieved from http://cpr.bu.edu/store/books/handbook-participatory-action-researchers

David, J., Zakus, L., & Lysack, C. L. (1998). Revisiting community participation. *Health Policy and Planning, 13*(1), 1–12.

Dubouloz, C., Egan, M., Vallerand, J., & von Zweck, C. (1999). Occupational therapists' perceptions of evidence based practice. *American Journal of Occupational Therapy, 53,* 445–453.

Dysart, A. M., & Tomlin, G. S. (2002). Factors related to evidence-based practice among US occupational therapy clinicians. *American Journal of Occupational Therapy, 56*(3), 275–284.

Elden, M., & Levin, M. (1991). Cogenerative learning: Bringing participation into action research. In W. F. Whyte (Ed.), *Participatory action research.* Thousand Oaks, CA: Sage.

Fawcett, S., Boothroyd, R., Schultz, J., Franciasco, V. T., Carson, V., & Bremby, R. (2003). Building capacity for participatory evaluation within community initiatives. *Journal of Prevention and Intervention in the Community, 26,* 21–36.

Fawcett, S. B., Seekins, T., Whang-Ramos, P., Muiu, C., & Suarez-Balcazar, Y. (1987). Involving consumers in decision-making. *Social Policy, 13*(6), 36–41.

Fine, M., & Asch, A. (1990). Disability beyond stigma: Social interaction, discrimination, and activism. In M. Nagler (Ed.), *Perspectives on disability* (pp. 61–74). Palo Alto, CA: Health Markets Research.

Freire, P. (1970). *Pedagogy of the oppressed.* New York, NY: Continuum. (30th Anniversary edition published in 2000 by Bloomsbury Academic)

Gordon, W. A. (1997). PAR: A realistic strategy for medical rehabilitation research? In B. Phillips-Tewey (Ed.), *Building participatory action research partnerships in disability and rehabilitation research.* Washington, DC: U.S. Department of Education, National Institute on Disability and Rehabilitation Research.

Hahn, H. (1990). The politics of physical difference: Disability and discrimination. In M. Nagler (Ed.), *Perspectives on disability* (pp. 118–123). Palo Alto, CA: Health Markets Research.

Higgs, J., & Titchen, A. (2001). Rethinking the practice-knowledge interface in an uncertain world: A model for practice development. *British Journal of Occupational Therapy, 64,* 526–533.

Katz, I., Hass, L., & Bailey, J. (1988). Attributional ambivalence and behavior toward people with disabilities. In H. Yuker (Ed.), *Attitudes toward persons with disabilities* (pp. 47–57). New York, NY: Springer.

Kielhofner, G. (2005a). Rethinking disability and what to do about it: Disability studies and their implications for occupational therapy. *American Journal of Occupational Therapy, 59,* 487–496.

Kielhofner, G. (2005b). Scholarship and practice: Bridging the divide. *American Journal of Occupational Therapy, 59,* 231–239.

Kielhofner, G. (2009). *Conceptual foundations of occupational therapy* (4th ed.). Philadelphia, PA: F.A. Davis.

Law, M. (Ed). (1998). *Client-centered occupational therapy.* Thorofare, NJ: Slack.

Litvak, S., Frieden, L., Dresden, C., & Doe, T. (1997). Empowerment, independent living research and participatory action research. In B. Phillips-Tewey (Ed.), *Building participatory action research partnerships in disability and rehabilitation research.* Washington, DC: U.S. Department of Education, National Institute on Disability and Rehabilitation Research.

Maxwell, N. (1992). What kind of inquiry can best help us create a good world? *Science, Technology, & Human Values, 17,* 205–227.

McCluskey, A. (2003). Occupational therapists report a low level of knowledge, skill and involvement in evidence-based practice. *Australian Occupational Therapy Journal, 50*(1), 3–12.

McCluskey, A., & Cusick, A. (2002). Strategies for introducing evidence-based practice and changing clinical behavior: A manager's toolbox. *Australian Occupational Therapy Journal, 49*(2), 63–70.

Metcalfe, C., Lewin, R., Wisher, S., Perry, S., Bannigan, K., & Moffett, J. K. (2001). Barriers to implementing the evidence base in four NHS therapies: Dietitians, occupational therapists, physiotherapists, speech and language therapists. *Physiotherapy, 87*(8), 433–441.

Meyerson, L. (1990). The social psychology of physical disability: 1948–1988. In M. Nagler (Ed.), *Perspectives on disability* (pp. 13–23). Palo Alto, CA: Health Markets Research.

Nyden, P., Figert, A., Shibley, M., & Burrows, D. (1997). *Building community: Social science in action*. Thousand Oaks, CA: Sage.

Oliver, M. (1990). *The politics of disablement*. London, England: MacMillan.

Park, P. (1993). What is participatory research? A theoretical and methodological perspective. In P. Park, M. Brydon-Miller, B. Hall, & T. Jackson (Eds.), *Voices of change: Participatory research in the United States and Canada* (pp. 1–19). Westport, CT: Bergin & Garvey.

Park, P. (1999). People, knowledge, and change in participatory research. *Management Learning, 30,* 141–157.

Peloquin, S. M., & Abreu, B. C. (1996). The academia and clinical worlds: Shall we make meaningful connections? *American Journal of Occupational Therapy, 50*(7), 588–591.

Prilleltensky, I., & Nelson, G. (2002). *Doing psychology critically: Making a difference in diverse settings*. Basingstroke, UK: Palgrave, MacMillan.

Reason, P., & Bradbury, H. (2013). *Handbook of action research: Participative inquiry and practice* (2nd ed.). London: Sage.

Riger, S. (2001). Working together: Challenges in collaborative research. In M. Sullivan & J. G. Kelly (Eds.), *Collaborative research: University and community partnerships* (pp. 25–44). Washington, DC: APHA.

Scaffa, M. E. & Reitz, S. M. (Eds.). (2014). *Occupational therapy in community based practice settings* (2nd ed.). Philadelphia, PA: F.A. Davis Company.

Schon, D. A. (1983). *The reflective practitioner*. New York, NY: Basic Books.

Selener, D. (1997). *Participatory action research and social change*. Ithaca, NY: Cornell Participatory Action Research Network, Cornell University.

Senge, P., & Scharmer, O. (2001). Community action research: Learning as a community of practitioners, consultants, and researchers. In P. Reason & H. Bradbury (Eds.), *Handbook of action research: Participative inquiry and practice*. London, England: Sage.

Suarez-Balcazar, Y., Davis, M., Ferrari, J., Nyden, P., Olson, B., Alvarez, J., . . . Toro, P. (2004). University-community partnerships: A framework & case study. In L. Jason, C. Keys, Suarez-Balcazar, Y., Taylor, R. R., & Davis, M. I. (Eds.), *Participatory community research: Theory and methods in action* (pp. 105–120). Washington, DC: American Psychological Association.

Suarez-Balcazar, Y., & Harper, G. (Eds.). (2004). *Empowerment and participatory and evaluation of community interventions: Multiple benefits*. New York, NY: Routledge.

Sudsawad, P. (2003, October 24). *Rehabilitation practitioners' perspectives on research utilization for evidence-based practice*. Paper presented at the American Congress of Rehabilitation Medicine conference, Tucson, AZ.

Taylor, R. R., Braveman, B., & Hammel, J. (2004). Developing and evaluating community services through participatory action research: Two case examples. *American Journal of Occupational Therapy, 58,* 73–82.

Thompson, N. (2001). *Theory and practice in human services*. Maidenhead: Open University Press.

Turnbull, A. P., & Friesen, B. J. (1997). Forging collaborative partnerships with families in the study of disability. In B. Phillips-Tewey (Ed.), *Building participatory action research partnerships in disability and rehabilitation research* (pp. 113–121). Washington, DC: U.S. Department of Education, National Institute on Disability and Rehabilitation Research.

Whyte, W. F. (1991). *Participatory action research*. Thousand Oaks, CA: Sage.

CHAPTER 31

Writing a Literature Review

Renée R. Taylor • Gary Kielhofner • Ellie Fossey

Learning Outcomes

- List the applications of a general (unsystematic) literature review.
- Identify the difference between a systematic and an unsystematic literature review.
- Define eight key strategies for effective scientific writing.
- Understand the fundamental questions that a literature review should address.
- Describe the role of critical appraisal in a literature review.

Introduction

During your career in occupational therapy, you may be required to write a literature review. For example, you may be required to write a review of the literature for a class you are taking. If you are working toward a master's or doctoral degree, a literature review is likely to be required as part of your preliminary field examinations, thesis, or dissertation. When conducting independent research, you will be required to write a literature review as part of the introduction for the manuscript you intend to publish, or for a book chapter or grant proposal. If you are managing a private practice or a rehabilitation unit in a health-care setting, you may be required to summarize the literature on a particular piece of equipment to be purchased or therapeutic practice to be supported by the unit.

In this chapter, you will learn the process of writing a literature review. A literature review is a critical evaluation of existing literature relevant to the topic under study (DePoy & Gitlin, 2011). A good literature review informs, evaluates, and integrates relevant existing literature (Thomas, 2000). If the literature review is done well, it will make apparent to the reader how the research represents a logical next step in building knowledge and/or how the research fills a critical gap in an area of knowledge (DePoy & Gitlin, 2011). It may also

inform the design of a study. Thus, in writing the literature review for a research paper, it is important to make sure that it is organized so as to tell a story or provide an argument that leads directly to the research question and study. A literature review that simply reports previous research may be inadequate in most cases. There are two types of literature reviews: systematic reviews and general literature reviews (unsystematic reviews).

A **systematic review** is an exhaustive and thorough research effort that focuses on assessing and evaluating the quality of all other research studies of a strictly defined scientific topic or question. Its focus is to eliminate bias in the review by using an objective and transparent methodological approach to information synthesis that can be replicated easily. In evidence-based medicine, systematic reviews of randomized controlled trials are considered the highest level of evidence available to determine the extent of support for a given treatment. In addition to medical or rehabilitation treatments, systematic reviews may also evaluate research about a given assessment tool, clinical test, adverse treatment effect, or social, economic, or behavioral intervention.

Systematic reviews are often data-driven, using statistical analyses to synthesize and quantitatively evaluate outcomes related to a given research question. Qualitative research methods may also be employed to synthesize and evaluate the evidence, provided that specific procedures for gathering, analyzing, and reporting the data are followed. The first step of a systematic review is to thoroughly search and collect all relevant literature on the topic. The second step is to check all of the articles against the preidentified criteria for relevance, inclusion, and exclusion. Additionally, the authors may choose to assign each study a rating of methodological quality according to the Preferred Reporting Items for Systematic Reviews and Meta-analyses (PRISMA) statement (http://www.prisma-statement.org) or to the standards of the Cochrane Collaboration (http://handbook.cochrane.org). At the University of London, the Evidence for Policy and Practice Information and

Coordinating Centre (EPPI-Centre) focuses on combining quantitative and qualitative approaches to conduct systematic reviews.

Another type of review by which a researcher may systematically collect and report evidence is referred to as a **scoping review**, or scoping study. This type of review focuses on the rapid collection of as much evidence as possible in a much broader clinical or policy-related area. In this case, the review might inform a range of study designs, and it does not address very specific questions or assess the quality of the studies that are included in the review. For those interested in undertaking a scoping review in a more rigorous manner, the steps described by Arksey and O'Malley (2005) may serve as a helpful resource.

By contrast, an **unsystematic review** is not typically considered to be a stand-alone work of research in itself (as a meta-analysis or other systematic review would be rendered). An unsystematic review does not adhere rigidly to a specific protocol (Sandelowski, 2008). It is a practical piece of writing that builds an evidence-based story, acting as a precursor to planned research or as an introduction to an executed study. An unsystematic review is at risk for more bias than a systematic review because its aim is to show how the existing literature progresses toward your topic (rather than to evaluate the methodological quality and level of evidence of that literature). In sum, the central aims of the general (unsystematic) literature review are to:

- Demonstrate advanced knowledge of the topic area;
- Establish the impact and relevance of the research question; and
- Build a rationale for future research and/or the proposed study to be conducted or reported.

This chapter is organized around creating a general literature review.

A precursor to writing a literature review is the underlying task of writing itself. Writing is absolutely necessary for research. Without it, one cannot garner the necessary approval and resources for research. More importantly, without writing, research is not shared with the scientific and professional community. For all practical purposes, an unpublished study could be considered never to have taken place. Therefore, anyone who wishes to do research must commit to the task of writing. Investigators have a wide range of reactions to the obligation of writing. Nonetheless, writing can be a satisfying culmination to the process of inquiry. It is, after all, an opportunity to share one's discovery.

When to Begin Writing

Your process of writing should begin when your topic is first conceived and should continue throughout the research process. If you are writing your literature review for the purpose of publication, you should seek to identify both the targeted journal or other venue for publication and the intended audience for a paper as soon as possible. Identifying the book or journal will provide the technical information (e.g., page limit, manuscript preparation format) necessary for preparing a final manuscript (see Box 31.1). The technical information can be found on the website of the journal or book publisher. For example, the *American Journal of Occupational Therapy* (AJOT) has a box on the journal's homepage titled "Authors and Reviewers" with a link to forms and guidelines. Identifying the audience means becoming familiar with answers to the following questions:

- Who is likely to read the literature review?
- What is their level and type of knowledge?
- What perspectives they are likely to bring to reading the review?

This information is essential not only to writing a review that will be understood by its intended audience, but also to its being considered appropriate for publication by the chosen journal or book. Also, it is valuable to read research papers from the journal or other chapters from the book in

---

BOX 31.1 Editorial Style for References

Every journal follows particular referencing and formatting guidelines, often termed the editorial style. Editorial style refers to the set of rules that are followed to ensure that material published in a particular journal is presented consistently.

The most common one used by occupational therapy and related social and behavioral science journals is the American Psychological Association's APA Style. Details about its Publication Manual (American Psychological Association, 2009), as well as information about self-teaching materials for learning APA Style and guidelines for citing electronic media and creating effective visual materials, can be found online at the website http://www.apastyle.org/

Before submitting a manuscript to a journal, one must become knowledgeable about the editorial style required by the journal and ensure that the manuscript submitted adheres to the format in all its details.

CASE EXAMPLE

For the past 10 years, Linda, a pediatric occupational therapist, has worked part time at a crisis nursery, where parents under severe stress may obtain temporary child care to reduce the risk of child abuse or neglect. The center also offers parenting skills, support, and training. Linda also serves at a local occupational therapy (OT) program as a fieldwork supervisor, and she is involved in coordinating continuing education events for her state OT association.

Over the years, Linda's expertise in working with toddlers with histories of physical abuse has become known. Despite periods of intense reflection about practice with this vulnerable population and having developed some unique and effective approaches to therapy, she has never had the courage to write about her experiences. However, she accepts yearly invitations to make verbal presentations to the OT students in the local program.

This year, Richard, a classmate of Linda's who is now a professor at the school they attended, contacted her. Richard is editing a book on pediatric occupational therapy, and he wants to include Linda as a coauthor of a chapter on therapeutic approaches to child survivors of abuse and neglect. Flattered but unsure of her abilities, Linda agrees and also invites a current student from the program to join them. When the two of them get together to discuss chapter contents, they agree that their first task is to write the chapter's introduction, which will provide a background of the literature in the area.

Because the book includes evidence-based practice approaches, Linda decides to include only peer-reviewed journal articles in the literature review, and she recommends that the student search the following bibliographic search engine databases at the university library: CINAHL, PsycINFO, and MEDLINE. They agree on three objectives to frame the online search: (1) To establish the impact of the topic, they will seek general epidemiological (i.e., prevalence and incidence) information about child abuse and neglect; (2) to demonstrate knowledge of the topic, they will seek information from a wide range of professional disciplines on rehabilitation approaches with children with a history of child abuse or neglect; and (3) to establish relevance of the topic to occupational therapists, they will seek information on rehabilitation approaches that are specific to occupational therapy.

After they assemble all of the literature for their unsystematic review, they read and organize it according to these three areas, propose a novel approach based on Linda's clinical experience, and end the chapter with a **case-composite example** from Linda's practice, an integrative discussion of the case in light of the existing literature, and suggestions for future research that incorporates Linda's approach. (A case-composite example is similar to an actual case example, but the client is de-identified such that there is no way to ever trace the details discussed about the person to an actual person. This requires altering the identity and some of the circumstances or characteristics of an actual case, or incorporating characteristics from other clients, hence the term "composite.")

---

which you intend to publish and papers on the same research topic.

The Writing Process

Writing research papers or book chapters is a skill that can be learned and maintained through deliberate and regular practice. It is valuable to learn this skill because it allows the individual to reflect on, contribute to, and communicate about the development of the science and practice in a particular field. This section describes strategies that can be used to become and remain an effective writer.

The Interrelated Tasks of Writing

Although writing is a creative process, it requires deliberate and disciplined management of several interrelated tasks (Brown, 1994). Figure 31.1 illustrates some of the range of tasks to be managed by the writer.

People often try to manage writing from the bottom up, that is, by focusing on the least complex tasks of writing shown at the bottom of Figure 31.1, such as grammar, language use, punctuation, and so forth. However, it is more effective to take a top-down approach to writing, attending to the more complex tasks earlier in the writing

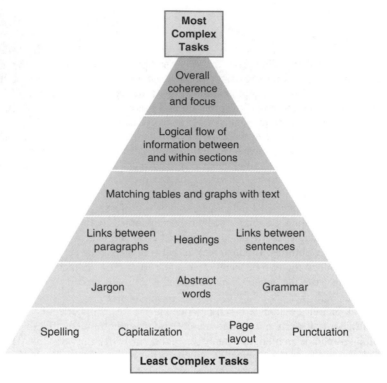

Figure 31.1   The hierarchy of tasks that writers need to master in managing the writing process. The least complex tasks are at the bottom of the pyramid. The most complex tasks are at the top. *(Adapted from Brown, 1994.)*

process. Doing so will tend to lead to a more coherent, readable, and engaging writing style.

Writing Strategies

In the following section, we describe eight key strategies for anyone who wishes to become an effective research writer:

1. Setting aside and structuring time for writing;
2. Discovering and developing one's own writing style and habits;
3. Writing for a particular audience;
4. Clarifying one's focus;
5. Mind-mapping and abstracting;
6. Finding one's story;
7. Drafting, sequencing, and rewriting; and
8. Seeking and using feedback.

Each of these strategies is briefly discussed.

Strategy 1: Setting Aside and Structuring Time for Writing

Writing takes time. Most writers find that they require large blocks of time to focus on writing.

Hence, there is no substitute for structuring one's schedule to include regular writing time. These blocks of time should be periods when one is alert and able to attend to the writing task. Scheduling writing in one's spare time, when one is tired or easily distracted, will only invite frustration. It can also be helpful to allocate less optimal or smaller blocks of time for the more mundane or concrete aspects of writing (i.e., those tasks nearer the bottom of Figure 31.1).

Strategy 2: Discovering and Developing One's Own Writing Style and Habits

Although some factors are essential to all writing, it is also a highly personal process. Individuals who are experienced and successful writers have paid attention to and developed their own writing style and habits. This includes consideration of such factors as what are optimal times and contexts for writing and what is the best way to organize resource materials.

Writing requires discipline. Anyone who has done substantial writing will admit that a key element is following through on planned time and making oneself focus during scheduled writing time. In scheduling writing times and tasks, one should take into consideration what times of the day/week are best for concentrating on the writing task and how long one can effectively write. Some people write better earlier in the day, whereas others prefer late at night. Some persons can write at a variety of times.

Writers should assess how long they can write optimally. Some people can write for only an hour or two. Others can write for an entire day. Some individuals require frequent breaks, whereas others want to stay focused throughout the writing. Knowing and respecting one's own writing patterns is vital. It is important to pay attention to when one gets the most writing done and when one has difficulty writing, and then plan one's schedule accordingly.

It is also useful to structure one's writing time. Some writers find it helpful to set short-term goals for the next hour or day, such as writing so many pages or finishing a particular section of a paper. Some people find it best to write for a period and then review what was written, revise, and go on to the next task. Once again, it is important to identify and use what works best.

An often underestimated element is finding the right context for writing. Scientific writing conjures up images of some quiet corner in a library, but such a context does not work for everyone. Some persons need quiet space; others write effectively with background noise or music. In the end, if a writer discovers ways to make the writing process enjoyable and fulfilling, it will require less effort to motivate oneself to write and the routine of writing will be easier to sustain (Fig. 31.2).

Most of the time, we write with resources that have been accumulated over time. These materials include such things as articles accumulated for a literature review, notes taken from reading, and boilerplates (i.e., previously written materials that are edited and incorporated into papers). Organizing these materials in ways that optimize one's writing style will facilitate efficient writing.

For instance, one of the authors of this chapter prefers to take notes on a laptop computer while reading and then uses those notes later when composing a chapter. This author tends to begin writing while reading. This author also typically works on several articles or chapters at a time and maintains a folder for each work in process in the computer. That way, notes, references, and other materials can be inserted in the folder whenever new information or new thoughts about a work in progress arise. When writing, the author takes all these resources and weaves them together into an organic document that generally gets revised multiple times, often quite dramatically, as it evolves into the final written manuscript.

Another of the authors prefers to first read, surrounded by hard copies of the readings, highlighting aspects of the readings that are important. Then, the author outlines the plan of the manuscript and proceeds to write the paper progressively from beginning to end, thinking carefully about each section of the manuscript as it is being written and doing most of the rewriting along the way. Once finished with a paper or manuscript, the author seeks feedback and then generally completes one overall rewrite before the paper is finished.

These differences in writing are matters of personal style that a new writer must discover through experimentation. Of course, writing style will also vary somewhat according to what one is writing, how familiar the topic is, and how tight a deadline one is facing. Respect for one's style, tempered with practical considerations of getting the task done, is a wise course.

When collaborating on papers, it is a good idea to discuss writing styles and figure out how they can be meshed over the course of working together. For example, one of us has found discussion, written comments, electronic editing, and time spent working together on the computer each to be effective at different stages in the process of writing collaboratively with colleagues. Sometimes, of course, this is not possible. For instance, this chapter was written without any face-to-face discussion among the authors. Each person took turns working on the manuscript, which was shared by e-mail.

Strategy 3: Writing for a Particular Audience

No literature review or research paper will be readily understood or interesting to everyone. Readers bring to a written piece their own training and knowledge and their sense of what is important. The sole purpose of writing is to communicate with readers. This may seem obvious, but it requires one to read one's writing from the imagined perspective of the reader. Writers, of course, understand their own writing because it is an outpouring of what they know. Readers, however, do not know what the writer knows, and thus the paper needs to be written and edited with the reader's perspective in mind.

Thus, the writing and rewriting process begins with a sense of one's audience, including the

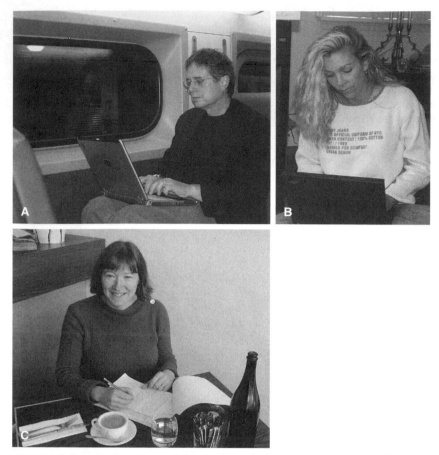

Figure 31.2   (A) Gary writes effectively in a variety of places and times. One of his most productive times for writing is during the daily commute to and from Chicago on the train. It provides over 2 hours a day of time away from interruptions. For him, the background noise helps him concentrate because he is unable to write in silence. (B) Renée writes best in a comfortable and quiet environment with large chunks of time. She needs relatively frequent short breaks. Writing in front of the fireplace in the winter or in a sunny spot in the yard in the summer works well for her. (C) Ellie writes drafts on the computer at home or work, but prefers to rework the structure of material, or edit it, on paper. Her favorite venues for editing are her local neighborhood cafés in Melbourne, with music and activity going on around her.

audience's knowledge base, interests, and expectations. Writers who do not consider their intended audience will inevitably be frustrated with rejected papers or requests for substantial rewriting. Hence, as previously noted, one should identify who one's audience is at the outset. Having done so, it is important to read one's own writing and rewriting from the perspective of that intended audience (Brown, 1994).

It takes some practice to develop this skill of reading your own work from another's perspective. Nonetheless, it is a skill worth cultivating. It can help to think of three or four specific people who are potential readers of your work and to write

and read your work with them in mind. It may also be useful to seek someone who represents that audience to give feedback, as a way of getting a sense of how the intended audience will approach your writing. In doing so, one should pay careful attention not only to the implications for a given paper, but also to how the person approaches the paper. This helps one develop the sense of what it means to pay attention to an audience.

Strategy 4: Clarifying One's Focus

Clarifying the main message of an intended paper will make the writing task more efficient and result in a paper that is easier for readers to understand (Brown, Rogers, & Pressland, 1993, 1994).

This advice sounds deceptively simple. Typically, writers find themselves with much more information than they can include in a single research report. Thus, they must make challenging decisions about what to include, what to leave out, and how to organize the information reported. Lack of clarity about the focus of a paper can create difficulty in making these decisions.

Strategy 5: Mind-Mapping and Abstracting

Based on their experiences of running workshops for researchers about how to write papers, Brown and his colleagues (1993, 1994) recommend two strategies that are helpful in creating a clear focus: mind-mapping to distill the main message and developing a working abstract as a framework for the first draft of a paper.

Mind-mapping and similar techniques, such as concept-mapping, involve generating and refining a visual representation of the ideas to be contained in a paper (Bihl-Hulme, 1985; Brown et al., 1994; Buzan & Buzan, 2000).

The process begins with laying out on paper a detailed free-form diagram of all the facts, ideas, thoughts, questions, and linkages that could go into a paper. One then identifies the most important parts of the mind-map by assigning priorities to the information contained in it (Brown et al., 1994). This process allows one to more readily see the relationships or connections between materials and to identify the material of most importance to the topic. Mind-mapping also helps to define the boundaries of a paper, letting one decide what not to include (Brown et al., 1994).

To further clarify the main message, it is often helpful to generate an initial draft of an abstract from the mind-map (see Box 31.2). This draft abstract functions as a mission statement that guides one's writing process. The contents may, indeed, go into the final abstract in some form, but the purpose of writing an abstract as part of this process is to make sure one has clear in one's own mind what is being written.

The use of outlines is often recommended as a tool for structuring written papers and organizing the material within them, but they can be difficult to create if you are not clear about what you intend to include in your literature review. Clarifying the main message and creating an initial draft of the abstract can provide the foundation for creating an outline. The priorities identified in the mind-map often yield the section headings and subheadings for an outline.

Strategy 6: Finding One's Story

Mind-mapping will not work for all writers, and it probably works better for visual thinkers. Other writers may find it more helpful to think about the paper as a story. A research paper basically involves telling the story of how one came up with the research question and went about answering it in the research process, then revealing the answers obtained.

In this case, one needs to identify the basic plot of the story. The plot involves a beginning, middle, and end that flow together into a whole. Each part of the writing contributes to the unfolding of the story.

To use this approach, one should write out the story in as few words as possible. In a sense, it's like creating the abstract. However, it is a good idea to create the story for a layperson. Imagine, for instance, how one would explain to a mother or to a friend what the paper is about. This requires the writer to pare down everything to a fairly simple storyline.

Once one is able to articulate the story in straightforward terms, deciding what to include and leave out is facilitated. Moreover, determining the best way to chunk the successive parts of the story and link them together becomes easier. As with the mind-mapping technique, one can create a more effective and integrated outline once one is clear about the underlying story.

Strategy 7: Drafting, Sequencing, and Rewriting

For most authors, writing typically involves a substantial number of drafts to communicate effectively with readers. Multiple drafts allow you to refine the content, to enhance the synthesis of ideas in a paper, and to improve the organization of information. This is because writing is itself a learning process. The more you learn about the topic, the more effectively you may write about it. Successive drafts tend to get better because you are more knowledgeable with practice.

Although there are different styles of writing and rewriting, redrafting different sections of the paper simultaneously, rather than one by one, often helps to achieve better structural and conceptual integration. This involves jumping from section to section and adding or deleting content as appropriate. This process also helps to ensure consistency in writing style and language use through the paper. Every paper should be read at least once as

BOX 31.2   Examples of Abstracts

Abstracts, like entire research reports, can vary in their format according to the methods used in the study. Following are two examples of abstracts. The first is from a quantitative study, and the second is from a qualitative study.

Abstract by Roche and Taylor (2005)

Existing studies have shown that individuals with chronic fatigue syndrome (CFS) demonstrate functional impairment in a number of domains related to occupational participation. Researchers have not yet explored whether coping styles may be associated with occupational participation in individuals with this condition. The aim of this study was to examine the effects of coping styles on occupational participation among adults with CFS. We hypothesized that occupational participation would be associated with coping strategies oriented toward information seeking and maintaining activity, and that this relationship would endure despite individual differences in illness severity. The study used a cross-sectional design to describe the associations between coping and occupational participation for 47 individuals diagnosed with CFS. Findings from linear regression analysis revealed that the coping style of maintaining activity was positively associated with occupational participation whereas accommodating to the illness was negatively associated. Implications of the findings for continued research and clinical practice in occupational therapy are discussed.

Abstract by Farnworth, Nitikin, and Fossey (2004)

Institutional environments are challenging settings in which to provide rehabilitation. This study describes the time use of a group of inpatients, the majority diagnosed with schizophrenia, in a secure forensic psychiatric unit in Australia. Time diaries, interviews, and field notes were collected over 5 weeks. Eight participants completed time diaries for 2 consecutive days, of whom five were also interviewed using the Occupational Performance History Interview-II.

Participants' time use was dominated by personal care and leisure occupations. In general, participants were dissatisfied with their time use, describing themselves as "bored" or "killing time." Many perceived that the environment created barriers to their participation in valued occupations, yet some also found occupations that provided solace, challenge, or connection with the outside world.

The findings indicate the importance of understanding individuals' unique occupational histories, interests, and skills to create opportunities to engage them in relevant occupations that utilize personal resources, as part of forensic rehabilitation programs, and the utility of the Occupational Performance History Interview-II in this context. Further research exploring patient and staff perspectives on the challenges of occupational programming in forensic settings and the longitudinal impact of such programming on inpatients' occupational functioning, health, and well-being is recommended.

a whole with an eye toward editing it to be a more integrated piece.

Strategy 8: Seeking and Using Feedback

Seeking feedback by having others read and comment on drafts of a paper can be very helpful. Writers always know more about what they want to say than do their readers. Consequently, when rereading your own work, it is easy to make mental assumptions and linkages that are not in the paper or apparent to the reader. Constructive feedback from someone else can help to identify assumed knowledge, missing links, and unanswered questions that a reader may have. Such feedback is extremely helpful for redrafting a paper.

There are different ways to get feedback on a paper. The following are some examples:

• Coaching from an experienced writer in your discipline/area of research (someone who knows the topic, as well as the intended audience and journal). This type of reviewer may provide feedback paragraph by paragraph on technical aspects of the writing, as well as on larger issues central to research.

• Participating in writing groups with peers. This process is helpful for developing overall writing skills because you not only receive feedback but also learn from reading and critiquing others' writing. Also, by mutually agreeing on deadlines for writing part or all of a manuscript, writers can help each other maintain discipline in writing.

• Asking for feedback from colleagues with differing disciplines or professional backgrounds who reflect the targeted audience. This type of feedback can be valuable in helping you step outside of familiar ways of presenting things and point out when papers are too full of jargon or insider perspectives. This type of feedback is especially useful when you are aiming for publication in an interdisciplinary journal.

An important form of feedback also comes as part of the review process following submission of a paper for consideration for publication. Written comments prepared by referees for authors are intended to provide constructive feedback about the content, structure, and presentation of the manuscript and to guide the authors in subsequent revision of their manuscripts. Revisions are almost always required, so being asked to make some revisions should not be taken by authors as an indication that a manuscript is of poor quality. Authors are well advised to pay careful attention to the referees' comments and recommendations in revising a manuscript.

If a journal decides not to accept a manuscript for publication, one should carefully examine the feedback. Rejection may mean the paper does not rise to the level of quality necessary for publication. It may mean that one needs to submit the paper to another journal. Generally, it is necessary also to revise the manuscript to address the new journal's style and format requirements, to ensure the writing "speaks" to the new readership, and to improve the manuscript on the basis of feedback from the previous submission. Attending carefully to the referees' feedback and seeking advice, or coaching, from colleagues with publishing experience can often be helpful at this stage.

Organizing the Components of Your Literature Review

The introduction to your literature review provides the context for what follows in the rest of the paper. In other words, it sets the scene by outlining:

- The area and topic;
- The impact or significance of the problem to society;
- The nature of the problem or issue being addressed by the review; and
- The relevance of the review to the professional and/or scientific community that is assumed to be the audience for the paper.

The introduction may also include a statement of the significance of the topic. Thomas (2000) suggests that a significance statement should be phrased along the following lines: "The problem I am studying affects lots of people in a particularly unfortunate way and/or costs a lot of money" (p. 35). The significance of a topic is the underlying reason that it was important to conduct a review of the topic. A second reason that a review of the literature is undertaken is to identify what is already known about a topic and the methods with which it is typically studied.

The major tasks in preparing and writing a literature review, therefore, are to locate, appraise, and then summarize the previous research relevant to the topic. You should address the issues and controversies that are raised in the literature and identify the gaps in the current knowledge base that provide the rationale for future research on the topic (i.e., the research study you are planning to conduct). Brown (1996) poses seven questions that should be answered in writing a review of literature:

1. Why is this topic important?
2. What is known about the topic?
3. What is unknown about this topic?
4. Why are some things unknown?
5. Why should the gaps be filled?
6. Which gaps does one propose to fill, and has one chosen them?
7. How does one propose to fill them?

If it is helpful in your approach to writing, the outline of your literature review may be structured around these questions.

In the literature review section of a research paper, it will not be possible to discuss the full scope and volume of literature on the research topic. The aim of a literature review is not to demonstrate the breadth and depth of the investigator's knowledge of the literature. Rather, the aim is to address the previously listed questions and, in so doing, to make apparent the underlying logic for undertaking a study of your topic.

Both accurate representation and **critical appraisal** of the literature are important to an effective literature review. Critical appraisal is an essential component of every literature review and a means of evaluating key aspects of the literature on a topic. Critical appraisal will:

- Identify the current trends and ways of thinking about the topic and how to research it;
- Identify the boundaries of the literature (e.g., what particular populations, settings, and perspectives were studied in the previous research?);
- Illuminate the gaps in the current knowledge base and the way in which it has developed;
- Evaluate the strengths and weakness of existing research approaches to studying the topic; and

- Make an argument for why any conflicting or differing research findings exist (if they exist).

DePoy and Gitlin (2011) suggest the following structure for organizing a literature review:

- Introduction, which includes defining the focus and scope of the review;
- Discussion of each specific concept, principle, or theory in the current literature on the topic;
- Brief overview of key studies, compared in parallel rather than serially, to achieve a critical appraisal of the current research;
- Integration of the work reviewed, identifying the relationships, inconsistencies among findings across studies, controversies, and gaps in the literature;
- Identification of the niche in the current knowledge base that your research fills; and
- Justification/rationale for the study and its design.

These components are typical of many literature reviews, but it should be remembered that the review is designed to characterize the content of literature that is relevant to the topic and that makes sense of the chosen question and research methods. Thus, there are instances in which the state of the literature, or the nature of the research question, may dictate a somewhat different structure. For example, if a study examines something for which little or no previous research is reported, the literature review may focus on providing the rationale for the importance of the topic area or extrapolate from literature that is only partly related to the research question. Also, some journals have formats that require literature to be succinctly reviewed as part of the introduction, rather than as a separate section. In these cases, the review may be structured differently, but it still needs to appraise the key literature of relevance.

Summary

In this chapter, we discussed the fundamental elements of writing a literature review. Specifically, we discussed both the usual content that goes into such a paper and the process of writing itself. As noted at the outset, many investigators thoroughly enjoy the writing process. Even those who find it very enjoyable know that good writing takes time and effort and requires personal discipline, persistence, and an openness to criticism and feedback.

Review Questions

1. Of all of the strategies for effective writing, which three are most important for you to keep in mind? Explain why this is the case.

2. What are three circumstances under which you might be required to write a general literature review?
3. What are the differences between a general literature review and a systematic literature review?
4. What are the fundamental components of a literature review?
5. What is the role of critical appraisal in a literature review?

REFERENCES

American Psychological Association. (2009). *Publication manual of the American Psychological Association* (6th ed.). Washington, DC: Author.
Arksey, H., & O'Malley, L. (2005). Scoping studies: Towards a methodological framework. *International Journal of Social Research and Methodology, 8* (1), 19–32.
Bihl-Hulme, J. (1985). Creative thinking in problem-based learning. In D. Bond (Ed.), *Problem-based learning in education for the professions* (pp. 177–183). Sydney, Australia: HERDSA.
Brown, R. (1994). The "big picture" about managing writing. In O. Zuber-Skerritt & Y. Ryan (Eds.), *Quality in postgraduate education—issues and processes* (pp. 90–109). London, England: Kogan Page.
Brown, R. (1996). *Key skills for writing and publishing research* (3rd ed.). Brisbane, Australia: Write Way Consulting.
Brown, R. F., Rogers, D. J., & Pressland, A. J. (1993). Righting scientific writing: Focus on your main message! *Rangelands Journal, 15*(2), 183–189.
Brown, R. F., Rogers, D. J., & Pressland, A. J. (1994). Create a clear focus: The "big picture" about writing better research articles. *American Entomologist, 40,* 144–145.
Buzan, T., & Buzan, B. (2000). *The mind map book* (3rd ed.). London, England: BBC Worldwide.
DePoy, E., & Gitlin, L. N. (2011). *Introduction to research: Multiple strategies for health and human services* (4th ed.). St. Louis, MO: C. V. Mosby.
Farnworth, L., Nitikin, L., & Fossey, E. (2004). Being in a secure forensic psychiatry unit: Every day's the same, killing time or making the most of it. *British Journal of Occupational Therapy, 67*(10), 430–438.
Roche, R., & Taylor, R. R. (2005). Coping and occupational participation in chronic fatigue syndrome. *Occupational Therapy Journal of Research, 25,* 75–83.
Sandelowski, M. (2008). Reading, writing and systematic review. *Journal of Advanced Nursing, 64*(1), 104–110.
Thomas, S. A. (2000). *How to write health sciences papers, dissertations and theses.* Edinburgh, Scotland: Churchill Livingstone.

RESOURCES

Brown, R. (1996). *Key skills for writing and publishing research* (3rd ed.). Brisbane, Australia: Write Way Consulting.
Hayes, R. L. (1996). Writing for publication: Solutions to common problems. *Australian Occupational Therapy Journal, 43,* 24–29.
Sandelowski, M. (2008). Reading, writing and systematic review. *Journal of Advanced Nursing, 64*(1), 104–110.
Thomas, S. A. (2000). *How to write health sciences papers, dissertations and theses.* Edinburgh, Scotland: Churchill Livingstone.

CHAPTER 32

Disseminating Research: Presenting, Writing, and Publishing

Gary Kielhofner • Ellie Fossey • Renée R. Taylor

Learning Outcomes

- Define the aims accomplished by disseminating research in occupational therapy.
- Understand the range of approaches to the dissemination of research.
- Discuss the process of peer review and why it serves as an important gauge of research rigor and quality.
- Differentiate between the needs of various stakeholders, such as funding agencies, consumers, advocacy groups, and academic audiences, in presenting research findings.
- List several options for dissemination that are available when the target audience includes consumers and advocacy groups.

Introduction

Research that is not publicly shared is incomplete. **Dissemination,** defined as the spoken or written distribution of research findings and their impact for scholarly and public consumption, is a key step in the research process, and thus before any investigation is undertaken, the researcher should plan ahead for how and when it will be shared.

Research is undertaken for the larger benefit of the scientific community and the public. Research dissemination communicates new knowledge to these constituencies. Moreover, when disseminating research, the investigator describes the research process so that peer scholars are able to evaluate its rigor and to replicate or build upon the study to advance science. Finally, dissemination shares knowledge with stakeholders so it can be used for practical ends (Mercier, Bordeleau, Caron, Garcia, & Latimer, 2004).

Participating in the discourse that advances research can, in turn, inform practice in a particular area. There is a growing emphasis in many sectors on assuring the utilization of research results. As a result, researchers are combining traditional concerns for scientific rigor with thinking about how successful outcomes would be applied within actual health-care settings (Peters, 2014). This growing emphasis on ensuring the practical impact of findings has underscored the importance of a comprehensive approach to dissemination. Such an approach helps ensure that the information generated through the research reaches the right audiences in a format that allows them to effectively use it to change and enhance their behavior and practices.

This chapter discusses the rationale, process, and range of mechanisms for disseminating research.

The Nature and Role of Dissemination

Dissemination refers to the processes by which researchers inform others within and beyond the scholarly community about their research process and what they have learned from it. As we will see, there are multiple ways that research can be disseminated. Each of these is suited to a particular audience and purpose.

In occupational therapy, the dissemination of research addresses the following aims:

- Making new information available to members of the profession to build and support evidence-based practice;
- Making information available to scholars in related disciplines who are doing research in the same or related areas so that they can incorporate and build upon the methods and findings;
- Permitting criticism and replication, each of which is necessary to the refinement and further development of professional knowledge;
- Making information available to consumers; and
- Making information available to entities and persons who fund and/or make decisions and policy that impact the availability and delivery of occupational therapy services.

CASE EXAMPLE

Tamica serves as a graduate research assistant for a study examining the effects of a unique type of graded physical conditioning on fatigue severity following breast cancer treatment. After several months of program implementation and data collection, Tamica has been assigned to conduct statistical analyses of the data and to plan a dissemination approach. Tamica conducts the analyses and shares them with Dr. Larsen. The findings suggest strong support for the study hypothesis, which is that the graded physical conditioning program is associated with lower self-reported fatigue severity and decreased evidence of muscle fatigue during and for 2 months following radiation therapy to the breast.

The principal investigator of the study, Dr. Larsen, has received a significant amount of funding for the study from the American Cancer Society. The fact that the funding source is a private, not-for-profit agency supported by donations from people with cancer, as well as their friends and families, should influence Tamica's dissemination plan. For this reason, Tamica recommends to Dr. Larsen a multipronged dissemination approach that includes publishing the findings in a peer-reviewed scientific journal, presenting the findings verbally for a lay audience at the CEO's Against Cancer National Meeting, presenting the findings verbally for a multidisciplinary audience at the American Association for Cancer Research, presenting the findings verbally at the American Occupational Therapy Association conference, posting an announcement about study findings on Dr. Larsen's university website, and working with media relations within her university to issue a press release. These approaches will ensure that academic audiences are made aware of the methodological details and findings, that the funding agency and its constituents are made aware of the impact of the funding on outcomes for people with cancer, and that rehabilitation professionals such as occupational therapists, as well as physicians and other health-care professionals, are made aware of the findings. Additionally, if the press release is successful and the findings make it into local or national news, there is an even greater opportunity that the findings will reach people with cancer, their caregivers, and their health-care professionals.

In planning and implementing a particular form of dissemination, one should always consider its purposes. Next, we briefly discuss each of the aims to which dissemination can be directed. It should be kept in mind that any particular act of dissemination has the potential to address more than one of these aims.

Making New Information Available to Members of the Profession

As discussed previously in this book, there is a professional obligation to base practice on evidence. Many different forms of evidence can inform practice; however, the most rigorous is generated through research. Most research conducted by occupational therapy (OT) researchers will have either direct or indirect implications for practice. By making their findings available, researchers are supporting their practitioner peers to provide services in line with evidence. In planning and reporting research, investigators should consider how their research can contribute to practice. Thus, a critical part of research dissemination is to discuss the practice implications of the findings. In the case example at the beginning of this chapter, Tamica wanted to ensure that the findings about the success of Dr. Larsen's unique approach to graded exercise were widely shared among practitioners specializing in breast cancer survivorship. Therefore, she arranged a number of in-service presentations at all of the hospitals with breast cancer survivorship within 100 miles of Dr. Larsen's laboratory, offering continuing education credits to a wide range of rehabilitation professionals in attendance. Additionally, she and Dr. Larsen submitted proposals to present findings at state and national conferences attended by a large number of practitioners, including the Tennessee Occupational Therapy Association conference and the American Occupational Therapy Association conference.

Making Information Available to Scholars in Related Disciplines

OT researchers conduct their investigations within an interdisciplinary context. First, occupational therapists mostly use research methods that were developed in other fields. Second, OT researchers are often investigating topics on which there is also interdisciplinary research. Further, even when therapists are investigating topics of specific interest to the profession, it is likely that their findings will have some relevance to members of other professions and disciplines.

Making one's research available to an interdisciplinary audience is an important way of participating in the discourse that advances research in a particular area. Reporting findings in an interdisciplinary context allows others to incorporate and build upon one's methods and findings. It is a way of returning something to the larger scientific community, from which the profession benefits. Moreover, the reputation of occupational therapists is enhanced when others encounter quality research conducted by them. Finally, disseminating findings in the interdisciplinary context informs others of the profession's particular perspective and concepts. Taking the example at the beginning of this chapter, Tamica and Dr. Larsen wanted to ensure that the findings from their study were shared with a broader audience of multidisciplinary rehabilitation professionals. To accomplish this aim, Tamica planned a two-pronged approach. First, they presented their findings to an academic audience at the annual conference of the American College of Rehabilitation Medicine. To reach physical therapy practitioners, they submitted a proposal to the annual convention of the American Physical Therapy Association. In both of these cases, they reviewed the guidelines for submission and, in some cases, made personal inquiries to the conference organizers to ensure that any overlap in content presented at one conference versus another one was permitted.

Permitting Criticism and Replication

One of the most demanding aspects of research is submitting to public scrutiny. Anyone who has submitted for review or published research is aware that such efforts almost assuredly generate feedback concerning the limitations and flaws of the research and its presentation. After one has worked hard for months or years to plan and implement research, it is not easy to hear others criticize it.

Nonetheless, this critique is an essential aspect of all research. By explicating how findings were generated, dissemination allows others to judge how much confidence they wish to place in the findings, given the limits and flaws in the particular research process. No investigation is ever perfect,

and it is important that others can objectively critique and learn from it. For example, before each one of her conference and in-service presentations, Dr. Larsen prepared Tamica to present certain limitations involving the research design, sample size, and assessments used for their graded exercise study just after the concluding slide of the presentation.

Dissemination is also important so that others can understand and replicate one's research. Replications are conducted to confirm whether similar results are obtained when studies are repeated by others and to test the generalizability of findings to different samples and situations. Subsequent research that fails to reproduce the earlier study's findings can help to illuminate flaws that were not apparent in the original research, or to distinguish the context-specific elements of the findings from those that are common across settings. When research findings are replicated by others, the scientific community places more confidence in them. Taking the Case Example from the beginning of the chapter, Tamica was careful to review the research protocol before each presentation she made so that she would be able to answer even the most detailed questions about the methodological approach to the graded exercise study. Because graded exercise is a topic of high impact and relevance in breast cancer rehabilitation, many researchers in the audience had questions about the methods and were eager to begin replication studies with women with different stages of breast cancer receiving different types of cancer treatment.

Making Information Available to Consumers and/or Participants

Consumers include persons who are receiving, or whose family members are receiving or may receive, OT services. Consumers also include advocacy and lobby groups that represent the interests of people in the community for whom the research has relevance. Research should be shared with consumers whenever it can enable them to make informed decisions about the need for and likely outcomes of services. This means that researchers should be willing to share research findings in ways that are accessible to consumers. Moreover, investigators are ethically obligated to provide information about research findings to agencies and/or individuals who participate in the research (Sieber & Tolich, 2013). For example, individual patients at the hospitals where Tamica gave in-service presentations and members of breast cancer survivor support groups within her geographical region represent the direct consumers of Tamica's research.

Making Information Available to Funding and Decision-Making Entities

Research can serve as a means of demonstrating the value of OT services. Such research has the potential of influencing persons to make affirmative decisions concerning reimbursing and making OT services available. For example, because the findings from Dr. Larsen's study ultimately made the national press, bringing reputational credit to the university and its affiliated medical center, she caught the attention of the hospital leadership, who noticed that she was an occupational therapist. The following year, a new budget line allowing for the hiring of one more occupational therapist specializing in cancer rehabilitation was added to the rehabilitation unit.

Peer Review

In most professional and virtually all scientific venues, one must submit the proposed poster, presentation, or journal article for peer review. **Peer review** is defined as a systematic approach to the review of a scientific work by others with expertise in the area being presented. The peer review process is used to ensure the quality of information disseminated and its suitability for the particular conference audience or journal readership.

Dissemination through peer-reviewed channels is essential to all research. Its importance is linked to the fact that the peer review process provides quality control. Presentations, posters, and published articles that have gone through a review process have been scrutinized. The peer review process assures that investigators have fully described their methods to allow evaluation of rigor and replication. It also serves to ensure that the claims about discovered knowledge made by the author(s) are warranted and that adequate attention is paid to the limitations of the study. Thus, peer review often improves the quality of the information presented about both the research process and findings to better serve those listening to, or reading, that information.

The Purpose of Reviews

Review procedures are intended to maintain the quality and standard of conferences and academic journals. For conference presentations and posters, this review process focuses on the quality and suitability of submitted abstracts (i.e., brief summaries of proposed presentations/posters) and is typically undertaken by an expert panel/committee responsible for selection of the program content.

In contrast, the review process for journal publication involves review of full-length research papers (also referred to as manuscripts) written and submitted to the journal by the researchers, which are then reviewed by designated members of the journal's editorial board or team of referees. For OT journals, peer review also ensures that published papers reflect and build on current thinking and developments within the field of occupational therapy.

Each journal has its own requirements for the format of papers, how many copies must be submitted, whether electronic copies are required/permitted, and so forth. These requirements are noted in the guide to authors, which can generally be found on the journal's website (if it has one) and/or in a copy of the journal itself. Journals ordinarily do not have deadlines. An exception is when a special issue of a journal is announced. Generally special issues of a journal focus on a given research topic, or method, and may involve one or more guest editors. These special issues are usually announced though a call for papers with a specified submission deadline.

Referees, the people who undertake reviews of papers submitted to journals, usually have experience in writing for publication, and they represent the broad range of professional backgrounds relevant to the journal's particular field. In occupational therapy, this means referees are likely to be occupational therapists and scholars in the field of occupational therapy and related fields who have the necessary publishing experience and expertise in particular practice areas and/or inquiry methods to review and constructively evaluate the types of work submitted for publication in OT journals.

Blind Review

Many, but not all, scientific/professional journals utilize blind review. Blind review means that the review procedure is undertaken by the referee(s) without the author(s) of a manuscript being identified to the referee(s). Blind review procedures are intended to foster fair evaluation of the quality and standard of the manuscript on its merits, by minimizing the extent to which knowledge of the authorship might influence opinions expressed by the referee about the work or bias the referee's judgment.

Consumer Review

Although less common than review by scientific/professional peers, consumer review is increasingly considered important and included for some dissemination venues. Consumer reviews offer the perspective of persons who participated in the study or those for whom the research is intended. Consumer review is intended to evaluate the relevance and applicability of research for consumer audiences, and facilitate its presentation in lay terms.

The Review Process

Peer review for journal articles requires submission of a full manuscript that is intended for publication. The manuscript will be forwarded to two to three reviewers whose expertise overlaps with the methodological and/or substantive content of the manuscript. Reviewers ordinarily are provided with detailed guidelines and forms for completing the review process and making recommendations about the disposition of the manuscript. Generally, reviewers are asked to make one of the following recommendations:

* Rejection,
* Invitation to make major revision and submit for re-review (in which case the revised manuscript is ordinarily re-reviewed by one or more of the original reviewers), or
* Acceptance pending minor or no revisions.

In addition to recommending disposition of the manuscript, reviewers generally provide detailed feedback, which provides the rationale for the recommendation and, when revisions are asked for, guidance to the author(s) of the manuscript as to the kind of revisions required.

The journal editor considers the reviewers' feedback, decides on a course of action, and then communicates to the author(s) whether the paper is rejected, invited to be resubmitted with revisions, or accepted with minor or no revisions. The editor ordinarily shares the outcome in a detailed letter, which provides the rationale and spells out any requested revisions.

Different journals have differing standards for and rates of manuscript acceptance. For extremely competitive journals, the majority of manuscripts submitted will be rejected. Authors who have had articles rejected from these top-tier journals often find their manuscripts accepted by less competitive journals. Experienced investigators choose the level of journal to which they originally submit papers based on their assessment of the quality and sophistication of their study as determined by such factors as design rigor, sample size, and degree of innovation.

In the case of papers that are accepted for publication, the most common experience of authors is to make fairly substantial revisions, which are then reexamined by reviewers and/or the editor. Anyone who wishes to publish research must be prepared to accept criticism and have a full measure of patience. After submitting a manuscript, one ordinarily waits 3 to 6 months for initial feedback. If revisions are required, a similar period after submission of the revised manuscript lapses before the author(s) receive the second round of feedback. Often at this stage the author must make additional (usually more minor) edits and submit a manuscript, which is then copyedited in most instances. Some months later, and prior to publication, the author ordinarily receives a galley proof (i.e., a facsimile of the article as it will appear in the journal), which must be checked for accuracy and returned with any corrections to the journal. A minimum of 6 months can be expected to elapse from the time of submission until publication, and more often the process takes upward of a year.

The process of review for conference presentations or posters begins with a call for abstracts with a deadline. Calls for papers and posters generally occur several months in advance of the conference. Authors are notified of the decision about whether their paper/poster is accepted well in advance of the conference. Each conference has its own rules for the length and content of an abstract. Some conferences publish abstracts of papers and posters that are selected for inclusion in a conference proceeding. Historically, abstracts were submitted on paper. Many conferences today use electronic formats, such as submission via a website.

Non-Peer-Reviewed Presentations and Publications

Not all of one's scholarly and scientific work requires publication in peer-reviewed venues. For example, an article tailored to a lay professional audience without specific expertise in the topic area is more appropriately published in a magazine or newsletter distributed by one's state or national professional organization. Non-peer-reviewed venues for dissemination also serve important roles. These venues include:

* Invited presentations,
* Continuing education,

- Books,
- Professional publications and newsletters,
- Nonprint materials containing information about research findings and their implications.

Each of these venues is described briefly in the following sections.

Invited Presentations

Conference organizers and academic and practice organizations and associations often invite outside speakers to present information generated from research. Although the specific content of these presentations is not peer reviewed, it is ordinarily the case that speakers (and sometimes their topics) are chosen because of the positive reputation of the quality of the speaker (and the research presented). Some invited presentations are associated with awards or honors, and the choice of speakers and topics is highly selective. Other venues, such as a routine research colloquium or "brown-bag" lunch presentations offered in an academic department, have open invitations for persons of varying levels of research accomplishment to present their work and obtain feedback. All of these venues, from the most prestigious to the routine, can be important opportunities for sharing information about research.

Continuing Education

Continuing education provides an important means of ensuring that professionals and researchers remain current in their knowledge and skills. The typical vehicle for continuing education is a workshop (ranging from a few hours to several days). Typically, one or more persons who are recognized experts will organize a program of sequential topics in a specific area of interest. Such workshops may provide opportunities for related studies to be presented and synthesized. Workshops are also an excellent venue for discussions of the practical challenges of doing research and the practice implications of findings.

Books

Books may or may not be peer reviewed, depending on the publisher and the topic. Additionally, the level of rigor of the peer review, including the backgrounds of the individuals selected to serve as reviewers for the book, varies greatly. This is, in part, due to the availability of people to review

books. Many scientists feel that their efforts are better placed reviewing journal articles because it keeps them closer to the cutting edge of developments in their respective fields. In some fields, it is common to report the results of research in a full book, necessitating peer review. It is not commonplace in occupational therapy. However, books do often describe, summarize, and synthesize research. For example, OT textbooks often make reference to research findings in discussing practice. In addition, books that present theoretical models typically describe the kinds of research that have been conducted to develop, apply, and test those models.

Professional Publications and Newsletters

A variety of professional magazines and newsletters can be useful resources for sharing research findings and their implications. *OT Practice*, published by the American Occupational Therapy Association, is one example of such a professional magazine. Although it does not feature the more technical discussions of research that appear in refereed journals, it can be an appropriate venue for discussing how research findings can be integrated into practice.

Newsletters are another appropriate vehicle for discussing the applied relevance of research. Some large institutional research programs and federal agencies that fund research also produce publications that share research findings. Finally, there are agencies whose purpose is to disseminate research. They produce a variety of publications that share research. Most of these venues secure articles by inviting authors to write, accepting contributed articles, and using in-house writers to compose articles. If there are not published guidelines for accepting contributed papers, this information can usually be obtained from the editor. In most cases, it is up to the editor of the publication to decide whether or not to include a particular topic or paper.

Websites Containing Information About Research Findings and Their Implications

With the growth of the Internet, a wide range of electronic sources now contain information related to research. These include sites specific

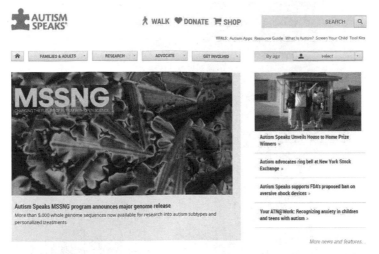

Figure 32.1   Information is often now disseminated on websites that are used by practitioners, patients, and caregivers, such as www.AutismSpeaks.org. *©2016 Autism Speaks Inc.*

to areas of research or even specific to individual research projects. Often, Web-based dissemination can serve both professional and other stakeholder audiences. Information can also be made available in different formats to suit these constituencies (Fig. 32.1).

Disseminating to Professionals and Scientists

The most common ways of disseminating research to professional and scientific peers occurs in the form of presentations and posters at conferences and journal publications. These can be either peer-reviewed or non-peer-reviewed venues. Peer-reviewed venues are more common for the presentation of the research methodology and findings. Non-peer-reviewed professional publications are generally more appropriate for emphasizing the significance of research findings for practice.

Dissemination mechanisms should be chosen to ensure that research findings are effectively communicated and utilized (Patton, 2008). Thus, it is important to consider:

- Who should know about the outcomes of this research?
- What information will be of most relevance to each of these various audiences (e.g., individuals, agencies, policymakers)?

- What will be the most effective mechanisms for sharing this information with them?

Verbal Presentations and Posters at Conferences

Professional and scientific conferences provide opportunities for investigators to share the process and results of recent research on a shorter timeline than publication. Conferences also provide a unique opportunity for members of the scientific/professional community to meet each other, discuss research informally, make connections, and share information that can benefit future research, as well as to interact with other stakeholders. The feedback that presenters receive can be helpful to preparation of a manuscript for publication. For these reasons, investigators frequently seek to present the results of their research first at conferences and later in published format.

Presentations

Presentations of scientific papers are usually brief (i.e., 10 to 30 minutes). Some time is ordinarily scheduled following presentations for brief public discussion. Verbal presentations are primarily an oral medium, so they rely on both the content of the presentation and its delivery by the presenter(s).

A good presentation is characterized by clarity, conciseness, and attention to the target audience. Generally, the quality of a presentation depends

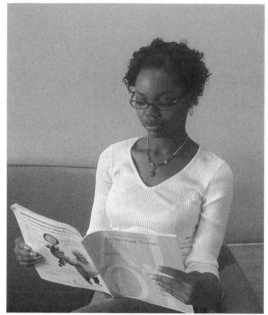

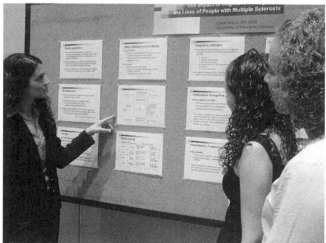

Figure 32.2   Researchers disseminate results in a variety of ways, including poster presentations at national professional conferences such as the annual meeting of the American Occupational Therapy Association, through publications in journals such as *American Journal of Occupational Therapy,* and through local media such as local news programs.

not only on the verbal content, but also on the graphic representation of the research. PowerPoint presentations are typical in modern conferences, and they may be supplemented with audience handouts. The use of these elements allows the presenter to emphasize major points, supplement verbal presentation with visual illustration, and provide attendees with information that goes beyond what can be presented within the time limit of the presentation (Fig. 32.2).

Scientific Posters

Poster presentations are ordinarily exhibited in a large room or hall that accommodates a number of posters simultaneously. Conference attendees view and select those they wish to read in detail. The authors are expected to be present during scheduled poster sessions, so they can further explain the content of their posters in response to questions. Posters may also be available for viewing

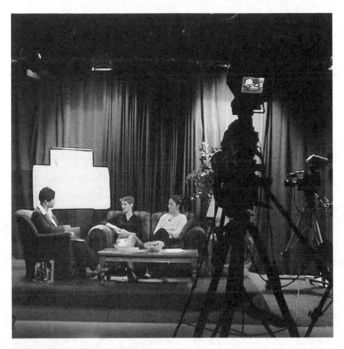

Figure 32.2 *Continued*

outside the scheduled poster session, depending on the conference rules.

The essential feature of a good poster is that the message is clear and understandable without the presenter and that it achieves a balance between words and graphics. A range of visual techniques can assist in presenting information in interesting and informative ways. These include, for instance, photographs; diagrams; tables; graphs; and layout methods, such as flowcharts and dot points.

Conference organizers typically provide specific guidelines about poster content, format, and size requirements. Familiarity with these requirements and attention to production design, clarity of content, colors, layout, and finishing are important to maximize effectiveness. It is important to be selective—that is, to include the key information to make the research understandable to the reader, but not to overload the poster with details.

Choosing a Poster or Verbal Format for Presentation

Choosing whether to orally present a paper or to present a poster at a conference involves several considerations. Generally, oral presentations are more competitive than posters, so depending on the overall level of acceptance rates for papers at a conference, one may consider the likelihood of having a verbal presentation versus a poster accepted. Poster sessions are also more likely to accept presentations of preliminary findings and research in process.

Posters are primarily a visual medium for sharing information. Poster presentations provide graphic and textual means to illustrate studies and their outcomes. They are particularly valuable for information that is best presented using schematic diagrams and flowcharts. The fact that a poster can be viewed at one's own pace and discretion may make it possible for others to better absorb the information than from verbal presentation. Because conference poster sessions involve face-to-face interaction, they tend to facilitate networking with others interested in related research.

Verbally presenting a paper allows one to share information with an audience in real time. For many investigators, it is the only time one shares research face to face with members of the scientific and professional community. Because much of research can involve long hours of private writing and interaction with others through written means, the verbal presentation is something many researchers value. Presentations are usually competitively selected, so the fact of presenting research gives it an air of authority. All in all, presentations are a time for researchers to engage in the most public aspect of the scientific process.

Peer-Reviewed Journal Publications

As discussed earlier in this chapter in the section on peer review, peer-reviewed journal publications represent the *sine qua non* in terms of disseminating one's scientific work to an audience of academic and research-oriented peers. Peer-reviewed journals, sometimes referred to as "refereed" journals, draw upon the expertise of researchers who have published extensively in a given topic area to review and opine in terms of the overall quality, relevance, impact, and methodological rigor of an article submitted by another researcher. These experts in a content area or discipline often comprise the editorial board of a given journal. Others are invited to review submitted articles on an ad-hoc basis, particularly if they have specific expertise in a narrow topic area with which editorial board members are less familiar.

Peer-reviewed journals vary in the extent to which they drill down to focused topics within a given subject area. Generally, peer-reviewed journals are specific either to a particular discipline and/or to a particular topic. For example, the *Scandinavian Journal of Occupational Therapy* is specific to the discipline of occupational therapy. It contains articles reflecting original research that contributes new knowledge on a wide range of topics within the discipline of occupational therapy. Alternatively, the *Journal of Stroke and Cerebrovascular Diseases* cuts across disciplines and contains articles specific to the topic of stroke and other cerebrovascular disorders.

Disseminating to Stakeholders

Historically, research dissemination focused on the scientific and professional communities through the kinds of means discussed earlier. There is increasing emphasis today on sharing research with various stakeholder audiences. **Stakeholders** refer to anyone outside the scientific and professional community who may be informed or influenced by the research findings either in their personal lives or in the exercise of their responsibilities. These include but are not limited to:

• Individuals and agencies that participate in the research,

• Consumers of health services for whom the research has relevance,
• Officials and agencies that make decisions and policies that might be informed by the research,
• Entities that address needs and/or fund services related to the research, and
• The general public, whose attitudes or behavior might be influenced by the research findings.

The avenues for disseminating research to these audiences are multiple. Major ones include:

• Procedures for sharing findings with the study participants;
• Public presentations to consumer and community groups and collaborating organizations;
• Reports to government and private agencies, legislative bodies, and public officials;
• Websites, targeted brochures, and other media for laypersons; and
• Releases to the popular press and media.

Each of these means offers opportunities to disseminate research to audiences beyond scholarly and professional communities. They are discussed next.

Sharing Information With Research Participants

Researchers have an ethical responsibility to disseminate information about research findings and outcomes with research participants (Sieber & Tolich, 2013). This responsibility is ordinarily not fulfilled by publication of results. Therefore, other dissemination mechanisms should be considered. One such mechanism for disseminating information to research participants is to prepare and send a written summary of the research findings to all participants and participating agencies. This approach has the advantages of being both low cost and time efficient, so it is particularly well suited to studies with large numbers of participants. Limitations of this approach are that it does not promote discussion about the potential uses of the research findings, nor does it enable participants to give feedback to the researchers.

Choosing the approach to disseminating to participants depends on the nature of the research process, the kind of information generated, and the audience being addressed. The following questions are helpful to consider in developing mechanisms for sharing information about research in these forums:

• What information from this research project could be helpful or useful to the research participants?

- What methods of information sharing are likely to facilitate respectful and sensitive communication with the research participants?
- What methods of information sharing are most likely to facilitate the research participants' understanding of this research?
- What methods of information sharing are likely to empower the research participants to engage with the material and identify its potential uses/implications for them?
- What resources are available for sharing the findings?

The use of technologies, such as e-mail, websites, and Internet discussion groups, has the potential to both efficiently disseminate research findings and enhance dialogue among researchers, participants, and relevant community groups about research. For this approach to be effective, use of these technologies must be widespread among the relevant stakeholder groups. Face-to-face meetings with participants, participating agencies, and community groups provide more targeted opportunities to discuss findings with relevant audiences and to gain feedback from them (McConnell & Kerbs, 1993).

Individually tailored feedback is labor intensive, but it is particularly useful in research involving performance-based assessments and disempowered or marginalized groups (Fossey, Epstein, Findlay, Plant, & Harvey, 2002). For example, in an Australian study involving participants with psychiatric disabilities, Fossey et al. (2002) developed and evaluated a process for sharing individual feedback with the participants about their occupational performance, based on results of the Assessment of Motor and Process Skills (AMPS) (Fisher, 2003). The investigators prepared written information for each participant, adopting a strengths-based approach in which the person's occupational performance strengths were described, and some ways in which these strengths could be used to overcome areas of difficulty were suggested. This written information was shared face to face, accompanied by verbal explanation. Participants reported that the focus of the feedback on strengths was helpful, and the verbal explanation was seen as essential to enabling their understanding and use of the written information.

Different research traditions have approached the issue of dissemination to stakeholders in different ways. For example, in the quantitative tradition, research tends to be viewed as the researcher's expertise, product, and property. Thus, providing feedback is usually viewed as a didactic process, in which the researcher gives information to stakeholders (Fossey et al., 2002). In contrast, qualitative research traditions, and particularly participatory inquiry approaches, view knowledge production as a shared process and findings as shared property. Feedback is considered integral to the research process, being a mechanism for ensuring validity and sharing power in the research relationship (Fossey et al., 2002; Guba & Lincoln, 1989; Patton, 2008). In participatory research, information sharing tends to be iterative, rather than unidirectional. Thus, sharing information with the research participants is an essential part of the research process.

Public Presentations to Consumer and Community Groups and Collaborating Organizations

Research findings may be shared with consumer groups through a variety of channels. One commonly utilized channel for presentation-based dissemination to consumers includes conferences and conventions hosted or co-hosted by consumer interest groups or by professional organizations that cater to consumer interest groups. For example, Penn State University collaborated with the Pennsylvania Department of Education and the Bureau of Special Education to offer a conference day open to patients, caregivers, and their families, during which research-based presentations were distinctly tailored to consumers attending the conference. Presentations were selected based on their relevance to patients and clinical utility. Similarly, the International Association of Psychosocial Rehabilitation Services (IAPSRS) in the United States and the Mental Health Services of Australia and New Zealand (MHS), respectively, run integrated conferences that foster mutual dissemination and learning opportunities for consumers, caregivers, and professional groups in the mental health field.

A second common means by which research findings may be disseminated to consumers is through more informal, direct presentations to consumers within their own organizations. For example, a researcher might give a presentation at a self-help group meeting, weekly staff meeting, or board meeting of a consumer organization with which he or she is collaborating. Alternatively, if the consumer group is not a research collaborator, research findings may be shared in a public presentation to inform the consumer/lobby group about findings that have relevant implications (e.g., for quality of life or service delivered).

Such presentations may also serve to forge new collaborative relationships with lobby groups and organizations. Recent advances of computer-based tele-health and tele-rehabilitation technologies also allow for public presentations of research findings to be disseminated through online broadcasting and DVDs.

Reports to Government and Private Agencies, Legislative Bodies, and Public Officials

It is not unusual for governmental agencies or bodies to ask for reports of research findings to use in their deliberations as they set policies and make laws. For example, the Office of the Surgeon General may request a report on the prevalence of a given health condition so that appropriate resources can be allocated for prevention. In addition, researchers can offer to make such reports available, even when they are not requested, as a means of facilitating public awareness about a key issue, or in an effort to advocate for increased support and funding for continued research and resources to address a given issue.

The following is an example of dissemination to a government body. The National Institutes for Disability and Rehabilitation Research funded a study to examine the impact of an alternative financing program for disabled persons to obtain loans to finance needed assistive technology. Under this study, two OT investigators, Hammel and Finlayson, developed a Web-based data management and outcomes system (Finlayson & Hammel, 2003; Hammel, Finlayson, & Lastowski, 2003) to study the impact of the program. They produced annual reports to inform U.S. congressional policymakers about the outcomes of their federal appropriations. The evidence they shared with Congress was used to justify sustaining and expanding the program funding allocation from $3.8 million in 2000 to $35.8 million in 2003. As with this example, dissemination to governmental agencies can have a significant impact in directly influencing policy-making and systems change.

Websites, Targeted Brochures, and Other Media for Laypersons

Research that leads to consumer-relevant information and products, such as educational curricula, resource directories, treatment tips, prevention guidelines, and frequently answered questions, can be made available to the public through linkable websites, printed brochures or booklets, and computer media. Printed materials are the most easily accessed by individuals capable of reading print, but they are also among the most expensive and time consuming to produce and distribute. Pen drives or simply disseminating a Web address on a small card offers the advantage of being readily convertible to accessible formats for persons with some kinds of disabilities (e.g., audio-translation by computer software for people with visual impairment). However, depending upon the setting, they may not yet be as appropriate for mass distribution as printed material because they require consumers to have access to computers and computer proficiency.

Websites are a common means of disseminating research-based information to consumers. Although development of a website requires training and knowledge in website design and construction, once developed, websites are relatively easy to maintain and update. All consumer-based websites need to be approved so that they are automatically accessible to individuals with visual and auditory impairments. The U.S. federal government and many state governments have specific laws in place to ensure that website content is accessible to persons with disabilities and ensure compatibility with other assistive technologies. WebXACT (formerly Bobby) is one example of a free online resource that may be used to check the compatibility of Web content with federal law. Examples of website barriers to accessibility include audio messages displayed in the absence of a written transcript (for those with hearing impairment) or pictures without written descriptions that can be broadcast through an audio device that describes the contents of that picture (for those with visual impairment). Approval can be accomplished by submitting the website address to the following website for approval: http://download.cnet .com/GoLive-Watchfire-WebXACT-extension/ 3000-2218_4-45589.html. Websites or webpages that are well designed and easy to navigate are easily accessible by any individual with access to a computer. They also offer the research a greater degree of visibility.

Releases to the Popular Press and Media

Everyone has read, heard on the radio, or seen on television reports of recent research findings considered to have importance for the general public. A number of strategies can be used to foster coverage of OT research in the popular media.

Most medical centers, colleges, and universities have marketing or "public relations" departments whose personnel are responsible for communicating with the press. Working with these communications personnel is typically the best strategy for getting media coverage of research. Nonetheless, individual researchers can directly contact local TV or newspaper health writers to inform them of newsworthy research findings. Sometimes, an investigator can foster the potential for media coverage by being responsive to lay requests for information.

Summary

This chapter covers the nature and role of dissemination in research and reviews a range of options for disseminating research. As stated at the outset, dissemination is an essential component of any inquiry. In this age of information, the options for sharing research are myriad. When the investigator takes seriously the obligation to disseminate to the various constituencies who have a right to know about and who could potentially benefit from awareness of the research, it is clear that substantial energy and time must be devoted to dissemination. Without this expenditure of effort, research will not realize its potential value and impact.

Review Questions

1. Why is it important to disseminate one's research findings to an academic audience?
2. What issues are considered during the process of peer review of a submitted journal article?
3. What are some examples of non-peer-reviewed dissemination outlets?
4. What are the advantages to disseminating one's research at a patient-oriented conference?

5. How might the dissemination of one's research findings enhance the reputation of the overall discipline of occupational therapy?
6. How might the dissemination of one's research findings affect decision-making among hospital administrators or others in public and private leadership positions (e.g., lawmakers and policymakers)?

REFERENCES

Finlayson, M., & Hammel, J. (2003). Providing alternative financing for assistive technology: Outcomes over 20 months. *Journal of Disability Policy Studies, 14*(2), 109–118.

Fisher, A. G. (2003). *AMPS Assessment of Motor and Process Skills, Volume 1: Development, standardization and administration manual* (5th ed.). Fort Collins, CO: Three Star Press.

Fossey, E., Epstein, M., Findlay, R., Plant, G., & Harvey, C. (2002). Creating a positive experience of research for people with psychiatric disabilities by sharing feedback. *Psychiatric Rehabilitation Journal, 25*(4), 369–378.

Guba, E. G., & Lincoln, Y. S. (1989). *Fourth generation evaluation.* Newbury Park, CA: Sage.

Hammel J., Finlayson, M., & Lastowski, S. (2003). Using participatory action research to create a shared assistive technology alternative financing outcomes database and to effect social action systems change. *Journal of Disability Policy Studies, 14*(2), 98–108.

McConnell, W. A., & Kerbs, J. J. (1993). Providing feedback in research with human subjects. *Professional Psychology: Research and Practice, 24*(3), 266–270.

Mercier, C., Bordeleau, M., Caron, J., Garcia, A., & Latimer, E. (2004). Conditions facilitating knowledge exchange between rehabilitation and research teams—a study. *Psychiatric Rehabilitation Journal, 28*(1), 55–62.

Patton, M. (2008). *Utilization-focused evaluation* (4th ed.). Thousand Oaks, CA: Sage.

Peters, D. H. (2014). The application of systems thinking in health: Why use systems thinking? *Health Research Policy and Systems, 12,* 1–6.

Sieber, J. E., & Tolich, M. B. (2013). *Planning ethically responsible research: A guide for students and internal review boards* (2nd ed.). Thousand Oaks, CA: Sage.

CHAPTER 33

Writing a Grant Proposal

Renée R. Taylor • Yolanda Suarez-Balcazar • Geneviève Pépin • Elizabeth White

Learning Outcomes

- Understand the need for grant funding in occupational therapy research.
- Choose the appropriate type of grant proposal for your research goals.
- Define the components of a successful grant proposal.
- Articulate the impact of a research study from multiple perspectives.
- Recognize the importance of building the right team of co-investigators.

Introduction

The most common mechanism for funding research is a grant. A **grant** is a specified amount of money given to an investigator via the investigator's host institution to undertake a specific research project. Grants may also include funding for development, educational, training, and/or evaluation projects that often have a research component. A grant application is a document that an investigator prepares to request the funding.

Depending on the funding agency or sponsor, grant funding can be achieved through different mechanisms. For example, in the United States, the National Institutes of Health (NIH) uses three types of funding venues to support researchers: grants, contracts, and cooperative agreements. Grants differ from contracts and cooperative agreements in that the investigator has more influence in deciding the research topic to be designed or developed and the accompanying methodological approach. With contracts, the government or private funder usually decides on and selects the research that fulfills the perceived need and then specifies detailed logistical or methodological requirements that an investigator is then asked to carry out. A cooperative agreement is similar to a grant, but the awarding institute or center and the researcher both have significant involvement in carrying out the activities of the project. Because most funding

agencies tend to utilize research grants as their primary funding source, this chapter focuses on describing the process of writing and applying for research grants. Information about contracts and cooperative agreements can be obtained from literature provided by individual funding agencies (see http://www.npguides.org/guide/index.html for resources). This chapter covers the nature of grant awards, what they fund, who provides them, and how to prepare a competitive grant application.

The Purpose of Grant Funding

The various agencies that provide grants do so to make possible a research project that might otherwise not occur. Thus, they often cover all or most of the expenses associated with the research study. Depending on the guidelines of the granting agency, grant funding may be used to cover:

- All or a certain percentage of team members' salaries;
- Tuition waivers and small monetary stipends to graduate research assistants;
- Supplies and equipment that are necessary for the conduct of the study (e.g., tests, mechanical devices for experiments, computers, printers, and relevant software);
- Incentives to participants; and
- The costs of ancillary needs such as telephone, postage, transportation, printing, and photocopy costs.

Some grants also cover indirect costs of doing the research, including, for example, space rental or maintenance, the cost of heating and air-conditioning, and electricity. These are referred to as indirect costs.

Major Types of Grants

There are four major types of grants that may be obtained by occupational therapy (OT) researchers:

CASE EXAMPLE

Donna recently completed a postdoctoral fellowship in occupational therapy and is now an assistant professor working toward tenure. Because she has chosen to join the faculty of a research-intensive university, it is important for her to produce research that is of high impact and importance to health care. Early in her career, she realized that high-impact studies require a substantial amount of research funding. Fortunately, she was part of a large grant-funded study in which she served as a project director during her postdoctoral research fellowship. The team conducted a randomized clinical trial to test the effects of a novel swallowing protocol for individuals with new, high-level spinal cord injury. The trial found that, compared with the usual swallowing protocol, the new protocol improved swallowing outcomes by 70% for those clients who were able to learn and practice it. However, adjusting for those who failed to comply with the protocol (i.e., study dropouts) brought the overall improvement rate down to 20%. The reasons why some clients were able to learn and practice the protocol and others failed were not investigated in the study.

Now that Donna is on her own, she decides to initiate an independent follow-up study that will not only test the replication of prior outcomes but will also answer the remaining question involving the low rates of compliance with the protocol. She reasons that this research question also has high impact because the protocol is highly effective, and yet people appear to have difficulty complying with it and tend to refuse it in the first stage (the protocol has three stages).

In reviewing possible funding sources, Donna chooses to apply, as principal investigator, for a grant from the Christopher & Dana Reeve Foundation. She chooses the Reeve Foundation because the foundation is specifically dedicated to advancing research involving spinal cord injury. She invites her former postdoctoral supervisor to serve as a co-investigator on the study because her former supervisor has done extensive research in the area and is well recognized for her scholarly reputation and contributions. Additionally, she invites as co-investigators the referring neurosurgeon and the chief speech therapist, who invented the original protocol, as well as a pharmacist to add different flavors and odors to the liquid used in the first stage of the protocol. She obtains letters of support from the president of the host hospital where the research will be performed and from the department heads or section chiefs of each of her co-investigators. Donna also builds some funding into the proposal for five graduate research assistants to implement the protocol and collect the data and for a biostatistician to serve as a consultant. The grant budget will provide partial salary coverage for Donna and her colleagues, and it will also cover the costs of the supplies and personnel to implement the protocol.

The central questions for the study are to test whether increased time spent to educate clients about the benefits of the protocol, increased one-on-one training and practice time with the therapist, and the introduction of incentives that include matching the client's preferred flavor and smell to the liquid used in the first stage of the protocol will increase compliance rates. A secondary objective is to replicate the successful outcomes of the original investigation.

Donna shares a draft of her proposal with her former postdoc supervisor, and she receives good feedback. She submits the proposal to the foundation and looks forward to receiving feedback from the reviewers.

1. Research grants;
2. Demonstration grants;
3. Training, educational, and professional development grants; and
4. Center grants.

Research Grants

Research grants allow investigators to address scientific questions that will contribute to knowledge in a given topic area. There are numerous kinds of studies that research grants tend to fund, but they can generally be classified into two major groups: basic (bench) science studies and applied science studies.

Basic science studies are typically narrow in focus. Rather than addressing a practical issue or clinical problem, basic science studies provide the necessary knowledge and background for later applied research. They are designed to generate knowledge about a particular theory or about a basic diagnostic, biological, behavioral, attitudinal, or emotional phenomenon. Basic science studies may include, but are not limited to, epidemiological studies, laboratory studies, and field observations.

Applied science studies aim to test the application of a particular theory to a practical life problem. Applied science studies may be used to develop new technologies or intervention approaches (e.g., rehabilitation strategies, such as the one described in the Case Example at the beginning of the chapter). Applied studies commonly involve evaluating the effectiveness of the application of one or more of these technologies or intervention approaches. A well-known example of an applied study is a clinical outcomes study (e.g., a randomized clinical trial) in which one or more technologies or intervention approaches are compared against a control condition to evaluate their efficacy in addressing a given clinical problem. Participatory research that seeks to empower individuals to transform their current skills, knowledge levels, or circumstances through education and social action is another example of applied research (see Chapter 30).

Demonstration Grants

The aim of a **demonstration grant** is to allow investigators to develop, expand, and evaluate a specific set of health-care services, a model program, or a particular methodological approach (Gitlin & Lyons, 2013). For example, some OT investigators use development grants to develop new assessments, interventions, new ways to disseminate health-care information, or assistive devices. Demonstration grants allow investigators to build on existing knowledge about the efficacy of a given approach to service or programming (Gitlin & Lyons, 2013). They typically involve some kind of program evaluation component that involves elements of research. These grants typically take place in settings seeking to expand or alter their services and those wanting to develop new programs that can serve as models for later replication in other settings. Demonstration grants may also be used to support the evaluation and modification of ongoing programs in clinical, industry, educational, and community settings.

Training, Educational, and Professional Development Grants

Training grants and **educational grants** are used to support professionals and students to develop or extend their knowledge or skills. These grants can be used to support professional activities that involve training and education (e.g., conferences or symposia). They can also be used to support the implementation of specialized academic programs. For example, a training grant can be issued to a university for the purpose of supporting first-generation undergraduate students from underserved groups who have a goal of pursuing graduate training in occupational therapy. Similarly, a **professional development grant,** sometimes referred to as a career development award, is used to enable an individual who is already employed in a professional capacity to begin a career in research or to further develop research-related skills and contributions.

Center Grants

Center grants are usually large grants; they are typically funded for about 5 years, with the possibility of competitive renewal. Center grants generally involve several related projects that incorporate research, development, implementation, training, and dissemination activities. Center grants also involve identifying multiple partners and collaborators, which might include several researchers from across the country and/or multiple agencies that have access to potential participants or want to participate in training and/or dissemination activities. For example, the second author of this chapter is one of the recipients of a grant from the Center for Capacity Building on Minorities With Disabilities at the University of Illinois at Chicago. This center grant was provided by a U.S. federal granting agency, the National Institute on Disability and Rehabilitation Research (#H133A040007), which is part of the U.S. Department of Education. As a result of this grant, the collaborative team developed a cultural competence conceptual framework for rehabilitation professionals (including occupational therapists), a training program, and an assessment instrument. The team provided multiple workshops and consultation to multiple institutions serving people of minority status with disabilities.

Although center grants often involve multiple collaborators and disciplines, they are focused and theme related. As such, all proposed research, development, or training activities are designed to make contributions to the advancement of knowledge, practice, and policies in a specific area. Overall, center grants are unique opportunities to develop state-of-the-art innovations and engage in multidisciplinary research, dissemination, and training activities.

Reasons to Apply for Grant Funding

In many academic settings, grant funding is vital to the daily operation and activities of the organization. Many clinics, clinical training programs, and academic departments would not exist in the absence of grant funding. Within the field of occupational therapy, grants support the refinement, advancement, and empirical study of education, theory, assessments, technologies, and services. Grant funding is also an indirect source of reputation-building and publicity for an organization and the occupational therapists involved.

For all of these reasons, grant funding is often an expectation of OT faculty members working in top research universities. Likewise, occupational therapists working in practice settings may be involved in writing grants. Such grants enable advancing, maintaining, and/or evaluating programs of service.

Grants also provide individual benefits to the investigators who receive them. They allow an investigator to have the resources to conduct a study that otherwise would not be possible. Or, they allow a study larger in scope and greater in impact than would otherwise be possible. Moreover, grants allow an investigator to work with a funding agency to produce peer-reviewed research that serves public, legislative, and/or private interests. Grants also allow an investigator to advance his or her career and work collaboratively with a research team that mutually enriches and supports the efficiency, productivity, and professional development of all of its members.

How Grants Get Funded

In most cases, grant funding occurs as a result of a rigorous review process, discussed in a later section of this chapter. One thing is certain: Grant funding does not occur in a vacuum. It requires the involvement of a number of entities, including:

- The investigator's sponsoring university, clinic, or home institution;
- Administrators within the funding agency (often referred to as project officers);
- Individuals charged to review the relevance and quality of the grant application (often referred to as peer reviewers or grant reviewers); and
- Individuals who take the feedback of project officers and reviewers and ultimately oversee the allocation of funds within a granting agency (e.g., agency trustees or a board of directors).

In addition to these individuals, investigators are wise to identify experienced colleagues, mentors, or hired reviewers to evaluate their ideas, methods, and eventual written grant proposal before it is submitted for formal review. When appropriate (e.g., when using research methodologies that emphasize consumer participation and representation), investigators should also involve and include prospective research participants in the grant writing and initial grant review and evaluation process.

The Process of Grant Writing and Application

Grant writing takes time and commitment as well as advance planning and preparation. In the grant writing and application process, the investigator must justify and plan the research, write and package the proposal to meet the requirements of the funding agency, gather institutional support and necessary collaborators or consultants, submit the proposal to the funding agency, and follow up with the funding agency once the grant has been submitted. A successful grant includes a good idea, knowledge of hot topics and current funding initiatives and policies, sophisticated understanding of research design and methods, a good track record, and patience.

Grant writing encompasses the following steps:

- Developing an idea;
- Evaluating and negotiating with the sponsoring institution;
- Identifying and enlisting support from co-investigators, consultants, and other future personnel;
- Selecting the appropriate funding agency, funding institute, and funding avenue;
- Knowing regulations, policies, and guidelines;
- Working with funding agency administrators;
- Identifying a theoretical basis for the study;
- Demonstrating expert knowledge of the topic area;
- Demonstrating good scholarship;
- Identifying specific aims;
- Developing hypotheses;
- Conducting pilot research;
- Choosing an appropriate and rigorous design;
- Ensuring an ethical design and methodological approach;
- Addressing logistical issues and obstacles in data collection up front;
- Planning analyses;
- Developing a timeline and evaluation plan;
- Developing a reasonable budget request;

- Obtaining letters of support; and
- Determining where to send the grant application.

Although these steps are presented and discussed sequentially, in reality, many of them are often performed simultaneously. Some steps will be left incomplete as others are initiated. The scramble to prepare a competitive application often requires substantial multitasking and cross-checking among all of the steps. Moreover, the order of the steps may vary depending on the funding source and the kind of competition to which one is applying. Nonetheless, in most cases, the steps discussed here will be required for preparing a grant proposal.

Developing an Idea: The Importance of Impact

The most critical aspect of preparing a grant proposal is developing a research idea that is significant and innovative enough to warrant funding. The extent to which a project answers a socially or medically significant need or question in a way that pushes the state of science and/or practice forward is referred to as **impact.** Agencies want to utilize their money wisely and parsimoniously. They want to be sure that studies have the potential to be of high impact in terms of understanding, preventing, reversing, or alleviating certain health conditions. Developing a grant proposal idea with the potential to be of high impact involves the following considerations:

- Defining impact,
- Taking into account policy documents and legislative initiatives;
- Matching the investigator's idea to the goals and priorities of the funding agency; and
- Building on existing contemporary scientific trends.

Often, one of the main challenges in evaluating one's idea in terms of impact involves knowing the ideology and funding priorities of the agency to which one is applying.

Defining Impact

Some agencies consider the severity, imminence, and potential for reversibility of a condition in determining their funding priorities and decisions. They may consider some diseases, chronic illnesses, or impairments to be more worthy of funding than others based on fatality rates or other characteristics of the disease or population. Other agencies may value certain methodological approaches over others. For example, an agency whose priority is to reduce and eradicate highly

prevalent diseases with high mortality rates may be more inclined to fund medically innovative research that involves biomarkers and/or aspects of the human genome over research that focuses on improving the quality of life of individuals living with the condition. Conversely, a different agency may be more inclined to fund research that focuses on empowerment and capacity-building for individuals with existing impairments. An added priority for many agencies is reducing health disparities. Such agencies will tend to fund researchers who work with participants who do not have adequate economic resources, educational and employment opportunities, and access to health care. Knowing these priorities can help a researcher determine how reviewers might evaluate a proposal in terms of its overall significance and potential for impact.

Taking Into Account Policy Documents and Legislative Initiatives

Being knowledgeable about politics, current events, and legislative initiatives can aid in determining whether a funding idea will be considered to be important and of high impact. Knowledge of legislative initiatives is particularly important when it comes to obtaining funding from federal agencies (Gitlin & Lyons, 2013). One can become familiar with legislative initiatives through funding-agency websites, government publications such as the *Federal Register* in the United States, and funding announcements distributed via e-mail distribution lists and other types of funding-agency listservs that one can join free of charge through the funding agency or institute of one's choice. If access to such a listserv is not immediately available or obvious on a funding-agency website, it is advisable to contact the program coordinator of a given institute or agency to inquire. At the broadest level, researchers can obtain knowledge about upcoming federal funding priorities by reading the daily newspaper, watching the news, and otherwise keeping current on issues in health-care policy through various media outlets.

Matching the Investigator's Idea to the Goals and Priorities of the Funding Agency

Investigators should always ensure that the research topic, population, and methodological approach reflect the goals and priorities of the funding agency to which they apply. A number of steps can be taken to effectively match a research idea to the agenda of the funding agency:

- Consult relevant Web-based and other resources (many of which are discussed in this chapter) to develop a preliminary working list of possible funding agencies to approach;
- Periodically scan the Web and other resources for program announcements and/or funding agencies that reflect one's area of interest;
- Consult with respected peers, mentors, and program officers to receive feedback about the match of funding agencies to the research idea; and
- Refine and define proposal ideas to match chosen potential agencies based on the information gathered.

Building on Existing Contemporary Scientific Trends

Most funding agencies keep relatively current in terms of their knowledge of methodological approaches that are contemporary and/or on the cutting edge of science. In addition, certain scientific trends tend to develop, and some gain a substantial amount of credibility and support within the research community. For example, recent trends within health-care research include:

- A focus on participatory approaches to program development, service provision, health disparities, and health-care reform;
- Transdisciplinary research (e.g., research that draws upon the expertise of professionals from a wide range of disciplines); and
- Translational research (e.g., studies that incorporate a range of approaches that span the basic and applied concerns).

Evaluating and Negotiating With the Sponsoring Institution

Before deciding to write a grant, investigators must identify and evaluate existing resources within their own institutions. Sponsoring institutions often have internal rules and regulations that govern the grant submission process, many of which involve budgetary and resource issues. For example, some sponsoring institutions specify a minimum requirement for indirect-cost support provided by a granting agency. Conversely, to award grant funding to an investigator, some funding agencies require a certain level of commitment of monetary or in-kind support (e.g., a certain percentage of cost-sharing or matching funds) from a sponsoring institution. It is important to clarify issues of resource allocation and administrative rules and regulations before a grant proposal is submitted so that all agreements are in place should a grant get funded.

Another important factor to consider during negotiations with a sponsoring institution is that grant writing takes time and commitment. Applicants will need support in the form of time allocated to writing and preparing the grant proposal and other types of support, such as access to secretarial, research assistant, and administrative support for such diverse things as conducting literature searches, gathering protocols and instruments, gathering letters of cooperation, preparing a budget, and making photocopies. The sponsoring institution should also be willing to release the applicant from other responsibilities (e.g., committee work, teaching) so he or she has the necessary time to construct a strong proposal.

Identifying and Enlisting Support From Co-investigators, Consultants, and Other Future Personnel

Most grant evaluation criteria include an assessment of the strengths and credentials of the various members of the investigative team. Thus, selection of the team members is critically important and requires thought and effort. Depending on the size of the study, research team members may include:

- Co-investigators/subcontractors,
- Consultants (e.g., biostatisticians),
- Grant staff,
- Student research assistants, and
- Volunteers.

Co-investigators (commonly paid as subcontractors unless they are housed within the same institution) are research personnel critical to conducting the study. They share responsibility for the intellectual contributions made to the development of the study idea, design, and methods and analyses, and they collaborate with the principal investigator in interpreting the findings and in accessing avenues for dissemination.

Co-investigators are typically senior-level scientists with the knowledge base, technical skills, publication history, and scientific reputation that support the central aims of the study and complement the credentials of the principal investigator and other collaborators. Increasingly, agencies expect a research team that reflects diverse and complementary disciplines.

Consultants are of similar status and complete similar functions as co-investigators. However, their role is often more circumscribed, and their contributions to the overall study are proportionally smaller than those of the co-investigators. Co-investigators and consultants are usually selected before a proposal is written, and they are always identified in the grant proposal. Most funding agencies require that they provide curricula vitae and written letters of support. In many cases, a subcontract agreement will be in place that allows for formal budgetary relationships to be established.

Other members of the research team, including grant staff, student research assistants, and volunteers, can be named once the grant has been funded. However, some reviewers look more favorably upon grant applications that identify key grant staff because it leaves an impression that the investigator has a stable research team. However, it is often not possible to name the more junior-level or secondary contributors up front.

Selecting collaborators involves deciding what intellectual and physical resources are needed to complete a study and determining who might be available to meet those needs (Gitlin & Lyons, 2013). Selecting strong collaborators will not only increase the likelihood of a positive review but will also ensure the overall success of the study.

Enlisting support from collaborators early in the grant writing process can be vital to idea development. In addition, collaborators may support activities such as grant writing, study implementation, and the write-up and dissemination of study findings.

Selecting the Appropriate Funding Agency, Funding Institute, and Funding Avenue

Being knowledgeable about the missions, values, and funding priorities of the different agencies that fund the kind of research one intends is vital. Sometimes, funding decisions are made even before the review process begins because the investigator has selected the wrong agency, funding institute, or funding avenue for the proposed project. Some of the more widely utilized funding sources that may be accessed by OT researchers and their collaborators include grants awarded by:

• Professional organizations,
• Private foundations,
• Self-help organizations,

• Grant competitions within university settings, and
• The federal government.

Grants Awarded by Professional Organizations

Grants awarded by professional organizations are useful resources for individuals seeking to advance the profession. As such, their scope is limited to projects within the singular discipline of occupational therapy, and typically funding is provided for tightly constructed, time-limited, and highly focused research studies, projects, or professional educational activities.

OT professional associations are increasingly becoming sources of funding. Information on OT professional bodies from the United States, Australia, Canada, the United Kingdom, and the World Federation of Occupational Therapy are outlined in the following sections. OT researchers in countries other than those mentioned here are encouraged to identify additional possible sources of funding within their own national professional bodies.

American Occupational Therapy Foundation. The American Occupational Therapy Foundation (AOTF) is a nonprofit organization whose mission is to advance OT research specifically as it informs clinical practice. AOTF is also focused toward efforts that increase public understanding of OT services. In conjunction with ongoing support from the American Occupational Therapy Association (AOTA), AOTF has provided nearly $4,000,000 in support for research grants and projects since 1965. In 2014, AOTF research expenditures totaled $542,229. Currently, AOTF and AOTA conjointly fund a research intervention grant program. This program is for early-stage or early-midcareer investigators with emerging funding histories who, for example, have not already received independent federal funding. Applications must demonstrate support from a named senior research mentor. A listing of intervention grant recipients may be found at http://www.aotf.org/scholarshipsgrants/aotfinterventionresearchgrantprogram/intervention researchgrantrecipients.

Gillette (2000) has published a 20-year history of research funding in occupational therapy that describes the various activities and awards made by AOTF and AOTA. A listing of grant opportunities and resources relevant to occupational therapists may be found on the AOTA website at http://www.aota.org/practice/researchers/funding.aspx.

In the United Kingdom, the UK Occupational Therapy Research Foundation (UKOTRF), a division of the College of Occupational Therapists, was launched in 2007, aiming to support research into occupation-focused interventions and to build research capacity within the profession. A sum of £100,000 is made available annually to support research proposals in two categories: a Research Priority Grant for research led by an experienced principal investigator in a priority area for the profession and two Research Career Development Grants to support members of the College in their doctoral or early postdoctoral research careers. The professional body also administers a range of small grants for members' research, education, and professional development activities, which are available on an annual basis. Awards arise both from restricted funds held by the College of Occupational Therapists (COT) and grants made available from companies and charitable organizations. Details are advertised on the website at http://www.cot.org.uk.

Occupational Therapy Australia Research Foundation. The Occupational Therapy Australia Research Foundation was founded in 2012. The aim of the foundation is to support occupational therapists and OT research that will contribute to improving the health and well-being of Australians. The foundation funds OT research that is consistent with the Australian Department of Industry, Innovation, Science, Research and Tertiary Education's National Research Priorities and the Australian Institute of Health and Welfare's National Health Priority Areas. The Occupational Therapy Research Foundation funds research grants, awards, and scholarships for Australian scholars. The Judith Marsham Farrell Research Grant is an example of a funding initiative supported by the foundation. This grant supports research in which the participants perform occupations to determine occupational participation and engagement for a human health condition.

Also, the foundation, in collaboration with the Board of Occupational Therapy Australia, presents Australian OT researchers whose contribution to the advancement of occupational therapy is exceptional with the Award of Fellow to the Occupational Therapy Australia Research Academy. Further information about the Occupational Therapy Research Foundation can be found on the Occupational Therapy Australia website at http://www.otaus.com.au/about/ResearchFoundation.

Canadian Occupational Therapy Foundation. The Canadian Occupational Therapy Foundation (COTF) is a nonprofit professional organization that works in tandem with the Canadian Association of Occupational Therapists (CAOT)

to develop mechanisms for granting awards to individuals and organizations for research, scholarship, and publication. A listing of current grant awards available through COTF may be found at http://www.cotfcanada.org/index.php/en/research-grants. COTF provides opportunities for OT researchers whose aim is to address the evolving needs of the OT community in Canada. COTF generates, receives, and maintains funds to support a broad range of research and scholarship in the field of occupational therapy.

With the support from CAOT and donations from individuals, corporations, organizations, and foundations, COTF provides four types of funding streams: Research Grants, Clinical Research Grants (awards are restricted only to OT clinicians), Scholarships Grants, and Provincial Awards. COTF's research expenditures in 2014 totaled $94,094.

World Federation of Occupational Therapists. Every 2 years, the World Federation of Occupational Therapists (WFOT) reviews applications for the Thelma Cardwell Foundation Award for Research and Education. This award supports any project aiming to enhance the development of occupational therapy in any way. The award does not support research projects for which funds could be sought from governmental agencies or other grant-giving foundations. The budget is restricted to include only coverage for equipment, maintenance, or technical assistance for an already approved research project. Thus, WFOT funding is best used to supplement other types of funding provided for a given study. More information about this grant award and evaluation criteria used to select applications can be found at http://www.wfot.org.

Grants Awarded by Private Foundations

Numerous private foundations support research, developmental, and educational activities. The mission and funding agenda of private foundations are as varied as the individual donors (e.g., Tiger Woods Foundation), families (e.g., Field Foundation of Illinois), and private industries (e.g., Procter & Gamble) that provide grants. Private foundation grants can range from small award amounts to awards in excess of US$1,000,000 for a single application. Topics for funding generally focus on, but are not limited to, community-based initiatives directed at improving communities; improving education; reducing conflict and violence; improving access and participation for individuals with disabilities; increasing job skills and employment for underserved, mentally ill, homeless, or adjudicated individuals; and reducing disease and disability and improving health outcomes for a wide range of populations and human conditions. In the following sections, a few private foundations of the thousands in existence around the world are described.

U.S. Foundations. The Robert Wood Johnson Foundation is the largest private philanthropy within the United States that is exclusively devoted to improving health and health care. This foundation has made basic science and applied research grant awards ranging from US$1,200 to US$50,000,000. Grants are announced through *calls for proposals* that are highly specific to the goals and agenda of the program that issues the call. Independent grants (i.e., unsolicited grant applications that reflect an investigator's unique ideas) can also be funded. Some of the foundation's interest areas are prevention and treatment of addictions, building human capital within the health-care workforce, health disparities, quality health care, and pioneering research that promotes fundamental breakthroughs in health and health care. More information about funding through the Robert Wood Johnson Foundation can be found at http://www.rwjf.org.

The John D. and Catherine T. MacArthur Foundation is a private, independent organization dedicated to promoting a lasting improvement in the human condition. The foundation awards grants in a wide range of areas pertaining to community and economic development, digital media and learning, arts and culture, juvenile justice, housing, and impact investments to help nonprofits achieve social goals. Although MacArthur provides funding to entities nationwide, in Chicago alone, the foundation has invested US$1.1 billion since 1978. More information about funding from the MacArthur Foundation can be found at http://www.macfound.org.

The Jacob & Valeria Langeloth Foundation is a private philanthropy that awards applied research grants in the area of health care (mainly to hospitals and other health-care facilities). In 2014, Langeloth awarded a total of US$4,579,242 in research funding. Current funding priorities include health care in correctional settings and projects focusing on chronic violence and community health. For more information about funding from the Langeloth Foundation, readers may access the foundation's website at http://www.langeloth.org.

In Australia, funding sources come from organizations and associations such as Multiple Sclerosis Australia Research, Arthritis Australia, Motor Neuron Disease Australia, Australian Rotary Health—Mental Health Grants, and the Victorian Women Benevolent Trust. Some organizations and associations will fund research projects over a few years, whereas others will support knowledge development in the form of postdoctoral and other fellowships. These organizations and associations provide specific information and clear guidelines on how to apply, what their priorities and areas of funded research are, what is and is not funded, and so forth. This information is essential when preparing an application to ensure that the type of research, its purpose and rationale, the team of researchers and other partners, the eligibility requirements, and how the application is prepared and presented meet the selection criteria.

Australian philanthropic organizations also support research and collaborations between organizations that have led to the development of different funding schemes. For example, the Ralph Lauren Pink Pony Campaign, an international initiative that supports access to support and health-care services for women with breast cancer, has an Australian branch administered by Cancer Australia. The Ralph Lauren Pink Pony seeding grants fund research that will benefit women with breast cancer in local communities in Australia.

Canadian Foundations. In Canada, most grants for OT-based research come from private organizations, charities, and associations such as the Alzheimer Society of Canada, the Canadian Cystic Fibrosis Association, the Parkinson Society of Canada, the Canadian Mental Health Association, or the Royal Canadian Legion Fellowship in Gerontology. Other important sources of funding come from each province's own funding agencies. Regardless of whether they are governmental or private, each has specific research interests, a mission, procedures for submitting a research project, and policies and criteria for funding. For example, in the province of Québec, the *Fonds de recherche en Santé du Québec* (http://www.frqs.gouv.qc.ca/en/) funds training awards, career awards, research grants, international collaborative programs, and research centers. The *Fonds de recherche Société et Culture du Québec* (http://www.frqsc.gouv.qc.ca/en/) is another funding agency that opens doors for occupational therapists concerned with social inclusion, diversity, and adaptation. It provides funding to scholars working in the areas of social sciences, the humanities, education, management, arts, and literature.

United Kingdom Foundations (Charities). In the United Kingdom, sources of grants for occupational therapists arise from a wide range of charities. This includes the Multiple Sclerosis Society

UK, Parkinson's UK, the Stroke Association, Arthritis Research UK, Age UK, and the Alzheimer's Society. Major research in the UK is funded by the Research Councils UK, which is a strategic partnership of the UK's seven Research Councils that aims to fund research that has an impact on the growth, prosperity, and well-being of the UK. The Research Councils of particular relevance to the research interests of occupational therapists include the medical, social sciences, and engineering councils. A further major funder of health-related research is the National Institute of Health Research, which provides a range of funding opportunities to support health research focused on the needs of patients and the public. Further research funding streams that can be accessed by occupational therapists may be found specific to one of the four UK countries: England, Wales, Scotland, and Northern Ireland.

Grants Awarded by Self-Help Organizations

Grants awarded by self-help organizations largely serve the interests of clients who have experienced or are experiencing a specific illness, trauma, or impairment, as well as their loved ones and their specialist health-care providers. As such, the scope of grants provided by self-help organizations is limited to projects that focus on a given condition or disease process. The size of grants awarded by self-help organizations is generally commensurate with the size of the membership and the amount of contributions made to a given organization. However, because self-help organizations are largely supported by small donations made by clients, their loved ones, and their health-care providers, they tend to make smaller or more mid-sized grant awards. There are thousands of self-help organizations that fund grants throughout the world.

One example is the American Heart Association (AHA), a multifaceted national self-help organization that has invested more than US$3.8 billion since 1949 to enhance knowledge about cardiovascular diseases and stroke. The AHA is a national volunteer organization within the United States whose mission is to improve cardiovascular health in all Americans and reduce cardiovascular death by 20% by the year 2020. The AHA's research program is guided by 12 essential elements developed by a broad group of stakeholders, including scientist volunteers, to guide the success of its research program. These elements are:

1. Develop innovative research models that integrate AHA research values.

2. Fund both investigator-initiated and strategically focused research.
3. Support research in all areas of cardiovascular and stroke science that support AHA's 2020 goals and overall mission.
4. Identify key questions that, if answered, could provide extraordinary impact in science and toward the overall mission.
5. Ensure funding mechanisms for investigators at all career stages and across disciplines.
6. Provide programs that, in addition to supporting the pursuit of research in question, facilitate the expansion of investigator skills.
7. Focus peer review on funding outstanding individuals, in addition to excellent science.
8. Clearly define and report research outcomes to all stakeholders.
9. Ensure that best practices are used for all governance and operational practices.
10. Ensure that all stakeholders—researchers, donors, and other volunteers—are involved as appropriate in research activities.
11. Fund research that could provide a return on investment to be funneled back to fund more future research.
12. Expand collaboration to leverage research dollars and outcomes.

(http://professional.heart.org/professional/ResearchPrograms/UCM_320223_AHA-Mission-Vision-and-the-12-Essential-Elements-Guiding-our-Research-Program.jsp)

More information about grant funding through the AHA can be located at http://professional.heart.org/professional/ResearchPrograms/UCM_316889_Research.jsp.

Grants and Grant Competitions Within University Settings

Two general types of grant competitions occur within university settings: limited internal competitions and seed grants. Limited internal competitions are made available to research-oriented universities by certain kinds of funding agencies (mostly federal agencies). These competitions involve two or more phases. The first phase occurs between faculty within the university to limit the number of applications from that university. Many limited internal competitions accept only one or two applications per university. The application that emerges as strongest and most relevant from the internal competition is the one that is selected.

Many university settings, particularly those with a research focus or emphasis, offer opportunities for faculty internal to the university to compete for small grants that are offered by the university itself. These grants are often referred to as seed grants. In large part, they are designed to provide funding (or other resources) to help an investigator collect pilot data for a later grant application to be submitted elsewhere, or to initiate a new line of research that is perhaps too novel to receive funding in a competitive environment outside of the university setting. The amount of funding available for these grants tends to be small, and usually funding is limited to only a few proposals. Information about limited internal competitions and seed grants is generally provided through a university research office.

Grants Awarded by Governments

Most countries, and often subjurisdictions such as states or provinces, have granting programs. These vary widely by country or jurisdiction. Major governmental funding bodies in the United States, Australia, Canada, and the United Kingdom are briefly reviewed in this chapter. Readers from other countries will want to investigate their national and local governmental sources of funding. Ordinarily, information is publicly available on websites and in official government publications. Nonetheless, it often takes substantial time and effort to learn all the mechanisms, rules, regulations, deadlines, and so on, that are part of government funding. Before applying for a government grant, one should become as familiar as possible with this type of information.

Federal Grants in the United States. A number of federal granting agencies have programmatic interest areas relevant to OT researchers in the United States. This section discusses those with the largest history of funding OT research. The National Institutes of Health (NIH) is the primary federal funding agency that supports medical research.

Most applications sent to NIH are investigator initiated. This means that the research idea (e.g., central aims of the research, topic area, study design, and methodology) is unsolicited and uniquely a product of the investigator's thinking. The investigator must be responsible for the planning, direction, and execution of the project. Despite the implicit intellectual liberties associated with this funding avenue, a caveat that many applicants forget is that their ideas still must incorporate concepts, aims, study populations, and methods that are considered of relevance to at least one of the various institutes or centers within NIH.

Opportunities for grant funding are announced in a number of ways. A Program Announcement (PA) is a formally prepared statement in writing that invites applications in a defined area of interest. A PA is not a guarantee that funds have been set aside to support the defined interest area, and applications are generally treated as being investigator initiated in all other respects. In a Request for Applications (RFA), NIH invites applications for a one-time competition in a specific topic area and describes an institute's initiative in a well-defined scientific area to stimulate research in an area of exceptionally high priority to the institute. In this case, the RFA does guarantee that a certain amount of funding has been set aside to support the defined interest area, and it specifies up front how many awards will be made. A Request for Proposals (RFP) is similar to an RFA except that an RFP involves a contractual relationship between the investigator and NIH, rather than a grant. RFAs and RFPs are dedicated mainly to problem-oriented research efforts that focus on disease-specific initiatives, particularly in the beginning stages of research.

NIH is comprised of 21 different institutes and six centers, each dedicated to a specific health-related topic area and mission. Some examples of NIH institutes that may be of particular relevance to OT researchers include, but are not limited to:

- The Eunice Kennedy Shriver National Institute on Child Health and Human Development (NICHD), which also houses the National Center for Medical Rehabilitation Research;
- The National Institute on Aging (NIA);
- The National Institute on Alcohol Abuse and Alcoholism (NIAAA);
- The National Institute on Drug Abuse (NIDA);
- The National Institute of Arthritis and Musculoskeletal and Skin Diseases (NIAMS);
- The National Institute of Mental Health (NIMH); and
- The National Institute of Neurological Disorders and Stroke (NINDS), among several others (see http://www.nih.gov/icd for a complete listing).

Specific research topics that represent strong interest areas for the NIH can be searched regularly by accessing the *NIH Guide for Grants and Contracts*, which can be found at http://grants.nih.gov/grants/guide/index.html.

Table 33.1, which was composed from information in several tables provided on the NIH website (http://grants1.nih.gov/grants/funding/funding_program.htm), describes some of the different types of grants awarded through the NIH that are relevant to OT researchers.

Agency for Healthcare Research and Quality. The Agency for Healthcare Research and Quality

Table 33.1 Selected* Funding Awards Made by the National Institutes of Health (NIH)

Award Type**	Brief Definition
NIH Research Grants	
NIH Research Project Grant Program (R01) http://grants1.nih.gov/grants/funding/r01.htm	An **R01** is typically a larger research grant award made to support a very well-defined and highly specific research project. R01s provide support to investigators for health-related research and development projects that coincide with the NIH mission. R01s can be funded for a period of 1 to 5 years and can total to more than US$2,000,000 for a full 5-year funding period.
NIH Small Grant Program (R03) http://grants1.nih.gov/grants/funding/r03.htm	An **R03** is a research grant award that provides limited funding for a short period of time. It can be used to fund pilot or feasibility studies; secondary analysis of existing data; small, self-contained research studies; development of research methodology; or the development of new technology.
NIH Academic Research Enhancement Award (AREA Grants) (R15) http://grants1.nih.gov/grants/funding/area.htm	AREA grants are small awards that support individual biomedical and behavioral science research projects that are conducted collaboratively by faculty and students in undergraduate institutions that are housed in schools that have not been major recipients of other types of NIH research grant funding.
NIH Exploratory/Developmental Research Grant Award (R21) http://grants1.nih.gov/grants/funding/r21.htm	An **R21** provides a limited amount of support for research projects, ideas, and methodologies that are exceptionally novel, potentially groundbreaking, or innovative.
NIH Clinical Trial Planning Grant Program (R34) http://grants1.nih.gov/grants/funding/r34.htm	The **R34** is a 1-year grant award that supports the development of Phase III clinical trials.
NIH Research Career Development Awards	
Mentored Research Scientist Development Award (K01) https://researchtraining.nih.gov/programs/career-development	The **K01** supports 3 to 5 years of an intensive, supervised, career development experience for an investigator entering a new area of research in a biomedical, behavioral, or clinical science.
International Research Scientist Development Award (KO1–IRSDA) https://researchtraining.nih.gov/programs/career-development	The **K01–IRSDA** supports U.S. postdoctoral biomedical, social, and behavioral scientists in newer stages of their research careers to conduct research or extend their current research into developing countries.
Independent Scientist Award (K02) https://researchtraining.nih.gov/programs/career-development	The **K02** award provides up to 5 years of salary support for newly independent scientists who can demonstrate a need for a period of intensive research focus that will enable them to expand their potential to make significant contributions to their selected area of research.
Senior Scientist Award (K05) https://researchtraining.nih.gov/programs/career-development	The **K05** provides salary support for up to 5 years for scientists of outstanding caliber who have demonstrated sustained, high-level productivity and whose expertise, research accomplishments, and contributions to the field are critical to the mission of the particular NIH center or institute.
Mentored Clinical Scientists Development Award (K08) https://researchtraining.nih.gov/programs/career-development	The **K08** supports specialized study for individuals with a health professions doctorate who want to gain independence as a laboratory or field-based researcher.
Mentored Patient-Oriented Research Career Development Award (K23) https://researchtraining.nih.gov/programs/career-development	The **K23** was designed to increase the number of clinicians trained to conduct high-quality patient-oriented clinical research. This area covers mechanisms of human disease, therapeutic interventions, clinical trials, and the development of new technologies.
NIH Small Business Funding Opportunities	
NIH Small Business Innovation Research Program (SBIR) http://grants1.nih.gov/grants/funding/sbir.htm	The SBIR program is designed to encourage U.S.-based small businesses to engage in research and development activities that have an impact on health and a potential for commercialization.

Table 33.1 Continued

Award Type**	Brief Definition
NIH Small Business Technology Transfer Research Program (STTR) http://grants1.nih.gov/grants/funding/sbir.htm	The STTR is similar to the SBIR program in that both programs seek to increase the participation of smaller businesses in federal research and development and to increase subsequent commercialization of technologies developed by this program within the private sector. One difference is that STTR program applicants are required to formally collaborate with a research institution.

*A more comprehensive listing of the numerous types of grant awards offered by the NIH can be found at http://grants1.nih.gov/grants/funding/funding_program.htm. Because the types of awards offered by NIH change periodically, readers are encouraged to access the website for the most updated information.

**Generally, the research awards (preceded by an "R") are designed to provide support for well-defined research and development projects. The research career development awards (preceded by a "K") provide support for new, mid-career, and senior scientists who are seeking to bring greater focus and/or knowledge. The small business awards promote the development and private commercialization of new technologies and promote collaboration between research scientists and small business owners.

(AHRQ) is a federal funding source within the U.S. Department of Health and Human Services Public Health Service dedicated to funding research that enhances the quality, appropriateness, and effectiveness of health-care services and service access. Topical areas of research cover the organization, financing, and delivery of health-care services; disease prevention; and the improvement of clinical health-care practices. Most of the large grants that AHRQ funds involve research projects, demonstration projects, program evaluations, and dissemination activities.

Because priorities are based on legislation, policies, and public need, areas of specific interest for AHRQ change regularly. AHRQ interest areas tend to be published in the form of RFPs, PAs, and notices. More information about current AHRQ funding opportunities can be accessed at http://www.ahrq.gov/funding/index.html.

In addition, announcements can be searched regularly by accessing the *NIH Guide for Grants and Contracts*, which can be found at http://grants.nih.gov/grants/guide/index.html.

United Kingdom. The purpose of funding for OT research in the United Kingdom is to both generate new knowledge and also to develop research capacity. Many research funders support interdisciplinary research, reflecting the team approach that is essential for effective social and health-care interventions. Among the most prestigious funding sources for social and health-care research in the United Kingdom are the government-funded research councils. The Medical Research Council (MRC) and the Economic and Social

Research Council (ESRC) invest in funding for high-quality, world-class research.

The National Health Service (NHS) is another highly regarded funding avenue within the United Kingdom. In England, the National Institute of Health Research funds a range of programs, including the NIHR Health Technology Assessment (HTA) Programme and Research for Patient Benefit Programme. In Scotland, the Chief Scientist Office, part of the Scottish Government Health Directorates, aims to support and increase the level of high-quality health research conducted in Scotland. Support for developing research that has a positive impact on the health, well-being, and prosperity of people living in Wales is provided by Health and Care Research Wales, whereas occupational therapists in Northern Ireland can access research funding support from the Northern Ireland Department of Health, Social Services and Public Health.

Within the United Kingdom, there has been recognition of the need to strengthen the research capacity of occupational therapists by supporting opportunities to undertake research and develop research careers (Creek & Ilott, 2002; Department of Health, 2000, 2005; Higher Education Funding Council for England, 2001; Ilott & White, 2001; Scottish Executive, 2004). As a result, increased funding is available for occupational therapists from sources such as the UK Occupational Therapy Research Foundation and the National Institute for Health Research (NIHR). The NIHR supports training in clinical and applied health research, including social care research, funding research activity that must have the potential to benefit patients and the public within 5 years of its completion. The NIHR offers personal training awards that occupational therapists can apply for, and these propose a career pathway that will facilitate the development of future research leaders in clinical settings. The prestigious NIHR Clinical Academic Training Pathway offers four levels of fully funded awards, from Masters in Clinical to Senior Clinical Lectureship. This competitive funding opportunity supports not only specific research projects but also efforts to build research capacity within nursing, midwifery, and the allied health professions.

In Australia, the National Health and Medical Research Council (NHMRC) supports health and medical research by funding basic science, clinical, public health, and health services research. The NHMRC has five categories of grants, and each category is divided into specific grant schemes: Grants to Create New Knowledge, Grants to Accelerate Research Translation, Grants to Build Australia's Future Capability, Work With Partners Grants, and Collaborative Grants (international activities). Each grant targets specific types of research, and generally, research undertaken by occupational therapists and OT scholars will be funded by the Grants to Create New Knowledge category under the Program Grants and Project Grants. Also, the Grants to Accelerate Research Translation category offers a variety of scholarships and fellowships of interest to OT researchers. More information about the NHMRC funding opportunities is available on the council's website at https://www.nhmrc.gov.au/.

The Australian Research Council (ARC) supports the highest-quality fundamental and applied research and research training in all fields of science, social sciences, and the humanities. It has a strong focus on supporting partnerships between researchers and community organizations, government, and industry. It also supports international collaborations. The ARC has different funding programs. The Discovery Programme primarily supports individual researchers or small teams. The Linkage Programme focuses on research outcomes achieved through partnerships. The Linkage Programme includes funding for ARC Centres of Excellence. The Centres of Excellence are based on significant collaborations and aim at developing exceptional expertise in research areas of national priority. Detailed information about the ARC and its funding schemes can be found on the council's website at http://www.arc.gov.au/welcome-australian-research-council-website.

Canada. Canada's major federal funding agency for health research is the Canadian Institute of Health Research (CIHR; http://www.cihr-irsc.gc.ca). The CIHR promotes research through an interdisciplinary structure made up of 13 institutes. Its philosophy rests on networks of researchers brought together to focus on specific and important health issues. Therefore, the CIHR's structure encourages partnerships and collaboration across sectors, disciplines, and regions. Some institutes of most relevance to occupational therapy include:

- Institute of Aging,
- Institute of Health Services and Policy Research,
- Institute of Human Development, Child and Youth Health,
- Institute of Musculoskeletal Health and Arthritis, and
- Institute of Neurosciences, Mental Health and Addiction.

Each institute focuses on a specific area and is open to research initiatives that range from fundamental biomedical and clinical research to research that focuses on cultural dimensions of health and environmental variables that affect well-being.

Summary of Grants

This section provided a brief overview of different types of funding agencies. These agencies represent numerous opportunities available to OT researchers and practitioners working in a wide range of academic, private, educational, and community-based settings. These opportunities change continually in conjunction with federal and private foundation health agendas and funding priorities. Each year, new foundations emerge that fund research related to health care, whereas others cease to offer funding opportunities related to health-care research.

Many research-oriented universities have formal or informal research development services or offices, which are geared toward disseminating funding opportunities like these and others to faculty and staff. In addition to university research development services, prospective grant applicants can subscribe to a wide range of publications and Web-based resources that allow access to updated information about funding agencies and priorities. Some of these links and guidelines for accessing information about private funding opportunities were provided in the section of this chapter on private foundation funding sources. For federal resources within the United States, the website http://www.grants.gov/web/grants/search -grants.html contains updated information about many types of funding announcements.

Knowing Regulations, Policies, and Guidelines

Because most funding agencies receive numerous applications for each funding cycle, and because grants involve (sometimes complex) financial arrangements between the agency and the applicant's home institution, all granting agencies rely heavily on policies and regulations that guide the application and award process and are generally uniformly upheld for all applicants.

Once an investigator is funded, many agencies have a number of requirements that must be met in order for the investigator to retain the funding award. Depending on the agency, examples may include providing periodic written progress reports that demonstrate that the research team members are completing the work that they promised to complete within the expected time frame, budget monitoring, or occasional audits to ensure that the research team is not spending the award money inappropriately or purchasing items that have not been approved within the budgetary guidelines. Investigators must take great care to follow guidelines like these, or an agency can and will discontinue funding. Grant writing and proposal preparation, administrative and budgetary maintenance, and the provision of periodic progress reports are not areas in which an investigator is permitted to cut corners or relax standards.

Working With Funding Agency Administrators

There are many different types of funding agency administrators. These may include, but are not limited to:

- Agency directors, advisory councils, and directorial boards (whose main job is to set agency funding priorities and provide ultimate oversight over the types of grants that receive funding),
- Referral officers (whose main job is to scan the titles and abstracts of grant applications and assign specific reviewers),
- Scientific review administrators (whose main job is to oversee the logistical, legal, and administrative aspects of the review process), and
- Project officers (whose main job is to guide applicants and grantees through the review and grant management processes).

The type of agency administrator with whom an investigator is likely to have the most contact is the project officer (or program officer). Project officers may be involved with a grant at all stages of its development and implementation. Generally, however, a project officer can educate an investigator about:

- The agency's funding priorities (i.e., the topic areas of most interest to the agency),
- The administrative aspects of applying for the grant (i.e., how to complete required forms and progress reports), and
- The review process (i.e., whether to resubmit an application and to what extent an investigator should respond to certain types of feedback from the reviewers).

More information about working with project officers in deciding whether to resubmit an application is provided later in this chapter.

Identifying a Theoretical Basis for the Study

High-quality research aims to evaluate the relevance of theory that underlies the research activities. In fact, one of the central reasons why many grant proposals receive poor scores from reviewers lies in the fact that the study is not well justified in terms of its relationship to a larger idea or system of ideas that support the central hypothesis. Theoretical justification is also a requirement for studies that focus on the development of an assessment, program, or other rehabilitation resource. Regardless of the nature of the study, a central theory must be closely linked and utilized to support the specific aims and methodology of the study.

For example, if one is designing a clinical trial that tests the efficacy of a given approach to rehabilitation, it would be expected that one would have based his or her approach to rehabilitation on an existing or emerging theory that defines the mechanisms that are expected to underlie the anticipated change.

Demonstrating Expert Knowledge of the Topic Area

For many granting agencies, one of the criteria by which a proposal is evaluated is the estimated expertise of the principal investigator and the research team. Level of expertise is typically judged according to a number of variables, including:

- Number of peer-reviewed publications in the area under study,
- Quality of the journals in which the articles are published,
- History of prior grant funding in the area under study,
- Evidence of specialized training and research mentorship in the area under study, and
- An established area of focus and a tradition of research.

One of the most important determinates of an investigator's expertise is the number and quality of publications that the investigator and research team members have in the area under study.

Another variable that is commonly evaluated is whether the investigator and/or other team members have a history of prior grant funding and participation on experienced research teams. A history of prior grant funding coupled with a consistent stream of high-impact publications emerging from prior grants are reasonable indicators that the investigator has experience successfully managing the intellectual, managerial, budgetary, and logistical challenges involved in carrying out a grant-funded study.

One of the most basic indicators of expertise, particularly for emerging research professionals, is evidence of an area of focus and a tradition of research (Taylor, Fisher, & Kielhofner, 2005). This most basic indicator overlaps with all of the other criteria mentioned in this section because developing an area of focus and a tradition of research necessarily involves receiving good training and mentorship in research and building a portfolio of evidence of ongoing research involvement in the area. For those just starting out, more information about how to establish an area of focus within occupational therapy and build a tradition of research can be found in Kielhofner (2002), and Kielhofner, Borrell, and Tham (2002). Before submitting any application for research, Gitlin and Lyons (2013) recommend conducting a self-evaluation to ensure one is ready to assume the role of principal investigator. The points that have been covered in this section can be used as a guide to this kind of self-evaluation.

One caveat is that it is important to recognize that the criteria used to evaluate an investigator's expertise are not uniformly applied within and across granting agencies. Some granting agencies issue classes of grant awards that are designed specifically to allow a new investigator or a clinician seeking to transition into a research role to develop his or her research skills in a given area. One contradiction to many of the criteria outlined in this section exists in some of the K-award funding (described in Table 33.3 later in this chapter) that is offered through the NIH. The purpose of the K awards is to support the professional development of researchers and prospective researchers at varied points within their research careers. The Mentored Research Scientist Development Award (K01) is one example of a K award that allows for newer researchers in a given area to receive funding for their research. The K01 requires a prospective investigator new to a given area of science to design a study and then obtain ongoing supervision and intensive training in his or her proposed area from an experienced researcher who serves as a career mentor for the investigator. The newer investigator is expected to accomplish the same research objectives as a more experienced researcher with the assistance of a mentor. In addition to professional development options offered to federal agencies, some private foundations and self-help organizations wanting to attract new investigators into an emerging or understudied area may place more value on an investigator's demonstrated interest in the research agenda and funding priorities of the agency than upon the investigator's preestablished track record of research in that area. Seed funding is also offered within many university settings to assist newer investigators in establishing an area of focus, a tradition of research, and a publication record.

Demonstrating Good Scholarship

One often unspoken but critical criterion for successful grant writing is to demonstrate good scholarship in writing and assembling the grant proposal. A grant proposal includes all of the elements of a research proposal (covered in Chapter 13), and possibly more, depending on the requirements of a given funding agency. For example, a funding agency might want a listing of the names and biographical information for as many key personnel and support staff participating in the research study as possible, up front, whereas a research proposal that is not being sent to a funding agency might not include such information. In any case, good scholarship is required in both the research proposal and the grant proposal, and this is indicated by:

- Organizing the proposal so that it adequately responds to each of the requested sections;
- Weaving a comprehensive and up-to-date literature review into various sections of the proposal;
- Including appropriate citations of prior, high-quality research in the area;

- Providing a well-reasoned and well-justified argument or rationale for the central aims and hypotheses;
- Presenting a meticulous and well-written document; and
- Obtaining mentorship, good advice, and peer reviews in advance of formal submission.

Because good scholarship is central to successful grant writing, the following section extends each of these points.

Organizing the Proposal So That It Adequately Responds to Each of the Requested Sections

One of the most basic aspects of grant writing that differentiates it from other forms of academic writing is that administrators and reviewers usually demand that the proposal follow a highly structured and organized format that is presented in the application instruction package. In addition to providing a highly organized structure for the proposal, some funding agencies assist applicants even further by asking them to organize the proposal in sections that perfectly mirror each of the criteria by which the proposal will be evaluated. Some agencies even provide questions that frame each section of the proposal to which the applicant is asked to respond. Most grant applications contain many or all of the following sections (Gitlin & Lyons, 2013):

- Title;
- Abstract;
- Introduction (including a literature review that reflects the background and significance of the problem, potential impact and feasibility of the study, theoretical foundation for the study, and general importance and relevance of the study to the scientific topic area);
- Specific aims (i.e., goals or objectives);
- Methods (including a research, evaluation, dissemination, and/or educational plan);
- Timeline and management plan (delineating roles and responsibilities of each research team member and time frames in which the work will be expected);
- Biographical information (i.e., biographical sketches and/or curriculum vitae for each member of the research team, illustrating credentials, level of expertise, and capacity to carry out the study);
- A summary of the resources and qualifications of the applicant's institution;
- A budget and budget narrative (justifying anticipated costs associated with the study);

- References (mirroring the citations provided in the text); and
- Appendices (containing consent forms, measures, treatment manuals and more detailed study protocols, fidelity rating scales, etc.).

Good scholars ensure that each of these sections is equally strong in terms of content and presentation.

Weaving a Comprehensive and Up-to-Date Literature Review Into Various Sections of the Proposal

Within any scientific tradition, it is critical to convey knowledge of the empirical findings that form the background of one's decision to develop and/or test a given concept, assessment, or intervention. A literature review should be utilized to accomplish the following objectives:

- Establish the need for the project and the significance of the problem to be addressed. For example, epidemiological research may be cited to describe the nature, course, prevalence, incidence, and long-term impact of a given condition on functioning.
- Provide evidence of the potential impact of the study. This may be accomplished by citing established unknowns or contradictions within the literature that need resolution.
- Provide evidence of the reliability, validity, and feasibility of the proposed study methods. This may be accomplished by citing studies that support an applicant's plans and provisions for recruiting and retaining an adequate number of subjects, by citing studies that have utilized similar methods of data collection, and by citing studies that attest to the reliability and validity of the measures, data collection methods, and statistical analyses to be used.
- Describe, explain, and provide evidence for the chosen theoretical foundation for the study.

In sum, the literature review should reflect both wide-ranging and highly specialized knowledge about the topic area proposed for study. Grant proposals are typically criticized if the background information, theoretical ideas presented, and rationale for the study are not well supported by an abundance of accurate citations of prior studies.

For proposals that are written in highly complex or controversial areas, it is not sufficient to cite studies that support only one side of a scientific argument. In most cases it is essential to cite representatives of both sides of the argument, provide an accurate and respectful summary of the work on each side, and then justify why one plans to take one side over another or explain how one's work will attempt to resolve the controversy. Refer to Chapter 31 for more information.

Including Appropriate Citations

Keeping updated and being knowledgeable about the work of important leaders and scientist peers in one's area of research is an ongoing but important process. The literature review must include not only broad-based and highly specific studies that justify the problem and explain the study approach, but also the most updated and cutting-edge work of key scientist peers working within the topic area. In some cases, important, not-yet-published preliminary findings from researchers willing to share their work privately can and should be included in the literature review to reflect the applicant's knowledge of evolving findings within the area closest to his or her field of study. For example, when applying for a successful grant that aimed to estimate the rates of nonrecovery from acute infectious mononucleosis in adolescents, the first author of this chapter included not-yet-published findings of adult rates of nonrecovery from a scientist leader within the same field of study.

Findings presented by other scientists at recent conferences or scientific meetings may also be used to support or provide background for an applicant's proposed work. In some cases, personal communications regarding key methodological issues, study feasibility issues, or other evidence of communication with leaders working in the same topical area is regarded positively (although cited work is always best). Having knowledge about the evolving and cutting-edge work in one's area demonstrates that an applicant is careful to remain absolutely current.

Providing a Well-Reasoned and Well-Justified Argument or Rationale for the Central Aims and Hypotheses

Another critical step in demonstrating good scholarship involves ensuring that one's proposal builds a logical justification for the central aims and hypotheses of the study. This rationale and justification must be articulated clearly and concretely in the proposal so that the reviewers are able to view the study as relevant and important to the field and link the background literature review to the aims and methods of the study. Building a rationale for the study may, for example, involve an explicit description of gaps or questions within the existing knowledge base that the study seeks to answer. See Chapter 11 for more information.

Presenting a Meticulous and Well-Written Document

Each application cycle, funding-agency administrators scan hundreds of proposals to determine whether they should be accepted for review. Subsequently, reviewers may be assigned to read or scan up to 20 to 30 proposals per meeting. For these reasons, it is important to write grant proposals in a clear, well-organized, and meticulous manner. Applicants must also ensure that their spelling is correct and that there are no careless typographical errors, formatting mistakes, or confusing and half-written sentences in the proposal. All of these errors can and do reflect poorly on the overall presentation of the proposal. See Chapter 32 for more information.

Obtaining Mentorship, Good Advice, and Peer Reviews in Advance of Formal Submission

Even if an applicant thinks he or she has made all possible provisions to ensure good scholarship in preparing a grant proposal, it is always wise to seek reviews or opinions from mentors or respected peers before formally submitting the proposal for review. The advice-seeking and opinion-gathering process should be initiated in the early stages of idea formulation and sustained throughout the writing process.

Conducting Pilot Research

Many funding agencies require an investigative team to have conducted preliminary research studies or pilot research that provides evidence for the feasibility and likelihood of success of the proposed research. The extent of pilot research or preliminary studies necessary depends on the requirements of the funding agency, the size of the proposed study, the research question, and the extent to which the collection of pilot data is economically and logistically feasible in the absence of grant funding. Pilot research is traditionally defined as a trial application of some, many, or all of the methods that a researcher plans to utilize in a larger, anticipated study using a smaller sample size. It can also include collection of data that helps demonstrate the need or value of the proposed project.

Thus, in grant writing, pilot research may be used to:

• Provide evidence of need for the study or intervention,
• Identify unanticipated logistical roadblocks in data collection,

- Test aspects of the reliability or validity of administering a given measure with a new population,
- Assess the feasibility of planned strategies for subject recruitment and retention, and
- Determine the likelihood of finding anticipated results in the larger study.

Choosing an Appropriate and Rigorous Design

Funding agencies and review groups vary widely in terms of what they consider to be appropriate and rigorous designs for research. Agencies that fund basic science studies and clinical research tend to value traditional experimental and quasi-experimental research designs, such as randomized controlled studies, epidemiological research, and prospective follow-up studies that utilize repeated measures designs. Agencies that fund research on health-care services and quality, innovative program development and program evaluation studies, and other forms of community-based research have a broader vision of what is considered to be an appropriate and rigorous design for a research study. In any case, it is important to ensure that the design chosen matches the central aims of the study, the resources (budget requested), and the sample size and is likely to produce the expected data.

For example, participatory approaches to research and approaches that are descriptive have become widely utilized in community-based research (see Chapter 30).

Qualitative research methodologies have also been incorporated. Over the past decade, occupational therapists and other medical and rehabilitation scientists have witnessed the incorporation of more of these designs into medical and rehabilitation research. See Chapter 12 for more information.

Ensuring an Ethical Design and Methodological Approach

A fundamental aspect of grant writing involves ensuring that the ethical guidelines established by one's home institution and the funding agency will be followed. All investigators are required to complete an institutional review board (IRB) application to ensure that all ethical issues have been considered to protect to the fullest extent possible the rights of participants.

In selecting designs and methodologies for grant-funded research studies, applicants must balance the demands of methodological rigor with the necessity to treat research subjects in an ethical manner and protect their rights to confidentiality.

For example, Taylor (2004) conducted a randomized clinical trial that examined the effectiveness of a rehabilitation program on quality of life using a sample of adults with chronic fatigue syndrome. Half of the sample (the treatment group) was assigned to receive the program immediately following recruitment, and the other half (delayed-treatment controls) was assigned to receive the program 1 year later. In a traditional randomized clinical trial, the investigator would not inform participants of their group assignment because expectancy effects might confound study findings. Specifically, delayed treatment controls would not be told they would be receiving the program 1 year later because their knowledge that they would eventually receive the program might bias their responses before, during, and after the program.

However, when the investigator developed the study in consultation with the ethics board, it was determined that all participants should be informed of their group assignment so that those in the delayed treatment control group knew that they would eventually be receiving the treatment. This approach triggered criticism about the violation of traditional randomization when the investigator submitted the findings from the study for publication. However, in this case, ethics demanded a less rigorous design in which all participants were informed of their group assignment.

When applicants are faced with ethical dilemmas in writing grant proposals, it is advisable to consult with ethics board representatives from the funding agency and from one's home institution (because both must approve the proposal before it is funded and conducted). In situations that are ambiguous or debatable, applicants should make it explicit within the grant proposal that alternative designs or methodologies were considered, and then justify why one approach was chosen over another. When complex situations arise, being explicit about ethical dilemmas demonstrates that an applicant has been thoughtful about these issues and opens the door for reviewers to support the selected approach or recommend alternatives. More detailed information and guidance about ethical considerations in OT research are provided in Chapter 14 of this text.

Addressing Logistical Issues and Obstacles in Data Collection Up Front

In addition to dilemmas involving competing ethical and methodological considerations, grant applicants often encounter dilemmas involving logistical and implementation issues. Expert reviewers are well aware that data collection that seeks to respond to a single research question can be approached from multiple methodological perspectives, and it can be completed in a wide range of settings. In applications that involve complex research questions that have the potential to be approached using a variety of different measures, methods, and/or statistical approaches to analysis, reviewers often look for evidence that an applicant is aware of and has considered the entire range of choices.

For example, in a proposed study that aimed to examine outcomes of an OT program for persons with HIV who were living in residential facilities, the investigators first considered a randomized clinical trial because it was ideally the most rigorous design for studying the outcomes of an intervention. However, in the grant proposal, the investigators, Kielhofner and Braveman (2001), made the following argument:

> Designing this study required us to deal with the following logistic constraints. Within a given facility, it would not be feasible to assign residents to different conditions. The model program will result in changes in the milieu of the facilities and cannot be implemented without contamination of control subjects in the same facility. Furthermore, once the intervention starts, it would be impossible for the facility to return to the control condition, for similar reasons. This rules out both a conventional randomized design at the level of the client and an interrupted times series design at the level of the facility.

The investigators then went on to propose their nonrandom control group design, describing statistical techniques that would be used to attenuate the effects of identified initial differences in the experimental and control groups. Because reviewers understood that the design proposed was the most rigorous design that could be implemented, given the circumstances of the study context, the grant was funded.

As in this case, a grant proposal should always:

- Make any study implementation dilemma explicit within the application and weigh the pros and cons of each approach or indicate why a more rigorous approach is not feasible, and
- Provide a rationale and justification for why the chosen approach was selected.

Planning Analyses

Most applications for research-related grants require investigators to specify how they plan to analyze the results and to describe in detail the statistical or qualitative methods that will be used. The data analysis plan is typically included in the methods section. In the case of quantitative studies, this section of the grant application is usually written by a statistical consultant or co-investigator with a high proficiency in mathematics and statistical methods.

For research studies that involve hypothesis testing, it is essential that all of the proposed statistical approaches represent an accurate and appropriate way to test the study hypotheses. In addition, each proposed statistical approach should correspond with each hypothesis listed. Each planned statistical approach should be described very clearly in lay terms in as much detail as possible. Any plans for the treatment of missing data and plans for troubleshooting other unanticipated complexities within the proposed data set should also be accounted for in this section.

Qualitative data analysis plans should be as complete as possible. However, if some of the analysis will depend on the unfolding research process, it should be specified how decisions about analysis will be made. If software for analysis is to be used, it should be noted. The analysis should clearly reflect the study question, be embedded in the specific qualitative approach to analysis, and reflect thorough efforts to maintain the trustworthiness of findings.

Developing a Timeline and Evaluation Plan

Most grant applications require a specific timeline of activities and when those activities are to be implemented, a detailed evaluation plan, and a description of performance indicators. Proposals ordinarily include:

- A detailed listing of all grant activities (e.g., from recruiting participants and sites to data collection, data analysis, and dissemination, etc.),
- When the specified activities will take place,
- Who will perform them, and
- The criteria by which they will be judged successfully completed (which is part of the evaluation plan, as presented in the following discussion).

Grant reviewers appreciate seeing a table with these elements included across the duration of the grant.

The evaluation plan ordinarily must include two separate levels of evaluation:

- A formative evaluation of all the activities proposed in the timeline (according to criteria included for successful performance as noted earlier), and

• A summative evaluation of the impact of the research study or training activity that the grant application has proposed.

Summative evaluation of the overall project usually involves specifying how one will determine the extent to which the aims and objectives proposed have been achieved and how they will be measured.

Many funders now require a project logic model to guide the evaluation process; it provides a visual representation of project goals, inputs, outputs, and outcomes (see Chapter 29 for a description of logic models). The logic model gives the researcher an overview of the outcomes of the project and also of the process of its implementation (or realization). Furthermore, it provides a framework that can serve as a reference point for the researcher to go back to and make sure that each step is achieved or that the proper adjustments are made.

Developing a Reasonable Budget Request

An important feature of any grant application is the budget request and budget narrative; together they justify the applicant's request for a certain amount of funding in each budget category. The budget narrative also provides the reviewers with a rough overview of the applicant's thinking about the logistical, timing, and implementation aspects of the study. In addition, the construction of the budget allows for the principal investigator and research team to anticipate and think through the personnel-related managerial and contractual aspects of the study.

Creating a budget up front allows the team to anticipate the amount of salaried release time from other duties that will be required by each team member to implement the grant. In addition, it allows for subcontract agreements to be negotiated between the principal investigator's sponsoring (home) institution and any other institutions that house the co-investigators in which certain study duties will be carried out.

Most funding agencies provide detailed instructions regarding the level of detail and budgetary planning that is required for documentation in an application. For example, some budget narratives can be so detailed that they specify the estimated number of study-related phone calls that will be made by each member of the research team, the estimated length of each call, and the estimated charge for each call. Other agencies and reviewers

may accept a more loosely written budget justification provided that the applicant is requesting what the reviewers and administrators consider to be a reasonable amount for each category. When possible, it is always advisable for an applicant to seek accounting consultation and assistance from an individual experienced in the assembly of a grant budget.

As outlined in an earlier section of this chapter (i.e., Selecting the Appropriate Funding Agency), funding agencies are highly diverse in terms of the amount of money they are willing to provide to support a single study or research group. The total amount of a grant award can range from $500 to well over $1,000,000 to support a single study. Despite this diversity, one characteristic that funding agencies have in common is that they all limit what they are willing to provide, and they all have regulations on how money can be spent in a given category. Thus, it is always wise to consult with a program officer if there are any questions about how much money can be requested in a single category or if there are other ambiguities regarding the budget in the application instructions. Generally, grant budgets for health-related research may be broken down into the following categories:

• Personnel and fringe benefits,
• Tuition waivers and training stipends for students,
• Consultants,
• Travel,
• Equipment,
• Supplies,
• Inpatient or outpatient costs,
• Subcontractual costs,
• Construction costs, and
• Other costs.

The costs for each category are generally added together in different combinations using a formula that subdivides the total into the following three categories:

• Total direct costs: This is defined by the sum of all or a certain combination of the categories in the previous list. (For example, a granting agency might define direct costs as the sum of all of the previously listed categories, excluding the costs of equipment and training stipends for students.)
• Indirect costs: Indirect costs cover basic infrastructure and operational costs involved in running a research study, such as office space, electricity, heating, and air-conditioning.
• Total budget request: This is the sum total of the direct and indirect costs across all years of the study.

Each funding agency has a different formula that is applied in the calculation of direct versus indirect costs. Many agencies put a cap on the percentage of indirect-cost funding that a sponsoring (home) institution can request in proportion to the total direct costs of a study. Some agencies do not allow a sponsoring institution to request any indirect costs because they expect an institution to provide the basic infrastructure support to operate the study. Under some circumstances, the percentage of indirect costs that an institution is permitted to extract from a grant is negotiated between the funding agency and the sponsoring institution.

Obtaining Letters of Support

Many funding agencies require letters of support to be appended to the grant application. Letters of support are formal testimonials that describe a collaborator's level of experience working in the research area, overall enthusiasm about the idea and/or methodological approach of the study, and planned role or contribution to the study. Letters of support are obtained from collaborators who intend to participate directly as members of the research team; from consumers who intend to serve in advisory capacities; and from collaborating sites such as community organizations, practice sites, or other individuals who intend to support the study in a more peripheral way (e.g., practitioners who have agreed to refer their patients to participate as subjects in the study). Letters of support are typically obtained from co-investigators, consultants, subcontractors, referral sources, and advisory board members.

After the Grant Has Been Submitted

The following subsections explain the critical processes and interactions that occur within the funding agency and between the program officers and the principal investigator after a grant has been submitted. It is important for investigators to have as much information about these processes as possible so that they better understand the details that contribute to a funding agency's decision to make a grant award. The three critical processes discussed in this section are:

- Review process,
- Grant scores and funding decisions, and
- Feedback and resubmission.

Understanding the Review Process

For most funding agencies and competitive grant applications, the outcome of the review process is the most critical determinant of whether an investigator's grant proposal will receive funding. In many agencies, the review process can take from several months to nearly a year to complete. During the review process, one or more individuals serving as representatives for the funding agency carefully scrutinize each application to determine whether it meets a set of prespecified criteria for funding.

Agencies differ in terms of these criteria. To a certain extent, these differences depend on the overall mission, values, or objectives of the funding source. Knowing as much as possible about the review process, evaluation criteria, and the individuals serving as reviewers is important in preparing as competitive an application as possible (Gitlin & Lyons, 2013).

Agencies differ in terms of the number of grant applications they receive and in terms of the numbers and kinds of individuals who are assigned to review a given application. For example, the U.S. Public Health Service, which includes the NIH and the AHRQ, receives and reviews approximately 40,000 grant applications per year. Because few proposals relative to this overall number are actually funded, the application process is highly competitive. Similarly, certain offices within the U.S. Department of Education have been known to fund only the top 4% of discretionary grant applications for certain competitions.

Because the review procedures for U.S. federal granting agencies tend to be more complex than those for other granting agencies, this section focuses on describing the review procedures for federal agencies (i.e., NIH, AHRQ, and the U.S. Department of Education). Private industry and foundations use many of the evaluation criteria and review procedures that are employed by federal agencies. Thus, the general ideas provided herein should be somewhat transferable for applications to other funding sources. However, it is important to keep in mind that all agencies will differ between and within themselves in terms of the evaluation criteria they designate as most important for an investigator to address for any given type of grant. Following application instructions to the letter and tailoring the proposal to each and every aspect of the evaluation criteria is the most critical aspect of preparing any grant proposal.

Many funding agencies adhere to a peer-review process in which reviewers are selected based on their expertise in a scientific area that matches that of the grant proposals being reviewed. Peer reviewers are typically selected based on a history of exceptional scholarship and achievement in the given area. The designation of peer reviewer does not mean that the investigator knows or works with the reviewer. In fact, many agencies have strict conflict-of-interest regulations against dual relationships or research collaborations between peer reviewers and applicants.

Usually, at least three reviewers are designated to provide a detailed review of a grant application. These reviewers are sometimes referred to as first, second, and third reviewers, for example. For some agencies, an additional group of as many as 20 other reviewers that comprise a review panel may be asked to score and give input on a single application. Often, this larger group of reviewers will skim the applications and base their scores on the reports given by the primary review group and on the contents of the discussion that followed those reports.

Some funding agencies assemble review panels that consist of both peer (professional) reviewers and lay reviewers or consumers. Lay reviewers may be members of the same community or population from which participants in the research project will be drawn (e.g., individuals with chronic fatigue syndrome from a wide range of work or professional backgrounds). Alternatively, they may be individuals who represent the voice of an even broader group of individuals of which the prospective participants may be a part (e.g., individuals with disabilities). Lay reviewers will inevitably read the application through different lenses than peer reviewers. It is important to know up front whether a lay reviewer will be reviewing the grant so that one will know whether his or her language and writing style should be tailored to a broader audience. Lay reviewers are usually charged with the same responsibilities and given as much power in the vote as peer reviewers regarding whether a given application should be funded.

If a grant received a fundable score as a result of the peer-review process, some granting agencies would employ a second tier of reviewers housed within the agency or closely linked to the agency (e.g., a board of directors) to make the final funding decision. For example, within the NIH, the National Advisory Council functions as an oversight board that consists of scientists and administrators. This board reviews each highly scored grant that has been recommended for funding to ensure that it provides adequate provisions for the protection of human subjects and that it is consistent with the overall policies, values, and vision of

the NIH. Similarly, the U.S. Department of Education has what is called a grants team that conducts an internal review of each highly scored grant to ensure that the reviewer's scoring sheets are correctly completed and to verify that the application meets all of the requirements of the program.

Criteria by which a grant application is judged vary widely. In many cases, evaluation criteria are provided in instructional format along with the initial grant application package. Some agencies have a rather rigid set of criteria by which an application is judged, whereas other agencies only offer general guidelines or do not offer much detail in the way of evaluation criteria. Examples of evaluation criteria set forth by the NIH and the U.S. Department of Education are provided in Tables 33.2 and 33.3, respectively.

The evaluation criteria presented in Tables 33.2 and 33.3 are simply examples, and they are not entirely comprehensive or exact. Even within a given agency, the evaluation criteria may change depending on the nature of the competition and the type of grant for which one is applying. Knowing and continually evaluating one's grant proposal against the published criteria for a given competition throughout the planning and writing process is fundamental to increasing the application's competitiveness. Just as evaluation criteria vary from agency to agency, so do approaches to scoring a grant proposal. More information about how applications are scored and how scores are typically interpreted is provided later in this chapter.

Interpreting Grant Scores in Light of Funding Decisions

Obtaining grant funding from most agencies is a highly competitive process. Agencies vary widely in their approaches to scoring grant applications. For example, the U.S. Department of Education scores applications such that high scores are given to the strongest applications and low scores to the weakest. Conversely, the NIH scores applications such that low scores are given to the strongest applications and high scores are given to the weakest. Applications that score above the 50th percentile based on preliminary review are generally not forwarded for formal review and are not scored. Within the NIH, this process is called *streamlining* because it is more time efficient and it facilitates a more detailed review of the stronger applications. Even though a review panel may assign a potentially fundable score to a grant application, it is not a guarantee that the application will be funded.

Table 33.2   Typical National Institutes of Health (NIH) Evaluation Criteria and Questions for Competing Research Applications*

Criterion	Types of Questions for Reviewers
Significance	• Is the scientific problem that the application addresses important? • Are the outcomes of the study likely to have a significant impact on existing scientific knowledge in this area? • How will this application advance existing knowledge, theoretical concepts, treatment approaches, or methodologies in this area?
Approach	• Is the study based on an overarching theory or conceptual framework? • Are the theory, design, methods, and statistical analyses cohesive and well developed? • Do they adequately reflect the specific aims and hypotheses of the study? • Is the proposed approach feasible and methodologically rigorous? • Does the investigator anticipate possible pitfalls or problems with the approach, and does he or she provide alternative ways of addressing those problems should they occur?
Innovation	• Does the study introduce new theoretical concepts, approaches, or methodologies? • How does the project challenge existing paradigms or seek to revise or reformulate existing treatments or methodologies?
Investigators	• Are the investigators and research team members sufficiently knowledgeable, experienced, and adequately trained to carry out the work of the proposed project?
Environment	• Does the scientific environment in which the study will take place provide adequate resources and increase the likelihood that the study will be successful? • Does the project involve useful and relevant collaborations between agencies or organizations? • Does the study take advantage of unique resources or equipment within the investigator's home institution?
Inclusions, budget, and protections	• Are the plans to include both men and women in the project adequate? • Are there adequate provisions for the recruitment and retention of individuals from minority groups? • Is the proposed budget reasonable given the amount of professional effort put forth, logistical requirements, methods, and length of the proposed study? • Are there adequate provisions in place for the protection of subjects participating in the research?

*Based on evaluation guidelines for reviewers provided at https://grants.nih.gov/grants/peer/critiques/rpg.htm.

Table 33.3   Examples of U.S. Department of Education General Evaluation Criteria for Grant Reviews

Criterion	Questions
Need for project	• Is the problem to be addressed of sufficient magnitude or severity? • How does the proposed project meet the need for services, identify gaps or weaknesses in existing services, and address those gaps? • How will the proposed project prepare personnel for fields in which shortages have been demonstrated?
Significance	• What is the national significance and likely impact of the proposed project in terms of improving employment? • How significant is the problem to be addressed by the project? • What is the potential contribution of the project to increased knowledge or understanding of rehabilitation or educational problems, issues, or effective strategies? • What is the likelihood that the project will result in system change or improvement? • How likely is the project to contribute to the development and advancement of theory, knowledge, and practices in the field of study? • How replicable will the program be in a variety of settings, and how generalizable will the findings be? • To what extent will the proposed project yield findings or products that will be utilized by other agencies or organizations? • How likely is it that the proposed project will build local capacity to provide, improve, or expand services? • Will the results be disseminated in ways that will enable others to use the information or strategies?

(continued)

Table 33.3 Continued

Criterion	Questions
Quality of the project design	• To what extent are the goals, objectives, and predicted outcomes clearly specified and measurable? • Is the project based on a specific and rigorous research design? • Does the design reflect up-to-date knowledge from research and effective practice? • Is the design appropriate for the needs of the target population, and is it likely to address those needs? • Is there a high-quality conceptual framework underlying the proposed research or demonstration activities? • Do the proposed activities add to a coherent and sustained program of research, training, or development in the field? • Do they add substantially to an ongoing line of inquiry? • Is the proposed design accompanied by a thorough, high-quality review of the literature, a quality plan for research activities/project implementation, and the use of appropriate theoretical and methodological tools to ensure successful achievement of the project objectives? • Will the design lead to replication of project activities or strategies? Are proposed development efforts accompanied by adequate quality controls and repeated testing of products? • Will the project build capacity and yield results that will extend beyond the funding period? • Does the proposed project represent an exceptional approach for meeting the priorities established for the competition and/or the statutory purposes and requirements? • To what extent will the project be coordinated with related efforts and establish linkages with both appropriate community, state, and federal resources and organizations providing services to the target population? • Does the project encourage consumer involvement? • Are performance feedback and continuous improvement integral to the design of the project? • What is the quality of the methodology to be employed in this project?
Quality of project services	• Are there strategies for ensuring equal access and treatment for eligible project participants who are members of groups that have traditionally been underrepresented based on race, color, national origin, gender, age, or disability? • Are the services to be provided by the project appropriate to the needs of the intended recipients or beneficiaries of those services? • Do entities that are to be served by any proposed technical assistance project demonstrate support for the project? • Do the services to be provided reflect up-to-date knowledge from research and effective practice? • What is the likely impact on the intended recipients of the services to be provided? • To what extent are the training or professional development services to be provided by the proposed project of sufficient quality, intensity, and duration to lead to improvements in practice among recipients of those services? • Will the training or professional development services alleviate the personnel shortages that have been identified? • Will the project lead to improvements in the academic achievement of students as measured against rigorous standards? • Will the project lead to improvements in the skills necessary to gain employment or build capacity for independent living? • To what extent will the project involve the collaboration of appropriate partners for maximizing the effectiveness of services? • To what extent are the services to be provided focused on those with greatest needs?
Quality of project personnel	• Will the investigator encourage applications for project staff positions from persons who are members of groups that have traditionally been underrepresented based on race, color, national origin, gender, age, or disability? • How qualified, trained, and experienced are the investigators, key project personnel, consultants, and subcontractors?

Table 33.3   Continued

Criterion	Questions
Adequacy of resources	• Are the facilities, equipment, supplies, and other resources from the applicant organization adequate? • Has each partner demonstrated commitment to the implementation and success of the project? • Is the budget adequate to support the proposed project? • Are the proposed costs reasonable in relation to the objectives, design, potential significance and benefit, and number of persons to be served? • Is there potential for continued support of the project by appropriate entities after federal funding ends? • Is there a potential for the incorporation of project purposes, activities, or benefits into the ongoing program of the agency after the funding period?
Quality of the management plan	• Is the management plan adequate to achieve the objectives of the project on time and within the budget? • Does the management plan include clearly defined responsibilities, timelines, and milestones for accomplishing project tasks? • Are the procedures for ensuring feedback and continuous improvement in project operations adequate? • Are the mechanisms for ensuring high-quality products and services from the project adequate? • Are time commitments from the investigators and other project personnel adequate to meet the objectives? • How will the applicant ensure that a diversity of perspectives is brought to bear in the operation of the proposed project, including those of parents, teachers, the business community, other disciplines, and consumers?
Quality of the project evaluation	• Are the methods of evaluation thorough, feasible, appropriate to the context within which the project operates, and appropriate to the goals, objectives, and outcomes of the project? • Do the methods of evaluation provide for examining the effectiveness of project implementation strategies? • Do the methods of evaluation include the use of objective performance measures that are clearly related to the intended outcomes of the project, and will they produce quantitative and qualitative data to the greatest extent possible? • Will project evaluation methods provide timeline guidance for quality assurance? • Will the evaluation provide guidance about effective strategies suitable for replication or testing in other settings?

*Based on guidelines adapted from evaluation guidelines for reviewers provided by the Education Department General Administrative Regulations, Part 75, Subpart D. A specific competition will typically use a subset of the types of questions listed in this table.

In conjunction with the requirement for additional evaluations of the overall relevance of the highly scored proposal to agency values and priorities, many agencies have cutoff points (often represented by percentile rankings) that determine which of the highly scored applications will be funded and which will not. For example, one agency may fund only the top 2% of applications for a given competition, whereas another agency may fund the top 15%. These cutoff points fluctuate depending on accounting formulas that are developed by each agency. These formulas typically incorporate the number of applications received for each funding cycle and the amount of money available from cycle to cycle. Many program officers are willing to provide investigators with information regarding percentile funding cutoffs once it becomes available.

Evaluating Feedback and Determining Whether to Resubmit the Proposal

After having worked numerous hours to write and assemble a grant proposal, receiving critical or negative feedback is a challenging process for even the most experienced grant writer. When a grant application is not funded, it is not only difficult to read feedback from reviewers, but at times it is also difficult to interpret it and decide whether others consider the proposal worthy of revision and resubmission. Some agencies, such as the U.S. Department of Education and the NIH, make the process of interpreting feedback somewhat easier by using a two-tier system. These agencies score and comprehensively evaluate only the stronger applications. Written feedback from the reviewers is forwarded only to investigators who achieved the higher scores. If an applicant's proposal is rejected but he or she receives written feedback from an agency, it indicates that the reviewers considered the application worthy of a detailed discussion regarding its merits and weaknesses.

In many cases, federal agencies consider applications that are streamlined (or not scored) as not salvageable because they are limited by major flaws. Such flaws may include ideas that lack significance or do not reflect the objectives of the funding agency, flaws in the design and methods, absence of an adequate theoretical basis, confusing or inconsistent aims and hypotheses, poor overall scholarship, and ethical or logistic problems (Gitlin & Lyons, 2013).

Proposals worthy of revision and resubmission include those that are given scores near the percentile cutoff for funding. In many cases, feedback will indicate that the reviewers were enthusiastic about the application and would encourage revision and resubmission. Sometimes reviewers will provide the applicant with questions to answer in the revised proposal or suggestions to address the concerns that have been raised. The program officer can often speak to the general level of enthusiasm about an application and can assist an applicant in deciding whether to revise and resubmit the grant application.

Summary

This chapter provides an orientation to the main kinds of funding opportunities for OT researchers. The authors explain the steps involved in writing and applying for grants that fund research studies and other research-related programs and initiatives. Twenty steps that the authors consider necessary for the attainment of grant funding are reviewed. The authors explain elements of grant writing that range from idea development to ensuring an appropriate review once a grant has been submitted. The authors then describe the review and evaluation process and explain how funding decisions are made. The chapter also provides information on how to revise and resubmit a grant proposal that was rejected. Explanations of international funding procedures and mechanisms available in the United Kingdom and Canada are provided, and examples that describe the process of obtaining different kinds of grant funding from different funding sources are presented.

Review Questions

1. What is an idea for a research study (or an existing example that you know of) that would have impact for the field of occupational therapy and would require grant funding to occur?

2. Daniel is a practicing occupational therapist with a professional doctorate (OTD). During his practice, he has developed several ideas for innovations to assist individuals with spinal cord injury in completing everyday activities. He wants to pursue research and development of these ideas, and he also wants to obtain a part-time academic position at a research-intensive university. He knows that he must obtain grant funding to do so. What is the most appropriate type of grant for Daniel to apply for? Explain your rationale.

3. What are the most important components of a successful grant proposal? Justify your perspective.

4. If you wanted to begin a research line in energy conservation and graded exercise for people with multiple sclerosis and you had not yet obtained grant funding in this area, how might you go about choosing a team of co-investigators? Whom would you invite to join your team? Justify your approach.

5. Ann recently received feedback after a review of a grant proposal she recently submitted. The grant was not funded, but she did receive a higher-than-average score. The main criticisms involved Ann's methodological approach, and she received some very detailed feedback from the reviewers. The reviewers did mention that the idea for the grant was of high impact. Would you advise Ann to resubmit? Why or why not?

REFERENCES

Creek, J., & Ilott, I. (2002). *Scoping study of occupational therapy research and development activity in Scotland, Northern Ireland and Wales.* London, England: College of Occupational Therapists.

Department of Health. (2000). *Meeting the challenge: A strategy for the allied health professions.* London, England: Author.

Department of Health. (2005). *Research governance framework for health and social care* (2nd ed.). London, England: Author.

Gillette, N. (2000). A twenty-year history of research funding in occupational therapy. *American Journal of Occupational Therapy, 54*(4), 441–442.

Gitlin, L. N., & Lyons, K. J. (2013). *Successful grant writing: Strategies for health and human service professionals* (4th ed.). New York, NY: Springer.

Higher Education Funding Council for England. (2001). *Research in nursing and allied health professions: Report of the Task Group 3 to HEFCE and the Department of Health.* Bristol, England: Author.

Ilott, I., & White, E. (2001). 2001 College of Occupational Therapists' research and development strategic vision and action plan. *British Journal of Occupational Therapy, 64*(6), 270–274.

Kielhofner, G. (2002). UIC's scholarship of practice. *OT Practice, 7*(1), 11–12.

Kielhofner, G., Borell, L., & Tham, K. (2002). Preparing scholars of practice around the world. *OT Practice, 7*(6), 13–14.

Kielhofner, G., & Braveman, B. (2001). Enabling self-determination for people living with AIDS. Department of Occupational Therapy, University of Illinois at Chicago. Grant proposal submitted to and funded by the National Institute of Disability and Rehabilitation Research, U.S. Department of Education (H133G020217-3).

Scottish Executive. (2004). Allied health professions research and development action plan. Edinburgh, Scotland: Scottish Executive.

Taylor, R. R. (2004). Quality of life and symptom severity for individuals with chronic fatigue syndrome: Findings from a randomized clinical trial. *American Journal of Occupational Therapy, 58,* 35–43.

Taylor, R. R., Fisher, G., & Kielhofner, G. (2005). Synthesizing research, education, and practice according to the scholarship of practice model: Two faculty examples. *Occupational Therapy and Health Care, 19,* 107–122.

RESOURCES

For Grant Writing

Gitlin, L. N., & Lyons, K. J. (2013). *Successful grant writing: Strategies for health and human service professionals* (4th ed.). New York, NY: Springer.

To Find a Potential Match Between a Private Source of Funding and an Idea/Project: United States

The Foundation Center: A nonprofit information clearinghouse and library that collects and disseminates information on more than 80,000 private foundations for organizations and individuals seeking information about grants. It is one of the most widely accessed search engines used by research development personnel to inform investigators of available funding opportunities and competitions. The Foundation Center can be accessed at http://www.foundationcenter.org.

Information About the Grant Review Process

Most funding agencies will have information on their grant review process posted on their websites. Detailed information about the review process within the NIH can be found at http://grants1.nih.gov/grants/peer/peer.htm

CHAPTER 34

Using Mixed-Methods Designs to Study Therapy and Its Outcomes

Mary A. Corcoran

Learning Outcomes

- Define a mixed-methods approach to research.
- List the major types of mixed-methods approaches.
- Discuss the four principles of mixed-methods designs.
- Differentiate the types of mixed-methods designs.
- Understand the importance of the integrity of methods.

Introduction

Historically, only two major research traditions have been widely recognized in the global scientific community. These traditions are known by a number of terms which fall into two broad categories, experimental (including post-positivist, experimental, and quantitative) and naturalistic (including constructivism, postmoderism, and qualitative). The quantitative–qualitative dichotomy may be most familiar because these terms differentiate the types of data primarily collected within each tradition. Other chapters in this text discuss these two traditions in detail and point out their differing epistemological modes (i.e., different underlying assumptions, focus, design, and methods of data gathering and analysis).

For years, scientists have informally combined designs or methods within or from both traditions. Usually, they do so by conducting a sidebar or secondary study within a larger one. These combinations are most often intended to generate in-depth information about the experiences or opinions of a group of people who have participated in an experimental study.

Mixed methods as a legitimate design approach began to gain wide attention in the 1980s after Denzin (1978) introduced the concept of triangulation. **Triangulation** refers to the practice of gathering data from a number of different sources

for the purposes of detaching the method of measurement from the phenomenon being measured. For example, if a social behavior emerges in an interview *and* is observed in action, this finding may be regarded as particularly salient because two different data sources independently confirm it. The concept of triangulation fit well with the new paradigm of pragmatism that was emerging and taking root at the same time (Howe, 1988).

Pragmatism holds that qualitative and quantitative traditions are compatible and can be successfully combined in the same design. However, the mixed-methods studies that followed were a hodgepodge of typologies, definitions, and procedures. Prominent methodologists have called for conceptualizing mixed methods as a third tradition separate from but equal to qualitative and quantitative traditions. They further support its development as a set of rigorous research tools for addressing complex questions.

The term **mixed methods** refers to a research design that integrates elements of both qualitative and quantitative methods so that the strengths of each are emphasized.[1] However, Tashakkori and Teddlie (2003) posit that mixed methods are more than just combinations of qualitative and quantitative procedures. Because qualitative and quantitative procedures stem from two separate (and in many ways, opposing) epistemologies, they must be combined as interdependent but separate procedures during data collection. This is usually accomplished by establishing one of the traditions (either qualitative or quantitative) as the core method. The underlying assumptions of the core method are prioritized and reflected in the study purpose, methodological decisions, and overall analytic approach. In implementing that portion of the study that is based on a secondary method, the investigator must guard against violating any

---

[1]Mixed methods should be distinguished from mixed designs, which are consistent with a quantitative tradition and involve "factorial designs in which the number of levels of the factors are not the same for all factors" (Vogt & Johnson, 2011, p. 233).

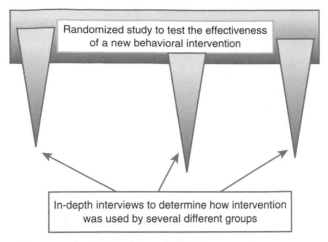

Figure 34.1   Illustration of a mixed-methods design.

of the assumptions of the core method while still maintaining the integrity of the secondary method. This requires careful planning and solid understanding of both traditions represented. During data analysis, the core method continues to dictate the overall approach, although data from the secondary method may be transformed and integrated with the data from the core method.

This relatively new approach to scientific inquiry is growing in popularity because of the flexibility it affords investigators (Creswell, Klassen, Plano Clark, & Smith, 2011). For example, a mixed methodologist has the ability to combine strict controls necessary for generalization with in-depth examinations of the study participants' experiences or perceptions on a particular topic. Figure 34.1 illustrates a typical mixed-methods approach that uses a combination of a controlled quantitative design with a qualitative naturalistic design. In this figure, traditional quantitative methods, such as experimental and quasi-experimental designs, can be conceptualized as the wide, shallow box. This box in Figure 34.1 represents the broad scope of experimental studies regarding a very narrow topic. The narrow but deep triangle represents the in-depth but highly focused approach of qualitative studies. In Figure 34.1, a primarily quantitative study to test the effectiveness of a new behavioral intervention also contains in-depth interviews that allow the investigator to understand more about the experiences of those individuals who participated in this efficacy study. The investigator may want to hear from several types of participants, including those who were able to incorporate behavioral changes in their lives, those who had difficulty doing so, and those who were unable to make changes called for in the intervention.

Investigators using such an approach can answer the question "*What is the effect of the intervention on X?*" and they can also gather information about how easy or difficult it was for participants to actually use the behavioral strategies from the intervention. This information can then be used to guide analysis, interpret the study findings, and refine the intervention in future trials.

There are many ways to merge quantitative and qualitative procedures in new and unique ways (Creswell et al., 2011). As research questions become more complex, mixed methods may emerge as a principal tradition in social science in years to come (Tashakkori & Teddlie, 2003). Mixed methods are particularly relevant for occupational therapy, a profession with firm foundations in a number of disciplines and that faces the challenge of blending many bodies of knowledge in the dynamic concept of occupation. Therefore, the purpose of this chapter is to introduce current thinking about mixed methods as a third methodological tradition with unique nomenclature, principles, designs, and procedures (Tashakkori and Teddlie, 2003) and to apply that tradition to occupational therapy.

Mixed Methods Nomenclature and Typologies

The overarching typology of research designs that includes mixed methods is known as multiple-methods designs (Tashakkori & Teddlie, 2003). **Multiple-methods designs** refer to use of two or more data collection strategies or methods

CASE EXAMPLE

Fibromyalgia is a complex syndrome involving chronic muscle and joint pain, fatigue, and tenderness in specific areas of the body known as tender points. Not much is known about its causes. One line of inquiry has involved the role of acute stress in precipitating autonomic activation and inflammation (Drummond & Willox, 2013). Other studies have found that continuing stress contributes to the intensity and frequency of symptoms via these and other multivariate mechanisms (Cleare, 2004). Carrying on a line of research from prior studies, Dr. Elsies plans to study variables that facilitate and interrupt return to work among women with fibromyalgia. Prior research suggests that women with fibromyalgia under work stress with physical capacity limits may have more difficulty continuing with work than others (Mannerkorpi & Gard, 2012). In contrast, having meaningful work, individual compensatory strategies, a favorable work environment, and social support outside of work facilitate continued engagement in work (Palstam, Gard, & Mannerkorpi, 2013). Based on this research, Dr. Elsies decides to explore the characteristics of women who do and do not sustain work within the health-care professions.

Dr. Elsies decides to apply a concurrent nested design in which she first conducts a descriptive epidemiological study to answer basic numerical questions and then conducts an in-depth, qualitative exploration of the personal and environmental characteristics of women with fibromyalgia who do and do not sustain work. Specifically, the descriptive quantitative data resulting from the epidemiological study will answer the following questions:

- What proportion of women with fibromyalgia work in a health-care profession?
- Are there certain types of health-care professions that are more sustainable for women with fibromyalgia than others?
- What psychological barriers exist within the health-care professions that prevent women with fibromyalgia from sustaining work? What psychological characteristics enable continued work?
- Do women identify infectious variables and other exposure-related risks as variables that prevent them from sustaining work?
- What physical barriers exist in terms of demands for physical functioning within the health-care professions that prevent women with fibromyalgia from sustaining work? Are there physical characteristics, such as fitness level or daily movement therapy, that allow for continued work?
- What barriers in women's familial and social environments outside of the workplace prevent continuing work? What familial and social variables enable continued work?
- What environmental barriers exist in terms of commuting time, climate, and other obstacles within and outside of the workplace? What facilitators exist within the environment?

After collecting data on these variables, Dr. Elsies then conducts individual in-depth interviews with each of the participants to uncover the answers to more informative questions regarding the sample of women's ability to continue work within the health-care professions. Such questions include:

- What do you find most motivating about your work? Least motivating?
- What personal strengths and coping mechanisms do you draw upon when you are having difficulty with fibromyalgia symptoms?
- Does physical activity outside of work enable or hinder your performance at work? In what types of physical activity do you engage outside of work? During work? Is there a tipping point of physical activity for you that makes the difference?
- In what ways are your family and friends encouraging of your continuing employment in your current work role? In what ways do they present difficulties for you in continuing in your current work role?

for a given research question. Multiple-methods designs can be further divided into two subcategories, multimethod designs and mixed-methods designs, which are defined in the following sections (Tashakkori & Teddlie, 2003, p. 11).

Tashakkori and Teddlie (2003) make the observation that quantitative research designs have enjoyed a long tradition of commonly understood and well-defined terms. This has provided the quantitative tradition with a common language as a basis for developing and describing methodologies. The qualitative research tradition has been working toward a common lexicon only for the past two decades but during that time has made great strides in identifying and defining key concepts.

Mixed methods, as a tradition in its "adolescence" (Tashakkori & Teddlie, 2003), has only begun to consider whether a common language is needed, and if so, what system of terms and definitions should be adopted. In their *Handbook of Mixed Methods in Social & Behavioral Research,* Tashakkori and Teddlie (2003) provide a glossary of terms that have been defined through consensus of several leading authors in the field and do not have alternative definitions. The serious student of mixed methods should be familiar with this new language.

Multimethod Designs

Multimethod designs incorporate two or more data collection techniques within only *one* tradition (qualitative or quantitative) (Tashakkori & Teddlie, 2003). For example, a study question regarding the effectiveness of an occupational therapy (OT) intervention may be best answered through a quantitative tradition, such as a randomized two-group design. However, an investigator using a multimethod approach may decide to triangulate his or her data with two different surveys to measure the dependent variable, independence in self-care. As shown in Figure 34.2, the dependent variable is measured by a self-report survey from the study participant and a proxy report from a caregiver.

Multimethod designs are powerful approaches to complex and nuanced research questions and an important strategy in the qualitative tradition for ensuring trustworthiness. However, because multimethod designs do not combine more than one research tradition, as do mixed-methods designs, competing philosophies and underlying assumptions are not an issue. Therefore, the remainder of this chapter is devoted to discussing the unique

methodological approach associated with mixed-methods designs.

Mixed-Methods Designs

In **mixed-methods designs,** qualitative and quantitative traditions are used simultaneously or consecutively in the methods section (Tashakkori & Teddlie, 2003). Extending the previous example, the investigator may suspect that an underlying cultural issue is mediating the effect of the intervention being tested. This investigator hypothesizes that the participants' culturally based definition of disability shapes the level at which they will enact the intervention procedures being studied.

A mixed-methods design could be used in this case. To implement such a design, the investigator might conduct an ethnography subsequent to the field experiment to develop a better understanding of the relationship between the definition of disability and self-care actions. By comparing Figures 34.1 and 34.2, one can see that the former is an illustration of a mixed-methods design (using methods from both the qualitative and quantitative traditions), whereas the latter illustrates a multimethod design (using more than one method to collect data within a single quantitative design).

Other authors have recommended more complex typologies. For instance, Newman, Ridenour, Newman, and DeMarco (2003) suggest that the typology be organized by research purpose rather than design type. Interested readers are encouraged to consult other texts for additional ways of systematically classifying mixed-methods designs, including Newman and Benz (1998), Tashakkori and Teddlie (1998, 2003), Creswell (2013), and Greene and Caracelli (1997).

Principles of Mixed-Methods Designs

Morse (2003) warns strongly against using the "muddling method" of combining models, which

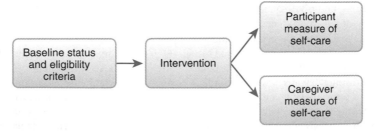

Figure 34.2 Illustration of a quantitative multimethod design.

involves simply tossing together methods and models without adequate consideration for issues of validity. For example, the investigator who combines ethnography with a field experiment must avoid changing the intervention midstream to reflect what he or she has learned from the participants, and runs the risk of being unable to maintain an unbiased and objective status. These actions might not be a problem in a qualitative tradition, but they introduce threats to validity in the quantitative portion of the study.

As with all traditions of research, decisions must be made based on the conceptual framework, purpose, and research question(s) of the study. This may be even more important when combining qualitative and quantitative traditions, which have diametrically opposed philosophies on several fundamental points, including the shape of the research process (linear versus spiral), the role of the investigator (objective versus subjective), and the type of logic used (deductive versus inductive). If not carefully planned, an investigator may find that a number of threats to validity have been introduced in the process of mixing methods and models.

Principles of Mixed-Methods Designs

Four principles are offered by Morse (2003) for a mixed-methods design, and these are discussed in the following sections.

Recognize the Theoretical Drive of the Project

Research projects fall broadly into two types of purpose: discovery or testing (i.e., inductive or deductive). Morse (1991) uses the term **theoretical drive** to refer to whether the main reasoning process required for the purpose of a project is inductive or deductive. The investigator must remain clear as to the type of inquiry and reasoning process driving the project and how each component fits the whole.

In a mixed-methods study, both quantitative and qualitative components are introduced. However, there can be only one theoretical drive, either inductive or deductive. The following example is used to illustrate these decisions in action. An investigator is interested in describing the ways in which people with traumatic brain injury (TBI) handle information about their diagnosis and medical history on the job. Do they disclose their head injury, and if so, to whom and how? If they do not disclose,

what barriers do they perceive as keeping them from doing so? The investigator plans to use both questionnaires and qualitative interviews drawing on both quantitative and qualitative traditions. This is obviously a project with a discovery basis, so an inductive drive is appropriate.

Adhere to the Methodological Assumptions of the Core Method

Respecting the **integrity of methods** (i.e., do not violate the assumptions, philosophical foundations, and procedures of the core method) seems like a simple message when introducing other secondary methods. In actual practice, respecting methodological integrity requires continually linking the unique philosophical foundations with the research question(s) and maintaining one method as dominant over the other.

When decisions are made throughout the project, the methodological integrity is always among the first considerations, but an investigator using a mixed-methods design cannot stop there. The investigator must begin with consideration for the integrity of the core method and then consider the implications of each decision for the integrity of the secondary method(s). Morse (2003) suggests keeping the core and secondary methods clear by using capital letters when referring to the core method (such as QUAL+ quan to denote a study that is primarily qualitative with a secondary quantitative component).

For example, an investigator is interested in knowing how a school-based intervention affects both the self-confidence of the participants and the legibility of their handwriting. The investigator decides to test intervention effects on the dependent variables in two ways, directly through a measure of self-confidence and handwriting samples of the participants and indirectly through a proxy open-ended interview with the teachers regarding these variables (self-confidence and legibility). The type of mixed design would therefore be written so as to designate that the study is quantitative with a deductive theoretical drive plus an additional qualitative method (proxy open-ended interview) used simultaneously (i.e., QUAN + qual). If the secondary quantitative investigation were to be conducted sequentially, the design would be written as QUAN → qual, such as in the case of interviewing only those individuals who dropped out of an experimental study. For an in-depth discussion of this principle and its use in several multiple-method studies, see Morse (2003).

Now, the investigator remains clear as to the order of each of the methods (quantitative and qualitative) and can make decisions that maintain the integrity of the core method. For example, the investigator using teachers' interviews to supplement direct observation and handwriting samples should gather the qualitative information at the same time that data are collected from the children. Even though it would be logistically easier to get all the teachers together once in a focus group for the purposes of collecting information on all the study participants, to do so would introduce a problem of comparing two different time frames for measuring the dependent variables.

Recognize the Role of the Imported Models to the Project

The core model of the project will determine the reasoning process of the entire project, but the secondary model must be understood to either supplement or inform the core model (Morse, 2003, p. 194).

Using the earlier example of a study of disclosure in the workplace among individuals with TBI, suppose the investigator notices midway through the investigation that individuals who appear to have an obvious residual physical impairment appear less reluctant to disclose. The investigator thus decided to pursue the heuristic that persons with less obvious impairments are more inclined to "pass" as nondisabled. However, this requires some kind of quantification of the extent to which a visible physical impairment is present. The investigator chooses a simple ordinal rating of:

- No obvious physical impairment,
- Marginally obvious physical impairment, and
- Obvious physical impairment.

The purpose of this secondary method is to further explore what is being discovered about individuals' perceptions regarding disclosure on the job. The project would be designated as QUAL→ quan with an inductive drive and a subsequent collection of quantitative data.

Work With as Few Data Sets as Possible

This principle refers to converting the data sets to forms that are consistent with the core method, when feasible. Converting data sets may not always make the most sense methodologically, especially in the sequential designs (secondary methods implemented subsequent to the core method) described later in the chapter. However, in concurrent designs (core and secondary methods implemented simultaneously), converting data sets can be a powerful way to approach analysis. That said, analysis of converted data sets must be approached carefully, however, to avoid violating the integrity of the core method. First, information about how to convert data sets is presented, followed by an example of the decision-making process involved when conducting the actual analysis.

Converting Data Sets. In a primarily inductive study, quantitative data from the secondary method should be **"qualitized"**—collected quantitative data types are converted to narratives that can be analyzed qualitatively (Tashakkori & Teddlie, 2003, p. 9). This is the approach used in the previous example when ordinal data were treated as a "code" for sorting and examining information about disclosure attitudes. In the qualitized data set, entire participant interviews are coded in terms of a quality (extent to which the physical impairment is obvious), which allows an investigator to sort all interview data according to whether the individual had obvious physical impairments or not. Conversely, in a primarily deductive study, qualitative data from the secondary method can be "quantitized"—that is, qualitative data types are converted into categorical or ordinal numerical codes that can be statistically analyzed (Tashakkori & Teddlie, 2003, p. 9). An example can be taken from the handwriting study mentioned earlier in which the investigator can code the teachers' open-ended interviews in terms of whether the students have high or low self-confidence. A numerical code is assigned to the teachers' reports (1 = teacher reports child has high self-confidence; 2 = teacher reports child has low self-confidence), and the data are entered into a statistical software program for analysis. Converting data not only serves to reduce the number of data sets that must be handled, but also integrates the data sets.

Maintaining Methodological Integrity When Working With Converted Data Sets. In a mixed-methods study, an investigator must adhere to the methodological assumptions of the core method when deciding how to approach analysis. The implications of these decisions can be subtle, as illustrated in the TBI study mentioned previously. In that study, the investigator has ordinal data for a subset of participants (remember, the researcher realized midway through the study that some participants may disclose based on how obvious their physical impairments were), which the researcher has qualitized. As a result, for this subset of the sample, the investigator can sort narrative information according to how obvious the physical impairments are and analyze the data to describe how the visibility of physical impairment interacts with the

Table 34.1 Summary of Mixed-Methods Designs

Name	Notation	Description
Sequential explanatory design	QUAN → qual	Explanation or prediction followed by in-depth description
Sequential exploratory design	QUAL → quan	In-depth description followed by explanation or prediction
Sequential transformative design	QUAN → qual **or** QUAL → quan	First-phase core method used to direct second-phase change in policy or action
Concurrent triangulation design	Qual + quan **or** Quan + qual	Neither tradition is designated as "core" or "secondary." Data from each are collected simultaneously.
Concurrent nested design	QUAL + quan **or** QUAN + qual	Either tradition is designated as core. Data from each are collected simultaneously.
Concurrent transformative design	Either of the concurrent notations above	Data collected through use of both traditions simultaneously. May or may not have a designated core method. Purpose is to direct a change in policy or action.

decision to disclose and other factors that influence thoughts about disclosure.

On the other hand, the investigator could decide to keep the ordinal data on the degree of residual physical impairment as numeric and quantitize the information on whether or not the person discloses (a dichotomous quantitative variable represented by 0 = does not disclose; 1 = discloses) in order to conduct a chi-square analysis. However, to do so could easily violate assumptions of the inductive theoretical drive by handling data analysis as though the purpose was deductive (i.e., testing the hypothesis of whether variable x is related to variable y). An inductive approach seeks to understand more about how differing levels of physical impairment interact with other factors to affect the way persons talk about disclosing, not to test a hypothesis about a specific relationship. Further, it is doubtful that the number of informants in a qualitative study would be large enough to adequately power a statistical test of the differences, so assumptions of even the supplemental component are violated.

Design Types in Mixed-Methods Designs

Creswell, Clark, Gutmann, and Hanson (2003) identify six major designs in mixed-methods research. These six designs can be organized into two larger categories:

- Sequential designs, and
- Concurrent designs.

Designs categorized as sequential introduce a secondary method subsequent to the core method. Designs in the concurrent category include secondary methods that are used simultaneously with the core method (Creswell et al., 2003). Each is described in more detail in the following sections and summarized in Table 34.1.

Sequential Explanatory Design

In a **sequential explanatory design,** an investigator first collects and analyzes core quantitative data used to explain or predict phenomena. This is followed by collection and analysis of in-depth information through the use of a qualitative tradition. The two approaches are analyzed separately. An example is a survey design to describe leisure performance patterns of adults who have survived a stroke that finds community access to be an identified issue, followed by in-depth interviewing of these individuals to fully describe their experiences.

Sequential Exploratory Design

A **sequential exploratory design** is identical to a sequential explanatory design except the sequence is reversed. The investigator first collects in-depth and nuanced information about a phenomenon using a qualitative tradition, followed by collection and analysis of quantitative data. Again, the two models are analyzed and interpreted separately. An example of a study using this type of design is a qualitative project to determine the meaning of caregiving for spouses of individuals with dementia, followed by development and testing of a survey based on the results of the qualitative core. The qualitative component informs the interpretation of the psychometric findings of the survey, including the solution that best fits the factor analysis.

Sequential Transformative Design

As with the two sequential designs described in the preceding text, there are two separate and subsequent phases of data collection and analysis (Creswell et al., 2003, p. 228). However, in a **sequential transformative design,** rather than the first model being the core model, either model, qualitative or quantitative, can be used as the core model. Moreover, the purpose of a sequential transformative design is to use a clearly identified theoretical perspective to direct the research question toward change in policy, action, or ideology (Creswell et al., 2003). An example of a transformative design is an evaluation component of a service program with the main purpose being feedback for improvement in the service.

Concurrent Triangulation Design

Creswell et al. (2003, p. 229) propose that a **concurrent triangulation design** is the most familiar of all six types; it is often the design that comes to mind when the term *mixed methods* is raised. As in all concurrent designs, both qualitative and quantitative data are gathered simultaneously, and results are validated by virtue of having been confirmed through multiple data collection techniques. Neither tradition is designated as core or secondary, which frees the investigator to pursue interesting developments as they occur. The disadvantage is the need to make decisions that maintain the methodological integrity of both traditions simultaneously. Data from all sources are integrated in the analysis phase of the study, when feasible.

An example of a concurrent triangulation design is a study that compared a self-report of caregiving strategies with an observation of caregiving in action (Corcoran, 2011). In this study, caregivers rated themselves on the Task Management Index Scale (TMIS) (Gitlin et al., 2002), which recorded the caregivers' report of the frequency with which specific strategies were used, such as "placing all items where they can be seen." Caregivers were then videotaped conducting a daily care task in which strategies on the TSMI may have been used. During a replay of the videotape, caregivers talked about their use of strategies in comparison to those reported on the TSMI, and these interviews were recorded and transcribed. During data analysis, the TSMI data were qualitized, and interviews were coded according to whether the frequency of caregiver use of strategies was above or below median for the sample. The investigator then was able to sort according to frequency of strategy use and examine both the videotapes and interview data for these two groups. In addition, the sample size was large enough that the investigator could also conduct a chi-square test to examine the relationship between use of strategies and overall approach to care (quantitized data that emerged from the interviews and videotapes). This provided an opportunity to examine the data from multiple perspectives and to triangulate use of caregiving strategies from three sources, one quantitative (TSMI) and two qualitative (videotape and follow-up interview). This triangulation procedure served to strengthen the trustworthiness of the study by corroborating data from several sources (Creswell, 2013).

Concurrent Nested Design

A **concurrent nested design** differs from a triangulation design only in terms of the predominance of one tradition over another. In a concurrent nested design, the primary tradition determines how data from the secondary tradition will be handled.

Creswell et al. (2003) propose that a nested design can serve many purposes. Two different traditions may be used to answer two different but related questions. Other studies may wish to measure aspects of the same phenomena at different levels. For instance, managerial focus groups may be used for in-depth understanding of personnel practices, but a survey is a better choice to describe workers' agreement with these practices. One very common use of concurrent nested designs is seen in quantitative studies that illustrate a particularly salient finding with a case study.

One example of concurrent nested design is particularly important for occupational therapy. Like many professions, occupational therapy is challenged to validate practice with efficacy studies and has been making good progress in doing so. However, too little attention is paid to measuring the level at which the tested intervention is actually delivered to study subjects as designed. Several authors have promoted the use of treatment implementation, or treatment fidelity, measures (Burgio et al., 2001; Lichstein, Riedel, & Grieve, 1994). Concurrent nested designs are very useful for devising strategies that collect valid treatment implementation data for the purposes of tracking the actual delivery, receipt, and enactment of an intervention as it was originally planned. Many issues can develop in an intervention study that threaten to change the treatment that is actually being tested. Problems with poorly defined protocols and lack of continual monitoring can result in a different form of the original intervention being delivered by each interventionist, such as changes over time as the interventionists gain more experience. Thus, each subject receives a different version of the original intervention plan. Further, subjects may actually receive and enact different versions of the intervention depending on their interpretation of what they are being told or shown. The result is that the investigator has little idea of what was actually being tested.

A concurrent nested design was used to measure and enhance treatment fidelity in Resources for Enhancing Alzheimer's Caregivers' Health 1 (REACH1), a large-scale, multisite study involving family caregivers of individuals with dementia (Schulz, Gallagher-Thompson, Haley, & Czaja, 2000; Wisniewski et al., 1999). In that study, each member of the research team was tested periodically for knowledge of relevant procedures (including those delivering the intervention), team meetings were analyzed for the level of understanding regarding the intervention, and each interventionist was evaluated on-site frequently to monitor adherence to the protocol. In addition, each study site was assessed in terms of the accuracy of the intervention manual and use of handouts to ensure the subjects actually received the intervention as designed. Finally, subject enactment of the intervention was assessed using a satisfaction survey that asked specifically the extent to which each component of the intervention was used (Burgio et al., 2001). Although time-consuming and associated with some additional costs, the treatment fidelity approach that used a concurrent nested design was vital to accurately interpreting and replicating the REACH1 intervention.

Concurrent Transformative Design

As with a sequential transformative design, the purpose of a **concurrent transformative design** is use of a theoretical perspective to enact change in a group or organization (Creswell et al., 2003, p. 230). Choices about the predominant tradition

and whether methods are nested or triangulated are made based on the degree to which the theoretical perspective is facilitated. Thus, a transformative design may take on the characteristics of either a nested or triangulated design, but the overall purpose is to promote change in the entity being studied. Participatory action research is usually based on a concurrent transformative design because the investigators use the methods necessary to give all stakeholders a voice in identifying the problem, developing a solution, and evaluating the outcome of implementing the solution.

Summary

This chapter examines mixed methods as a flexible, yet rigorous approach to complex study problems that defy study with more traditional approaches. Mixed methods are used to strengthen the study and compensate for the weaknesses inherent in designs from both qualitative and quantitative traditions. Topics studied as part of occupational therapy seem well suited to the design types (sequential and concurrent) described in this chapter. Further, use of mixed methods is recommended as one way to ensure the treatment fidelity of OT interventions.

Review Questions

1. What is the mixed-methods approach to research?
2. What are the major types of mixed-methods approaches?
3. What are the four principles of mixed-methods designs?
4. How are the different types of mixed-methods designs applied to research?
5. Why is it important to uphold the integrity of methods when conducting mixed-methods research?

REFERENCES

Burgio, L., Corcoran, M. A., Lichstein, K. L., Nichols, L., Czaja, S., Gallagher-Thompson, D. E., . . . Ory, M. (2001). Judging outcomes in psychosocial interventions for dementia caregivers: The problem of treatment implementation. *The Gerontologist, 41,* 481–489.

Cleare, A. J. (2004). Stress and fibromyalgia—what is the link? *Journal of Psychosomatic Research, 57*(5), 423–425.

Corcoran, M. A. (2011). *Caregiving Styles: A cognitive and behavioral typology associated with dementia family caregiving. The Gerontologist,* 51(4), 463–472.

Creswell, J. W. (2013). *Research design: Qualitative, quantitative, and mixed methods approaches* (4th ed.). Thousand Oaks, CA: Sage.

Creswell, J. W., Clark, V. P., Gutmann, M. L., & Hanson, W. E. (2003). Advanced mixed methods research designs. In A. Tashakkori & C. Teddlie (Eds.),

Handbook of mixed methods in social & behavioral research (pp. 209–240). Thousand Oaks, CA: Sage.

Creswell, J. W., Klassen, A. C., Plano Clark, V. L., Smith, K. C. for the Office of Behavioral and Social Sciences Research. (2011). *Best practices for mixed methods research in the health sciences.* Retrieved from https://obssr-archive.od.nih.gov/mixed_methods_research/

Denzin, N. K. (1978). The logic of naturalistic inquiry. In N. K. Denzin (Ed.), *Sociological methods: A sourcebook* (pp. 6–28). New York, NY: McGraw-Hill.

Drummond, P. D., & Willox, M. (2013). Painful effects of auditory startle, forehead cooling and psychological stress in patients with fibromyalgia or rheumatoid arthritis. *Journal of Psychosomatic Research, 74*(5), 378–383.

Gitlin, L. N., Winter, L., Dennis, M., Corcoran, M., Schinfeld, S., & Hauck, W. (2002). Strategies used by families to simplify tasks for individuals with Alzheimer's disease and related disorders: Psychometric analysis of the task management strategy index. *The Gerontologist, 42,* 61–69.

Greene, J. C., & Caracelli, V. J. (1997). *Advances in mixed-method evaluation: The challenges and benefits of integrating diverse paradigms* (New Directions for Evaluation, No. 74). San Francisco, CA: Jossey-Bass.

Howe, K. R. (1988). Against the quantitative-qualitative incompatibility thesis or dogmas die hard. *Educational Researcher, 17,* 10–16.

Lichstein, K. L., Riedel, B. W., & Grieve, R. (1994). Fair tests of clinical trials: A treatment implementation model. *Advances in Behavior Research and Therapy, 16,* 1–29.

Mannerkorpi, K., & Gard, G. (2012). Hinders for continued work among persons with fibromyalgia. *BMC Musculoskeletal Disorders, 13,* 96.

Morse, J. M. (1991). Approaches to qualitative-quantitative methodological triangulation. *Nursing Research, 40*(2), 120–123.

Morse, J. M. (2003). Principles of mixed methods and multimethod research design. In A. Tashakkori & C. Teddlie (Eds.), *Handbook of mixed methods in social & behavioral research* (pp.189–208). Thousand Oaks, CA: Sage.

Newman, I., & Benz, C. R. (1998). *Qualitative-quantitative research methodology: Exploring the interactive continuum.* Carbondale, IL: Southern Illinois University Press.

Newman, I., Ridenour, C. S., Newman, C., & DeMarco, G. M. P. (2003). A typology of research purposes and its relationship to mixed methods. In A. Tashakkori & C. Teddlie (Eds.), *Handbook of mixed methods in social & behavioral research* (pp. 167–188). Thousand Oaks, CA: Sage.

Palstam, A., Gard, G., & Mannerkorpi, K. (2013). Factors promoting sustainable work in women with fibromyalgia. *Disability and Rehabilitation, 35*(19), 1622–1629.

Schulz, R., Gallagher-Thompson, D. E., Haley, W., & Czaja, S. (2000). Understanding the intervention process: A theoretical/conceptual framework for intervention approaches to caregiving. In R. Schulz (Ed.), *Handbook of dementia caregiving interventions* (pp. 33–60). New York, NY: Springer.

Tashakkori, A., & Teddlie, C. (1998). *Mixed methodology: Combining the qualitative and quantitative approaches* (Applied Social Research Methods, No. 46). Thousand Oaks, CA: Sage.

Tashakkori, A., & Teddlie, C. (2003). *Handbook of mixed methods in social & behavioral research.* Thousand Oaks, CA: Sage.

Vogt, W. P., & Johnson, B. (2011). *Dictionary of statistics and methodology* (4th ed.). Thousand Oaks, CA: Sage.

Wisniewski, S., Belle, S., Coon, D., Marcus, S., Ory, M., Burgio, L., . . . Schulz, R. (1999). The resources of enhancing Alzheimer's caregiver health (REACH) project design and baseline characteristics. *Psychology and Aging, 18,* 375–384.

RESOURCES

DePoy, E., & Gitlin, L. N. (2011). *Introduction to research: Understanding and applying multiple strategies* (4th ed.). St. Louis, MO: C. V. Mosby.

Newman, I., & Benz, C. R. (1998). *Qualitative-quantitative research methodology: Exploring the interactive continuum.* Carbondale, IL: Southern Illinois University Press.

Schwandt, T. A. (2007). *The Sage dictionary of qualitative inquiry* (3rd ed.). Thousand Oaks, CA: Sage.

Tashakkori, A., & Teddlie, C. (2003). *Handbook of mixed methods in social and behavioral research.* Thousand Oaks, CA: Sage.

Vogt, W. P., & Johnson, B. (2011). *Dictionary of statistics and methodology* (4th ed.). Thousand Oaks, CA: Sage.

Creating Outcomes Research for Evidence-Based Practice

Pimjai Sudsawad

Learning Outcomes

- Understand the research-to-practice gap in occupational therapy.
- Describe the barriers to generating evidence-based practice from outcomes research in occupational therapy.
- Apply the diffusion of innovations theory to an existing outcomes study in occupational therapy.
- List three desirable characteristics of research evidence in occupational therapy.
- Provide an example of a research study that demonstrates clinical significance, ecological validity, and social validity.

Introduction

Evidence-based practice (EBP), which includes research on practice outcomes, was defined in a foundational work as the conscientious, explicit, and judicious use of current best evidence in making decisions about the care of individual patients (Sackett, Rosenberg, Gray, Haynes, & Richardson, 1996). Despite the general consensus on the importance of using EBP as a practice approach, there are both facilitators and barriers to the uptake of EBP in occupational therapy (Thomas & Law, 2013). A number of barriers make it difficult to implement EBP in real practice situations. Difficulty implementing EBP is certainly not unique to occupational therapy. Other rehabilitation professions, such as physical therapy, face similar issues (Jette, 2012).

EBP involves, when available, using research evidence as a basis for practice decisions. However, a number of studies with occupational therapy (OT) practitioners indicate that practitioners prefer and continue to use other sources of information more often than research evidence when making practice decisions (Bennett et al., 2003; Dubouloz, Egan, Vallerand, & von Zweck, 1999; Sudsawad, 2004; Sweetland & Craik, 2001). To execute EBP effectively, research evidence has to be used by practitioners. Research articles in professional and interdisciplinary journals have been the main sources of the most current evidence for OT practitioners, particularly studies of intervention effectiveness. Research evidence that relates to the needs of the practice community and is understandable to the practitioners is conceivably more likely to be used than evidence that does not have those characteristics.

Practitioners often report difficulties when attempting to use information from research articles for practice. Several difficulties have been identified both in nursing and in rehabilitation, such as:

- The lack of someone to help translate findings into practice (Champion & Leach, 1989),
- Failure to make clear the implications for practice in the research presentation (Funk, Champagne, Tornquist, & Wiese, 1995),
- Difficulties with how research is communicated in publications (Kajermo, Nordström, Krusebrant, & Björvell, 2000),
- Practitioners' lack of skills in interpreting research evidence (Law & Baum, 1998),
- Difficulty understanding statistical analyses as presented (Parahoo, 2000), and
- Perceived lack of relevance, ease of application, or orientation of the research literature to professional practice (Campbell, 1996; Di Fabio, 1999; Dubouloz et al., 1999).

With such difficulties, it is understandable why practitioners would be reluctant to use research evidence for EBP.

Just because research evidence is generated and disseminated does not mean that it will be used or that it is usable. Snell (2003) observed that researchers tend to define the problems and test the solutions apart from practitioners, typically use different terminology, and have a discrepancy in perspectives and goals. Nonetheless, most discussions of EBP focus on practitioners, who are expected to learn the skills essential to

CASE EXAMPLE

Marissa's OT program requires her to design and propose a research study that bridges the research-to-practice gap. To achieve this outcome, the proposed research study must demonstrate clinical significance, ecological validity, and social validity as they pertain to the field of occupational therapy. Marissa's neighbor, Myrna, whom she always admired, experienced a stroke in her early 50s. The stroke left her with left-sided weakness, a facial droop, and difficulty with word pronunciation. At the time of her stroke, Myrna was a stay-at-home mother to her two high-school-aged children, and she loved to shop at charity shops and second-hand stores when the family traveled to larger towns and cities. Now in her 60s, Myrna is a successful shop owner in the small town of Rice Lake, Wisconsin. She enjoys selling second-hand clothing, jewelry, and handbags at her shop; is an avid walker; and loves playing with her six grandchildren. Myrna has always attributed her ability to recover from her stroke to her occupational therapist, who inspired her participation in rehabilitation by allowing her to engage in what was volitional (Kielhofner, 2008) (i.e., buying second-hand goods at a discount) by taking her to various second-hand stores, charity shops, and garage sales as part of the treatment process.

It was Myrna's story that prompted Marissa to apply to OT school. Appropriately, Marissa chooses to propose a study of the application of Kielhofner's (2008) Model of Human Occupation (MOHO) to return-to-work outcomes among stroke survivors. Marissa will recruit from the inpatient rehabilitation unit 50 clients who were working full time and subsequently experienced hemiplegic stroke. She will follow their work engagement for a 24-month period. Twenty-five clients will be assigned to MOHO-based treatment with an emphasis on return to work. The remaining 25 will be assigned to usual-care occupational therapy. Return-to-work outcomes on three MOHO assessments will be collected at the end of each client's treatment period. The study hypothesis is that those receiving MOHO-based therapy emphasizing return to work will be more likely to return to work earlier and to sustain employment for a longer period of time because MOHO-based treatment comprehensively emphasizes the dimensions of volition, habituation, performance capacity, and environment when considering a client's return to work. Marissa explains that this study is relevant to practice because all OT practitioners face the ongoing dilemma of engaging clients to work toward goals that have personal meaning and relevance to their daily life roles.

The MOHO and its corresponding work assessments offer appropriate tools to facilitate and measure return to work as an OT outcome. For example, the Work Environment Impact Scale (WEIS) (Moore-Corner, Kielhofner, & Olson, 1998) measures characteristics of the environment that facilitate and inhibit work performance and satisfaction, including the need for accommodation. The Worker Role Interview (WRI; Braveman et al., 2005) measures the role of psychosocial and environmental variables as they affect a client's return to work and role as a worker. The Assessment of Work Performance (AWP; Sandqvist, Lee, & Kielhofner, 2010) measures how effectively and appropriately a client executes work-related skills and performs work-related activities.

For her capstone, Marissa concludes that a study of this nature would have clinical significance because the expectation is that clients undergoing MOHO treatment will experience meaningful change as they resume their work roles. The study would have ecological validity because the research outcomes would be relevant to the reality that clients face upon completion of rehabilitation: the need to return to work. Finally, the study would have social validity because there is a need within the workplace and within the broader national and world economies for people to resume their work roles as soon as possible following the experience of impairment.

using research information in its current form. Little emphasis has been placed on researchers and their role in the research application and utilization process.

Researchers certainly share responsibility for bridging the gap between research and practice. Researchers need to:

- Examine how research is being created,
- Consider its applicability and usability for practice,
- Be open to a different paradigm of creating research evidence, and
- Produce outcomes research that can be used for EBP.

Ottenbacher, Barris, and Van Deusen (1986) first raised the issues of research characteristics that could create impediments to OT practitioners' use of research for practice. They pointed out the problems with using group statistics to determine treatment effectiveness because even if statistically significant differences are found, clinically relevant information cannot be inferred. They also pointed out the difficulties in duplicating the intervention strategies reported in research articles within a clinical environment. They called for both researchers and practitioners to be concerned with the effectiveness with which information generated through research is disseminated and incorporated into practice. Their observations and suggestions are certainly still timely today.

In the following sections, the diffusion of innovations theory is introduced as the framework to help identify desirable characteristics of research evidence that could facilitate its use for EBP. The concepts of social validity, ecological validity, and clinical significance are presented as vehicles that can help to create those desirable characteristics when applied to the design and implementation of outcomes research in occupational therapy. The discussion in this chapter specifically pertains to the creation of clinical outcomes research that is intended to guide practice decisions regarding treatment interventions.

Identifying Desirable Characteristics of Research Evidence

As explained throughout this text, it is paramount that the evidence of successful outcomes for a given intervention reflects a high level of innovation and relevance. Ensuring innovation and relevance leads to the perception that the intervention being tested will have wide application in practice and broad impact in terms of advancing the science within the specific topical area of study. Thus, when thinking about testing the outcomes of an intervention, two ideas apply. The first is diffusion of innovations. This is a framework that provides a structure for planning. The second idea emphasizes the need to be strategic in considering which aspects of a research innovation should be disseminated and applied within the practice community (and/or public writ large). Both of these ideas are discussed further in the following sections.

Diffusion of Innovations

The **diffusion of innovations** (Rogers, 2003) framework identifies the process and influencing factors in communicating an innovation (defined as an idea, practice, or object that is perceived as new). This framework has been used widely in fields such as business, marketing, and public health. There are four main elements in the diffusion of an innovation:

- The innovation,
- The communication channels,
- Time, and
- The social systems.

The most influential of these elements for the diffusion of an innovation is the characteristics of the innovation itself, which accounts for 49% to 87% of the variance in predicting its adoption rate (Rogers, 1995).

As identified by Rogers (2003), there are five characteristics of an innovation that could either facilitate or hinder the adoption of an innovation, delineated as follows:

- **Relative advantage:** The degree to which an innovation is perceived as better than the idea it supersedes. The degree of relative advantage may be measured in many terms (economic, prestige, convenience, satisfaction, etc.), and the greater the perceived relative advantage of an innovation, the more rapid its rate of adoption will be.
- **Compatibility:** The degree to which an innovation is perceived as being consistent with the existing values, past experiences, and needs of the potential adopter. An idea that is incompatible with the values and norms of the social system will not be adopted as rapidly as an innovation that is compatible.
- **Complexity:** The degree to which an innovation is perceived as difficult to understand and use. The innovations that are readily comprehended

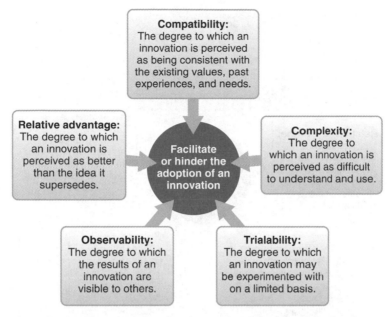

Figure 35.1 Characteristics of an innovation influencing its adoption.

by most potential adopters will be adopted more rapidly, whereas the others that are perceived as more complicated will be adopted more slowly.
- **Trialability:** The degree to which an innovation may be experimented with on a limited basis. If new ideas can be tried on a small scale, they will generally be adopted more quickly.
- **Observability:** The degree to which the results of an innovation are visible to others. The easier it is for individuals to see the results of an innovation, the more likely they are to adopt.

As shown in Figure 35.1, these characteristics are factors that influence the extent to which the innovation will be adopted and used.

Application of Desirable Characteristics of an Innovation to Research Evidence

Research evidence fits the definition of an **innovation** because it represents new ideas and/or practice. Therefore, the diffusion of innovations framework can be used to examine characteristics that, if present, would likely make research evidence be received more favorably by its potential users. In this case, the potential users of interest are OT practitioners who would like to use research evidence as a basis for decision-making in practice. The diffusion of innovations framework can be applied to research characteristics as follows:

- First, research must be perceived as containing stronger evidence than other sources so that it is viewed as having a relative advantage over other kinds of evidence.
- Second, the design and conduct of research must be consistent with the existing values, past experiences, and the needs of practitioners and/or OT consumers to increase compatibility.
- Third, research must be presented in ways that make it easy to understand and use to reduce complexity.
- Fourth, the intervention investigated must be easily implemented in the clinical setting to increase the level of trialability.
- Last, the research outcomes must demonstrate changes/improvement with a magnitude that is obvious to anyone, including the practitioners, to increase observability.

Based on the diffusion of innovations framework, these characteristics can be conceptualized as factors that influence the extent to which practitioners will use research findings for EBP, as shown in Figure 35.2.

Initial findings suggest that practitioners accept research evidence as stronger than other kinds of evidence (Sudsawad, 2004). It appears that OT researchers should place an immediate focus on other characteristics to ensure that OT outcomes research is produced such that it is most relevant to practice. Considering the scarcity of the resources available for OT research, it seems unwise to use those resources to create outcomes research that

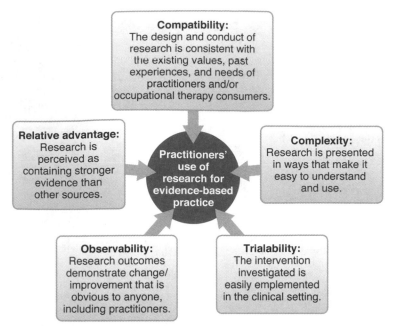

Figure 35.2   Characteristics of outcomes research influencing practitioners' use of research for evidence-based practice.

does not lend itself to use in practice. Creating outcomes research that is acceptable and usable for practitioners is the most important contribution OT researchers can make toward evidence-based practice.

Concepts and Methods to Fulfill the Desirable Characteristics of Research Evidence

In the following sections, the concepts of social validity, ecological validity, and clinical significance are introduced and their methods discussed in relation to the five desirable characteristics of research information as delineated earlier. Researchers can use these concepts as guides to creating research that is likely to be used in EBP.

These concepts should be used as a supplement to the usual consideration of rigor in the design and conduct of outcome research because scientific rigor in and of itself is not sufficient to make research evidence usable in practice. It is essential that OT investigators also consider other characteristics to make outcomes research maximally relevant for its use in EBP.

Social Validity

Wolf (1978), who first proposed the concept of **social validity,** referred to it as something of social importance. According to Wolf (1978), researchers should ask three questions to assess the social validity of outcomes research concerning goals, procedures, and outcomes:

- Goals: Are the goals of the intervention being investigated really what society wants?
- Procedures: Are the intervention techniques used acceptable to the consumers, or do they cost too much (e.g., in terms of effort, time, discomfort, ethics, or the like)?
- Outcomes: Are the consumers satisfied with the intervention outcome, both with predicted change and with unpredicted side effects?

The terms **society** and **consumers** include anyone who may be involved with and affected by the intervention process and outcome, including the OT clients, their caregivers, their parents and teachers (in the case of children), community members, disability groups, and others.

There are a variety of methods for operationalizing the social validity concept (e.g., Foster & Mash, 1999; Hawkins, 1991; Kazdin & Matson, 1981; Kendall & Grove, 1988; Schwartz & Baer, 1991). However, this discussion focuses on verification with consumers as a method for establishing social validity.

Schwartz and Baer (1991) identified four different types of consumers who can be approached to determine social validity:

- Direct consumers,
- Indirect consumers,
- Members of the immediate community, and
- Members of the extended community.

Direct consumers are the primary recipients of the intervention. **Indirect consumers** are those who purchase the intervention for someone else or are strongly affected by the behavioral changes targeted in the intervention, but they are not its recipients. **Members of the immediate community** are those who interact with the direct and indirect consumers on a regular basis, usually through close proximity in work, school, or social situations. The **members of the extended community** include those who probably do not know or interact with the direct and indirect consumers but who live in the same community. The point of this delineation is that a few different groups of consumers are available to socially validate the goals, procedures, and outcomes. To strengthen the social validity, more than one consumer group's opinion and perspective may be sought at the same time.

Social validity can be implemented from the initial conception of the research to the conclusion of the study. OT researchers can seek the appropriate study topic/research questions (*goals*) by seeking to learn about the topics of interest to practitioners and/or what type of evidence is needed in practice situations. In addition, researchers can include OT clients to help identify appropriate treatment goals.

The following is an example of verifying the relevance of research questions/treatment goals. O'Brien et al. (2000) conducted a study to investigate the effectiveness of an OT intervention designed to improve playfulness in children. In this study, information obtained from initial home visits and parent interview were used to determine the area of concern for each child and set up the treatment goal (rather than determining the goal based on the researchers' own opinion).

A study's intervention (procedures) can be developed such that the reality of practice is taken into consideration. Then, if the intervention studied is found to be effective, practitioners can use it. The acceptability of the intervention can also be verified with service consumers because if consumers find the intervention unacceptable, they may choose not to receive or cooperate with the intervention.

Before the intervention, researchers can verify with the clients that the intervention outcomes (outcomes) chosen are important outcomes from their perspective. The social validity of outcomes can also be verified after the intervention by asking clients whether they are satisfied with the outcomes obtained. Practitioners can also help to identify the types of outcomes that may be relevant to their clients.

The following is an example of verifying the social appropriateness of the intervention procedures and social importance of the outcomes. Schilling, Washington, Billingsley, and Deitz (2003) conducted a study to investigate the effects of using therapy balls as seating on in-seat behaviors and legible word productivity of students with attention deficit-hyperactivity disorder (ADHD). They used the social validity methods to verify both the appropriateness of the intervention and the importance of the outcome. The researchers asked teachers, students in the class who were classmates of the study's participants (and also using therapy balls as seating in the classroom at the same time as the study's participants), and the participants themselves to complete a questionnaire to determine whether they observed improvement in performance in the actual classroom setting. The teacher answered questions concerning whether she saw the improvement in students' performance. The students answered questions about whether they saw improvement of their own performance. To verify the acceptability of the intervention, students were also asked whether they preferred using the therapy ball to sitting on chairs, and they were given an opportunity to put in writing their opinion of sitting on balls in the classroom.

Relationship Between Social Validity and Desirable Characteristics of Research Evidence

Involving both the consumers and the practitioners in the process of determining research questions/treatment goals, intervention procedures, and intervention outcomes when conducting research studies should increase compatibility—the degree to which research information is perceived as being consistent with the existing values, past experiences, and needs of OT practitioners—either through addressing the consumers' needs (which is the matter of interest to practitioners) or taking into consideration the practitioners' input based on actual practice situations, or both. In addition, investigating intervention methods that are realistic for implementation in practice settings and acceptable by consumers should increase trialability—the degree to which information obtained from research studies can be implemented in practice settings.

Ecological Validity

Ecological validity is related to the social importance of research outcomes; it is the degree to which results obtained in controlled experimental conditions are related to those obtained in naturalistic environments (Tupper & Cicerone, 1990). What a person can do in the artificial experimental environment is not necessarily what the person does or can do in his or her everyday environment. Similarly, the interaction between an individual's abilities (or disability) and unique environmental demands will yield different performances (Sbordone, 1996).

Choosing an ecologically valid outcome also partly relates to the social validity aspect of the outcome. Not only should the outcome measure represent performance in a real-life environment, it should also reflect the performance that the clients, their significant others, or their peers consider to be important and those with which they are satisfied.

Moseley and colleagues (2004) assessed the ecological validity of walking speed measurement after a traumatic brain injury (TBI) of three clinical gait tests in predicting walking performance in three natural environments (a corridor in a brain injury rehabilitation unit, a parking lot of a metropolitan shopping center, inside a metropolitan shopping center). They found that for participants with TBI, the agreement between the speed used in the clinical gait tests and the natural environments was poor. Sudsawad, Trombly, Henderson, and Tickle-Degnen (2001) assessed the ecological validity of a standardized handwriting assessment and found that the level of handwriting performance of children with various degrees of handwriting illegibility bore almost no relationship with the children's performance in classroom setting as rated by teachers.

Another aspect of ecological validity relates to the standardized test instruments used for assessment of outcomes. Franzen and Wilhelm (1996) indicated two general aspects of ecological validity in assessment:

- **Verisimilitude,** which is the similarity of the data collection methods in the test to tasks and skills required in the free and open environment, and

- **Veridicality,** which is the extent to which test results reflect or can predict phenomena in the open environment or "real world."

Verisimilitude is important in the design of assessment instruments, but once an instrument is designed, veridicality becomes more important (Franzen & Wilhelm, 1996). To achieve ecological validity, a test must provide information that is relevant to the person's functioning in daily life, not simply be representative of a hypothetical construct or even a neurological syndrome (Silver, 2000). If a standardized test is to be used as a measurement instrument in outcomes research, it should have some evidence of ecological validity, Better yet, real-life performance should be used as a basis to demonstrate the intervention effectiveness in natural settings whenever possible because there is no guarantee that a test (or a number of tests) will predict performance in a natural setting.

The following studies are examples of how real-life performance can be incorporated into outcomes studies. In a study of the dose–response effects of a medication for ADHD, Evans et al. (2001) used everyday tasks in normal classroom activities as dependent measures, including note-taking quality, quiz and worksheet performance, written language usage and productivity, teacher ratings on task and disruptive behavior, and homework completion. The researchers believed that the measures of behavior and academic performance were needed to assess medication response, rather than using laboratory tasks as proxy measures of academic functioning, because past research had showed little correspondence between performance on such tasks and classroom academic performance.

In a study comparing the effectiveness of three interventions for stuttering plus a control group, Craig et al. (1996) measured the participants' stuttering frequency and speech rate not only during conversations in the clinic with the clinician, but also in two other relevant contexts: performance during a telephone conversation with a family member or friend and face-to-face conversation with a family member or friend in the home environment.

In another study investigating the effectiveness of oral–motor sensory treatment, Gisel, Applegate-Ferrante, Benson, and Bosma (1996) measured oral–motor skills through the administration of a standardized feeding assessment during observations at lunch/snack time in the children's accustomed room with the person who was the child's regular feeder.

Relationship of Ecological Validity to the Desirable Characteristics of Research Evidence

Choosing study outcomes that represent actual performance in real-life settings can positively contribute to the use of research evidence for practice. Demonstrating the effect of an intervention in terms of ability or performance in a natural context will help to increase compatibility of research information for OT practitioners because such outcomes reflect the profession's philosophy of enabling clients to be able to engage in an occupation. Presenting the outcomes in everyday terms should also reduce the perceived complexity of the information drawn from research evidence because such outcomes can be easily related and understood. Finally, the results of an intervention are more likely to be perceived as easily observed because outcomes are something that can be readily seen by normal observation as opposed to the abstraction of test scores, hence providing increased observability of research evidence.

Clinical Significance

Clinical significance refers to the practical value or the importance of the effect of an intervention, that is, whether it makes a real difference in everyday life to the clients or to others with whom the clients interact (Kazdin, 1999). Statistical significance, although necessary to verify that any changes observed in a study are not likely the result of chance, does not ensure that such changes are meaningful for clients' real-life performance. Therefore, statistical significance is an insufficient index for the usefulness of an intervention to improve everyday function. The fact that a treatment effect was probabilistically not "due to chance" is not adequately informative to the practice community (Saunders, Howard, & Newman, 1988). Not surprisingly, agencies and policymakers increasingly demand evidence about real-world effects of interventions to invest resources in them (Czaja & Schulz, 2003). Nonetheless, the concept of clinical significance has not been implemented consistently in rehabilitation outcomes research (Sudsawad, 2004) or in medical research (Chan, Man-Son-Hing, Molnar, & Laupacis, 2001).

Authors have presented different ways to demonstrate the clinical significance of treatment outcomes, including both statistical and nonstatistical methods. The more suitable method that researchers can use to demonstrate clinical significance for their study will depend on many factors, such as:

- The study area,
- The study sample,
- The nature of the treated condition, and
- The nature of the expected treatment outcomes.

Some of the proposed methods to demonstrate clinical significance include:

- The use of effect sizes to demonstrate the magnitude of change;
- Using measures of risk potency, such as odds ratio, risk ratio, relative risk reduction, risk difference, and number needed to treat (NNT);
- Comparing both group and individual performance to normative data (Jacobson & Traux, 1991; Kazdin, 1977; Kendall & Grove, 1988);
- Using meta-analysis for a pooled effect size from several studies that is compared with normative data (Nietzel & Trull, 1998);
- Showing that the studied intervention eliminates symptoms/impairments that the intervention is intended to eliminate;
- Demonstrating that the researched intervention enables clients to meet role demands, increases the level of functioning in everyday life, and/or achieves change in quality of life;
- Incorporating subjective judgments of change by the clients, their significant others, or people who interact with the clients in their natural environments; and
- Documenting satisfaction with the treatment results, including input obtained from the client, his or her significant others, or even professionals who are not part of the research team (e.g., a child's regular occupational therapist, teacher, classroom assistant).

Using statistical methods to determine clinical significance (the first four bullet points in the previous list) is important to improve the quality of evidence. These methods, however, do not provide information on the impact of the intervention on the client's everyday life, and they generate information at a level of abstraction that does not correspond to the everyday world of practice. Focusing on elimination of symptoms/impairments or normative comparison, although useful in some contexts, may not be applicable to many areas of OT services. Often, the goal of OT intervention is to maximize the client's ability to participate in everyday living as much as possible, although not necessarily in ways typical of the "normal" population.

Making use of client input (and the input of others with whom the client is associated) on the client's performance in natural contexts is a comprehensive approach. For example, assessing a client's satisfaction with the change in his or her performance in everyday activities meets the criteria for social validity, ecological validity, and clinical significance. This strategy includes the consumer's perspective and opinion, measures real-life everyday function, and ensures that the change achieved is substantial such that it is satisfactory to the client. On the other hand, if the increased functioning in everyday life is based only on the researcher's observation, it may meet the criteria of ecological validity and clinical significance, but it may not have equally strong social validity.

Relationship of Clinical Significance to Desirable Characteristics of Research Evidence

Applying the concept of clinical significance to demonstrate a meaningful change in everyday function can increase the compatibility of research information with the ultimate goal of OT intervention, which is to positively affect clients' everyday lives. Demonstrating change in ways that are related to everyday functions can also help to decrease the complexity of research information from practitioners' perspectives. They can relate to this type of outcome as evidence of treatment effectiveness more readily than to statistical significance. Clinical significance of treatment outcomes that demonstrate an impact on the study participants' everyday life functioning also increases the observability of findings.

Application of the Diffusion of Innovations Framework in OT Research

OT researchers can use the diffusion of innovations framework as a guide, and the social validity, ecological validity, and clinical significance as tools, to create outcomes research that is appealing to practitioners. This approach has the potential to bridge the gap between research and practice because it emphasizes designing, conducting, and reporting research with the ultimate goal of creating information that is actually related to and usable in real-life practice. The following kinds of questions can be used to guide the design and implementation of outcomes studies:

- Is the topic of the study what the practitioners/ service consumers are interested in or need to know about?

- Is the intervention investigated in the study practical enough to be implemented in practice settings if found to be effective?
- Is the intervention procedure acceptable to the practitioners/service consumers?
- Is the treatment outcome to be measured in the study what practitioners and/or consumers consider to be an important outcome?
- Does the intervention outcome represent performance of daily activities in natural contexts?
- Does the method chosen to measure change/ improvement demonstrate an impact on or make a difference in the client's everyday life function?

The use of social validity, ecological validity, and clinical significance concepts simultaneously to design and conduct outcomes research, aimed to increase its usability for practice, was termed the **social validation model** in a recent investigation (Sudsawad, 2004). Based on responses received from more than 900 practitioners in occupational therapy, physical therapy, and speech–language pathology, there was strong support for the use of the social validation model in rehabilitation outcomes research. The majority of practitioners indicated that it was either important or very important that research evidence possesses the key elements included in the questions just listed. They also indicated that doing so would either likely or very likely increase their use of research information for practice.

Summary

It is imperative that OT researchers create research evidence that not only meets the standards of scientific rigor but also has utility in everyday practice. Moreover, in the current climate of limited available resources, OT researchers are well advised to produce outcomes research that is relevant and applicable to OT practice. By doing so, researchers will make an important contribution to the progression of evidence-based practice.

Review Questions

1. What is an example of an OT research study that widens the research-to-practice gap?
2. What is an example of an OT research study that bridges the research-to-practice gap?
3. What are the barriers to generating evidence-based practice from outcomes research in occupational therapy?
4. How does the diffusion of innovations theory provide a framework for the translation of outcomes research to evidence-based practice?

5. What are the three desirable characteristics of research evidence in occupational therapy?

REFERENCES

Bennett, S., Tooth, L., McKenna, K., Rodger, S., Strong, J., Ziviani, J., Mickan, S., & Gibson, L. (2003). Perceptions of evidence based practice: A survey of Australian occupational therapists. *Australian Occupational Therapy Journal, 50,* 13–22.

Braveman, B., Robson, M., Velozo, C., Kielhofner, G., Fisher, G., Forsyth, K., & Kerschbaum, J. (2005). *The Worker Role Interview (WRI).* Chicago, IL: Model of Human Occupation Clearinghouse, University of Illinois at Chicago.

Campbell, T. W. (1996). Systemic therapy practice and basic research. *Journal of Systemic Therapy Practice, 15*(3), 15–39.

Champion, V. L., & Leach, A. (1989). Variables related to research utilization in nursing: An empirical investigation. *Journal of Advanced Nursing, 14,* 705–710.

Chan, K. B. Y., Man-Son-Hing, M., Molnar, F. J., & Laupacis, A. (2001). How well is the clinical importance of study results reported? An assessment of randomized controlled trials. *Canadian Medical Association Journal, 165*(9), 1197–1202.

Craig, A., Hancock, K., Chang, E., McCready, C., Shepley, A., McCaul, A., . . . Reilly, K. (1996). A controlled clinical trial for stuttering in persons aged 9 to 14 years. *Journal of Speech and Hearing Research, 39,* 808–826.

Czaja, S. J., & Schulz, R. (2003). Does the treatment make a real difference? The measurement of clinical significance. Translating psychosocial research into practice: Methodological issues. *Alzheimer's Care Quarterly, 4*(3), 229–240.

Di Fabio, R. P. (1999). Myth of evidence-based practice. *Journal of Orthopaedic and Sports Physical Therapy, 29,* 632–634.

Dubouloz, C-J., Egan, M., Vallerand, J., & von Zweck, C. (1999). Occupational therapists' perceptions of evidence-based practice. *American Journal of Occupational Therapy, 53,* 445–453.

Evans, S. W., Pelham, W. E., Smith, B. H., Bukstein, O., Gnagy, E. M., Greiner, A. R., . . . Baron-Myak, C. (2001). Dose-response effects of methylphenidate on ecologically valid measures of academic performance and classroom behavior in adolescence with ADHD. *Experimental and Clinical Psychopharmacology, 9,* 163–175.

Foster, S. L., & Mash, E. J. (1999). Assessing social validity in clinical treatment research: Issues and procedures. *Journal of Consulting and Clinical Psychology, 67,* 308–319.

Franzen, M. D., & Wilhelm, K. L. (1996). Conceptual foundations of ecological validity in neuropsychological assessment. In R. J. Sbordone & C. J. Long (Eds.), *Ecological validity of neuropsychological testing* (pp. 91–112). Delray Beach, FL: GR Press/St. Lucie Press.

Funk, S. G., Champagne, M. T., Tornquist, E. M. & Wiese, R. A. (1995). Administrators' views on barriers to research utilization. *Applied Nursing Research, 8,* 44–49.

Gisel, E. G., Applegate-Ferrante, T., Benson, J., & Bosma, J. F. (1996). Oral-motor skills follow a sensory mortar therapy in two groups of moderately dysphagic children with cerebral palsy. *Dysphagia, 11,* 59–71.

Hawkins, R. P. (1991). Is social validity what we are interested in? Argument for a functional approach. *Journal of Applied Behavior Analysis, 24,* 205–213.

Jacobson, N. S., & Traux, P. (1991). Clinical Significance: A statistical approach to defining meaningful change in psychotherapy research. *Journal of Consulting and Clinical Psychology, 59,* 12–19.

Jette, A. (2012). 43rd Mary McMillan Lecture: Face into the storm. *Physical Therapy, 92,* 1–27.

Kajermo, K. N., Nordström, G., Krusebrant, Å., & Björvell, H. (2000). Perceptions of research utilization: Comparisons between healthcare professionals, nursing students and a reference group of nurse clinicians. *Journal of Advanced Nursing, 31,* 99–109.

Kazdin, A. E. (1977). Assessing the clinical or applied importance of behavior change to social validation. *Behavior Modification, 1,* 427–452.

Kazdin, A. E. (1999). The meanings and measurement of clinical significance. *Journal of Consulting and Clinical Psychology, 67,* 332–339.

Kazdin, A. E., & Matson, J. L. (1981). Social validation in mental retardation. *Applied Research in Mental Retardation, 2,* 39–53.

Kendall, P. C., & Grove, W. M. (1988). Normative comparisons in therapy outcome. *Behavioral Assessment, 10,* 147–158.

Kielhofner, G. (2008). *Model of Human Occupation: Theory and application* (4th ed.). Philadelphia, PA: WoltersKluwer.

Law, M., & Baum, C. (1998). Evidence-based practice occupational therapy. *Canadian Journal of Occupational Therapy, 65,* 131–135.

Moore-Corner, R., Kielhofner, G., & Olson, L. (1998). *The Work Environment Impact Scale (WEIS).* Chicago, IL: Model of Human Occupation Clearinghouse, University of Illinois at Chicago.

Moseley, A. M., Lanzarone, S., Bosman, J. M., van Loo, M. A., de Bie, R. A., & Hassett, L. (2004). Ecological validity of walking speed assessment after traumatic brain injury: A pilot study. *Journal of Head Trauma Rehabilitation, 19,* 341–348.

Nietzel, M. T., & Trull, T. J. (1998). Meta-analytic approaches to social comparisons: A method for measuring clinical significance. *Behavioral Assessment, 10,* 159–169.

O'Brien, J., Coker, P., Lynn, R., Suppinger, R., Paerigen, T., Rabon, S., . . . Ward, A. T. (2000). The impact of occupational therapy on a child's playfulness. *Occupational Therapy in Health Care, 12*(2/3), 39–51.

Ottenbacher, K. J., Barris, R., & Van Deusen, J. (1986). Issues related to research utilization in occupational therapy. *American Journal of Occupational Therapy, 40,* 111–116.

Parahoo, K. (2000). Barriers to, and facilitators of, research utilization among nurses in Northern Ireland. *Journal of Advanced Nursing, 31,* 89–98.

Rogers, E. M. (1995). *Diffusion of innovations* (4th ed.). New York, NY: The Free Press.

Rogers, E. M. (2003). *Diffusion of innovations* (5th ed.). New York, NY: The Free Press.

Sackett, D. L., Rosenberg, W. M. C., Gray, J. A. M., Haynes, R., & Richardson, W. S. (1996). Evidence based medicine: What it is and what it isn't? *British Medical Journal, 312,* 71–72.

Sandqvist, J., Lee, J., & Kielhofner, G. (2010). *The Assessment of Work Performance (AWP).* Chicago, IL: Model of Human Occupation Clearinghouse, University of Illinois at Chicago.

Saunders, S. M., Howard, K. I., & Newman, F. L. (1988). Evaluating the clinical significance of treatment effects: Norms and normality. *Behavioral Assessment, 10,* 207–218.

Sbordone, R. J. (1996). Ecological validity: Critical issues for the neuropsychologist. In R. J. Sbordone & C. J. Long (Eds.), *Ecological validity of neuropsychological testing* (pp. 15–41). Delray Beach, FL: GR Press/St. Lucie Press.

Schilling, D. L., Washington, K., Billingsley, F. F., & Deitz, J. (2003). Classroom seating for children with attention deficit hyperactivity disorder: Therapy balls versus chairs. *American Journal of Occupational Therapy, 57,* 534–541.

Schwartz, I. S., & Baer, D. M. (1991). Social validity assessments: Is current practice state of the art? *Journal of Applied Behavior Analysis, 24,* 189–204.

Silver, C. H. (2000). Ecological validity of neuropsychological assessment in childhood traumatic brain injury. *Journal of Head Trauma Rehabilitation, 15,* 973–988.

Snell, M. E. (2003). Applying research to practice: The more pervasive problem? *Research and Practice for Persons With Severe Disabilities, 28*(3), 143–147.

Sudsawad, P. (2004). *Developing a social validation model for effective utilization of disability and rehabilitation research.* Project summary submitted to the National Institute of Disability and Rehabilitation Research, U.S. Department of Education, Grant # H133F020023.

Sudsawad, P., Trombly, C. A., Henderson, A., & Tickle-Degnen, L. (2001). The relationship between the Evaluation of Children's Handwriting (ETCH) and teachers' perception of handwriting legibility. *American Journal of Occupational Therapy, 55,* 518–523.

Sweetland, J., & Craik, C. (2001). The use of evidence-based practice by occupational therapists who treat adult stroke patients. *British Journal of Occupational Therapy, 64,* 256–261.

Thomas, A., & Law, M. (2013). Research utilization and evidence-based practice in occupational therapy: A scoping practice. *American Journal of Occupational Therapy, 67*(4), e55–65.

Tupper, D., & Cicerone, K. (1990). Introduction to the neuropsychology of everyday life. In D. Tupper & K. Cicerone (Eds.), *The neuropsychology of everyday life: Assessment and basic competencies* (pp. 3–18). Boston, MA: Kluwer Academic.

Wolf, M. M. (1978). Social validity: The case for subjective measurement or how applied behavior analysis is finding its heart. *Journal of Applied Behavior Analysis, 11,* 203–214.

RESOURCES

Kazdin, A. E. (1999). The meanings and measurement of clinical significance. *Journal of Consulting and Clinical Psychology, 67,* 332–339.

Rogers, E. M. (2003). *Diffusion of innovations* (5th ed.). New York, NY: The Free Press.

Sbordone, R. J. (1996). Ecological validity: Critical issues for the neuropsychologist. In R. J. Sbordone & C. J. Long (Eds.), *Ecological validity of neuropsychological testing* (pp. 15–41). Delray Beach, FL: GR Press/St. Lucie Press.

Wolf, M. M. (1978). Social validity: The case for subjective measurement or how applied behavior analysis is finding its heart. *Journal of Applied Behavior Analysis, 11,* 203–214.

Glossary

A

A–B design: The most common single-subject design upon which all others are built. The A indicates a baseline phase, and B indicates a treatment (or intervention) phase.

A–B–A or **withdrawal design:** This is a type of withdrawal design in which there is a minimum of three phases, a baseline phase (A), an intervention phase (B), and then the intervention is withdrawn to return to the baseline phase (A). Conversely, the design may proceed as having an intervention (B), a baseline (A), and an intervention (B).

A–B–A–B design: In this single-subject design, the baseline and intervention phases reverse twice so that subjects are exposed to both conditions twice.

A–B–C successive intervention design: With this design, a second intervention is introduced in the C phase.

Abstract: A concise summary (typically between 150 and 250 words) of key aspects of the study.

Active reading: A key early step in the analysis process by which the reader interacts with the data by making notes in reaction to what is read.

Adequacy of the data: Measure indicating that enough data will be available to provide a rich description of the phenomena of interest.

Alternating-treatments design: These single-subject designs involve the fast alternation of two or more different interventions or conditions. They may be used to compare the effects of intervention and no intervention, or they may be used to compare the effects of two or more distinct interventions.

Alternative hypothesis: Specifies a relationship between variables that is not due to chance; also referred to as the research hypothesis.

Analytic memos: Longer annotations in the margins of a document. Rather than serving primarily an indexing function, memos are methodological and analytic notes from which explanations and findings are built. Although these memos may start as notes in the margin, they commonly become longer and more complex as analysis proceeds. Analytic memos are the raw material for later interpretation and findings.

Analytical approach (or statistical analysis): Section in the research paper that describes how the information or data collected in the study were coded, scored, summarized, analyzed, and interpreted.

Analytical preciseness: A means of evaluating the quality of qualitative research that is defined by congruence between study data, findings, interpretations, theoretical linkages, and conclusions drawn.

Ancestry method: Type of retrieval approach in which the reviewer gathers information by tracking citations from one study or research report to another.

Anecdotal evidence: Stories based on nonspecific observations, personal interviews, or other public statements.

Animal welfare: Involves protecting the physical and emotional well-being of animals that are being used in research.

APA format: Guidelines from the American Psychological Association that give a very specific order in which an entire research article is presented, as well as how the contents of a study are reported and described and the references are styled.

Applied research: Investigations that seek to solve some practical problem or to generate information specifically to inform practice.

Appropriateness: The identification of participants who will best inform the researcher about the phenomena under inquiry.

Assessment research: An approach to assuring the dependability (reliability and validity) of evaluation of the measures that are used to test deficits, strengths, progress, and setbacks in therapy. Also referred to as psychometric research.

Assessments: Specific method, instrument, strategy, or tool used as a part of an evaluation process or to gather data for a study.

Audit trail: A systematically maintained set of documentation, typically including all data generated in the study, explanations of all concepts and models that shaped the study design, explanations of procedures used in data collection and analysis, notes about technical aspects of data collection and analysis as well as decisions taken throughout the study to refine data-collection procedures and interpretations, personal notes and reflections, and copies of all instruments and interview protocols used to collect study data.

B

Basic experimental design: The most rigorous type of group comparison study.

Basic research: Investigations undertaken for the purposes of understanding some phenomenon or testing a model or theory that explains some phenomenon.

Beneficence: The principle requiring that human subjects research minimize risk to the greatest extent possible and maximize the potential for benefits to be gained from the research (either for the individuals participating in the research or from the knowledge that will be gained).

BESD (binomial effect size display): A statistical measure of effect size that converts the *r*-statistic into a percentage comparison of improvement between groups.

Between-subjects design: Studies that compare two groups of subjects who are expected to change in different ways at different rates or that compare one group that is expected to change with another that is not.

Bias: Type of prejudiced consideration or judgment.

Bibliographic searches: Method for retrieving evidence for a meta-analysis using the same terms as descriptors or keywords that may produce different results depending on the database searched.

Biomechanical theory: Describes a client's capacity to engage in movement that is functional.

Biometry and physiological measures: Objective means of assessing any range of variables that involve physical, biological, or physiological functioning.

Biostatisticians: Professionals who are learned in understanding and conducting advanced statistical analyses that concern multiple variables and multiple levels of analysis.

Blinding: A methodological control used to increase the rigor of a study and eliminate bias caused by knowing the condition or group to which a subject was assigned. It refers to the process of not informing participants of the condition to which they were assigned.

Boolean connectors: Connectors such as "and," "or," or "not" that are used to combine codes in complex electronic search processes.

Boolean logic: A form of algebra in which all values are determined as either true or false.

Browsing: Entering terms into a search engine, either according to a preplanned approach or an inductive, evolving approach; it can be structured or serendipitous.

C

Case-comparison design: A type of design used to find out if some specific variable from the past discriminates between people who today have a disease (or disability) and people who do not. Also known as *case-control design* and *case-referent design*.

Case-composite example: Similar to an actual case example, but the client is de-identified such that there is no way to ever trace the details discussed about the person to an actual person. This requires altering the identity and some of the circumstances or characteristics of an actual case or incorporating characteristics from other clients, hence the term *composite*.

Case-control design: A retrospective design that compares people who have and have not developed a disease in terms of an independent variable.

Case-control study: An observational epidemiological comparison of one group of subjects with a common diagnosis or problem (cases) with another group of subjects without this diagnosis or problem (controls). Cases and controls are compared in terms of the relationship of disease status and the presence, absence, or frequency/degree of that attribute to the disease.

Case-referent design: A type of design used to find out if some specific variable from the past discriminates between people who today have a disease (or disability) and people who do not. Also known as *case-control design* and *case-comparison design*.

Case report: A structured description of a novel approach to assessment and/or intervention with a single client or a small number of clients.

Case-series study: A longitudinal study of case-report information from a single group of subjects who were given a similar intervention.

Case study: A qualitative design in which researchers obtain and reveal information about a phenomenon from a single subject under study by gathering in-depth information.

Case-study research: Type of research in which an investigator studies the effects of an intervention on a single individual over time with no control; it is not considered to be randomized and also represents a lower level of evidence.

Categorical scale: Defines two or more discrete categories within a variable.

Ceiling effect: This lack of responsiveness occurs where the sample's scores are already so high on the scale that little improvement is possible.

Center grants: Grants that generally involve several related projects that are tied together by a single theme or focus. They incorporate research, development, implementation, training, and dissemination activities.

Citation searching: Involves looking at the bibliographic citations or references at the end of articles.

Classical test theory: A set of psychometric approaches that aim to define and improve the reliability of assessments and predict other outcomes, such as item difficulty or the score of a test-taker on a given variable.

Classicism: Reasoning that if pure logic was used to connect the natural world to scientific knowledge, then scientific knowledge could be demonstrated to be true.

Clinical expertise: The proficiency and judgment that individual practitioners acquire through experience.

Clinical reasoning research: Research that examines how occupational therapists identify problems and make treatment decisions.

Clinical significance: The demonstration of meaningful change in everyday function. This can increase the compatibility of research information with the ultimate goal of occupational therapy intervention, which is to positively affect clients' everyday lives.

Cluster randomized controlled trial: A special kind of randomized controlled trial in which clinical sites are randomly assigned to arms (conditions of the independent variable), as opposed to randomly assigning individual participants.

Cluster sampling: A probability-based sampling method in which groups or programs, rather than individuals, are selected, and every member of that group or program is invited to participate in the study.

Cochrane levels-of-evidence model: Model that considers three criteria to determine the credibility of findings from a treatment or intervention: strength of the evidence, size of the effect, and relevance of the evidence.

Code directory: Includes operational definitions and inclusion and exclusion criteria, or instructions about circumstances under which the code should or should not be applied.

Cohort design: A design used in developmental research in which a sample of participants is followed over time and repeated measures are taken at certain intervals to describe how the variable(s) under study have changed.

Collaborating mode: The application of a theoretical concept consistent with Taylor's Intentional Relationship Model. It is enacted in therapy when a therapist chooses to allow a client total control over the tasks and activities of therapy.

Collaboration: A theoretical concept defined uniquely in Taylor's Intentional Relationship Model as shifting all control of the therapy process to the client.

Colloquium: A summary of research papers by a panel of specialists that is typically followed by a question-and-answer session with the audience.

Communality: Describes the context in which research occurs. This context involves a community of scientists who consider how research in a given area should be conducted, who scrutinize individual studies, and who collectively arrive at judgments about what conclusions should be drawn about a body of research findings.

Community-building approaches: This defines a set of approaches to needs assessment in which the focus is on the community and on fostering development of a collective to promote social change.

Comparative need approach: This approach assumes that the baseline group actually needs the programs and services that the complex provides, and that they are receiving them in the correct amount.

Compatibility: One of the five determinants of an innovation that may facilitate or hinder its adoption. It refers to the degree to which an innovation is perceived as being consistent with the existing values, past experiences, and needs of the potential adopter. An idea that is incompatible with the values and norms of the social system will not be adopted as rapidly as an innovation that is compatible.

Complexity: One of the five determinants of an innovation that may facilitate or hinder its adoption. It refers to the degree to which an innovation is perceived as difficult to understand and use. The innovations that are readily comprehended by most potential adopters will be adopted more rapidly, whereas those that are perceived as more complicated will be adopted more slowly.

Computer-assisted qualitative data analysis (CAQDA): Using a computer and specialized software to assist with the management and analysis of qualitative data.

Concept: A definition or label for a phenomenon.

Concept contraction: A process used to focus the retrieval of data into a more conceptually consistent, relevant, and manageable set of information.

Concept expansion: The process of broadening a search topic to include all its relevant dimensions; often originates from a specific item of information, or a small set of such items.

Conceptual labels: Words or short phrases that serve as a kind of tag for segments of text, categorically describing information the segments contain. They eventually evolve into a list of index codes used to label and retrieve segments of text that relate to a common theme.

Concerns report method: An approach to needs assessment that draws on focus groups, survey research, and analytic strategies that originate in discrepancy modeling.

Concurrent nested design: A mixed-methods design where the primary tradition determines how data from the secondary tradition will be handled.

Concurrent transformative design: A mixed-methods design that involves the use of a theoretical perspective to enact change in a group or organization. Choices about the predominant tradition and whether methods are nested or triangulated are made based on the degree to which the theoretical perspective is facilitated. A transformative design may take on the characteristics of either a nested or triangulated design, but the overall purpose is to promote change in the entity being studied.

Concurrent triangulation design: The most commonly used mixed-methods design approach in which both qualitative and quantitative data are gathered simultaneously. Results are validated by virtue of having been confirmed through multiple data collection techniques. Neither tradition is designated as core or secondary, which frees the investigator to pursue interesting developments as they occur.

Concurrent validity: An approach to establishing criterion validity that refers to evidence that the assessment under development or investigation concurs or covaries with the result of another assessment that is known to measure the intended construct or with another criterion. Concurrent validity is often the method of choice when there is an existing "gold standard" assessment.

Confidence interval: Often used when evaluating effect size. A statistical range that tells us the lower and upper limits of the true effect size in the population.

Conflict of commitment: Issues that may prevent researchers from expending their full energy and effort for their primary employment and, in particular, for discharging research obligations.

Conflict of interest: A situation in which the researcher derives personal benefit from the research at the expense of subjects and/or the institution in which the research is being conducted.

Confounding variable: Extraneous influences that might lead to an incorrect conclusion about the influence of the independent variable on the dependent variable.

CONSORT (Consolidated Standards of Reporting Trials) Statement: CONSORT provides a checklist of essential items that should be included in a randomized controlled trial.

Construct: An abstract idea that exists in the absence of quantification.

Construct validity: The capacity of an assessment to measure the intended underlying construct. It defines whether an assessment measures the phenomenon that it is believed to measure, and it is the ultimate objective of all forms of empirically assessing validity.

Consumers: Includes anyone who may be involved with and affected by the intervention process and outcome, including the occupational therapy clients, their caregivers, their parents and teachers (in the case of children), community members, disability groups, and others. Also known as *society*.

Contamination effect: An unanticipated confound in which subjects in an experimental condition share aspects of a treatment with subjects in a control condition, influencing outcomes for subjects in the control condition.

Content analysis: The use of existing documents and a specialized analytic approach. The raw material of content analysis may be any form of communication or text, although written forms are most common. Historically, content analysis emphasized systematic, objective, and quantitative counts and descriptions of content derived from researcher-developed categories. Today, content analysis can be exclusively numeric or exclusively interpretive—largely dependent on the theoretical traditions dominant within the researcher's discipline.

Content validity: The adequacy with which an assessment captures the domain or universe of the construct it aims to measure.

Contextual and environmental assessments: Assessments that measure aspects of physical, social, educational, or work-related settings in which subjects perform daily life occupations.

Continuous scale variable: May assume any value along a continuum that is defined by a given range.

Control group: An experimental condition to which a group of subjects is assigned as a basis for comparison with the experimental group.

Controlled-language term: A term that matches language that has been preprogrammed into the database.

Convenience sampling: The most problematic, yet widely used nonprobability method to obtain subjects. Convenience sampling is the use of volunteers or easily available subjects such as a group of students in a program or clientele in a clinic.

Convergence: The principle that two measures intended to capture the same underlying trait should be highly correlated.

Correlated-samples tests: Term used to describe related-samples tests.

Correlational research: Type of research that aims to demonstrate relationships between variables under study.

Correlational research design: Descriptive research that aims to demonstrate relationships between variables under study.

Corresponding author: The author of an article who has agreed to receive and respond to any correspondence regarding the article.

Counterbalanced design: A design starts off like a basic experiment, in which participants are randomly assigned to as many groups as there are conditions of the independent variable, but each group then goes on to experience both conditions of the independent variable. Also known as a *crossover design.*

Counterbalancing of the dependent variables: This is where the different variables are experienced in different sequences, so each dependent variable sometimes occurs early in the testing protocol and sometimes late.

Criterion referencing: Making judgments or interpretations of a score with reference to what is considered adequate or acceptable performance.

Criterion standard: Also referred to as the gold standard, the criterion standard is a method of correctly defining the dependent variable that is recognized as the ideal way to measure that variable in the field of study. Thus, in selecting a data collection procedure for the dependent variable, the investigator asks if there is a consensus in the field concerning the best way to measure or categorize that variable.

Criterion validity: Involves collecting objective evidence about the validity of an assessment. It refers to the ability of an assessment to produce results that concur with or predict a known criterion assessment or known variable.

Critical appraisal: An essential component of every literature review and a means of evaluating key aspects of the literature on a topic.

Critical modernism: Argues that theories progress by becoming better at the particular way they make sense of the world.

Critical theory: Epistemology where researchers take the stance that knowledge (and theory) is not universal and absolute. Instead, it starts with the basic premise that social reality is embedded and constructed in specific historical times and places, and that it is produced and reproduced by people.

Critically appraised paper: When a single study is appraised as the "best" available evidence, the outcome is a critically appraised paper.

Critically appraised topic: A short summary of evidence on a topic of interest, usually focused around a clinical question.

Crossover design: This design begins like a basic experiment, in which participants are randomly assigned to as many groups as there are conditions of the independent variable. But each group then goes on to experience both conditions of the independent variable.

Cross-sectional design: Often used in developmental research, design in which the investigator collects data at one time point from a sample that is stratified. Compares different types of persons in terms of some immediately measurable dependent variable. In this design, the researcher does not manipulate the assignment of subjects to groups, as in experiments. This kind of independent variable is sometimes called an organismic variable or a variable consisting of preexisting conditions.

D

***d*-statistic:** A commonly cited statistical measure of effect size. It describes the effectiveness of an intervention as ranging between 0 (negligible effect) and > 1.00 (very large effect).

Data: The information collected from participants in the study.

Data analysis: Involves manipulating the data to answer the research question.

Data analysis approach: Describes how you will organize and scrutinize your data to test whether your original aims or hypotheses were accomplished.

Data checking: Running frequency distributions and measures of central tendency and variability on each of the individual variables in the analysis file to check for missing or out-of-range values.

Data cleaning: The process of correcting data entry errors.

Data coding: Translating participant responses into numerical values to facilitate statistical analysis.

Data collection approach: Describes how and where data will be elicited from the subjects.

Data fabrication: A research integrity issue in which an investigator makes up her or his own data.

Data management: The logistical, reflective, and behind-the-scenes processes and infrastructure that allow a researcher to produce high-quality information to address the study questions and describe how and what has been done during a study accurately and comprehensively.

Deductive: Phase of research where predictions are derived from existing theory to see if those predictions hold in the natural world.

Deductive processes: Thought process of making use of existing concepts and knowledge, including wisdom received from others while growing up as human beings, and professional training.

Deductive reasoning: Deriving predictions from existing theory to see if those predictions hold in the natural world.

Degrees of freedom: The number of independent observations in a sample, subtracting the number of parameters that must be estimated from the sample data.

Delayed-treatment control group: A type of control group in which subjects are put on a waiting list and then receive the treatment in a period of time after the treatment group has already received the treatment.

Demonstration grant: This type of grant allows investigators to develop, expand, and evaluate a specific set of health-care services, a model program, or a particular methodological approach.

Dependability: Indicates the extent to which a measure is estimated to be reliable and valid.

Dependent-samples tests: Term used to describe related-samples tests.

Dependent variable: The outcome variable in a hypothesized relationship between two or more variables.

Descendency search: Type of retrieval approach using the Science or Social Science Citation Indexes (Web of Science).

Descriptive case study: An in-depth description of the experiences or behaviors of a particular individual or a series of individuals.

Descriptive research: This approach takes advantage of naturally occurring events or available information to generate new insights through inductive processes. Consequently, descriptive investigations often serve an exploratory purpose.

Descriptive statistics: A means of summarizing the characteristics about a single sample of clients (rather than generalizing or making inferences about a larger population of clients from which that sample was derived).

Design: Part of the method section of a research proposal that describes the type of study that was developed and the way in which a research question or problem will be examined.

Developmental research: A type of research that seeks to describe patterns of growth or change over time within selected segments of a population.

Dichotomous scale: Defines two discrete categories within a variable.

Diffusion of innovations: Theory that is introduced as the framework to help identify desirable characteristics of research evidence that could facilitate its use for evidence-based practice.

Direct consumers: The primary recipients of the intervention.

Discussion: A section of the research proposal that provides an overview of study aims and findings.

Dissemination: Defines the manner by which research findings are shared with others.

Divergence (or discriminant validity): An approach to demonstrating construct validity. It is designed to measure whether different traits show patterns of association that discriminate between them.

Domain analysis: The critical process of selecting and adding pieces of information through interview and observation and analyzing it for further discovery.

Double-blind study: When researchers choose for not only subjects to be blinded but for themselves not to know what condition a subject is in until the study is over and findings have been analyzed.

Dropouts: Individuals who drop out of a study, which is also referred to as attrition; particularly likely in long-term experiments. Participants drop out because they lose interest over time, find the experiment to be burdensome or uncomfortable, become ill in ways that are not relevant to the experiment, die, or move away.

E

Ecological validity: The social importance of research outcomes; it is the degree to which results obtained in controlled experimental conditions are related to those obtained in naturalistic environments.

Educational grants: Grants that are used to support professionals and students to develop or extend their knowledge or skills. They may be used to support professional activities that involve training and education (e.g., conferences or symposia) or to support the implementation of specialized academic programs and collaborations, which might include several researchers from across the country. Also called training grants.

Effect size: Name given to a family of indices that measure the magnitude of a treatment effect. Unlike significance tests, these indices are independent of sample size. They are calculated by taking the difference between control and experimental group means and dividing that difference by the standard deviation of the scores of both groups combined.

Emic: Refers to an insider perspective in qualitative research.

Empiricism: Means that scientific knowledge emerges from and is tested by observation and experience.

Epistemology: The broad arena of philosophy concerned with the nature and scope of knowledge.

Epoche: The first phase of phenomenological research.

Ethical approval: Ensures the safety and ethicality of a research proposal.

Ethical responsibility: Involves being aware of the need to engage in research by staying up to date with practice developments and innovations that are supported by careful and systematic research. This ensures that clients receive the appropriate level of care.

Ethical review: A process designed to protect subjects from harm, ensure that subjects' effort and any risk involved are warranted by the study's importance, and ensure that subjects freely give informed consent to participate.

Ethnographic designs: A type of research derived from sociology that focuses on the social definitions and meanings of behavior or other phenomena.

Ethnography: A qualitative design that focuses on the social definitions and meanings of behavior or other phenomena.

Evidence-based practice: An approach to practice that assumes the active application of current research findings to inform practice decisions and treatment options.

Exclusion criteria: The characteristics that will prohibit the subject from being an appropriate candidate for the study.

Expectancy effects: Possible psychological effects of knowing one is receiving a treatment on actual treatment outcomes.

Experience-based practice: Practice based primarily on experience.

Experimental design: The most rigorous type of group comparison study that tests if-then statements and provides evidence about probable causality. Two or more groups of participants are randomly assigned to different levels (or experimental conditions) of one or more independent variables.

Experimental group (or groups): Subjects in experimental groups receive the treatment condition of primary interest.

Experimental report: A structured report of findings from a research investigation.

Experimenter bias: A type of bias that erroneously influences outcomes. It occurs when the researcher is testing a treatment that he or she believes will be effective and therefore expects the treatment to be effective.

Experimenter expectancy: Occurs when a researcher expects that subjects will have a better outcome due to having received the treatment or therapy.

Expert opinion: A person or convened group of people having specialized knowledge about a topic based on education, experience, or certain achievements that are not possessed by the average person.

Expressed need: This refers to demand for a service, either through current use or waiting lists.

External clinical evidence: Findings from high-quality clinically applied research studies within the field's scientific literature.

External validity: The extent to which we may generalize a research finding to different persons, settings, or times.

F

Fabrication: Generating fictitious data or findings and reporting them as if they were discovered during a research study.

Face validity: Means that an assessment has the appearance of measuring an underlying construct.

Factor analysis: An approach to demonstrating construct validity that examines a set of items that make up an assessment and determines whether there are one or more clusters of items.

Falsification: Involves changing or distorting data, data collection procedures, or research findings to portray the desired findings rather than the actual ones.

Federated searching: Using metasearch engines that allow the user to input a single set of search terms into the search interface that will be sent to many different information sources.

Felt need: This refers to want, with or without actions to obtain that which is wanted.

Fidelity: Fidelity defines the degree to which an intervention is loyal to itself in terms of the intended content and process of the intervention.

Fidelity measures: Used in intervention studies to ensure that the therapists abide by the intended treatment protocol.

Field studies: Studies that occur outside of the laboratory and in a naturalistic setting in which investigators seek to gain an insider's view of the phenomena under study through intensive and extended immersion.

Floor effect: A lack of responsiveness that occurs when the scores on a variable are so low that little change or improvement is expected.

Focus group: A group discussion conducted by an investigator who serves as a moderator, guiding the discussion by introducing questions, usually from a written set of questions or topics.

Focus-group interviews: Interviews conducted with a small group of people on a specific topic; typically, four to six people participate in the interview, which lasts about 1 to 2 hours.

Follow-up procedures: Typically involve assessments undertaken after subjects have completed the intervention to follow their reaction to the intervention over time.

Follow-up study: A study of the long-term effects of an intervention.

Formative evaluation: A beginning aspect of program evaluation used to assess the extent to which actual programming matches that which was planned and the extent to which programming and services address the identified needs of the target population.

Formative research: Research into the processes by which an intervention creates change. Also known as *process research*.

Frequency (*f*): Describes the number of counts within a category. Frequencies are used to summarize nominal and ordinal-scale variables.

Frequency distribution: A means of describing data in terms of "counts" within each level or category of a variable.

G

Gaining access: The entry point into a qualitative inquiry, which affects the selection of subjects.

Grant: A specified amount of money given to an investigator via the investigator's host institution to undertake a specific research project.

Grant proposal: Document written to request funding for research.

Gray literature: Information that is not published or available in usual formats such as journals.

Grounded theory: A qualitative design that attempts to generate a theoretical understanding of a phenomenon by extracting meaning from social interactions.

Group comparison designs: Designs that test hypotheses by comparing groups of subjects.

H

Hawthorne effect: Occurs when subjects change their behavior because they know they are being observed.

Heuristic relevance: A means by which the quality of qualitative research is evaluated.

High-status informant data: Data from interviews with high-status informants who are articulate, reflective, and observant.

Historically controlled study: Compares a group that received an intervention (treatment group) to a group that did not receive the intervention (control group).

Human subject: A person who is invited and consents to participate in any kind of research (i.e., information gathering and sharing).

Hypothesis: A prediction about the relationship between variables within a population; a structured statement of anticipated results of a research study.

Hypothesis testing: Defines the process by which outcomes or significant differences found in a study reflect true outcomes or are due to chance or error.

I

Impact: The extent to which a project answers a socially or medically significant need or question in an innovative way that pushes the state of science and/or practice forward.

Incidence: A descriptive epidemiological estimate that is concerned with how many persons have onset of a condition during a given span of time.

Inclusion criteria: The traits that the researcher has identified as characterizing the population.

Independent samples test: A test performed on variables from two or more different sample groups. Also known as a *between-subjects test.*

Independent samples t-test: Compares the means from two independent groups or samples.

Independent variable: The variable thought to influence the outcome in a hypothesized relationship between variables.

In-depth interviews: Interviews that are most often conducted in face-to-face situations with one individual, with a goal of delving deeply into a particular event, issue, or context.

Index codes: Text codes added to data that are the result of multiple readings through the data in which descriptive conceptual labels become more systematic and consolidated.

Indirect consumers: Those who purchase the intervention for someone else or are strongly affected by the behavioral changes targeted in the intervention, but they are not its recipients.

Inductive: Phase of research where explanations and theories are generated from specific observations of the natural world.

Inductive approach: Approach to research analysis that allows findings to emerge from the raw data that has been collected, without the restraints imposed by stricter methodologies or preestablished theories.

Inductive processes: Thought process often used in qualitative research where investigators use observation to see in new ways and build up new ideas.

Inductive reasoning: Generating explanations and theory from specific observations of the natural world.

Inferential statistics: A means of making inferences about a population or larger group of people based on the sample, which represents a small portion of the larger group.

Information queries: Words or phrases that are entered into the interface of online information retrieval tools.

Informed consent: A process in which potential human subjects learn about the purpose of the study and what is being asked of them as participants and subsequently decide whether or not to participate.

Innovation: New ideas and/or practice.

Inscribing social discourse: Looking beyond the words and descriptions of interview subjects to understand more fundamental conceptualizations of how people experience what they do; it represents a deliberate act to ensure that interactional details are fully captured.

Institutional affiliation: Designates the name, location, and nature of the place where the authors were working when the study was conducted.

Institutional review board (IRB): A mechanism for regulatory oversight that exists within a university, medical center, or other industry in which one or more committees of informed individuals review research proposals to ensure that the study is safe and ethical for all participants.

Integrity of methods: Not violating the assumptions, philosophical foundations, and procedures of the core method. Respecting methodological integrity requires continually linking the unique philosophical foundations with the research question(s) and maintaining one method as dominant over the other.

Intention-to-treat analysis: A statistical approach to the treatment of missing data in which dropouts are sought out for outcomes testing even if they discontinued the intervention to which they were assigned and even if they ended up experiencing the opposing intervention (the other condition of the independent variable).

Internal consistency: The extent to which the items that make up an assessment covary or correlate with each other.

Internal validity: The extent to which we may infer that an explanation for a particular phenomenon is true or a specific intervention or action has caused an effect (or outcome).

Interrater reliability: The ratings of more than one rater on a single assessment of a single subject are compared to estimate the ability of the assessment to be rated consistently across users.

Interval scale: A scale of measurement of data according to which the differences between values can be quantified in absolute but not relative terms and for which any zero is merely arbitrary—for instance, dates are measured on an interval scale because differences can be measured in years.

Interval scale variable: A scale in which the intervals between values are equivalent.

Interview schedule: The written form or guide to be used by the interviewer in a face-to-face interview.

Interviewer training: Teaching technical skills on how to ask the interview questions and the use of follow-up probes to elicit more detailed explanations; it also includes training on appropriate behaviors needed to gain entry into the research context.

Interviews: Structured, semistructured, or unstructured question-and-answer sessions that allow a researcher to collect information that leads to a broader, more holistic, or more integrative view of a subject's impairment or life situation.

Introduction: Part of a published peer-reviewed article that describes prior studies in the topic area and provides background evidence

justifying the relevance and need for the study at hand.

J

Justice: The principle of justice requires that the research impose the burden of risk and the potential for benefit upon the same groups of people.

K

Key informant interviews: Interviews with individuals considered to be influential, prominent, and/or well-informed people in an organization or community.

Key words: Four or five terms from an article that capture the main topics covered by the article but are distinct from the words used in the title; they are usually placed immediately following the abstract.

Keyword: Key terms assigned to articles, including the title, author, subject, and abstract fields, that are used as search terms in database search engines.

Keyword searching: Using one or more keywords to retrieve information from a database.

Known groups method: An approach to establishing construct validity that involves identifying subjects who are demonstrated to differ on the characteristic the assessment aims to measure.

L

Level of an independent variable: An experimental condition that reflects the degree to which the variable is introduced to the subject.

Level of evidence: The extent of methodological rigor applied before asserting the conclusion that the intervention was effective.

Level-of-evidence model: Major criteria used to evaluate the rigor, relevance, effect, and quality of research.

Level of evidence of the study design: One determinant of the strength of evidence of a quantitative research study. This is an estimate of certainty that the identified evidence is a true measure of the benefits of an intervention.

Level of significance or "alpha": Typically set at .05 in occupational therapy studies. This means that researchers are willing to accept a 5% chance that they will find an effect by chance when there really is no true effect.

Limitations section: Part of the discussion section of a research article in which researchers acknowledge any flaws in study design, procedures, measures, and/or analyses, or any variables that were not examined, that could have limited the interpretation and generalizability of the findings.

Literature review: A practical piece of writing that builds an evidence-based story, acting as a precursor to planned research or as an introduction to an executed study; sometimes referred to as an *unsystematic review.*

Logic models: These are typically presented in graphical or figure form. The visual image portrays relationships between resources (inputs), activities, outputs (deliverables), and outcomes (impacts), and they are used for program planning or program evaluation.

Logical positivism: The belief that research allows theory to progress toward truth through testing hypotheses that support or reject theory.

Logical reasoning: Used to systematically link knowledge to what the knowledge is supposed to explain. This occurs through the process of inductive and deductive reasoning.

Longitudinal approach: The same sample is repeatedly measured at planned intervals over time.

Longitudinal study: A study in which subjects are tracked over time.

Low-status informant data: Data that emerge from interviews with individuals who are not as articulate and may not be held in high regard by community members; these informants may even hold a minority viewpoint.

M

Management plan: A description of the major tasks necessary to complete the project, who will do them, and when they will be done.

Management plan and project timeline: The specific tasks that will need to be done over the course of an entire project and when these tasks need to be completed.

Mean: The most widely utilized and reliable measure of central tendency. It is another way of defining the average score among all of the scores in the sample. The mean is calculated by dividing the sum of all of the scores (or values) in the sample by the total number of clients (or possibilities) in the sample.

Measure: Specific method, instrument, strategy, or tool used to gather data for a study. Also known as *assessment.*

Measurement approach: Describes the means by which the data were collected.

Measurement error: Represents the general degree of error present in measurement.

Measures: A part of the method section of a research proposal that describes the assessments and other data collection devices that will be used to collect data.

Mechanism-based reasoning: A lower level of evidence in quantitative research defined by studies that involve an inference from findings related to individual mechanisms to claims that an intervention leads to a particular outcome.

Mechanisms of change: The processes by which an intervention creates change in a client.

Median: Reflects the middle position in a set of ordered or ranked scores.

MEDLINE: An abstracted search engine containing peer-reviewed journal articles from the fields of biomedicine, public health, behavioral sciences, and bioengineering.

Member check: The researcher approaches study participants to describe, cross-check, and thereby validate qualitative findings and interpretations.

Members of the extended community: Includes those who probably do not know or interact with the direct and indirect consumers but who live in the same community.

Members of the immediate community: Those who interact with the direct and indirect consumers on a regular basis, usually through close proximity in work, school, or social situations.

Memos: Margin notes containing not only index labels, but also longer annotations.

Memoing: Writing notes and memos through which the investigators can record impressions about the data, methodological insights, and developing interpretations and theory.

Meta-analysis: A comprehensive study that summarizes the findings of several individual studies to answer scientific (and clinical) questions. This summary includes statistical data that reflect a best estimate of the cumulative evidence for the explanation of a mechanism or outcome in occupational therapy.

Metadata: Data about data that are new text and/or graphic products created by the researcher to represent key themes, constructs, and relationships that emerge from and are applied to a body of qualitative data.

Metasearch engines: Provide a single search interface for a cluster of individual search engines.

Method: The second part of a peer-reviewed research article that describes in detail the approach that the researchers used to answer a particular practice question or solve a practice problem.

Methodological congruence: A means of evaluating the quality of qualitative research that refers to the extent of rigor in documentation, procedures, and ethics and the extent to which methods would be able to be replicated by another researcher.

Methods section: Encompasses the research design, sample, population, sampling approach, subject retention plan, assessments or measures, procedures, ethical review, and approval.

Mind-mapping: A means of generating and refining a visual representation of the ideas to be contained in a paper.

Misconduct: Fabrication, falsification, plagiarism, or other practices that seriously deviate from those that are commonly accepted within the scientific community for proposing, conducting, or reporting research.

Mixed-methodological study: One that incorporates both quantitative and qualitative methodological approaches.

Mixed methods: A research design that integrates elements of both qualitative and quantitative methods so that the strengths of each are emphasized.

Mixed-methods designs: A subtype of multiple methods designs in which qualitative and quantitative traditions are used simultaneously or consecutively in the methods section.

Mode: Defined as the score that occurs with the highest frequency in the data set.

Model of Human Occupation (MOHO): Describes how occupations are motivated, supported by habits and roles, and performed within social and physical environments.

Modernism: Replaced the concern for absolute truth with concern for how to correct errors in knowledge. Modernists envisioned science as a process of testing and verification of the theory created through inductive reasoning.

Multigroup cohort design: The researcher matches a sample that has a hypothesized risk factor to a sample that does not. Then the researcher picks a future point in time (or a series of points if using repeated measures) to see whether the hypothesized risk factor truly predicts the disease or disability.

Multimethod designs: A subtype of multiple-methods design that incorporates two or more data collection techniques within only one tradition (qualitative or quantitative).

Multiple-baseline design: Single-subject design that requires repeated measures of at least three baseline conditions that typically are implemented concurrently, with each successive baseline being longer than the previous one.

Multiple-baseline design across behaviors: A multiple-baseline design in which the same treatment variable is applied sequentially to separate behaviors in a single participant.

Multiple-baseline design across participants: A multiple-baseline design in which one behavior is treated sequentially across matched participants.

Multiple-baseline design across settings: This is a multiple-baseline design in which the same behavior or behaviors are studied in several independent settings.

Multiple-methods designs: The use of two or more data collection strategies or methods for a given research question.

Multiplicity: This is the result of having too many dependent variables. It defines the increase in type I error due to multiple statistical tests on the same participants.

N

Narrative inquiry: Seeks to understand how people construct storied accounts of their and others' lives and of shared events.

Narrative reviews: A synthesis of aggregated investigations from individual quantitative research studies.

Naturalistic observation: Refers to quantitative research that takes place in natural settings.

Nazi Doctors Trials: Following World War II, a tribunal identified numerous experiments that had been conducted in the "interests" of science, which represent horrific abuses of human beings.

Needs assessment research: An assessment approach that involves identifying the needs of broader groups of people to develop or modify services, programs, and policies and their respective goals.

Nesting: Allows Boolean search-term relationships to be combined with each other in a search query to improve control over the set of retrieval items.

Network sampling: Method in which initially identified subjects provide names of others who may meet the study criteria. Also known as *snowball sampling*.

Nominal scale: A scale with two or more categories that represent named classifications and are not ordered in relationship to one another. Used to classify characteristics such as gender. In this case numbers are used to identify a specific category (e.g., 1 = female; 2 = male). In nominal scales, numbers have no meaning other than identifying the category or characteristic to which a person belongs.

Nonconcurrent multiple-baseline design across individuals: A multiple-baseline design whereby different individuals are studied at different times. With this design, the researcher predetermines baseline lengths and randomly assigns these to participants as they become available.

Nonequivalent control-group design: Study design in which more than one comparable group is observed, at least one of which does not receive the intervention.

Nonexperimental designs: Studies that are purely descriptive or observational in which variables that are thought to be associated with one another are analyzed statistically.

Nonexperimental group comparison designs: Study designs that lack the degree of control achieved by experimental designs; sometimes called *quasi-experimental designs* or *nonrandom designs*.

Nonparametric statistics: A statistical method wherein the data are not required to fit a normal distribution.

Nonrandomized comparison group design: Study design that is similar to an experimental design, but it uses convenient preexisting groupings as the method of assigning participants to conditions of the independent variable, as opposed to randomization. This is also called a *nonrandomized trial* when the dependent variable is a valued health outcome.

Nonrandomized controlled cohort study: A study of subsamples from a given population who differ in terms of the extent to which they have been, are being, or will be exposed to something hypothesized to influence the outcome of a given impairment.

Nonresponse bias: Bias in survey findings because the views of respondents selected for the sample who elect not to respond are not represented.

Normal distribution: Defines an average or "norm" within a sample of people and describes successive deviations from that norm.

Normative need: A need that is defined by professionals and experts rather than by members of the community themselves.

Normative research: A type of study undertaken in order to establish usual or average values for specific variables.

Norm-referenced measures: Measures that are standardized according to statistical norms established within certain groups of people.

No-treatment control group: A control condition in which subjects are either naïve to any treatment for their particular impairment or have independently withdrawn from or have been deliberately withdrawn from treatment for purposes of the study.

Null hypothesis: The assumption that an intervention (or other experimental manipulation) has had no effect.

Nuremberg Code: One of the earliest U.S. codes regarding the ethical conduct of research that was written during the Nazi Doctors Trials.

O

Observability: One of the five determinants of an innovation that may facilitate or hinder its adoption. It refers to the degree to which the results of an innovation are visible to others. The easier it is for individuals to see the results of an innovation, the more likely they are to adopt.

Observation: Method of investigation that requires careful watching, listening, and recording of events, behaviors, and objects in the social setting chosen for study. The observation record, frequently referred to as *field notes*, is composed of detailed nonjudgmental, concrete descriptions of what has been observed.

Observational approach: Data collection method used to answer questions related to performance or behavior in real time; does not require the participant to reflect upon and recount his or her personal experience.

Observer bias: A bias that erroneously influences outcomes. It occurs when the researcher is looking for a physical cue or behavior to occur during an observation that follows a particular intervention or treatment.

Observer presence or characteristics: A bias effect in a study where the observer may have an impact on the behavior or information provided by the client.

Occupational science: Development of a basic science concerned with the study of occupation.

One-group posttest-only design: Type of study where a single group of subjects receives an occupational therapy treatment and then a posttest is given to determine whether the treatment was successful.

One-way analysis of variance (ANOVA): Allows the researcher to test differences between three or more means (or levels) of a single independent variable.

Operational multiplicity: The fact that a particular concept or construct may be operationally defined in a variety of ways across different studies.

Operationalizing a construct: Refers to assigning a concrete means of defining an abstract idea, such as a measurement.

Opinion paper: An essay containing novel or controversial information about a topic of broad impact within a profession.

Ordinal scale: A categorical variable in which the numbers representing the different categories are ordered or ranked in a linear way from least to greatest or from greatest to least.

Organismic variable: A type of variable that is part of the organism. It is often referred to as a *fixed variable*, a *nonmanipulated variable,* or a *variable consisting of preexisting conditions.*

Outcome variable: The outcome variable in a hypothesized relationship between two or more variables.

Outcomes research: An approach to research concerned with the results (success/failure) of occupational therapy techniques and approaches.

P

p-**value:** A statistic that tells whether a finding was significant or not; used as a cutoff point to determine the extent to which a conclusion about a sample reflects a true difference within the larger population, versus the conclusion being due to error or chance.

Paired samples t-tests: Compare the means from a single group of clients, typically at two points in time.

Panel discussion: A small group of people with special expertise who are typically seated together at the front or in the center of the presentation room. Interactive discussion among panel members and between panel members and audience members typically takes place.

Paper presentation: A brief verbal presentation by a single researcher or group of researchers that follows a similar structure to a peer-reviewed journal article.

Parallel forms reliability: Involves administration of the alternative forms to subjects at the same time.

Parametric statistics: A branch of statistics that assumes that sample data come from a population that follows a probability distribution based on a fixed set of parameters.

Participant identifier: Numeric or alphanumeric code (e.g., A-001) that is used in place of the participant's name on all documents pertaining to that individual.

Participant-observer: A researcher who is also a member of the group of persons being observed.

Participants: Part of the method section of a research article that describes the social and demographic characteristics of the sample and the criteria by which the individuals in the study were selected for participation.

Participation: An overall approach to inquiry and a data gathering method. To some degree, all qualitative research has a participatory element. Participation demands first-hand involvement in the social world chosen for study.

Participatory action research (PAR): An approach to research used to confront pressing social problems. Although PAR can be combined with quantitative designs, it most often employs qualitative research strategies.

Participatory approaches: In this set of approaches to needs assessment, the underlying assumption is that knowledge is power, and that knowledge development within a community will lead to social action.

Participatory research: An approach that involves the participants as co-creators and co-investigators who shape the research questions, methods, and outcomes while at the same time transforming themselves and others within their immediate contexts in significant and enduring ways.

Pearson correlation test: The most commonly used measure of association in statistics. According to this test, the strength of the association between two variables is represented as an *r*-value and ranges from $r = -1$ to $+1$.

Peer debriefing: The process of using multiple researchers to analyze data, which provides a mechanism for contrary views to arise and receive careful review.

Peer review: Defined as a systematic approach to the review of a scientific work by others with expertise in the area being presented.

Peer-reviewed journal: A professional journal in which submitted articles are rigorously evaluated by members of an editorial board who have expertise in research methods and in the topic area under study

Peer-reviewed journal article: A research article that has undergone intensive review by at least two other professionals who would be considered peers of the authors in a given field of study.

Percentage values: Calculated by dividing the frequency (or number of counts within a category) by the total number of eligible counts within the sample.

Performance measures: Data collection method in which a subject performs certain behaviors or tasks in a laboratory or clinical area using standard equipment, allowing the researchers to measure performance in the task.

Per-protocol analysis: An approach to the treatment of missing data in an experiment in which dropouts are excluded, with the rationale that inclusion of dropouts only causes random error and increases the chances of a type II error.

Phenomenology: A qualitative design that focuses on how subjects experience and make sense of their immediate worlds.

Philosophical orientation: The preference toward approaching knowledge and knowledge development in occupational therapy from a particular ideological perspective.

Phrase matching: Using a particular string of text during a database search to reduce the quantity of retrieved items by increasing specificity.

Placebo: A substitute for the condition or treatment that is intended to have an effect but in reality has no effect.

Placebo control groups: Groups of subjects receiving a placebo condition.

Placebo effect: The perception or experience that a treatment has been successful even if no treatment or a placebo (fake) treatment is being applied.

Placebo treatment: A fake treatment that is designed to deceive the participant into thinking he or she is receiving a treatment,

but the placebo actually has no effect on the desired outcome.

Plagiarism: Using another writer's ideas, methods, results, writing, or work without credit to the origin, thereby taking personal credit for it falsely.

Poster presentations: Experimental reports or case studies that are presented on a single poster with at least one author standing beside it to engage in discussion with the viewers.

Postmodernism: Set of ideas in which scientific knowledge is no more privileged than any other source of knowledge.

Postulate: A logical statement or rule that specifies relationships between concepts.

Practice theory research: An approach to research that explains problems that therapists address and justifies approaches to solving them that are used in therapy.

Precision: Exactness of an assessment (i.e., the extent of its ability to discriminate differing amounts of a variable). The more precise an assessment is, the finer is its ability to discriminate between different amounts.

Predictive validity: An approach to establishing criterion validity that involves generating evidence that an assessment is a predictor of a future criterion.

Preexisting documents: Existing documents such as medical records.

Pretest-posttest design: An approach to summative evaluation involving an observation before and after the intervention has taken place.

Pretest-posttest nonequivalent group designs: Type of study in which subjects end up in different groups as a matter of convenience.

Prevalence: Defined as a proportion of a total population of people who have a particular health-related condition.

Principles of Belmont: The three principles are respect for persons, beneficence, and justice.

Probabilistic equivalence: Although the treatment and control groups are not equal in terms of all variables, any differences between the two groups are likely to be based on chance rather than on some systematic pattern or variation.

Probability: The likelihood that a predicted outcome or event will actually occur or the degree to which an event will occur in a series of observations.

Procedures: The procedures section of the research proposal that outlines what will happen in the study, the order in which it will happen, and the timeline according to which it will happen.

Process research: Research into the processes by which an intervention creates change. Also known as *formative research*.

Professional development grant: Grant used to enable an individual who is already employed in a professional capacity to begin a career in research or to further develop research-related skills and contributions. Sometimes referred to as a *career development award*.

Professional responsibility: A therapist's obligation to use research to enhance the quality of decision-making.

Program development: The systematic design, planning, and implementation of new services, innovations, or initiatives.

Program evaluation: A process documenting the impact of a newly developed or existing intervention or program of services.

Program planning: An early aspect of program evaluation that involves determining the type of service to be provided, enumerating resources needed to provide the services, characterizing the population, and identifying how the services/program will be delivered.

Project-based methods: Methods used to enhance qualitative research, including daily operational procedures that help to minimize errors in all processes related to data collection, data storage, and data management.

Project information: The information about the process of data collection (e.g., recruitment processes and outcomes, progress on data collection, coding, entry and cleaning, status of data storage and security, and documentation of decisions) that will make it easier for the investigator to describe what he or she has done during the course of the study when it is time to disseminate the study findings.

Prolonged engagement: The period of time spent in the field observing the phenomenon of interest.

Proximity connectors: Connectors used in a complex electronic search process that allows for the analysis of spatial relationships between coded segments.

Psychometric research: An approach to assuring the dependability (reliability and validity) of evaluation of the measures that are used to test deficits, strengths, progress, and setbacks in therapy. Also referred to as *assessment research*.

Psychometric studies: Specifically designed to investigate the properties of clinical assessment tools or data collection instruments intended for use in research.

PsycINFO: An abstracted search engine containing peer-reviewed journal articles from the field of psychology and related fields.

PUBMED: A free-access search engine that contains articles from MEDLINE in addition to book chapters and other types of publications.

Purposive sampling: The deliberate selection of individuals by the researcher based on certain predetermined criteria (usually stated as inclusion and exclusion criteria).

Q

Qualitative analysis: Understanding meanings, processes, people, and people's thoughts and actions through the interpretation of people's words.

Qualitative data analysis: Encompasses a range of approaches to the management and analysis of qualitative data.

Qualitative research: Broad term for approaches to developing new knowledge that have as their main goal the naturalistic discovery, identification, and description of basic features of the worlds people live in and their experiences of those worlds. Qualitative methods are used when it's important to learn more about the kinds of features that are present and to determine the salient contents and meanings of a phenomenon.

Qualitative research methods: Approaches to program evaluation involving observational methods, such as participant observation and direct observation, and other strategies such as interviews with key stakeholders, focus groups, and public forums.

Qualitized: Collected quantitative data that are converted to narratives to be analyzed qualitatively.

Quality of the evidence: One criterion for evaluating the level of evidence in a quantitative research study. Involves the extent to which the researchers minimize bias in the study design by controlling for variables that could bias the results or the interpretation of results.

Quantitative research: An approach to research characterized by objectivity. Researchers create and test theory using standardized and predetermined designs, measures, sampling approaches, and procedures.

Quasi-experimental design: These types of designs are similar to experimental designs, but they rely upon random selection from a convenience sample, and subjects are familiar with the condition to which they have been assigned.

Querying: Part of the process of information retrieval that **involves** seeking matches to a particular text phrase matching or keyword.

Quota sampling: Used when different proportions of subject types are needed so that there is appropriate representation in the sample that may not be attainable with purposive or convenience sampling.

R

r-statistic: Referred to as Pearson's r or as a correlation coefficient. The r-statistic is a direct measure of effect size used when paired quantitative data are available.

Random assignment: Subjects are assigned to treatment versus control groups without knowledge of the groups to which they are being assigned.

Random error: An error that may occur by chance when administering an assessment.

Random sampling: Means that each member or element of the population can theoretically have an equal chance of being selected for the sample.

Random selection: Subjects are aware of the condition to which they are being selected to participate.

Randomization: Considered to be the cornerstone of quantitative research. It balances both the measured and unmeasured characteristics that affect the outcomes of a study, allows for masking, and provides a basis for inference.

Randomized controlled trial (RCT): An experiment wherein an important health outcome is the dependent variable, a clinical intervention is part of the independent variable, and research participants are recruited and randomly assigned over time as they become available. Also referred to as a *randomized trial* or *randomized clinical trial.*

Range: The range defines the difference between the lowest and highest values for a given variable.

Rater bias: May occur when the rater translates the information obtained into a classification or rating. In this situation, any number of characteristics of the rater may introduce error. Rater characteristics that might result in error include demographic characteristics, experience, training, or theoretical orientation of the rater.

Ratio scale: An interval scale in which distances are stated with respect to a rational zero.

Ready-reference searching: Part of the process of information retrieval that is typically very specific, and usually resolved through a closed-ended search process.

Recruitment and retention methods: Describe the means by which the authors were able to locate, access, enroll, and retain their sample over time and through the course of the study.

Recruitment approach: Describes how you will gain participation from subjects in your study.

Reflexivity: A deliberate and systematic process of self-examination.

Regression toward the mean: Defined as the tendency for extreme scores to be followed with scores that are more average.

Related-samples test: Defined as when a statistical test is being performed on variables from the same sample group. Other names include correlated-samples tests, paired-samples tests, within-subjects tests, and dependent-samples tests.

Relative advantage: One of the five determinants of an innovation that may facilitate or hinder its adoption. It refers to the degree to which an innovation is perceived as better than the idea it supersedes. The degree of relative advantage may be measured in many terms (economic, prestige, convenience, satisfaction, etc.), and the greater the perceived relative advantage of an innovation, the more rapid its rate of adoption will be.

Relevance of the evidence: A means of evaluating the quality of quantitative research. It refers to the degree to which the instrument used to measure the effectiveness (or harmfulness) of an intervention is an appropriate and useful measure for the people and problem under study.

Reliability: Refers to whether a given instrument provides stable information across different circumstances.

Reliability coefficient: Defines the ratio of the variance of the true score to the total variance observed on an assessment.

Reliability of data: Measures to ensure that the accuracy of information collected was not unduly affected by any extraneous circumstances surrounding data collection. Reliability is typically concerned with how accuracy may be affected by circumstances of data collection (i.e., who collects data, what kind of instrument is used to collect the data, and how and when the data were collected).

Repeated-measures design: When the expected outcome of an experiment is measured repeatedly over the course of the experiment.

Replicability: Refers to the ability of others to repeat the research question and methodological approach of a given study and, by so doing, arrive at the same findings and conclusions.

Research: The means by which the profession generates evidence to test and validate its theories and to examine and demonstrate the utility of its practice tools and procedures.

Research advocate: One who supports research by finding knowledge gaps, generating relevant questions, identifying research priorities, and lobbying professional leaders.

Research aims: Describes the purpose of the study or what it intends to accomplish. Also known as *specific aims.*

Research collaborator: One who joins with others in a supportive role to assist in the production of research.

Research consumer: An individual who utilizes research to solve problems and/or inform decisions.

Research design: The specific strategies that the investigator will use to answer the question or questions that guide the research (or to test a hypothesis where a hypothesis is included).

Research-emergent profession: A profession that has lacked a consistent history and infrastructure to support individuals who conduct research.

Research grants: Grants that allow investigators to address scientific questions that will contribute to knowledge in a given topic area.

Research hypothesis: Clearly written statement of the expected results of quantitative study.

Research methodology: A broad category that includes selecting and applying a research design, defining sample groups from a given population, applying an approach to assessment or data collection, and choosing how the data will be analyzed to produce findings.

Research problem: A broadly defined gap in knowledge.

Research producer: An individual with a high level of research-related expertise who can function independently as a research leader.

Research proposal: A written plan that organizes the research process in terms of a literature review, the research questions, and the research methodology that will be applied.

Research question: A narrow, focused, and specific question intended to generate knowledge to help close a gap.

Respect for persons: The most basic of the three principles of Belmont; asserts that human persons must be respected in terms of their right to self-determination.

Respondent: Person responding to a survey.

Response bias: Bias in survey findings introduced because those who responded may have been more likely to respond because they agree with or are interested in the study topic.

Responsiveness: Also referred to as sensitivity, responsiveness is the capacity of the dependent variable to show small but meaningful increments of change over time.

Results: A section of the research article that contains the statistical findings or qualitative summarization resulting from the data analyses that were conducted.

Retention plan: Specifies how you will maintain participation from the subjects in your study over time.

Rigor: Means that investigators carefully follow rules, procedures, and techniques that have been developed and agreed upon by the scientific community.

Roundtable discussions: Discussion among a group of individuals with expertise in a given area who raise and respond to questions that are focused on a specific topic.

Running head: An abbreviated title in a research article, placed at the top of each page, that reminds readers of the title as they read through the study, which is one among many within a printed journal volume.

S

Sample: A group of people selected from a larger population of people sharing one or more characteristics under study. The sample group of people is intended to reflect the characteristics under study within the larger population.

Sample size: The number of observations or replicates to include in a statistical sample.

Sampling approach: Describes the characteristics that the subjects who are actually participating in your study will have (e.g., age), criteria by which people will be included versus excluded, and what interventions they might be eligible to receive in the study.

Sampling error: Represents the difference between the values obtained by the sample and the actual values that exist in the population.

Sampling population: The population from which your sample is drawn.

Saturation: The point in the data collection period when the researcher is gaining little or no new information.

Scale of measurement: Explains the rule of logic that defines how numbers are used to describe variation in people, objects, or events.

Scholarship of practice: Defines a dynamic and flexible dialectic between empirical and theoretical knowledge.

Scoping review: This type of review focuses on the rapid collection of as much evidence as possible in a much broader clinical or policy-related area. In this case, the review might inform a range of study designs (rather than a single design), and it does not address very specific questions or assess the quality of the studies that are included in the review. Also referred to as a *scoping study*.

Search terms: Items used in search queries that connect the intended topic to text in information items that are retrieved.

Selection bias: Subjects self-selecting into a study or condition out of self-interest, or a researcher's bias in assigning certain subjects to a specific condition.

Self-report measures: Written instruments on which subjects are asked to record information. They typically ask the subject to self-reflect on his or her experience or needs and select the best option from a finite number of categories or to provide an open-ended explanation as a response.

Semantic connectors: Connectors used in a complex electronic search process that allow for the creation of semantic relationships, or relationships between meanings, that indicate hierarchical or other types of relationships between codes.

Semistructured interviews: Interviews that provide some structure by using a combination of fixed-response and open-ended questions.

Sensitivity: Refers to the ability of an assessment to detect the presence of a problem or condition when it is present.

Sensory integration: Describes how sensations are received and organized neurologically to produce human behavior.

Sequential exploratory design: Type of study in which the investigator first collects in-depth and nuanced information about a phenomenon

using a qualitative tradition followed by collection and analysis of quantitative data.

Sequential exploratory design: A mixed-methods design in which an investigator first collects and analyzes in-depth information through the use of a qualitative tradition, then collects and analyzes core quantitative data used to explain or predict phenomena. The two approaches are analyzed separately.

Sequential transformative design: A mixed-methods design where either model, qualitative or quantitative, can be used as the core model. Moreover, the purpose of a sequential transformative design is to use a clearly identified theoretical perspective to direct the research question toward change in policy, action, or ideology.

Serendipitous browsing: A random process of information retrieval in which the searcher travels a nonlinear path to information.

Significance testing: Involves testing the null hypothesis that an intervention (or other experimental manipulation) has had no effect. Significance testing tells us whether the effect of an intervention is greater than 0.

Single-group design: An approach to summative evaluation that includes one observation after the intervention has taken place.

Single-subject design: Study design that follows the logic of experimentation but examines the impact of interventions on single subjects who serve as their own controls.

Single-subject research: Defines a group of related methodological approaches that involve in-depth analyses of the behaviors of a single research subject or of a relatively small group of subjects that is considered collectively, serving as their own controls.

Skepticism: The idea that any assertion of knowledge should be open to doubt, further analysis, and criticism.

Social constructivism: A viewpoint that pervades postmodern thought. It asserts, in essence, that all knowledge, including scientific knowledge, is socially constructed and, therefore, relative.

Social desirability bias: Occurs when subjects change their behavior toward what they perceive as more socially desirable within the situation because they know they are being observed.

Social validation model: Refers to the use of social validity, ecological validity, and clinical significance concepts simultaneously to design and conduct outcome research, aimed to increase its usability for practice.

Social validity: Research that is of social significance in which the goals align with what society wants, the procedures or interventions are acceptable and affordable to consumers, and the outcomes predict satisfactory change without unpredicted or unwanted side effects.

Society: Includes anyone who may be involved with and affected by the intervention process and outcome, including occupational therapy clients, their caregivers, their parents and teachers (in the case of children), community members, disability groups, and others. Also known as *consumers.*

Specific aim: A statement that describes the purpose of a study or what it intends to accomplish. Also known as *research aim.*

Specificity: The ability of an assessment to produce negative results when the problem or condition is not present.

Split-half reliability: Occurs when investigators divide the items of a questionnaire into two smaller questionnaires (usually by dividing it into odd and even items, or first half–last half) and then correlates the scores obtained from the two halves of the assessment to test the reliability of the entire measure.

Stakeholder: Any individual (or group of individuals) who has something to gain or lose from the project, inquiry, or intervention being conducted.

Standard deviation: Defined as the average variability of individual scores from the mean.

Standard normal distribution: Assumes that the norm has a zero point and that the deviations from zero occur symmetrically, in units of one standard deviation at both the positive and negative ends of the possible range of choices.

Standardization: Refers to specifying a process or protocol for administering the assessment.

Standardized interventions: Interventions that follow a structured format and do not deviate from implementation guidelines.

Standardized tests: Contrived cognitive or motor tasks that are administered and scored under strictly standardized conditions and typically generate norm-referenced or criterion-referenced scores.

Statement of impact: An important statement made early in the introduction of a published, peer-reviewed journal article. It references data (typically prevalence rates or findings about the severity or functional impact and other consequences of a problem or impairment) that point to the importance of the topic under study.

Statistical conclusion validity: Defines the extent to which an independent variable and dependent variable are related (or covary).

Statistical power: The likelihood of finding a significant difference between groups or association between variables when one exists.

Statistical precision: A criterion in evaluating the quality of rigor in a quantitative study. It refers to the accuracy with which an outcome or effect of the intervention was measured and estimated using appropriate statistical analyses.

Statistical significance: Determined by a finding from a statistical test meeting the probability cutoff of $p < 0.05$ or $p < 0.01$.

Statistics: The means by which data are collected, organized, analyzed, and presented to serve the various objectives of a research study.

Stratified sampling: Similar to a simple random sample, but the selection is from identified subgroups in the population.

Strength of the evidence: One criterion determining the level of evidence of a quantitative research study. It is further determined by three criteria: level of evidence of the study design, quality of evidence, and statistical precision.

Structured browsing: A preplanned process of information retrieval in which the searcher uses a list of topics and a sub-list of more specific topics

Structured interviews: Interviews that include questions and response categories that are virtually all predetermined.

Study design: Describes the method or experimental strategy with which the research question was approached.

Subject pool: Refers to those who are identified as eligible to participate in the study.

Subject searching: An iterative and ongoing information-seeking process that involves successive steps to arrive at information that is a close-as-possible match to the information being sought.

Summative evaluation: An outcomes approach to program evaluation that provides information about the extent to which a program achieves the objectives for which it was developed.

Survey research: A method of inquiry characterized by collecting data using structured questions to elicit self-reported information from a sample of people.

Survey studies: Nonexperimental designs undertaken to investigate unknown characteristics of a defined population.

Symposia: Collections of research papers tied together by a common theme.

Systematic errors: Consistent or predictable errors; they occur when an assessment misestimates the true score by a consistent amount and in the same direction (too low or too high).

Systematic review: An exhaustive and thorough research effort that focuses on assessing and evaluating the quality of all other research studies of a strictly defined scientific topic or question. Its focus is to eliminate bias in the review by using an objective and transparent methodological approach to information synthesis that can be replicated easily.

Systematic sampling: Considered equivalent to random sampling as long as there is no reoccurring pattern or order in the listing.

T

Technical rationality: Idea that practical activity is derived seamlessly from basic knowledge.

Test-retest reliability: Measures the ability of an assessment to remain stable over time in what it aims to measure. This is estimated when data from a single assessment are gathered from the same group of subjects on two or more occasions within a short time frame. Also known as *stability*.

Theoretical connectedness: A means of evaluating the quality of qualitative research. Defines the extent to which the theoretical constructs and their relationships with one another were validated by the data, clearly defined, comprehensive, and linked to a new or existing occupational therapy conceptual practice framework or map.

Theoretical drive: Whether the main reasoning process required for a project is inductive or deductive.

Theory: A network of explanations; it provides concepts that label and describe phenomena and postulates that specify relationships between concepts.

Theory-practice gap: A known gap in communication and collaboration between scholars whose work focuses on the ideas that ground occupational therapy (theory) and the observed actions of therapists whose work focuses on the actual implementation of practice (practice).

Three-phase model: A tool that can be used to facilitate the planning of a needs assessment. It operates as a checklist of steps and activities that must be achieved over the different stages of a needs assessment.

Time-series designs: Type of study in which subjects remain in a single group and are studied at various time points before and after the experimental manipulation.

Title page: The first part of a published, peer-reviewed article that typically contains the title, the running head, the authors, and the institutions with which the authors are affiliated.

Training grants: Grants that are used to support professionals and students to develop or extend their knowledge or skills. They may be used to support professional activities that involve training and education (e.g., conferences or symposia). They can also be used to support the implementation of specialized academic programs and collaborators, which might include several researchers from across the country. Also called *educational grants*.

Transformative research: A broad classification for inquiry that is designed specifically to bring about change in some practical situation or a specific context.

Trialability: One of the five determinants of an innovation that may facilitate or hinder its adoption. It refers to the degree to which an innovation may be experimented with on a limited basis. If a new idea can be tried on a small scale, it will generally be adopted more quickly.

Triangulated study: A research design that integrates elements of both qualitative and quantitative methods so that the strengths of each are emphasized.

Triangulation: Refers to the use of two or more strategies to collect and/or interpret or analyze information for the purposes of detaching the method of measurement from the phenomena being measured.

Truncation: Refers to inserting a character, instead of a letter, into a word to expand the word's reach during the search process.

Tuskegee experiments: A series of experiments that led to public outcry and the implementation of human subjects regulations on research.

Two-group posttest-only design: Type of study that offers slightly more rigor than the one-group posttest-only design; it allows the researcher to test whether a certain therapy or other action led to a desired outcome by allowing for a direct comparison between a group of subjects receiving the therapy and one not receiving the therapy.

Two-group posttest-only randomized experiment: The most basic experimental design in which subjects are randomly assigned to either a treatment group or the no-treatment control group.

Two-group pretest-posttest randomized experiment: Type of study that is identical to the two-group posttest-only randomized experiment; the only difference is the addition of a pretest before the treatment is offered.

Type I error: Involves reporting a significant relationship between variables when there really is no relationship.

Type II error: The failure to find and report a significant relationship between variables when the relationship actually exists.

U

Unit of analysis: Refers to the subject of analysis in the study.

Univariate research designs: Studies in which data are collected on a single variable or a series of single variables and then characterized with descriptive statistics

Unstructured interviews: Interviews that resemble guided conversations. Such interviews typically include a relatively short list of "grand tour" general questions (sometimes referred to as an interview guide), and interviewers generally respect how interviewees frame and structure their responses.

Unsystematic review: A practical piece of writing that builds an evidence-based story, acting as a precursor to planned research or as an introduction to an executed study.

Usual care: Describes the current standard-of-care situation (as opposed to an intervention, which is typically added to usual care or in some cases replaces usual care).

Usual-care control group: A control condition in which subjects continue to receive what is considered to be the usual standard of care for their particular impairment.

V

Validity: Refers to whether an instrument measures what it is intended to measure.

Validity of data: Measures to determine whether the data collected actually represent the variable under study. Empirical assessment of validity focuses on such factors as the extent to which items used to quantify a variable coalesce together and whether the instrument's scores converge with measures of variables that are theoretically related to the variable the instrument intends to measure.

Variable: A means of labeling or giving meaning to a set of characteristics (represented by numbers) that are expected to vary among the clients being studied.

Variance: The extent to which individual subjects in the sample deviate or drift away from the mean.

Veridicality: The extent to which test results reflect or can predict phenomena in the open environment or "real world."

Verifiability: Refers to sufficient explication of a study so that others may understand the methodological approach in detail and how the study conclusions were generated.

Verisimilitude: The similarity of the data collection methods in the test to tasks and skills required in the free and open environment.

Volition: An aspect of Kielhofner's Model of Human Occupation. Volition drives occupational performance and participation and is comprised of three elements: the client's interests (the sense of preference toward an occupation), personal causation (the sense of ability to perform an occupation), and values (the sense of personal and societal importance of the occupation).

Vulnerable populations: Those who do not have the capacity to consent to participate in research or who may be pressured into participating for the wrong reasons.

W

Wait-list control-group design: This is sometimes called a delayed-treatment control. Those at the top of a waiting list for an intervention are assigned to an intervention, and those at the bottom of the list serve as the control group. After the completion of the study, those at the bottom of the list receive the intervention, so this design is favored for humanitarian reasons.

Within-subjects tests: Term used to describe related-samples tests.

Index

Note: Page numbers followed by the letter f refer to figures, those followed by the letter t refer to tables.

A

A-B design, in single-subject research, 360
 case example, 362f
 variation of, 362–363, 362f
A-B-A design, in single-subject research, 362f, 363
A-B-C design, in single-subject research, 362–363, 362f
Absolute truth, positivistic science and, 27–28
Abstract, 38–39
 defined, 38
 purpose of, 42
 of research paper, 443, 444
 sample, 39f
Accepted practices, in human subject research, 154
Active reading of data, 219
Activity Card Sort (ACS), in factor analysis, 289
Administrative records, 407t
Advocates, research, 73
Agency for Healthcare Research and Quality (AHRQ), grants funded by, 186, 470, 472
Allegations, in human subject research, mechanisms for resolving, 156
Alternating-treatments design, in single-subject research, 367–369
 example of, 368f
 strengths and weaknesses of, 369
Alternative hypotheses, statistical, 337
American Journal of Occupational Therapy, 36, 36f
American Occupational Therapy Foundation, grants awarded by, 466–467
Analogue scales, visual, in data collection, 304
Analytical approach, 44
Analytical approach section, 41
Ancestry method, 347
Anecdotal evidence, 59
Animal welfare, 155–156
Animal-assisted therapy research, 87–88
ANOVA (one-way analysis of variance), 340–341
APA format, 37
Applied research, 21–22
Argument presented in grant proposal, 477
Aristotle, scientific philosophy of, 26, 26f, 27
Artificiality, in long-term experimental research projects, 259
Assessment for data collection, 140–141
Assessment research, 7
Assessor, need relative to, 399
ATLAS.ti® software, 215, 215f, 216f

Attention-deficit hyperactivity disorder, therapy ball study in, 361, 362, 362f
Audience
 academic, qualitative analyses reports for, 241–242
 specific, report writing for, 441–442
 stakeholder, research dissemination among, 456–459
Audit trail, qualitative data quality associated with, 209–210
Australia, international regulations governing research in, 145t
Authorship
 policies governing, 156–157
 responsible, in human subject research, 156–157

B

Backup protocols, in data management, 327
Basic research, 20–21
Behavioral management case example, 48–49
Behaviors, multiple-baseline designs across, 363, 365f
Belmont principles, 147–148
Beneficence, in human subject research, 147–148
Between-subjects designs, 51
Between-subjects test, 338
Bias
 in data collection instrument reliability inter-rater, 283–284, 284t
 rater, 283
 defined, 207
 management of, in qualitative research, 207
 nonresponse, 375
 response, 375
 sampling, examples illustrating, in quantitative research, 168
 selection, 128
 social desirability, 200
Bibliographic citation analysis, 105–106
Bibliographic citation database(s)
 CINAHL, 112
 conduction of online searches in, 104, 105f
 journals and websites, 112
 OT SEARCH, 112–113
 subject searches, 103–104
 World Wide Web, 103
Bibliographic search, 347
Binomial effect size display (BESD), 54
Biomechanical theory, 83
Biometry, in data collection, 306
Biostatistician, 331
Blind review, in research dissemination, 450

Blinding of participants
 defined, 13
 double-blind study, 252
 in experimental designs, 124
 purpose of, 252
 for quality of evidence, 53
Books, dissemination of information through, 452
Boolean connectors, in computer-assisted qualitative data systems, 224
Boolean logic, in literature searches, 108–109, 108f
Bradshaw's categories of need, 399t
Brochures, targeted, research dissemination to, 458
Browsing, online, 102
Budget
 in grant applications, 480–481
 research study, 142

C

Canada
 Canadian Occupational Therapy Foundation, grants awarded by, 467
 government grants, 473
 international regulations governing research in, 145t
 private foundation grants, 468
Case comparison design, 270
Case reports, 36
Case sensitivity, in literature searches, 109
Case studies, descriptive, 248–249
Case-composite example, 439
Case-control design, in quantitative research, 270–271, 270f
Case-control study, 52
Case-series study, 52
Case-study research, 53, 130
Catalogs, public access to, online, 103
Categorical scale, 332
Causality, probable, in experimental quantitative research, 249–250
Ceiling effect, 253
Census figures, in needs assessment process, 407t
Center grants, 462
Central tendency, measure(s) of, 336
 mean as, 336
 median as, 336
 mode as, 336
Challenges, in qualitative analysis, 231–232
CINAHL, as information resource, 104, 112
CIRRIE, as information resource, 104
Citation(s)
 in grant applications, 477
 in human subject research, 157
 searching, 105–106

single theory, choosing and applying, 81–83
Odds ratio, used in meta-analysis studies, 353t
Office of Research Integrity (ORI), 153, 155–156
One-group posttest-only design, 126, 126f
One-group pretest–posttest design, 120f, 127, 127f
One-way analysis of variance (ANOVA), 340–341
Online information retrieval, process of, 102–104
Online questionnaires, advantages and disadvantages of, 377t
Online search strategies, by subject, 103–104
Open-ended interviews, in needs assessment process, 407t
Open-ended questions
  vs. fixed-response questions, 202t
  formulation of, 381–382
Operational multiplicity, 346
Opinion, vs. data, 96
Opinion papers, 36
Oral presentation
  at conferences
    non-peer-reviewed, 452
    peer-reviewed, 451
  of qualitative analyses, 241
Ordinal scale
  in data collection, 277t, 278
  formatting questions for, 385
  of measurement, 332–333
Organismic variable, 263
OT SEARCH, 112–113
Outcome research
  creation of, relevant for evidence-based practice, 498–506. See also Evidence-based practice (EBP)
  in support of practice, 8
Outcome variable, 332

P

p value, 337
Paired-samples test, 338
Paired-samples *t*-test, 340, 341t
Panel discussion, 44
Paper data storage, of human subject research, 154
Paper presentation, 44
Parallel forms of reliability, 281
Parametric statistics, 338, 339t
Participant(s)
  feasibility and preferences, in research method selection, 132–133
  in multiple-baseline design research, 364–366, 365f, 366f
  participant-observer, 56
  participants section, published ans presented research, 40
  in qualitative research
    appropriateness of, 173–174
    determining number of, 176
    strategies for selection of, 175–176

in quantitative research
  issues affecting selection of, 162–163
  representation, 164
in research studies
  availability of information to, 449–450
  dropout of, 259
  ID sheets for, 324, 325f
  identifiers of, 322–324
  protection of, 145–149
  recruitment of, 92–93
  respect of, 147
  tracking of, 322–324, 323f
Participation, in gathering qualitative data, 198–199
  defined, 196
  example of, 197–198
  key activities using, 199–200
Participatory action research (PAR)
  conduction of, 185–186
  contributions of, 186
  defined, 185
  resources on, 186
Participatory needs assessment approach, 404–405, 405t
Participatory research, 424–434
  approach to, 426–427
  challenges of, 434
  consumer voice in, 426
  defined, 424, 426–427
  forms, 427
  implementation of, principles in, 427–428
  knowledge-creation and evaluation in, 429–432, 431f
  need for, 426
  partnerships, 428f
  research-practice gap in, 426
  stakeholder's voices in, 429, 430t
  step(s) in, 432–434, 432f
    analysis and planning as, 433
    critical reflection and analysis as, 432–433
    data collection as, 433–434
    design choice as, 433–434
    developing service strategies as, 433
    implementing action as, 434
    reflection and utilization as, 434
  in support of practice, 8–9
Pearson correlation test, 338–340
Peer debriefing, in gathering qualitative data, 209
Peer review
  conference presentations, 451
  defined, 450
  of grant applications, 477
  of journal articles, 451, 456
  purpose of, 450
  in research dissemination, 450–451
    at conferences, oral presentations and posters and, 451, 453–456, 454f–455f
  importance of, 450
  integrity, 158
  journal publications, 456
  process of, 451

Peer-reviewed journal articles, 36–42, 451, 456
  abstract, 38–39, 39f
  appendices, 42
  defined, 36–37, 102
  discussion, 41–42
  figures, 42
  introduction, 39–40
  method, 40–41
  references, 42
  results, 41
  sequence of sections, 37f
  tables, 42
  title page, 37–38, 38f
Peer-reviewed journal, defined, 101–102
Percentage values of data, 335–336, 335t
Performance measurements
  administration of, 305
  in data collection, 305
Performance sites for research, 92
Per-protocol analysis, 265
Personal style and habits, in report writing, 440–441
Person-Environment-Occupation-Performance (PEOP) model, 79
Personnel preparation, for data collection, 310
Phase lengths, in single-subject research, 370
Phenomena under study
  in descriptive research, 246–247
  in qualitative research, 15, 182
  in quantitative research, 31
Phenomenological research, 3f
Phenomenology
  defined, 131
  in qualitative research, 190–191
    conduction of, 191–192
    contributions of, 192
    defined, 14, 190
Philosophical foundations, of scientific inquiry, 25–33. See also Scientific inquiry, philosophical foundation(s) of
Philosophical orientation, 30
Phrase matching, 102
Phrases, in literature searches, 109
Physiological drive, need as, 398
Pilot research, in grant applications, 477–478
Piloting questionnaire, in survey research, 386–387
Placebo, 17
Placebo control group, 17, 125
Placebo effect, 53, 123
Placebo treatment, 124
Plagiarism, in research, 155–156
Planning analyses, in grant applications, 479
Policy(ies)
  documentation, in data management, 315–316
  governing authorship, 156–157
  governing integrity, in human subject research, 155
  in grant applications, 464
Political orientation, of needs assessment, 397–398, 397f